OPHTHA GY

T0210199

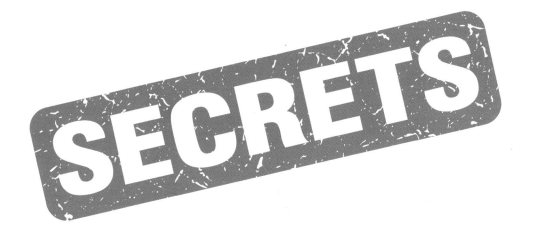

FIFTH EDITION

OPHTHALMOLOGY

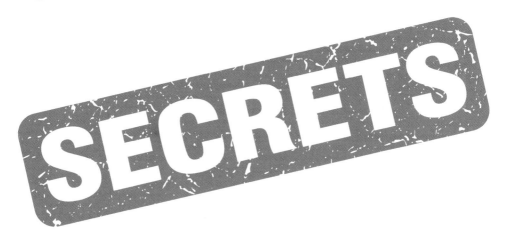

SECRETS

JANICE A. GAULT MD, FACS
Associate Surgeon
Cataract and Primary Eye Care
Wills Eye Hospital
Philadelphia, Pennsylvania

Assistant Professor
Ophthalmology
Thomas Jefferson University Hospital
Philadelphia, Pennsylvania

ELSEVIER

Elsevier
1600 John F. Kennedy Blvd.
Ste 1800
Philadelphia, PA 19103-2899

OPHTHALMOLOGY SECRETS, FIFTH EDITION ISBN: 9780323661881

Copyright © 2023 by Elsevier, Inc. All rights reserved.

Notice

Previous editions copyrighted 2016, 2007, and 2002.

Content Strategist: Marybeth Thiel
Senior Content Development Manager: Laura Schmidt
Content Development Specialist: Kristen Helm
Publishing Services Manager: Shereen Jameel
Project Manager: Aparna Venkatachalam
Design Direction: Bridget Hoette

Printed in India

Last digit is the print number: 9 8 7 6 5 4 3 2

Working together
to grow libraries in
developing countries

www.elsevier.com • www.bookaid.org

To Caroline Anna, William Henry, and Eliza Avery
Janice A. Gault

PREFACE

In putting together this book, my hope is that the question-and-answer "Socratic method" format recreates how a large portion of clinical medical education takes place, on rounds, in clinic, and in testing formats. I hope it answers questions you find when seeing patients in your practices daily and you can refer to it easily and often.

I greatly appreciate the efforts of the many talented contributors who have shared their wisdom and experiences to create this book and update the subsequent editions. I have received much positive feedback on the first four editions of this book, among residents and fellows here at Wills Eye Hospital and elsewhere. I hope that clinicians and students will continue to enjoy this new edition and find it valuable.

Janice A. Gault, MD, FACS

CONTRIBUTORS

Usiwoma Abugo MD
Howard University Hospital
Washington, DC

Brandon D. Ayres MD
Attending Physician
Cornea
Wills Eye Hospital
Philadelphia, Pennsylvania

Augusto Azuara-Blanco MD, PhD
Professor of Ophthalmology
Centre for Public Health
Queen's University Belfast,
Belfast, Great Britain

Honorary Consultant Ophthalmologist
Ophthalmology
Belfast Health and Social Care Trust,
Belfast, Great Britain

Robert S. Bailey MD
Director and Attending Surgeon
CPEC
Wills Eye Hospital,
Philadelphia, Pennsylvania

Upneet Kaur Bains MD
Assistant Professor of Ophthalmology
Ophthalmology
Lewis Katz School of Medicine at Temple University,
Philadelphia, Pennsylvania

Vincent F. Baldassano MD
Doctor
Ophthalmology
Geisinger Eye Institute,
Danville,
Philadelphia, Pennsylvania

Caroline R. Baumal MD, FRCSC
Professor, Vitreoretinal Surgery
New England Eye Center
Tufts University School of Medicine,
Newton, Massachusetts

Edward H. Bedrossian BA, MS, MD
Attending Surgeon
Ophthalmic Plastic & Reconstructive Surgery
Wills Eye Hospital,
Philadelphia, Pennsylvania

Clinical Professor of Ophthalmology
Ophthalmology
Temple University School of Medicine,
Philadelphia, Pennsylvania

Director, Ophthalmic Plastic and Reconstructive Surgery
Ophthalmology
Temple University School of Medicine,
Philadelphia, Pennsylvania

Paramjit K. Bhullar MD
Ophthalmology
Duke University School of Medicine,
Durham, North Carolina

Jurij R. Bilyk MD
Attending Surgeon
Skull Base Division, Neuro-Ophthalmology Service
Wills Eye Hospital,
Philadelphia, Pennsylvania

Professor of Ophthalmology
Thomas Jefferson University Hospital,
Philadelphia, Pennsylvania

Jeffrey P. Blice MD
Clinical Professor
Ophthalmology
Storm Eye Institute Medical
Univeristy of South Carolina,
Charleston, South Carolina

Michael J. Borne MD
Founding Partner
Mississippi Retina Associates,
Jackson, Mississippi

Steven E. Brooks MD
Professor
Ophthalmology
Columbia University,
New York, New York

David G. Buerger MD
Clinical Instructor of Ophthalmology
Ophthalmology
University of Pittsburgh,
Pittsburgh, Pennsylvania

Alan N. Carlson MD
Professor of Ophthalmology
Duke University School of Medicine,
Durham, North Carolina

Corneal Specialist, Ophthalmologist
Duke University Eye Center,
Durham, North Carolina

Marc S. Cohen MD
Associate Professor of Ophthalmology
Thomas Jefferson University Hospital,
Philadelphia, Pennsylvania

Mary Jude Cox MD
Instructor
Glaucoma
Wills Eye Hospital,
Philadelphia, Pennsylvania

Ophthalmologist
Eye Physicians,
Voorhess, New Jersey

Kristin M. DiDomenico MD, FCPP
Comprehensive Ophthalmology
Cataract and Primary Eye Care
Wills Eye Hospital,
Philadelphia, Pennsylvania

John Donald Dugan MD
Attending Surgeon
Cataract and Primary Eye Care
Wills Eye Hospital,
Philadelphia, Pennsylvania

Jacob Starr Duker MD
Fellow Physician
Ophthalmology
Ophthalmic Consultants of Boston,
Boston, Massachusetts

Ralph Conrad Eagle MD
Director
Department of Pathology
Wills Eye Hospital,
Philadelphia, Pennsylvania

Mitchell S. Fineman MD
Attending Surgeon
Retina Service
Wills Eye Hospital,
Philadelphia, Pennsylvania

Associate Professor of Ophthalmology
Thomas Jefferson University,
Philadelphia, Pennsylvania

Janice A. Gault MD, FACS
Associate Surgeon
Cataract and Primary Eye Care
Wills Eye Hospital,
Philadelphia, Pennsylvania

Assistant Professor
Ophthalmology
Thomas Jefferson University Hospital,
Philadelphia, Pennsylvania

Roberta E. Gausas MD
Associate Clinical Professor
Ophthalmology
University of Pennsylvania Perelman School of Medicine,
Philadelphia, Pennsylvania

Kenneth B. Gum MD
Traverse City Eye
Traverse City, Michigan

Shipra Gupta MD
PGY3 Resident
Ophthalmology
University Hospitals-Case Medical Center,
Cleveland, Ohio

Sadeer B. Hannush MD
Attending Surgeon
Cornea Service
Wills Eye Hospital,
Philadelphia, Pennsylvania

Professor of Ophthalmology
Department of Ophthalmology
Sidney Kimmel Medical College at Thomas Jefferson University,
Philadelphia, Pennsylvania

Jeffrey D. Henderer MD
Dr. Edward Hagop Bedrossian Chair
Department of Ophthalmology
Lewis Katz School of Medicine at Temple University,
Philadelphia, Pennsylvania
Professor

Department of Ophthalmology
Lewis Katz School of Medicine at Temple University,
Philadelphia, Pennsylvania

Terry Kim MD
Professor of Ophthalmology
Duke University School of Medicine
Duke University Eye Center,
Durham, North Carolina

Kendra A. Klein MD
Ophthalmology
Associated Retina Consultants,
Phoenix, Arizona

Nicole A. Langelier
Scheie Eye Institute
University of Pennsylvania Health System
Philadelphia, Pennsylvania

Joseph I. Maguire MD
Assistant Professor
Ophthalmology
Wills Eye Hospital, Thomas Jefferson University Hospital,
Philadelphia, Pennsylvania

Marlene R. Moster MD
Professor
Ophthalmology
Thomas Jefferson School of Medicine,
Philadelphia, Pennsylvania

Glaucoma
Wills Eye Hospital,
Philadelphia, Pennsylvania
OPP Vantage,
Bala Cynwyd, Pennsylvania

Mark L. Moster MD
Director, Neuro-Ophthalmology Fellowship
Neuro-Ophthalmology
Wills Eye Hospital,
Philadelphia, Pennsylvania

Professor
Neurology and Ophthalmology
Sidney Kimmel Medical College of Thomas Jefferson University,
Philadelphia, Pennsylvania

Leonard B. Nelson MD, MBA
Co-Director
Pediatric ophthalmology and ocular genetics
Wills Eye Hospital,
Philadelphia, Pennsylvania

Scott E. Olitsky MD, MBA
Professor
Ophthalmology
UMKC,
Kansas City, Missouri

Joshua Paul MD
Resident
Ophthalmology
Temple University Hospital,
Philadelphia, Pennsylvania

Robert B. Penne MD
Clinical Professor
Ophthalmology
Sydney Kimmel Medical College Thomas Jefferson University,
Philadelphia, Pennsylvania

Director, Ophthalmic Plastic Surgery Department
Wills Eye Hospital,
Philadelphia, Pennsylvania

Attending Surgeon
Ophthalmology
Lankenau Hospital,
Wynnewood, Pennsylvania

Julian D. Perry MD
Physician
Ophthalmology
Cole Eye Institute,
Cleveland, Ohio

Irving Raber MD, F.R.C.S. (C)
Attending Surgeon
Cornea Service
Wills Eye Hospital,
Philadelphia, Pennsylvania

Ehsan Rahimy MD
Vitreoretinal Surgeon
Ophthalmology
Palo Alto Medical Foundation,
Palo Alto, California

Christopher J. Rapuano MD
Chief
Cornea Service
Wills Eye Hospital,
Philadelphia, Pennsylvania

Professor of Ophthalmology
Sidney Kimmel Medical College
Thomas Jefferson University,
Philadelphia, Pennsylvania

Carolyn S. Repke MD
Assistant Surgeon
Cataract and Primary Eye Care
Wills Eye Hospital,
Philadelphia, Pennsylvania

Physician partner
Vantage Eye Care, Philadelphia Eye Associates Division,
Philadelphia, Pennsylvania

Douglas J. Rhee MD
Professor and Chair
Ophthalmology & Visual Sciences
Case Western Reserve University School
  of Medicine,
Cleveland, Ohio

Director
University Hospitals Eye Institute,
Cleveland, Ohio

Lorena Riveroll-Hannush MD
Clinical Coordinator
Cataract and Cornea Associates,
Langhorne, Pennsylvania

Ex-Adscrito
Servicio de Cornea
Hospital Para Evitar la Ceguera en Mexico,
Mexico City, Mexico DF

Warren Robinson BS
Pharmacist
Temple University Hospital,
Philadelphia, Pennsylvania

Tal J. Rubinstein MD
Assistant Professor
Ophthalmology
Ophthalmic Plastic Surgery, Albany Medical Center,
Albany, New York

Brooke D. Saffren BS
Bradway Scholar Research Fellow
Pediatric Ophthalmology and Ocular Genetics
Wills Eye Hospital,
Philadelphia, Pennsylvania

OMS-IV
Philadelphia College of Osteopathic Medicine,
Philadelphia, Pennsylvania

Jonathan H. Salvin MD
Pediatric Ophthalmology
Division of Ophthalmology
Nemours/A.I. duPont Hospital for Children,
Wilmington, Delaware

Clinical Associate Professor
Ophthalmology and Pediatrics
Sydney Kimmel College of Medicine,
Philadelphia, Pennsylvania
Department of Pediatric Ophthalmology
Wills Eye Hospital,
Philadelphia, Pennsylvania

Bruce M. Schnall MD
Associate Surgeon
Pediatric Ophthalmology
Wills Eye Hospital,
Philadelphia, Pennsylvania

Carol L. Shields MD
Director
Ocular Oncology Service
Wills Eye Hospital,
Philadelphia, Pennsylvania

Jerry A. Shields MD
Wills Eye Hospital
Oncology
Wills Eye Hospital,
Philadelphia, Pennsylvania

Andrew P. Shyu MD
Resident Physician
Ophthalmology
Temple University Hospital,
Philadelphia, Pennsylvania

George L. Spaeth BA, MD
Esposito Research Professor
Glaucoma
Wills Eye Hospital/T. Jefferson University,
Philadelphia, Pennsylvania

Archana Srinivasan MD
Fellow
Neuro ophthalmology
Wills eye hospital,
Philadelphia, Pennsylvania

Richard E. Sutton MD, PhD
Professor
Section of Infectious Diseases, Department of Medicine
Yale School of Medicine,
New Haven, Connecticut

Nancy G. Swartz MS, MD, FACS
Director of Facial Rejuvenation
Myrna Brind Center of Integrative Medicine
Thomas Jefferson University Hospital,
Philadelphia, Pennsylvania

Associate Surgeon
Neuro-Ophthalmology Service
Wills Eye Hospital,
Philadelphia, Pennsylvania

Clinical Associate
Ophthalmology
University of Pennsylvania School of Medicine,
Philadelphia, Pennsylvania

Instructor
Ophthalmology
Thomas Jefferson University Medical College,
Philadelphia, Pennsylvania

Janine G. Tabas MD
Ophthalmologist
Kay, Tabas, Niknam & DiDomenico Ophthalmology Associates,
Bala Cynwyd, Pennsylvania

Ophthalmologist
Cataract and Primary Eye Care
Wills Eye Hospital,
Philadelphia, Pennsylvania

William S. Tasman MD
Ophthalmologist
Retina Service
Wills Eye Hospital,
Philadelphia, Pennsylvania

Richard Tipperman MD
Attending Surgeon
Cataract Surgery
Wills Eye Hospital,
Philadelphia, Pennsylvania

Sydney Tyson MD, M.P.H
Attending Surgeon
Cataract and Primary Eyecare Service
Wills Eye Hospital,
Philadelphia, Pennsylvania

Neil Vadhar MD
Fellow
Cornea
Wills Eye Hospital,
Philadelphia, Pennsylvania

Priya Sharma Vakharia MD
Physician
Ophthalmology
Retina Group of Washington,
Greenbelt, Maryland

James F. Vander MD
Attending Surgeon
Retina Service
Wills Eye Hospital,
Philadelphia, Pennsylvania
Clinical Professor

Ophthalmology
Thomas Jefferson University,
Philadelphia, Pennsylvania

Nandini Venkatswaran MD
Ophthalmologist; Cataract, Cornea, and Refractive
    Surgeon
Massachusetts Eye and Ear,
Boston, Massachusetts

Clinical Instructor of Ophthalmology
Harvard Medical School,
Boston, Massachusetts

Tamara R. Vrabec MD
Ophthalmology
Geisinger Medical Center,
Danville, Pennsylvania

Clinical Professor
Ophthalmolgoy
Temple University Hospital,
Philadelphia, Pennsylvania

Lauren B. Yeager MD
Assistant Professor of Ophthalmology
Ophthalmology
Columbia University Irving Medical Center,
New York, New York

CONTENTS

TOP 100 SECRETS XV
Janice A. Gault and James F. Vander

CHAPTER 1	CLINICAL ANATOMY OF THE EYE 1
	Kenneth B. Gum

CHAPTER 2	ANATOMY OF THE ORBIT AND EYELID 7
	Edward H. Bedrossian Jr.

CHAPTER 3	OPTICS AND REFRACTION 10
	Janice A. Gault

CHAPTER 4	COLOR VISION 22
	Mitchell S. Fineman

CHAPTER 5	OPHTHALMIC AND ORBITAL TESTING 29
	Kendra A. Klein and Caroline R. Baumal

CHAPTER 6	VISUAL FIELDS 50
	Janice A. Gault

CHAPTER 7	THE RED EYE 65
	Janice A. Gault

CHAPTER 8	CORNEAL INFECTIONS 77
	Paramjit Bhullar, Nandini Venkateswaran, Alan N. Carlson, and Terry Kim

CHAPTER 9	OPHTHALMIA NEONATORUM 90
	Janine G. Tabas and Kristin M. DiDomenico

CHAPTER 10	TOPICAL ANTIBIOTICS AND STEROIDS 94
	Christopher J. Rapuano and Richard E. Sutton

CHAPTER 11	DRY EYES 103
	Janice A. Gault

CHAPTER 12	CORNEAL DYSTROPHIES 112
	Sadeer B. Hannush and Lorena Riveroll-Hannush

CHAPTER 13	KERATOCONUS 121
	Irving Raber

CHAPTER 14	REFRACTIVE SURGERY 130
	Neil Vadhar and Brandon D. Ayres

CHAPTER 15	GLAUCOMA 143
	Mary J. Cox and George L. Spaeth

CHAPTER 16	ANGLE-CLOSURE GLAUCOMA 151
	George L. Spaeth

CHAPTER 17	SECONDARY OPEN-ANGLE GLAUCOMA 168
	Janice A. Gault

CHAPTER 18	MEDICAL TREATMENT OF GLAUCOMA 173
	Joshua Paul, Upneet Bains, Warren Robinson, and Jeffrey D. Henderer

CHAPTER 19	TRABECULECTOMY SURGERY 181
	Marlene R. Moster and Augusto Azuara-Blanco

CHAPTER 20   TRAUMATIC GLAUCOMA AND HYPHEMA   191
Douglas J. Rhee and Shipra Gupta

CHAPTER 21   CATARACTS   201
Richard Tipperman

CHAPTER 22   TECHNIQUES OF CATARACT SURGERY   205
Sydney Tyson

CHAPTER 23   COMPLICATIONS OF CATARACT SURGERY   211
John D. Dugan Jr. and Robert S. Bailey Jr.

CHAPTER 24   AMBLYOPIA   218
Lauren B. Yeager and Steven E. Brooks

CHAPTER 25   ESODEVIATIONS   223
Brooke D. Saffren, Scott E. Olitsky, and Leonard B. Nelson

CHAPTER 26   MISCELLANEOUS OCULAR DEVIATIONS   228
Janice A. Gault

CHAPTER 27   STRABISMUS SURGERY   235
Bruce M. Schnall

CHAPTER 28   NYSTAGMUS   239
Andrew P. Shyu and Jonathan H. Salvin

CHAPTER 29   THE PUPIL   244
Archana Srinivasan and Mark L. Moster

CHAPTER 30   DIPLOPIA   248
Tal J. Rubinstein and Julian D. Perry

CHAPTER 31   OPTIC NEURITIS   255
Archana Srinivasan and Mark L. Moster

CHAPTER 32   MISCELLANEOUS OPTIC NEUROPATHIES AND NEUROLOGIC DISTURBANCES   259
Janice A. Gault

CHAPTER 33   TEARING AND THE LACRIMAL SYSTEM   265
Nancy G. Swartz and Marc S. Cohen

CHAPTER 34   PROPTOSIS   270
David G. Buerger

CHAPTER 35   THYROID EYE DISEASE   274
Robert B. Penne

CHAPTER 36   ORBITAL INFLAMMATORY DISEASES   279
Nicole A. Langelier, Usiwoma Abugo, and Roberta E. Gausas

CHAPTER 37   PTOSIS   283
Carolyn S. Repke

CHAPTER 38   EYELID TUMORS   289
Janice A. Gault

CHAPTER 39   UVEITIS   294
Tamara R. Vrabec, Caroline R. Baumal, and Vincent F. Baldassano Jr.

CHAPTER 40   TOXIC RETINOPATHIES   311
Priya Sharma Vakharia

CHAPTER 41   COATS' DISEASE   319
James Vander and William S. Tasman

CHAPTER 42   FUNDUS TRAUMA   325
Jeffrey P. Blice

CHAPTER 43   AGE-RELATED MACULAR DEGENERATION   335
James F. Vander and Joseph I. Maguire II

CHAPTER 44   RETINOPATHY OF PREMATURITY   341
James F. Vander

CHAPTER 45   DIABETIC RETINOPATHY   347
James F. Vander

CHAPTER 46   RETINAL ARTERIAL OBSTRUCTION   354
Jacob Duker

CHAPTER 47   RETINAL VENOUS OCCLUSIVE DISEASE   359
Ehsan Rahimy

CHAPTER 48   RETINAL DETACHMENT   366
James F. Vander and Michael J. Borne

CHAPTER 49   RETINOBLASTOMA   373
Carol L. Shields

CHAPTER 50   PIGMENTED LESIONS OF THE OCULAR FUNDUS   379
Carol L. Shields and Jerry A. Shields

CHAPTER 51   OCULAR TUMORS   386
Ralph C. Eagle, Jr.

CHAPTER 52   ORBITAL TUMORS   397
Jurij R. Bilyk

INDEX   403

TOP 100 SECRETS

Janice A. Gault and James F. Vander

These secrets summarize the concepts, principles, and most salient details of ophthalmology.

1. The goal of refractive correction is to place the circle of least confusion on the retina.

2. To find the spherical equivalent of an astigmatic correction, add half the cylinder to the sphere.

3. Recheck if the axial length measures less than 22 mm or more than 25 mm or if there is more than a 0.3-mm difference between the two eyes. For each 1 mm in error, the intraocular lens (IOL) power calculation is off by 2.5 diopters (D). Recheck keratometry readings if the average K power is <40 D or >47 D or if there is a difference of more than 1 D between eyes. For every 0.25-D error, the IOL power calculation is in error by 0.25 D.

4. According to Kollner's rule, retinal diseases cause acquired blue-yellow color vision defects, whereas optic nerve diseases affect red-green discrimination.

5. A junctional scotoma is a unilateral central scotoma associated with a contralateral superotemporal field defect and is caused by compression of the contralateral optic nerve near the chiasm.

6. False-negative errors cause a visual field to appear worse than it actually is. False-positive errors cause a visual field to look better than it actually is.

7. Lesions anterior to the optic chiasm cause unequal visual acuity, a relative afferent papillary defect, and color abnormalities. The optic disc may also have asymmetric cupping and pallor.

8. A drop of 2.5% neosynephrine is a simple test to distinguish between episcleritis (these vessels will blanch) and scleritis (these vessels do not)—two entities with very different prognoses and evaluations. Because 50% of patients with scleritis have systemic disease, referral to an internist is necessary for further evaluation.

9. Immediately irrigate any patient with a chemical ocular injury from an alkali or an acid, even before checking visual acuity. Normalize the pH before examining the patient to prevent further damage to the eye.

10. Rule out uncontrolled hypertension or blood dyscrasias in patients with recurrent subconjunctival hemorrhages.

11. A corneal ulcer is infectious until proven otherwise. You are never wrong to culture an ulcer; any ulcer not responding to therapy should be recultured.

12. Systemic treatment is necessary for gonococcal, chlamydial, and herpetic neonatal conjunctivitis because of the potential for serious disseminated disease. The mother and her sexual partners must be evaluated for other sexually transmitted diseases, including HIV.

13. Treatments that are effective for prophylaxis of gonococcal and chlamydial neonatal conjunctivitis include 1% silver nitrate, 0.5% erythromycin, and 1% tetracycline. Silver nitrate is rarely used, however, because of its potential for causing chemical conjunctivitis.

14. Topical steroids may promote herpetic keratitis if viral shedding is coincident with administration.

15. Steroid-induced increases in intraocular pressure occur in about 6% of patients on topical dexamethasone. This risk is higher in patients with known glaucoma or a family history of glaucoma.

16. Patients may be symptomatic with dry eye even with a normal slit lamp exam.

17. Ask about gastric bypass procedures in patients who have recent severe dry eye with no discernible cause. Vitamin A deficiency may be the reason. Similarly, patients after gastric bypass may present with Wernicke-Korsakoff syndrome (nystagmus, diplopia, ptosis, and mental confusion) due to vitamin B_1 deficiency.

18. If a patient presents with symptoms consistent with recurrent corneal erosion syndrome but no findings on slit lamp exam of the same, look for an underlying dystrophy, specifically epithelial basement membrane dystrophy.

19. If a patient with a corneal dystrophy is undergoing corneal transplantation but also has a clinically significant cataract, consider staging the cataract extraction a few months after the corneal transplant, offering the patient the advantage of better IOL power calculation and postoperative refractive result. Alternatively, Descemet's stripping endothelial keratoplasty, which does not alter corneal contour, may be combined with cataract surgery with a more predictable refractive outcome.

20. Corneal opacification in a neonate has a differential diagnosis of STUMPED: sclerocornea, trauma, ulcers, metabolic disorder, Peter's anomaly, endothelial dystrophy, and dermoid.

21. Most patients with keratoconus can be managed successfully with contact lens wear. Corneal transplantation is very successful in treating patients whose visual needs are not satisfied with glasses or contact lens correction, although corneal crosslinking may prevent keratoconus from progressing, thus preventing the need for a transplant.

22. As many as 30% to 50% of individuals with glaucomatous optic nerve damage and visual field loss have an initial intraocular pressure measurement less than 22 mm Hg.

23. The treatment of both primary open-angle glaucoma and low-tension glaucoma aims to preserve vision and quality of life through the lowering of intraocular pressure.

24. When evaluating a patient with angle-closure glaucoma, it is important to look at the fellow eye. Except for cases of marked anisometropia, the fellow eye should have a similar anterior chamber depth and narrow angle. If it does not, consider other nonrelative papillary block mechanisms of angle closure.

25. Patients with sporadic inheritance of aniridia need to be evaluated for Wilms' tumor, as it is found in 25% of cases.

26. Allergy from topical medications can present months to years after starting the drop.

27. If a patient's glaucoma continues to worsen, even with seemingly reduced intraocular pressure during office visits, think of noncompliance.

28. Before trabeculectomy surgery, identify high-risk patients in whom sudden hypotony should be avoided: those with angle-closure glaucoma, shallow anterior chambers, very high preoperative intraocular pressure, elevated episcleral venous pressure, or high myopia. Hemorrhagic choroidals and expulsive hemorrhages are more likely.

29. Patients with traumatic ocular injuries must be evaluated for systemic injuries as well.

30. Posterior fractures most commonly occur in the posteromedial orbital floor.

31. Patients recovering from a traumatic hyphema are at increased risk for glaucoma and retinal detachments in the future. They need ongoing ophthalmic evaluation for the rest of their lives.

32. Always check the pressure in the contralateral eye in a patient with ocular trauma. Asymmetrically low intraocular pressure may be an important clue to a possible ruptured globe.

33. Complete systemic evaluation by a pediatrician is mandatory for any infant with a congenital cataract.

34. Patients must have a documented functional interference in quality of life from a visual standpoint before cataract surgery is indicated.

35. Glare testing can reveal significant functional visual problems even in patients with excellent visual acuity on Snellen testing.

36. Amblyopia is a diagnosis of exclusion. If amblyopia is associated with an afferent pupillary defect, a lesion of the retina or optic nerve should be suspected and ruled out.

37. The critical period of visual development is from birth through age 6 to 7 years. Amblyopia is most successfully treated during this time. However, treatment can be successful at older ages with good compliance. Atropine penalization can be as effective as patching.

38. Early treatment for congenital esotropia gives the best chance for the development of binocular vision. Be certain that a patient with a partial accommodative esotropia is wearing the maximum tolerated hyperopic prescription.

39. Check the light reflex test and cover test to determine if a true deviation exists. If the light reflex is in the appropriate place and there is no refixation on cover testing, the patient is orthophoric.

40. A young patient with asthenopia should be evaluated for exophoria at near (convergence insufficiency) as well as for their cycloplegic refraction for undercorrected hyperopia (accommodative insufficiency).

41. Any patient with chronic progressive external ophthalmoplegia needs an electrocardiogram to rule out heart block. These patients may need a pacemaker to prevent sudden death.

42. A patient with acute onset of any combination of third, fourth, fifth, and sixth cranial nerve palsies; extreme headache; and decreased vision must be immediately placed on intravenous steroids and referred to neurosurgery for pituitary apoplexy.

43. The signs of endophthalmitis typically appear 1 to 4 days after strabismus surgery and include lethargy, asymmetric eye redness, eyelid swelling, and fever.

44. Before evaluating for strabismus, make sure patients with double vision have binocular diplopia. Strabismus does not cause monocular diplopia.

45. Always consider myasthenia gravis and thyroid eye disease in patients presenting with diplopia and normal pupils.

46. When performing surgery on both oblique and rectus muscles, hook the obliques first.

47. In a recess–resect procedure, the recession should be done first.

48. If a patient has a significant deviation in primary gaze or an abnormal head posture, strabismus surgery is indicated in most incomitant strabismus cases.

49. Try for fusion of all patients with nystagmus. Aim for exophoria with fusion.

50. Smoking is a controllable risk factor for thyroid eye disease.

51. All patients with optic neuritis should experience some improvement in vision. However, 5% of patients who presented with visual acuity of less than 20/200 were still 20/200 or less at 6 months.

52. An abnormal magnetic resonance imaging (MRI) in a patient with optic neuritis is the strongest predictor of developing multiple sclerosis (MS). Fifty-six percent of patients with optic neuritis and a white matter lesion on MRI will develop MS within 10 years.

53. The closer a patient stands to a visual-field testing screen, the smaller the field should be. This is helpful in determining a malingering patient.

54. Any patient suspected of giant cell arteritis should immediately be started on high doses of steroids to prevent involvement of the other eye even if the temporal artery biopsy cannot be done beforehand.

55. Dacryocystitis must be treated emergently to prevent cellulitis or intracranial spread of the infection.

56. Computed tomography (CT) scanning is superior to MRI in most cases of orbital disease owing to better bone–tissue delineation.

57. The most common cause of unilateral or bilateral proptosis is thyroid eye disease (Graves ophthalmopathy). Most patients with thyroid-related ophthalmopathy (TRO) will not require surgery for their disease; it will burn out with time.

58. The most common cause of unilateral proptosis in children is orbital cellulitis.

59. A child with rapidly progressive proptosis, inferior displacement of the globe, and upper eyelid edema should have immediate neuroimaging followed by an orbital biopsy to rule out rhabdomyosarcoma.

60. Suspect TRO in patients with nonspecific redness and inflammation of the eyes even if there is no history of a systemic thyroid imbalance.

61. Myositis, a nonspecific inflammation of an extraocular muscle, can be distinguished from thyroid-associated ophthalmopathy (TAO) by the location of muscle inflammation. TAO demonstrates thickening of the muscle belly, but only myositis shows thickening of the tendon insertion as well.

62. Persistent proptosis and progression of orbital infection while on intravenous antibiotics for orbital cellulitis should prompt a repeat CT scan to rule out an orbital abscess.

63. The sinuses are the most common source of an orbital infection. The ethmoid sinus is the most frequent culprit as its lateral wall is the thinnest orbital wall, the lamina papyracea.

64. Surgical drainage should be undertaken in orbital cellulitis if sinuses are completely opacified, response to antibiotics is poor by 48 to 72 hours, vision decreases, or an afferent pupillary defect presents.

65. Mild ptosis associated with miosis and neck or facial pain should raise suspicion of a carotid artery dissection, prompting an urgent workup.

66. Acute ptosis and ocular misalignment mandate a careful evaluation of the pupil to rule out pupil-involving third-nerve palsy. A dilated pupil requires neurologic evaluation for a compressive aneurysm.

67. Basal cell carcinoma is the most common malignant eyelid tumor. It has a 3% mortality rate because of invasion into the orbit and brain via the lacrimal drainage system, prior radiation therapy, or clinical neglect.

68. Squamous cell carcinoma may metastasize systemically.

69. Keratoacanthomas often resolve spontaneously but should be removed surgically if near the lid margin to prevent permanent deformity.

70. Rule out sebaceous cell carcinomas in a patient with a recurrent chalazion in the same spot.

71. Young patients with xanthelasma should be evaluated for diabetes mellitus and hypercholesterolemia.

72. All patients who have anterior uveitis must have a dilated examination to exclude associated posterior segment disease.

73. Consider masquerade syndromes in the very young, the elderly, and in patients who have uveitis that does not respond to treatment. Uveitis in patients with acquired immunodeficiency syndrome is almost invariably part of a disseminated systemic infection. Lymphoma may masquerade as retinitis.

74. Never aspirate subretinal exudates for diagnostic purposes in a patient with potential Coats disease, unless retinoblastoma has been absolutely ruled out. It may take as long as 1 to 2 years for exudation to clear after successful treatment of the abnormal peripheral retinal vessels.

75. The five trauma-related breaks are horseshoe tears, operculated tears, dialyses, retinal dissolution, and macular holes.

76. The globe is most likely to rupture at the limbus, underneath a rectus muscle, or at a previous surgical site.

77. A break in the Bruch membrane is necessary for a choroidal neovascular membrane to form.

78. Age-related macular degeneration (ARMD) is the leading cause of legal blindness in the Western world. The leading epidemiologic risk factors for ARMD are increasing age, smoking, and genetic predisposition.

79. Threshold disease of retinopathy of prematurity (ROP) is five contiguous or eight cumulative clock hours of stage 3 ROP in zone I or II in the presence of plus disease.

80. When ROP reaches the Early Treatment for Retinopathy of Prematurity (ETROP) Study Type 1 (high-risk disease), indirect laser photocoagulation dramatically reduces the risk of blindness.

81. Newborns weighing less than 1500 g at birth and/or born at or before 28 weeks' gestational age should be screened for ROP at 4 to 6 weeks after birth or 31 to 33 weeks postconceptual age and followed until the retinal vascularization has fully matured.

82. The most common cause of vision loss in diabetic retinopathy is macular edema.

83. Neovascularization of the iris is an ominous finding in proliferative diabetic retinopathy and requires prompt treatment with panretinal photocoagulation, intravitreal anti–vascular endothelial growth factor (VEGF) injections, or both.

84. Clinically significant macular edema is defined as one of the following: retinal thickening within 500 μm of the center of the fovea, hard yellow exudate within 500 μm of the fovea and adjacent retinal thickening, or at least one disc area of retinal thickening, any part of which is within one disc diameter of the center of the fovea. It is based on fundus exam and is NOT related to visual acuity or optical coherence tomography findings.

85. Most central retinal artery obstructions are thrombotic; most branch retinal artery obstructions are embolic. Systemic disease must be ruled out in any patient with retinal artery obstruction.

86. First-line treatment for macular edema from retinal venous occlusive disease is intravitreal anti-VEGF injections. However, there is an emerging role for intravitreal corticosteroid treatment, especially in refractory cases.

87. In patients with central retinal venous occlusions, argon laser photocoagulation is indicated only when neovascularization develops; it is not for prophylaxis.

88. Perform iris examination and gonioscopy before dilation in a patient with a central retinal vein occlusion. Neovascular glaucoma is the most feared complication of a central retinal vein occlusion.

89. Branch and central retinal venous occlusions are classified as ischemic or nonischemic. Patients with ischemic occlusions lose vision primarily from macular edema. Vision loss in nonischemic occlusions is due to macular nonperfusion, vitreous hemorrhage, tractional retinal detachments, and neovascular glaucoma.

90. The classic symptoms of a retinal break are flashes and floaters. Pigmented cells or blood in the vitreous strongly suggests the possibility of a retinal break. Risk factors for rhegmatogenous retinal detachment (RRD) include previous cataract surgery, lattice degeneration, myopia, trauma, family history, and fellow eye with a history of an RD.

91. Pneumatic retinopexy for an RRD should be avoided if patients are at high risk of significant vitreoretinal traction, that is, early PVR, highly elevated flap tears, multiple tears, lattice degeneration, or sizable vitreous hemorrhage.

92. Retinoblastoma is the leading eye cancer in children. About 98% of children with retinoblastoma in the United States and developed nations survive owing to early detection and proper management.

93. Most children with unilateral retinoblastoma have a somatic mutation and are managed with enucleation or intra-arterial chemotherapy.

94. Most children with bilateral retinoblastoma have a germ-line mutation and are managed with intravenous or intra-arterial chemotherapy.

95. The presence of dilated, tortuous episcleral blood vessels warrants a complete exam to rule out an underlying ciliary body or peripheral choroidal tumor.

96. Ultrasound findings of low to medium internal reflectivity and collar-button shape can confirm the diagnosis of a choroidal melanoma and differentiate it from other choroidal lesions.

97. Uveal melanomas with epithelioid cells have a poorer prognosis. Seventy percent of uveal metastases are from breast or lung cancer.

98. Most periocular lymphomas are B cell, extranodal marginal zone lymphoma, also known as mucosal-associated lymphoid tissue lymphoma.

99. Management of orbital lymphoma is largely based on two factors: the particular histologic subtype and the stage of disease.

100. Based on recent data, the treatment of choice for optic nerve sheath meningioma is stereotactic radiotherapy.

CHAPTER 1

CLINICAL ANATOMY OF THE EYE

Kenneth B. Gum

GENERAL

1. Name the seven bones that make up the bony orbit and describe which location is most prone to damage in an orbital blow-out fracture.
   The seven orbital bones are the frontal, zygoma, maxillary, sphenoid, ethmoid, palatine, and lacrimal. A true blow-out fracture most commonly affects the orbital floor posteriorly and medially to the infraorbital nerve. The ethmoid bone of the medial wall is often broken.

2. Which nerves and vessels pass through the superior orbital fissure? Which motor nerve to the eye lies outside the annulus of Zinn, leaving it unaffected by retrobulbar injection of anesthetic?
   The superior orbital fissure transmits the third, fourth, and sixth cranial nerves, as well as the first division of the fifth cranial nerve, which has already divided into frontal and lacrimal branches. The superior ophthalmic vein and sympathetic nerves also pass through this fissure. The fourth cranial nerve, supplying the superior oblique muscle, lies outside the annulus. This position accounts for residual intorsion of the eye sometimes seen during retrobulbar anesthesia (Fig. 1.1).

3. A 3-year-old is referred for evaluation of consecutive exotropia after initial bimedial rectus recessions for esotropia performed elsewhere. A review of the operative notes discloses that each muscle was recessed 4.5 mm for a 30-prism diopter deviation. Unfortunately, the child had mild developmental delay and presents with a 25-prism diopter exotropia. You decide to advance the recessed medial rectus of each eye back to its original insertion site. Where is this site in relation to the limbus? Identify the location of each of the rectus muscle insertion sites relative to the limbus.
   Reattach each medial rectus muscle 5.5 mm from the limbus. Insertion of the inferior rectus is 6.5 mm from the limbus, the lateral rectus is 6.9 mm from the limbus, and the superior rectus, 7.7 mm. The differing distances of

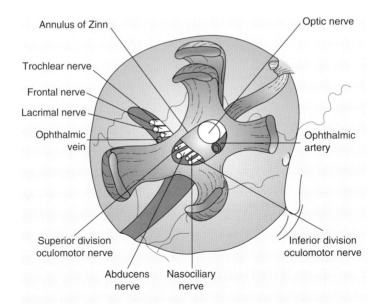

Fig. 1.1 The annulus of Zinn and surrounding structures. (From Campolattaro BN, Wang FM: Anatomy and physiology of the extraocular muscles and surrounding tissues. In Yanoff M, Duker JS, editors: *Ophthalmology*, ed 2, St. Louis, 2004, Mosby.)

rectus-muscle insertions from the limbus make up the spiral of Tillaux. An important caveat in developmentally delayed children is to postpone muscle surgery until much later, treating any amblyopia in the interim. Early surgery frequently leads to overcorrection.

4. What is the most common cause of both unilateral and bilateral proptosis in adults?
Thyroid orbitopathy is the most common cause. Many signs are associated with thyroid eye disease, which is probably caused by an autoimmune reactivity toward the epitope of thyroid-stimulating hormone receptors in the thyroid and orbit. The order of frequency of extraocular muscle involvement in thyroid orbitopathy is as follows: inferior rectus, medial rectus, lateral rectus, superior rectus, and obliques. There is enlargement of the muscle belly with sparing of the tendons.

5. You have just begun a ptosis procedure. A lid crease incision was made, and the orbital septum has been isolated and opened horizontally. What important landmark should be readily apparent? Describe its relation to other important structures.
The orbital fat lies directly behind the orbital septum and directly on the muscular portion of the levator (Fig. 1.2). A separate medial fat pad often herniates through the septum in later years.

6. To what glands do the lymphatics of the orbit drain?
There are no lymphatic vessels or nodes within the orbit. Lymphatics from the conjunctivae and lids drain medially to the submandibular glands and laterally to the superficial preauricular nodes.

7. What is the orbital septum?
The septum is a thin sheet of connective tissue that defines the anterior limit of the orbit. In the upper lid, it extends from the periosteum of the superior orbital rim to insert at the levator aponeurosis, slightly above the superior tarsal border (see Fig. 1.2). The lower lid septum extends from the periosteum of the inferior orbital rim to insert directly on the inferior tarsal border.

8. A 70-year-old patient presents with herpes zoster lesions in the trigeminal nerve distribution. Classic lesions on the side and tip of the nose increase your concern about ocular involvement. Why?
This sign, called Hutchinson's sign, results from involvement of the infratrochlear nerve. The infratrochlear nerve is the terminal branch of the nasociliary nerve, which gives off the long ciliary nerves (usually two) that supply the globe.

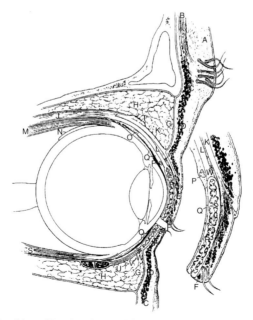

Fig. 1.2 Schematic cross-section of the eyelids and anterior orbit. A, Skin; B, frontalis muscle; C, orbicularis muscle (orbital portion); D, orbicularis muscle (preseptal portion); E, orbicularis muscle (pretarsal portion); F, orbicularis muscle (muscle of Riolan); G, orbital septum; H, orbital fat; I, superior transverse ligament; J, levator muscle; K, levator aponeurosis; L, Müller's muscle; M, superior rectus muscle; N, superior oblique tendon; O, gland of Krause; P, gland of Wolfring; Q, conjunctiva; R, tarsus; S, inferior rectus muscle; T, inferior oblique muscle; U, inferior tarsal muscle; V, capsulopalpebral ascia; W, peripheral arterial arcade. (From Beard C: *Ptosis*, ed 3, St. Louis, 1981, Mosby.)

9. Where is the sclera the thinnest? Where are globe ruptures after blunt trauma most likely to occur?

    The sclera is thinnest just behind the insertion of the rectus muscles (0.3 mm). Scleral rupture usually occurs opposite the site of impact and in an arc parallel to the limbus at the insertion of the rectus muscles or at the equator. The most common site of rupture is near the superonasal limbus.

10. Describe the surgical limbus and Schwalbe's line.

    The surgical limbus can be differentiated into an anterior bluish zone that extends from the termination of Bowman's layer to Schwalbe's line, which is the termination of Descemet's membrane. The posterior white zone overlies the trabecular meshwork and extends from the Schwalbe's line to the scleral spur.

11. You are preparing to do a laser trabeculoplasty. Describe the gonioscopic appearance of the anterior chamber angle.

    The ciliary body is a visible concavity anterior to the iris root. The scleral spur appears as a white line anterior to the ciliary body. Above this are the trabecular meshwork and canal of Schlemm. For an argon laser trabeculoplasty, treatment is applied to the anterior trabecular meshwork. For a selective laser trabeculoplasty, the aiming beam straddles the entire trabecular meshwork.

12. After a filtering procedure, your patient develops choroidal effusions. Explain the distribution of these fluid accumulations based on uveal attachments to the sclera.

    The uveal tract is attached to the sclera at the scleral spur, the optic nerve, and the exit sites of the vortex veins. The fluid dissects the choroid from the underlying sclera but retains these connections.

13. Describe the structure of Bruch's membrane. Name two conditions in which defects develop in this structure spontaneously.

    The Bruch's membrane consists of five layers: internally, the basement membrane of the pigment epithelium, the inner collagenous zone, a central band of elastic fibers, and the outer collagenous zone; externally, the basement membrane of the choriocapillaris. Pseudoxanthoma elasticum and myopia may cause spontaneous defects in this membrane, making the patient prone to development of choroidal neovascularization.

KEY POINTS: BRUCH'S MEMBRANE

1. Composed of five layers.
2. Spontaneous breaks can occur in pseudoxanthoma elasticum and myopia.
3. Defect in Bruch's membrane in age-related macular degeneration may lead to the exudative form.
4. Trauma may cause a break in the membrane, leading to a choroidal neovascular membrane.

14. Less laser power is required for photocoagulation in darkly pigmented fundi. What determines this pigmentation?

    The pigmentation of the fundus seen ophthalmoscopically is largely determined by the number of melanosomes in the choroid. The darker macular area results from taller pigment epithelial cells that contain more and larger melanosomes than the periphery.

15. What is the blood–retinal barrier?

    The inner blood–retinal barrier consists of the retinal vascular endothelium, which is nonfenestrated and contains tight junctions. The outer blood–retinal barrier is the retinal pigment epithelium. Bruch's membrane is permeable to small molecules.

16. Name the 10 classically described anatomic layers of the retina and the cells that make up the retina.

    The retina may be divided into 10 layers, starting just above the choroids and extending to the vitreous:
    - Retinal pigment epithelium
    - Outer segments of the photoreceptors
    - External limiting membrane
    - Outer nuclear layer
    - Outer plexiform layer
    - Inner nuclear layer
    - Inner plexiform layer
    - Ganglion cell layer
    - Nerve fiber layer
    - Internal limiting membrane

    Within these layers lie the photoreceptors, horizontal cells, bipolar cells, amacrine cells, retinal interneurons, ganglion cells, and the glial cells of the retina, Müller cells.

17. **Which retinal layer is referred to as the fiber layer of Henle in the macular region?**
    The outer plexiform layer, which is made up of connections between photoreceptor synaptic bodies and horizontal and bipolar cells, becomes thicker and more oblique in orientation as it deviates away from the fovea. At the fovea, this layer becomes nearly parallel to the retinal surface and accounts for the radial, or star-shaped, patterns of exudate in the extracellular spaces under pathologic conditions causing vascular compromise, such as hypertension.

18. **What are three clinically recognized remnants of the fetal hyaloid vasculature?**
    Mittendorf's dot, Bergmeister's papilla, and vascular loops (95% of which are arterial).

19. **A patient presents with a central retinal artery occlusion and 20/20 visual acuity. How do you explain this finding?**
    Fifteen percent of people have a cilioretinal artery that supplies the macular region. Thirty percent of eyes have a cilioretinal artery supplying some portion of the retina. These are perfused by the choroidal vessels, which are fed by the ophthalmic artery and thus are not affected by central retinal artery circulation.

20. **Where do branch retinal vein occlusions occur? Which quadrant of the retina is most commonly affected?**
    Branch retinal vein occlusions occur at arteriovenous crossings, most commonly where the vein lies posterior to the artery. The superotemporal quadrant is most often affected because of a higher number of arteriovenous crossings on average.

21. **Discuss the organization of crossed and uncrossed fibers in the optic chiasm.**
    Inferonasal extramacular fibers cross in the anterior chiasm and bulge into the contralateral optic nerve (Willebrand's knee). Superonasal extramacular fibers cross directly to the opposite optic tract. Macular fibers are located in the center of the optic nerve. Temporal macular fibers pass uncrossed through the chiasm, whereas nasal macular fibers cross posteriorly. However, in albinism, many temporal fibers also cross.

22. **Describe the location of the visual cortex.**
    The visual cortex is situated along the superior and inferior lips of the calcarine fissure. This area is called the striate cortex because of the prominent band of geniculocalcarine fibers, termed the stria of Gennari after its discoverer.

23. **What is the most likely anatomic location of pathology associated with downbeat nystagmus?**
    Downbeat nystagmus is usually indicative of cervicomedullary structural disease. The most common causes are Arnold-Chiari malformation, stroke, multiple sclerosis, and platybasia. Any patient with this finding should have neuroimaging studies done.

24. **A patient presents with a chief complaint of tearing and ocular irritation. As she dumps the plethora of eyedrops from her purse, she explains that she has seen seven different doctors and none has been able to help her. The exam shows mild inferior punctate keratopathy but a normal tear lake and normal Schirmer's test. Of interest, she had blepharoplasty surgery 6 months previously. What is the diagnosis?**
    You are already patting yourself on the back as you ask if the irritation is worse in the morning or evening. She replies emphatically that it is much more severe upon awakening. You ask her to close her eyes gently and see 2 mm of lagophthalmos in each eye. This is a frequently overlooked cause of tearing in otherwise normal eyes.

25. **During orbital surgery, a patient's lacrimal gland is removed. Afterward, there is no evidence of tear deficiency. Why not?**
    Basal tear production is provided by the accessory lacrimal glands of Krause and Wolfring. Krause's glands are located in the superior fornix, and the glands of Wolfring are located above the superior tarsal border. They are cytologically identical to the main lacrimal gland.

26. **Describe the anatomy of the macula and fovea.**
    The macula is defined as the area of the posterior retina that contains xanthophyllic pigment and two or more layers of ganglion cells. It is centered approximately 4 mm temporal and 0.8 mm inferior to the center of the optic disc. The fovea is a central depression of the inner retinal surface and is approximately 1.5 mm in diameter.

27. **Fluorescein angiography typically shows perfusion of the choroid and any cilioretinal arteries prior to visualization of the dye in the retinal circulation. Why?**
    Fluorescein enters the choroid via the short posterior ciliary arteries, which are branches of the ophthalmic artery. The central retinal artery, also a branch of the ophthalmic artery, provides a more circuitous route for the dye to travel, resulting in dye appearance in the retinal circulation 1 to 2 seconds later.

28. **Explain why visual acuity in infants does not reach adult levels until approximately 6 months of age, based on retinal differentiation.**
    The differentiation of the macula is not complete until 4 to 6 months after birth. Ganglion cell nuclei are initially found directly over the foveola and gradually are displaced peripherally, leaving this area devoid of accessory

neural elements and blood vessels as neural organization develops to adult levels by age 6 months. This delay in macular development is one factor in the inability of newborns to fixate, and improvement in visual activity parallels macular development.

29. **A neonate presents with an opacification in her left cornea. What is the differential diagnosis?**

Neonatal cloudy cornea usually falls into one of the following categories (which can easily be recalled by using the mnemonic *STUMPED*): sclerocornea, trauma, ulcers, metabolic disorder, Peters' anomaly, endothelial dystrophy, and dermoid.

30. **Describe the innervation of the lens.**

The lens is anatomically unique because it lacks innervation and vascularization. It depends entirely on the aqueous and vitreous humors for nourishment.

31. **Describe the innervation of the cornea.**

The long posterior ciliary nerves branch from the ophthalmic division of the trigeminal nerve and penetrate the cornea. Peripherally, 70 to 80 branches enter the cornea in conjunctival, episcleral, and scleral planes. They lose their myelin sheath 1 to 2 mm from the limbus. The network just posterior to the Bowman's layer sends branches anteriorly into the epithelium.

32. **What are the three layers of the tear film? Where do they originate?**
   - The *mucoid layer* coats the superficial corneal epithelial cells and creates a hydrophilic layer that allows for spontaneous, even distribution of the aqueous layer of the tear film. Mucin is secreted principally by the conjunctival goblet cells but also from the lacrimal gland.
   - The *aqueous layer* is secreted by the glands of Kraus and Wolfring (basal secretion) and the lacrimal gland (reflex secretion). The aqueous layer contains electrolytes, immunoglobulins, and other solutes, including glucose, buffers, and amino acids.
   - The *lipid layer* is secreted primarily by the meibomian glands and maintains a hydrophobic barrier that prevents tear overflow, retards evaporation, and provides lubrication for the lid/ocular interface.

33. **What are the differences in the structure of the central retinal artery and retinal arterioles?**

The central retinal artery contains a fenestrated internal elastic lamina and an outer layer of smooth muscle cells surrounded by a basement membrane. The retinal arterioles have no internal elastic lamina and lose the smooth muscle cells near their entrance into the retina. Hence, the retinal vasculature has no autoregulation.

34. **Where is the macula represented in the visual cortex?**

Macular function is represented in the most posterior portion at the tip of the occipital lobe. However, there may be a wide distribution of some macular fibers along the calcarine fissure.

35. **What is macular hole formation?**

Macular hole formation is a common malady that can result in rapid loss of central vision. Approximately 83% of cases are idiopathic, and 15% are due to some sort of trauma.

36. **Describe the stages of macular hole formation as proposed by Gass, as well as the changes in our understanding of the disease process since the development of optical coherence tomography (OCT).**

Gass's theory proposed that the underlying causative mechanism was centripetal tangential traction by the cortical vitreous on the fovea. He also proposed the following stages:
   - **Stage 1a:** Tractional elevation of the foveola with a visible yellow dot.
   - **Stage 1b:** Enlargement of the tractional detachment with foveal elevation. A yellow ring becomes visible.
   - **Stage 2:** Full-thickness retinal defect less than 400 μm.
   - **Stage 3:** Full-thickness retinal defect larger than 400 μm.
   - **Stage 4:** Stage 3 with complete posterior vitreous detachment.

OCT analysis has revealed that some patients have perifoveal vitreous detachment with a remaining attachment of the fovea. Occasionally, patients may develop an intraretinal split with formation of a foveal cyst. This cyst may evolve into a full-thickness hole with disruption of the inner retinal layer and opening of the foveal floor. These findings suggest a complex array of both anterior–posterior and tangential vector forces as an etiology for molecular hole formation.

BIBLIOGRAPHY

American Academy of Ophthalmology: Basic and clinical science course, section 2, San Francisco, 1993–1994, American Academy of Ophthalmology.

Burde RM, Savino PJ, Trobe JD: Clinical decisions in neuro-ophthalmology, St. Louis, 1985, Mosby.

Fine BS, Yanoff M: Ocular histology, ed 2, Hagerstown, MD, 1979, Harper & Row.

Gass JDM: Stereoscopic atlas of macular diseases, ed 4, St. Louis, 1997, Mosby.

Guyer DR, Yannuzzi LA, Chang S, et al.: Retina-vitreous-macula, Philadelphia, W.B. 1999, Saunders.

Jaffe NS: Cataract surgery and its complications, ed 5, St. Louis, 1990, Mosby.

Justice J, Lehman RP: Cilioretinal arteries: a study based on review of stereofundus photographs and fluorescein angiographic findings, Arch Ophthalmol 94:1355–1358, 1976.

Miller NR: Walsh and Hoyt's clinical neuro-ophthalmology, vol 1, ed 4, Baltimore, 1982, Williams & Wilkins.

Spaide RF: Optical coherence tomography: interpretation and clinical applications, Course #590, AAO Annual Meeting, Chicago, 2005.

Stewart WB: Surgery of the eyelid, orbit, and lacrimal system. Ophthalmology monographs, vol 1, San Francisco, 1993, American Academy of Ophthalmology.

Weinberg DV, Egan KM, Seddon JM: The asymmetric distribution of arteriovenous crossing in the normal retina, Ophthalmology 100: 31–36, 1993.

ANATOMY OF THE ORBIT AND EYELID

Edward H. Bedrossian Jr.

CHAPTER 2

ORBIT

1. Name the bones of the orbit (Fig. 2.1).
   - **Medial wall:** Sphenoid, ethmoid, lacrimal, maxillary
   - **Lateral wall:** Zygomatic, greater wing of the sphenoid
   - **Roof:** Frontal, lesser wing of the sphenoid
   - **Floor:** Maxillary, zygomatic, palatine

2. What are the weak spots of the orbital rim?
   - Frontozygomatic suture
   - Zygomaticomaxillary suture
   - Frontomaxillary suture

3. Describe the most common location of blow-out fractures.
   The posteromedial aspect of the orbital floor.

4. What is the weakest bone within the orbit?
   The lamina papyracea portion of the ethmoid bone.

5. Name the divisions of cranial nerve V that pass through the cavernous sinus.
   - Ophthalmic division (V1)
   - Maxillary division (V2)

6. What is the annulus of Zinn?
   The circle defined by the superior rectus muscle, inferior rectus muscle, lateral rectus muscle, and medial rectus muscle.

7. What nerves pass through the superior orbital fissure but outside the annulus of Zinn?
   Frontal, lacrimal, and trochlear nerves.

8. What structures pass through the optic canal?
   The optic nerve and ophthalmic artery.

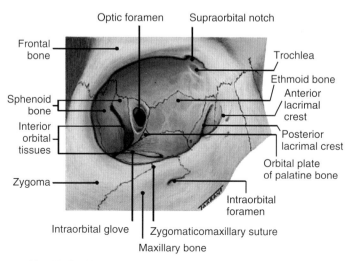

Fig. 2.1 Anatomy of the orbit. (From Kanski JJ: *Clinical ophthalmology: a systematic approach*, ed 7, London, 2011, Elsevier.)

EYELID

9. List the factors responsible for involutional entropion.
   - Lower lid laxity
   - Override of the preseptal orbicularis oculi muscle onto the pretarsal orbicularis oculi muscle
   - Dehiscence/disinsertion of the lower lid retractors
   - Orbital fat atrophy

10. Describe the sensory nerve supply to the upper and lower eyelids.
    - The ophthalmic nerve (V1) provides sensation to the upper lid.
    - The maxillary nerve (V2) provides sensation to the lower lid.

11. What are the surgical landmarks for locating the superficial temporal artery during temporal artery biopsies?
    The superficial temporal artery lies deep to the skin and subcutaneous tissue but superficial to the temporalis fascia.

12. What structures would you pass through during a transverse blepharotomy 3 mm above the upper eyelid margin?
    - Skin
    - Pretarsal orbicularis muscle
    - Tarsus
    - Palpebral conjunctiva (Fig. 2.2)

13. What is meant by the phrase *lower lid retractors*?
    The lower lid retractors consist of the capsulopalpebral fascia and the inferior tarsus muscle. The capsulopalpebral fascia of the lower lid is analogous to the levator complex in the upper lid. The inferior tarsus muscle of the lower lid is analogous to the Müller's muscle in the upper lid.

14. What structures would be cut in a full-thickness lower-lid laceration 2 mm below the lower tarsus?
    - Skin
    - Preseptal orbicularis oculi muscle
    - Conjoint tendon (fused orbital septum and lower lid retractors)
    - Palpebral conjunctiva

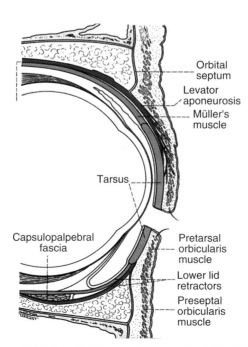

Orbital septum

Levator aponeurosis

Müller's muscle

Tarsus

Capsulopalpebral fascia

Pretarsal orbicularis muscle

Lower lid retractors

Preseptal orbicularis muscle

Fig. 2.2 Eyelid structures. (From Kanski JJ: *Clinical ophthalmology: a systematic approach*, ed 5, New York, 2003, Butterworth-Heinemann.)

15. What structures would be cut in a full-thickness lower-lid laceration 6 mm below the lower tarsus?
    - Skin
    - Preseptal orbicularis oculi muscle
    - Orbital septum
    - Fat
    - Lower lid retractors (capsulopalpebral fascia and inferior tarsus muscle)
    - Conjunctiva

16. Discuss the bony attachments of the Whitnall's superior suspensory ligament.
    Medially, it attaches to the periosteum of the trochlea. Laterally, the major attachment is to the periosteum at the frontozygomatic suture. It also sends minor attachments to the lateral orbital tubercle.

17. What structure separates the medial fat pad from the central (also called the preaponeurotic) fat pad in the upper eyelid?
    The superior oblique tendon.

18. Lester Jones divided the orbicularis oculi muscle into three portions. Name them.
    - Orbital portion
    - Preseptal portion
    - Pretarsal portion

19. What portions of the orbicularis oculi muscle are important in the lacrimal pump mechanism?
    The preseptal and pretarsal portions.

20. Describe the insertion of the lateral canthal tendon.
    The lateral canthal tendon inserts onto Whitnall's orbital tubercle that lies posterior to the lateral orbital rim.

BIBLIOGRAPHY

Anderson R, Dixon R: The role of Whitnall's ligament in ptosis surgery, Arch Ophthalmol 97:705–707, 1979.
Bedrossian Jr EH: Embryology and anatomy of the eyelids. In Tasman W, Jaeger E, editors: Foundations of clinical ophthalmology, 1998, Lippincott Williams & Wilkins, pp 1–22.
Bedrossian Jr EH: Surgical anatomy of the eyelids. In Della Rocca RC, Bedrossian EH Jr, Arthurs BP, editors: Ophthalmic plastic surgery: decision making and techniques, Philadelphia, 2002, McGraw-Hill, pp 163–172.
Duane TD: Duane's foundations of clinical ophthalmology, United States, 1998, Lippincott.
Dutton J: Atlas of clinical and surgical orbital anatomy, Philadelphia, 1994, W.B. Saunders.
Gioia V, Linberg J, McCormick S: The anatomy of the lateral canthal tendon, Arch Ophthalmol 105:529–532, 1987.
Hawes M, Dortzbach R: The microscopic anatomy of the lower eyelid retractors, Arch Ophthalmol 100:1313–1318, 1982.
Jones LT: The anatomy of the lower eyelid, Am J Ophthalmol 49:29–36, 1960.
Lemke B, Della Rocca R: Surgery of the eyelids and orbit: an anatomical approach, Norwalk, CT, 1990, Appleton & Lange.
Lemke B, Stasior O, Rosen P: The surgical relations of the levator palpebrae superioris muscle, Ophthal Plast Reconstr Surg 4:25–30, 1988.
Lockwood CB: The anatomy of the muscles, ligaments and fascia of the orbit, including an account of the capsule of tenon, the check ligaments of the recti, and of the suspensory ligament of the eye, J Anat Physiol 20;1–26, 1886.
Meyer D, Linberg J, Wobig J, McCormick S: Anatomy of the orbital septum and associated eyelid connective tissues: Implications for ptosis surgery, Ophthal Plast Reconstr Surg 7:104–113, 1991.
Sullivan J, Beard C: Anatomy of the eyelids, orbit and lacrimal system. In Stewart W, editor: Surgery of the eyelids, orbit and lacrimal system, American Academy of Ophthalmology Monograph No. 8, 1993, Oxford University Press, pp 84–96.
Whitnall SE: The levator palpebrae superioris muscle: the attachments and relations of its aponeurosis, Ophthalmoscope 12:258–263, 1914.
Whitnall SE: The anatomy of the human orbit and accessory organs, London, 1985, Oxford Medical Publishers.

CHAPTER 3

OPTICS AND REFRACTION

Janice A. Gault

1. **What is the primary focal point (F₁)?**

   The primary focal point is the point along the optical axis at which an object must be placed for parallel rays to emerge from the lens. Thus, the image is at infinity (Fig. 3.1).

2. **What is the secondary focal point (F₂)?**

   The secondary focal point is the point along the optical axis at which parallel incoming rays are brought into focus. It is equal to 1/lens power in diopters (D). The object is now at infinity (Fig. 3.2).

3. **Where is the secondary focal point for a myopic eye? A hyperopic eye? An emmetropic eye?**

   The secondary focal point for a **myopic** eye is anterior to the retina in the vitreous (Fig. 3.3A). The object must be moved forward from infinity to allow the light rays to focus on the retina. A **hyperopic** eye has its secondary focal point posterior to the retina (Fig. 3.3B). An **emmetropic** eye focuses light rays from infinity onto the retina.

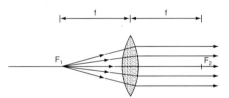

Fig. 3.1 The primary focal point (F₁), which has an image at infinity. (From Azar DT, Strauss L: Principles of applied clinical optics. In Albert DM, Jakobiec FA, editors: *Principles and practice of ophthalmology*, vol 6, ed 2, Philadelphia, 2000, W.B. Saunders, pp 5329–5340.)

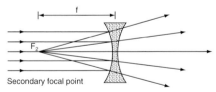

Fig. 3.2 The secondary focal point (F₂), which also has an object at infinity. (From Azar DT, Strauss L: Principles of applied clinical optics. In Albert DM, Jakobiec FA, editors, *Principles and practice of ophthalmology*, vol 6, ed 2, Philadelphia, 2000, W.B. Saunders, pp 5329–5340.)

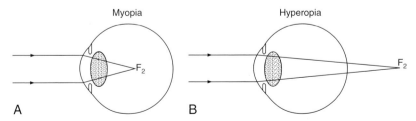

Fig. 3.3 A, The secondary focal point of a myopic eye is anterior to the retina in the vitreous. **B,** In hyperopia, the secondary focal point is behind the retina. (From Azar DT, Strauss L: Principles of applied clinical optics. In Albert DM, Jakobiec FA, editors: *Principles and practice of ophthalmology*, vol 6, ed 2, Philadelphia, 2000, W.B. Saunders, pp 5329–5340.)

4. What is the far point of an eye?
The term *far point* is used only for the optical system of an eye. It is the point at which an object must be placed along the optical axis for the light rays to be focused on the retina when the eye is not accommodating.

5. Where is the far point for a myopic eye? A hyperopic eye? An emmetropic eye?
The far point for a **myopic** eye is between the cornea and infinity. A **hyperopic** eye has its far point beyond infinity or behind the eye. An **emmetropic** eye has light rays focused on the retina when the object is at infinity.

6. How do you determine which lens will correct the refractive error of the eye?
A lens with its focal point coincident with the far point of the eye allows the light rays from infinity to be focused on the retina. The image at the far point of the eye now becomes the object for the eye.

7. What is the near point of an eye?
The near point is the point at which an object will be in focus on the retina when the eye is fully accommodating. Moving the object closer will cause it to blur.

8. Myopia can be caused in two ways. What are they?
- **Refractive myopia** is caused by too much refractive power owing to steep corneal curvature or high lens power.
- **Axial myopia** is due to an elongated globe. Every millimeter of axial elongation causes about 3 D of myopia.

9. The power of a proper corrective lens is altered by switching from a contact lens to a spectacle lens or vice versa. Why?
Moving a minus lens closer to the eye increases effective minus power. Thus, myopes have a weaker minus prescription in their contact lenses than in their glasses. Patients near presbyopia may need reading glasses when using their contacts but can read without a bifocal lens in their glasses (see question 45). Moving a plus lens closer to the eye decreases effective plus power. Thus, hyperopes need a stronger plus prescription for their contact lenses than for their glasses. They may defer bifocals for a while. The same principle applies to patients who slide their glasses down their nose and find that they can read more easily. They are adding plus power. This principle works for both hyperopes and myopes.

10. What is the amplitude of accommodation?
The total number of diopters that an eye can accommodate.

11. What is the range of accommodation?
The range of clear vision obtainable with accommodation only. For an emmetrope with 10 D of accommodative amplitude, the range of accommodation is infinity–10 cm.

12. How does a diopter relate to meters?
A diopter is the reciprocal of the distance in meters.

13. What is the near point of a 4-D hyperope with an amplitude of accommodation of 8?
The far point is 25 cm (¼ D) behind the cornea. The patient must use 4 D of accommodation to overcome hyperopia and focus the image at infinity on the retina. Thus, he or she has 4 D to accommodate to the near point, which is 25 cm (¼ D) anterior to the cornea. However, when wearing a +4.00 lens, he or she has the full amplitude of accommodation available. The near point is now 12.5 cm (⅛ D).

14. What is the near point of a 4-D myope with an amplitude of accommodation of 8?
The far point is 25 cm (¼ D) in front of the eye. The patient can accommodate 8 D beyond this point. The near point is 12 D, which is 8.3 cm (¹/₁₂ D) in front of the cornea.

15. When a light ray passes from a medium with a lower refractive index to a medium with a higher refractive index, is it bent toward or away from the normal?
It is bent toward the normal (Fig. 3.4).

16. What is the critical angle?
The critical angle is the incident angle at which the angle of refraction is 90 degrees from normal. The critical angle occurs only when light passes from a more dense to a less dense medium.

17. What happens if the critical angle is exceeded?
When the critical angle is exceeded, total internal reflection is the result. The angle of incidence equals the angle of reflection (Fig. 3.5).

18. Give examples of total internal reflection.
Total internal reflection at the tear–air interface prevents a direct view of the anterior chamber. To overcome this limitation, the critical angle must be increased for the tear–air interface by applying a plastic or glass goniolens to the surface. Total internal reflection also occurs in fiber-optic tubes and indirect ophthalmoscopes.

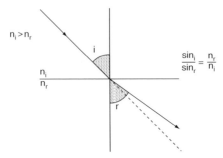

Fig. 3.4 When light passes from a medium with a lower refractive index (n_i) to a medium of higher refractive index (n_r), it slows down and is bent toward the normal to the surface. Snell's law determines the amount of bending. Here, i is the angle of incidence, and r is the angle of refraction. (From Azar DT, Strauss L: Principles of applied clinical optics. In Albert DM, Jakobiec FA, editors: *Principles and practice of ophthalmology*, vol 6, ed 2, Philadelphia, 2000, W.B. Saunders, pp 5329–5340.)

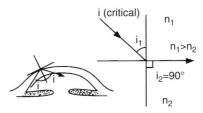

Fig. 3.5 Total internal reflection occurs when the critical angle is exceeded. (From Azar DT, Strauss L: Principles of applied clinical optics. In Albert DM, Jakobiec FA, editors: *Principles and practice of ophthalmology*, vol 6, ed 2, Philadelphia, 2000, W.B. Saunders, pp 5329–5340.)

19. What is the formula for vergence?

$$U + P = V,$$

where U is the vergence of light entering the lens, P is the power of the lens (the amount of vergence added to the light by the lens), and V is the vergence of light leaving the lens. All are expressed in diopters. By convention, light rays travel left to right. Plus signs indicate anything to the right of the lens, and minus signs indicate points to the left of the lens.

20. What is the vergence of parallel light rays?
    The vergence of parallel light rays is zero. Parallel light rays do not converge (which would be positive) or diverge (which would be negative). Light rays from an object at infinity or going to an image at infinity have zero vergence.

21. What is the image point if an object lies 25 cm to the left of a +5.00 lens?
    Everything must be expressed in diopters: 25 cm is 4 D (1/0.25 m). Because the image is to the left of the lens,

$$U = -4\ D$$
$$P = +5\ D$$
$$-4 + 5 = 1$$

The vergence of the object is +1 D. Converted to centimeters, the object lies 1 m to the right of the lens ($^1/_1$ D = 1 m = 100 cm).

22. Draw the schematic eye, labeling power in diopters (δ), nodal point (np), principal point, f and f', refractive index (n'), and respective distances.
    See Fig. 3.6.

23. How is the power of a prism calculated?
    The power of a prism is calculated in prism diopters (Δ) and is equal to the displacement in centimeters of a light ray passing through the prism measured 100 cm from the prism. Light is always bent toward the base of the prism. Thus, a prism of 15 Δ displaces light from infinity 15 cm toward its base at 100 cm.

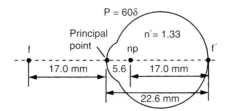

Fig. 3.6 The reduced schematic eye. (From Azar DT, Strauss L: Principles of applied clinical optics. In: Albert DM, Jakobiec FA, editors: *Principles and practice of ophthalmology*, vol 6, ed 2, Philadelphia, 2000, W.B. Saunders, pp 5329–5340.)

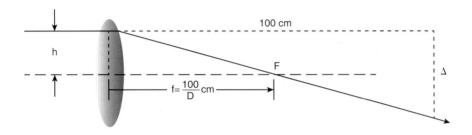

By similar triangles: $\dfrac{\Delta}{h} = \dfrac{100}{\dfrac{100}{D}}$

Δ	$=$	h	x	D	
Prism diopters		cm		Diopters	Prentice's rule

Fig. 3.7 Prismatic effect of a lens according to Prentice's rule. Δ is the induced prism (measured in prism diopters), *h* is the distance from the optical center in centimeters, and *D* is the power of the lens in diopters. (Reproduced, with permission, from Meltzer DW, *Basic and Clinical Science Course: Section 3: Optics, Refraction, and Contact Lenses*, American Academy of Ophthalmology, 1992.)

24. What is Prentice's rule?

$$\Delta = hD$$

The prismatic power of a lens (Δ) at any point on the lens is equal to the distance of that point from the optical axis in centimeters (*h*) multiplied by the power of the lens in diopters (δ). It follows that a lens has no prismatic effect at its optical center; a light ray will pass through the center undeviated (Fig. 3.7).

25. How is Prentice's rule used in real life?
In a patient who has anisometropia, the reading position may cause hyperdeviation of one eye owing to the prismatic effect.

KEY POINTS: HOW TO ALLEVIATE SYMPTOMATIC ANISOMETROPIA

1. Contact lenses
2. Lowering optical centers
3. Slab-off

26. How can the prismatic effect be alleviated?
   - Contact lenses move with the eye and allow patients to see through their optical center, preventing the prismatic effect.
   - Lowering the optical centers decreases the *h* of Prentice's rule.
   - Slab-off (removing the prism inferiorly from the more minus lens) helps to counteract the prismatic effect.

27. How does Prentice's rule affect the measurement of strabismic deviations when the patient is wearing glasses?

Plus lenses decrease the measured deviation, whereas minus lenses increase the measured deviation. The true deviation is changed by approximately 2.5 D%, where D is the spectacle power. Plus lenses have the base of the prism centrally, whereas minus lenses have the base of the prism peripherally.

28. Bifocals can cause significant problems induced by the prismatic effect. What is the difference between image jump and image displacement?

- **Image jump** is produced by the sudden introduction of the prismatic power at the top of the bifocal segment. The object that the patient sees in the inferior field suddenly jumps upward when the eye turns down to look at it. If the optical center of the segment is at the top of the segment, there is no image jump. Image jump is worse in glasses with a round-top bifocal because the optical center is far from the distance lens optical center. A flat-top bifocal is better because the optical center is close to the distance optical center.
- **Image displacement** is the prismatic effect induced by the addition of the bifocal and the distance lenses in the reading position. Image displacement is more bothersome than image jump for most people. A flat-top lens is essentially a base-up lens, whereas a round-top lens is a base-down lens. A myopic distance lens has base-up prismatic power in the reading position; thus, image displacement is worsened with a flat-top lens. The prism effects are additive. Similarly, a hyperopic correction is a base-down lens in the reading position; thus, a round-top lens makes image displacement an issue.

29. Should a hyperope use a round-top or flat-top reading lens?

A plus lens will have significant image displacement with a flat-top lens. Image displacement is lessened with a round-top lens. Although image jump will be present, it is the less disturbing of the two.

30. Should a myope use a flat-top or round-top reading lens?

A round-top lens has significant image displacement with a minus lens. A flat-top lens minimizes image displacement and image jump. Of course, a blended bifocal renders these issues moot.

31. What is the circle of least confusion?

Patients with astigmatism have two focal lines formed by the convergence of light rays. The first focal line is nearer the cornea and created by the more powerful corneal meridian. The second focal line is farther away, created by the less powerful meridian. The circle of least confusion is the circular cross-section of the Sturm's conoid, dioptrically midway between the two focal lines (Fig. 3.8). The goal of refractive correction is to choose a lens that places the circle of least confusion on the retina.

32. What is the spherical equivalent of $-3.00 + 2.00 \times 125$?

Take half the cylinder (-1.00) and add it to the sphere ($+1.00 - 3.00 = -2.00$). The spherical equivalent is -2.00 sphere.

33. Change the following plus cylinder refraction to the minus cylinder form: $-5.00 + 3.00 \times 90$.

First, add the sphere and cylinder to each other ($-5.00 + 3.00 = 2.00$). Then change the sign of the cylinder, and add 90 degrees to the axis. Thus, the minus cylinder form is $-2.00 - 3.00 \times 180$.

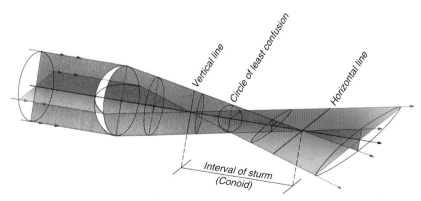

Fig. 3.8 The circle of least confusion. (From Azar DT, Strauss L: Principles of applied clinical optics. In Albert DM, Jakobiec FA, editors: *Principles and practice of ophthalmology,* vol 6, ed 2, Philadelphia, 2000, W.B. Saunders, pp 5329–5340.)

34. After large superior incision extracapsular cataract surgery, a patient has the following refraction: +1.00 + 3.00 × 100. Does the patient have with-the-rule or against-the-rule astigmatism?
With-the-rule astigmatism is corrected with a plus cylinder at 90 degrees (±15 to 20 degrees). Against-the-rule astigmatism is corrected with a plus cylinder at 180 degrees (±15 to 20 degrees). The patient has with-the-rule astigmatism.

35. How should you proceed with the patient's care?
Check the remaining sutures. Cutting the 11:00 suture will relax the wound and decrease the amount of astigmatism.

36. What if another patient has a refraction of +2.00 − 2.00 × 90 after large superior incision extracapsular cataract extraction? Where should you cut the suture?
Changing the refraction to the plus cylinder form, you see that the patient is plano + 2.00 × 180 and has against-the-rule astigmatism. You cannot cut any sutures to relax the astigmatism. The only option is to do a relaxing incision of the cornea, but it is likely that the patient will tolerate glasses, especially if the refraction is close to the preoperative correction. Also, check the preoperative keratometry. The patient may have had against-the-rule astigmatism before surgery. However, if the large incision is temporal, cutting the suture at 180 degrees will decrease the corneal astigmatism.

37. Thick lenses have aberrations. List them.
- **Spherical aberration:** The rays at the peripheral edges of the lens are refracted more than the rays at the center, thus causing night myopia. The larger pupil at night allows more spherical aberration than the smaller pupil during daylight.
- **Coma:** A comet-shaped blur is seen when the object and image are off the optical axis. Coma is similar to spherical aberration but occurs in the nonaxial rays.
- **Astigmatism of oblique incidence:** When the spherical lens is tilted, the lens gains a small astigmatic effect that causes curvature of the field (i.e., spherical lenses produce curved images of flat objects). This effect is helpful in the eye because the retina has a similar curvature (Fig. 3.9).
- **Chromatic aberration:** Each wavelength has its own refractive index; the shortest wavelengths are bent the most (Fig. 3.10).
- **Distortion:** The higher the spherical power, the more significantly the periphery is magnified or minified in relation to the rest of the image. A high plus lens produces pincushion distortion; i.e., straight lines in the periphery bulge toward the center. A high minus lens produces barrel distortion, i.e., straight lines bend outward from the center.

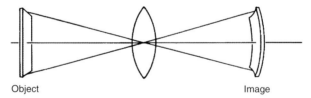

Object   Image

Fig. 3.9 The aberration caused by the astigmatism of oblique incidence is helpful in the eye because the curvature of the field that it induces is almost identical to the retinal curvature.

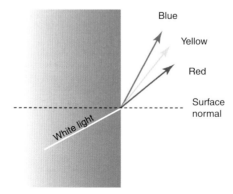

Fig. 3.10 Because each wavelength has a different refractive index, light passing through a prism will reveal the characteristic visible spectrum. (Reproduced, with permission, from Meltzer DW, *Basic and Clinical Science Course: Section 3: Optics, Refraction, and Contact Lenses,* American Academy of Ophthalmology, 1992.)

38. Are red or green light rays refracted more by a plus lens?
The shorter green rays are bent more than the longer red rays. This distinction causes chromatic aberration and is the basis for the red–green duochrome test. Green rays are focused 0.50 D closer to the lens than red rays. When a corrected myopic patient is fogged to prevent accommodation, the red letters should be clearer than the green. Slowly add more minus in 0.25 increments until the green and red letters are equal in clarity. This technique prevents overcorrection of myopia.

39. A myopic patient tilts his glasses to see in the distance. What does this tell you?
The patient is using the principle of astigmatism of oblique incidence to strengthen the power of his or her glasses. He or she needs a refraction. Tilting a minus lens induces a minus cylinder with axis in the axis of tilt. Tilting a plus lens induces a plus cylinder with axis in the axis of tilt. A small amount of additional sphere of the same sign is induced as well.

40. What measurements are necessary in determining the intraocular lens implant calculation?
Axial length in millimeters and keratometry readings in diopters. The desired postoperative refraction is also necessary. Newer formulas also use corneal size (white to white diameter), lens thickness, effective lens position, and anterior chamber depth. Most calculations are done on computers rather than manually as done in the past. For each lens used, specific constants determined by the manufacturer are necessary to insert into the formulas (i.e., A constant).

41. How does an axial error that is incorrect by 0.1 mm affect the intraocular lens calculation?
For every 0.1 mm error, the calculation is affected by 0.25 D. Recheck the A-scan if the axial length is less than 22 mm or more than 25 mm or if there is more than a 0.3-mm difference in the measurement between the two eyes.

42. How does an error in keratometry readings affect the intraocular lens calculation?
For every error of 0.25 D, the calculation is in error by 0.25 D. Recheck the keratometer measurements if the average corneal power is less than 40 D or more than 47 D. Also check if there is a difference of more than 1 D in the average keratometer readings between eyes.

43. What is the formula for transverse magnification?
Also known as linear or lateral magnification, transverse magnification equals $I/O = v/u$, where I is the size of the image, O is the size of the object, v is the distance from the lens to the image, and u is the distance of the object from the lens. All are measured in millimeters.

44. What is the formula for axial magnification?
Axial magnification is the square of the transverse magnification. Magnification along the visual axis causes distortion in three-dimensional images.

45. What is the effect of axial magnification on accommodative requirements for a given near-viewing distance?
Hyperopes must accommodate more through glasses than through contact lenses because the stronger plus prescription required in the contact lens provides more axial magnification of the image compared with the prescription for glasses. Conversely, myopes must accommodate less through glasses than through contact lenses. This effect can be clinically significant in early presbyopic years. The effect is greatest with high refractive errors. For example, a -5.00 myope may be able to read without bifocal glasses but require reading glasses with contact lenses. Conversely, a hyperope may be able to forego reading glasses with contact lenses but need bifocal glasses.

46. What is angular magnification?
Angular magnification is the magnification of a simple magnifier, such as viewing something with an eye or a single lens. Magnification is $D/4$, where D is the power of the lens used.

47. What is the magnification of a direct ophthalmoscope?
The examiner uses the optics of the patient's eye as a simple magnifier. Estimating the power of the eye as $+60$ D, the magnification is $15\times$. Thus, the retina appears 15 times larger than it is.

48. Does an astronomic telescope form an upright or an inverted image?
It forms an inverted image, which has few uses in ophthalmic optics.

49. Does a Galilean telescope form an upright or an inverted image?
It forms an upright image, which is used often in ophthalmic optics. An aphakic eye corrected with spectacles or a contact lens is an example. The eyepiece is the aphakic eye estimated to be -12.50 D, and the objective is the corrective lens.

50. What is the magnification formula for a telescope?

$$\text{Magnification} = \text{D eyepiece} / \text{D objective}$$

This formula applies to both astronomic and Galilean telescopes. For the aphakic eye with a spectacle correction of $+10.00$ D, the magnification is 1.25, or 25%. For a contact lens, this translates to $+11.75$ D, accounting for the vertex distance of 10 mm. Magnification now is 1.06, or 6%. Thus, aniseikonia with a contact lens is better tolerated than aniseikonia with glasses if the patient needs less powerful correction in the other eye.

51. When using the direct ophthalmoscope, which patient provides the larger image of the retina—the hyperope or the myope?

The myope functions as a Galilean telescope and provides extra magnification. The eyepiece (spectacle lens) is a minus lens, and the objective (the patient's own lens) is a plus lens. The hyperope functions as a reverse Galilean telescope and provides minification in comparison. In this situation, the eyepiece is a plus lens, and the objective is a minus lens.

52. What do you need to determine the best low-vision aid for a patient?

Best refraction, visual acuity, visual field, and practical needs of the patient.

53. What are the advantages and disadvantages of using a high add in a bifocal for a low-vision aid?

The advantages include a large field of view. Disadvantages include a short reading distance, as well as significant cost.

54. What are the advantages and disadvantages of using a high-power single-vision lens as a low-vision aid?

High-power single-vision lenses come in monocular and binocular forms. They also afford a large field of view but have a short reading distance.

55. How do you estimate the strength of plus lens needed to read newspaper print without accommodation?

The reciprocal of the best Snellen acuity is equal to the plus power of the lens required. For example, if a patient can read 20/60, a +3.00 D will suffice. The reciprocal of the diopter power gives the reading distance (i.e., 33 cm).

56. What adjustment is necessary when a binocular high-power single-vision lens is used?

Base in prisms to augment the natural ability to converge. Otherwise, patients develop exotropia at near when looking through high plus lenses.

57. What are the advantages and disadvantages of handheld magnifiers for low-vision aids?

Handheld magnifiers have a variable eye-to-lens distance and are easily portable. They enjoy a high rate of acceptability. However, they have a small field of view when the lens is held far from the eye and are difficult to manipulate by patients with tremors and arthritis. A stand magnifier may be more useful for such patients.

58. What are the advantages and disadvantages of using loupes as a low-vision aid?

Loupes are essentially prefocused telescopes. They allow a long working distance and keep the hands free. But they have a small field of view, have a limited depth of field, and are expensive.

59. The devices mentioned thus far are for magnifying at near. What is available for distance aids?

The only magnifying device for distance is a telescope. Telescopes are monocular or binocular and can be handheld or mounted on glasses. They also have an adjustable focus. Unfortunately, they have a restricted field of view (approximately 8 degrees). Thus, the object of regard may be difficult to find.

60. Do convex mirrors add plus or minus vergence?

Convex mirrors, like minus lenses, add minus vergence. Concave mirrors, like plus lenses, add plus vergence. Plane mirrors add no vergence.

61. What is the reflecting power in diopters of a mirror?

$D = 2/r$, where r is the radius of curvature. The focal length is one-half the radius.

62. What instrument uses the reflecting power of the cornea to determine its readings?

The keratometer uses the reflecting power of the cornea to determine the corneal curvature. The formula is $D = (n - 1)/r$, where D is the reflecting power of the cornea and n is the standardized refractive index for the cornea (1.3375).

63. How much of the cornea is measured with a keratometer?

Only the central 3 mm. A peripheral corneal scar or defect may be missed by using a keratometer instead of corneal topography.

64. Why does a keratometer use doubling of its images?

A keratometer doubles its images to avoid the problems of eye movement in determining an accurate measurement. Doubling is done with prisms.

65. What is a Geneva lens clock?

A Geneva lens clock is a device to determine the base curve of the back surface of a spectacle. It is often used clinically to detect plus cylinder spectacle lenses in a patient used to minus cylinder lenses. It is specifically calibrated for the refractive index of crown glass. A special lens clock is available for plastic lenses.

66. **Do you measure the power of spectacles in a lensometer with the temples toward you or away from you?**
The distance is measured with the temples facing away from you as if the patient were wearing them facing you (back vertex power). The add is measured with the temples pointing toward you (front vertex power). You must measure the difference between the top and the bottom segments, especially if the patient has a highly hyperopic prescription. However, if the patient has a blended bifocal, you can often read the power etched into the lens if you use a magnifier or hold it the lens up to a bright light.

67. **If you obtain "with" movement during retinoscopy, is the far point of the patient in front of the peephole, at the peephole, or beyond the peephole?**
It is beyond the peephole. The goal is neutralization of the light reflex so that the patient's far point is at the peephole. The light at the patient's pupil fills the entire space at once. More plus must be added to the prescription to move the far point to neutralization. "Against" movement means that the far point is in front of the peephole; more minus must be added to move the far point to neutralization.

68. **What does a pachymeter measure?**
It measures the corneal thickness or anterior chamber depth.

69. **How does the Hruby lens give an upright or inverted image?**
A Hruby lens is -55 D and gives an upright image. The Goldman lens is -64 D and also provides an upright image. The Volk 90 D lens provides an inverted image.

70. **Why does the indirect ophthalmoscope provide a larger field of view than the direct ophthalmoscope?**
The condensing lens used with the indirect ophthalmoscope captures the peripheral rays to give a field of view of 25 degrees or more depending on the lens power used. The direct ophthalmoscope does not use the condensing lens and thus provides only a 7 degree field of view.

71. **What are the wavelengths of the spectrum of visible light?**
The range is from 400 nm for violet light to 700 nm for red light. Anything shorter than 400 nm is considered ultraviolet, and anything longer than 700 nm is in the infrared spectrum.

72. **Antireflective coatings on spectacle lenses are based on what principle?**
Interference. Antireflective coatings use destructive interference. The crest of one wavelength cancels the trough of another.

73. **What is the most effective pinhole diameter?**
A pinhole diameter of 1.2 mm neutralizes up to 3 D of refractive error. A 2-mm pinhole neutralizes only 1 D. An aphakic patient may need a $+10$ D lens in addition to the pinhole to obtain useful visual acuity.

74. **When is a cycloplegic refraction indicated?**
- For patients younger than 15 years, especially if they have strabismus. Make sure to measure the deviation before cycloplegia.
- For hyperopes younger than 35 years, especially if they experience asthenopia.
- For patients with asthenopia suggestive of accommodative problems.
Note: Check accommodative amplitudes and any reading adds before cycloplegia.

75. **Which cycloplegic agent lasts the longest? The shortest?**
- Atropine can last for 1 to 2 weeks. Watch for toxic effects in small children and elderly patients. Tropicamide (Mydriacyl) lasts 4 to 8 hours and is not strong enough for cycloplegia in children. One or two diopters of hyperopia may remain. Cyclogyl lasts 8 to 24 hours; homatropine, 1 to 3 days; and scopolamine, 5 to 7 days.

76. **What are the signs and symptoms of systemic intoxication from cycloplegic medications? How are they treated?**
Signs and symptoms of systemic intoxication include dry mouth, fever, flushing, tachycardia, nausea, and delirium. Treatment includes counteraction with physostigmine.

77. **When is it important to measure the vertex distance in prescribing glasses?**
Measure the vertex distance when the patient has a strong prescription of more than ±5.00 D. Tables are available to adjust the prescription accordingly.

78. **What is the threshold for prescribing glasses in a child with astigmatism?**
When visual acuity is not developing properly, as noted by amblyopia or strabismus, give the full correction. Children tolerate full correction better than adults. Most often, amblyopia or strabismus occurs with at least 1.50 D of astigmatism. Anisometropia that presents with 1.00 D or more of hyperopic asymmetry also requires full correction.

79. **What may cause monocular diplopia?**
- Corneal or lenticular irregularity, i.e., dry eye, corneal scarring, cataract
- Decentered contact lens

- Inappropriate placement of reading add
- Transient sensory adaptations after strabismus surgery
- Distortion from retinal lesions (rare)

80. **What conditions may give a false-positive reading with a potential acuity meter?**
    Macular scotomas in a patient with amblyopia or retinal disease, such as age-related macular degeneration, may give a false-positive reading. Acute macular edema also may elevate the reading, but the elevation disappears with chronic edema. An irregular corneal surface can falsely improve the potential acuity; however, wearing a contact lens may help.

81. **What do you check when patients complain that their new glasses are not as good as their previous pair?**
    - Ask specifically what the complaint is: Distance reading? Near problems? Asthenopia? Diplopia? Pain behind the ears or at the nose bridge from ill-fitting glasses?
    - Read the new and old glasses on the lensometer and compare. Make sure that the old glasses did not have any prism. Check the patient for undetected strabismus with cover testing.
    - Refract the patient again, possibly with a cycloplegic agent if the symptoms warrant.
    - Check the optical centers in comparison with the pupillary centers.
    - Check whether the reading segments are in the correct position—level with the lower lid.
    - Make sure that the new glasses fit the patient correctly.
    - Check whether the old glasses were made with plus cylinder by using the Geneva lens clock.
    - Check whether the base curve has changed with the Geneva lens clock.
    - Find out if the material for the new lenses is the same as the old lenses.
    - Evaluate the patient for dry eye.
    - If the patient has a high prescription, check the vertex distance. Often, it is easier to refract such patients over their old pair of glasses to keep the same vertex distance.
    - Check the pantoscopic tilt. Normally, the tilt is 10 to 15 degrees so that when the patient reads, the eye is perpendicular to the lens. If the tilt is off, especially in relation to the old glasses, the patient may notice.
    - With postoperative glasses, evaluate for diplopia in downgaze due to anisometropia.
    - Perhaps the add is too strong or too weak. Check the patient using trial lenses and reading material.
    - Sometimes, if the diameter of the lens is much larger in the newer frames, the patient notices significant distortion in the peripheral lens. Encourage a small frame. However, too small a frame can make progressive bifocals very difficult. It is best to keep a frame size fairly consistent over the years.
    - Did the patient change bifocal types? Round top, flat top, executive style, and progressives all require different adaptations. Patients often have trouble when changing styles.
    - Above all, try to test the new prescription in trial frames with a walk around the office. You do not want to go through this process again.

82. **If after repeat refraction the patient suddenly develops more hyperopia than you previously noted, what do you look for?**
    Look for a cause of acquired hyperopia, such as a retrobulbar tumor, central serous retinopathy, posterior lens dislocation, or a flattened cornea from a contact lens.

KEY POINTS: CAUSES OF MONOCULAR DIPLOPIA

1. Corneal or lenticular irregularity
2. Decentered contact lens, intraocular implant, or refractive surgery
3. Inappropriate placement of reading add
4. Sensory problems after strabismus surgery
5. Retinal lesions (very rare)

83. **What if the patient has more myopia than previously noted?**
    Check the cycloplegic refraction to make sure that it is true. Acquired myopia may be caused by diabetes mellitus, sulfonamides, nuclear sclerosis, pilocarpine, keratoconus, a scleral buckle for retinal detachment, and anterior lens dislocation.

84. **What about acquired astigmatism?**
    Lid lesions such as hemangiomas, chalazions, and ptosis may cause acquired astigmatism. A pterygium or keratoconus may reveal a previously undetected astigmatism. And, of course, healing cataract wounds may change the previous astigmatism.

85. If the astigmatism has changed and the patient has difficulty with tolerating the new prescription, what are the options?

    If the astigmatism is oblique, try rotating the axis toward 90 degrees or toward the old axis. The astigmatic power may be reduced, but keep the spherical power the same. Sometimes, a gradual change in prescription over time may allow the patient to adapt. For example, if a patient's prescription is $-3.00 + 2.00 \times 110$, a possibility is $-2.50 + 1.00 \times 90$. The spherical equivalent of -2.00 D has been maintained.

86. What does laser stand for?

    Laser is an acronym for light amplification by stimulated emission of radiation.

87. To steepen a contact lens fit, do you increase the diameter of the lens or the radius of curvature?

    Increasing the diameter of the lens or decreasing the radius of curvature will steepen the lens (Fig. 3.11). This information is useful for lenses that fit too tightly.

88. How many seconds of arc does the "E" on the 20/20 line of the Snellen eye chart subtend?

    It subtends 5″. The Snellen eye chart measures the minimal separable acuity.

89. When the Jackson cross is used to define the astigmatic axis, is the handle of the lens parallel to the axis or 45 degrees from it?

    It is parallel. To define the astigmatic power, the handle is 45 degrees to the axis. Define the axis before the power.

90. A 25-year-old patient has a manifest refraction of $+0.50$ OU and complains of asthenopia. What do you do?

    Check the patient's accommodative amplitude and look for an exophoria at near to evaluate for convergence insufficiency. Then do a cycloplegic refraction to check for undercorrection. On exam, the amplitude of accommodation is 3 D OU. Because this value is low for a young person, suspect undercorrection of hyperopia. Indeed, the cycloplegic refraction is $+2.50$ OU. The patient has accommodative spasm. Try giving one-half of the cycloplegic findings. Sometimes atropine is needed to break the spasm so that the patient can accept the stronger prescription.

91. What instrument is useful to measure the accommodative amplitude?

    Accommodative amplitude is measured with the Prince rule.

92. A 35-year-old man has 20/40 uncorrected vision. With $+0.50$ glasses, he is 20/20. He will remain 20/20 with a $+1.50$ manifest refraction. With cycloplegia, he has a refraction of $+4.00$. Define absolute hyperopia, facultative hyperopia, manifest hyperopia, and latent hyperopia.

    • **Total hyperopia:** Found by cycloplegia, $+4.00$
    • **Manifest hyperopia:** Found without cycloplegia; more plus will blur vision, $+1.50$

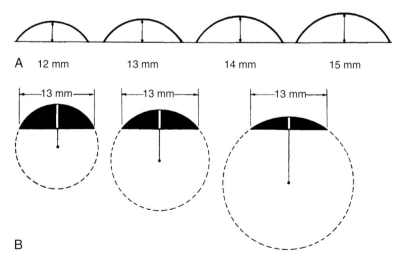

A   12 mm   13 mm   14 mm   15 mm

B

Fig. 3.11 A, When the radius of curvature is kept constant while the diameter of the contact lens is increased, the fit steepens. **B,** Conversely, increasing the radius of curvature while maintaining the same diameter allows a flatter fit. (Reproduced, with permission, from Meltzer DW, *Basic and Clinical Science Course: Section 3: Optics, Refraction, and Contact Lenses*, American Academy of Ophthalmology, 1992.)

- **Latent hyperopia:** Total minus manifest hyperopia, +2.50
- **Absolute hyperopia:** The minimal correction that the patient needs to see distances, +0.50
- **Facultative hyperopia:** Manifest minus absolute hyperopia; compensation accomplished by accommodation, +1.00

BIBLIOGRAPHY

American Academy of Ophthalmology: Basic and clinical science course, San Francisco, 2012, American Academy of Ophthalmology.
Milder B, Rubin ML: The fine art of prescribing glasses without making a spectacle of yourself, ed 3, Gainesville, FL, 2004, Triad Publishing.
Rubin ML: Optics for clinicians, ed 3, Gainesville, FL, 1993, Triad Publishing.

CHAPTER 4

COLOR VISION

Mitchell S. Fineman

1. **What are photons?**
   Atoms consist of a nucleus (composed of protons and neutrons) and electrons that revolve around the nucleus in orbits of more or less fixed diameter. An electron can move to a higher orbit if it receives energy from an external source (e.g., heating). However, it remains in the higher orbit for only one-hundred-millionth of a second. As it falls back to its original lower orbit, it releases its excess energy by emitting a small "packet" of energy called a quantum or a photon.

2. **Describe the physical properties of photons.**
   In a vacuum, all photons move at the speed of light. As they travel, they vibrate, causing measurable electric and magnetic effects (wave properties). The farther an electron falls to reach its original lower orbit, the greater its frequency of vibration, and the shorter its wavelength (λ), which is the straight-line distance a photon moves during one complete vibration. Frequency and wavelength are related by the formula $f = c/\lambda$, where f is the frequency of vibration, λ is the wavelength, and c is the speed of light. Thus, f and λ are inversely proportional (i.e., as frequency increases, wavelength decreases). For example, γ-rays have a very high frequency and a very short wavelength, and radio waves have a very low frequency and a rather long wavelength.

3. **What is the electromagnetic spectrum?**
   Light, x-rays, γ-rays (gamma rays), and radio waves are all forms of electromagnetic energy. When photons (quanta) are classified according to their wavelength, the result is the electromagnetic spectrum. The photons with the longest wavelengths are radio and television waves; those with the shortest are γ-rays. The photons we see (visible light) are near the middle of the spectrum.

4. **Why can we "see" light, but not other types of electromagnetic energy?**
   The rods and cones of the retina (photoreceptors) contain pigments that preferentially absorb photons with wavelengths between 400 and 700 nm (a nanometer is a billionth of a meter) and convert their energy into a neuronal impulse that is carried to the brain. Wavelengths longer than 700 nm and shorter than 400 nm tend to pass through the sensory retina without being absorbed (Fig. 4.1).

5. **What is the light spectrum?**
   Photons can be classified not only by their wavelength but also by the sensation they cause when they strike the retina. Photons of the shortest wavelengths that we can see are perceived as blue and green; those of longer wavelengths are perceived as yellow, orange, and red.

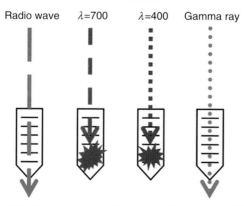

Retinal pigments <u>catch</u> photons

Radio wave λ=700 λ=400   Gamma ray

Fig. 4.1 Photoreceptors are stimulated only by certain wavelengths of light.

6. How does a prism break white light into the colors of the rainbow?
Photons travel at the speed of light in a vacuum, but if they enter a denser medium, such as glass, their wavelength and speed decrease. The frequency of vibration remains the same. The shorter the wavelength, the more the speed is decreased. For example, one can imagine two photons traveling through a vacuum, one of wavelength 650 nm and the other of wavelength 450 nm. As long as they remain in a vacuum, they keep pace with one another. When they strike the glass perpendicularly, the 450-nm photon is slowed down more than the 650-nm photon. If they enter the glass obliquely, their paths are bent in proportion to how much their speed is slowed. In other words, the shorter the wavelength, the greater the bending. The blue is bent more and is separated from the red.

7. How do rods differ from cones?
Both rods and cones are photoreceptors. These retinal cells initiate the process of vision. Rods function best when the eye is dark-adapted (i.e., for night vision). They cannot distinguish one color from another. Cones, on the other hand, function when the retina is light-adapted (i.e., for day vision).

8. What are the visual pigments?
There are four visual pigments: rhodopsin, which is present in rods, and the three cone pigments. All visual pigments are made up of 11-*cis* retinal (vitamin A aldehyde) and a protein called an opsin. When a photon is absorbed, the 11-*cis* retinal is converted to the all-*trans* form and is released from the opsin, initiating an electrical impulse in the photoreceptor that travels toward the brain. The eye then resynthesizes the rhodopsin and the reaction repeats.

9. Describe the three cone pigments.
Our ability to distinguish different colors depends on the fact that there are three different kinds of cone pigment. All visual pigments use retinal, but each has a different opsin. The function of the different opsins is to rearrange the electron cloud of retinal, thereby changing its ability to capture photons of different wavelengths. Red-catching cones (R cones) contain erythrolabe, which preferentially absorbs photons of long wavelengths. It is best stimulated by 570-nm photons but also absorbs adjoining wavelengths. Blue-catching cones (B cones) contain cyanolabe, which absorbs the shortest wavelengths best. Its maximal sensitivity is at 440 nm. Green-catching cones (G cones) contain chlorolabe, which is most sensitive to the intermediate wavelengths. Its maximal sensitivity is at 540 nm.

10. How does the sensation of light get to the brain?
The electrical signals initiated by absorption of photons by the photoreceptors are transmitted to bipolar cells and then to ganglion cells. Horizontal and amacrine cells modify these messages. For example, if a cone is strongly stimulated, it sends inhibitory messages by way of a horizontal cell to neighboring cones, thereby reducing "noise" and sharpening up the message the brain receives. Bipolar cells send similar inhibitory messages by way of amacrine cells. The axons of ganglion cells bundle together to form the optic nerve, which carries information to the brain. In the brain, there is thought to exist a "hue center" (Fig. 4.2), which adds up the information from the different color channels and determines which color we see. In general, the hue we see depends on the relative numbers of photons of different wavelengths that strike the three different cones.

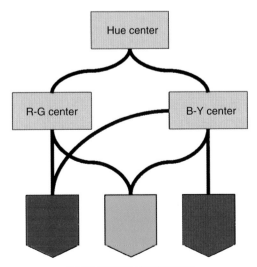

Fig. 4.2 Illustration of the hue center.

11. **What three attributes are necessary to describe any color?**
To accurately describe any color, one must specify three attributes: hue, saturation, and brightness.

12. **What is hue?**
Hue is synonymous with "color" and is the attribute of color perception denoted by blue, red, purple, and so forth. Hue depends largely on what the eye and brain perceive to be the predominant wavelength present in the incoming light. In simplest terms, this means that if light of several wavelengths strikes the eye and more light of 540 nm is present than is light of other wavelengths, we will see green.

13. **What is saturation?**
Saturation (chroma) corresponds to the purity or richness of a color. When all the light seen by the eye is the same wavelength, we say that a color is fully saturated. Vivid colors are saturated. If we add white to a saturated color, the hue does not change, but the color is paler (desaturated). For example, pink is a desaturated red.

14. **What is brightness?**
Brightness (luminance, value) refers to the quantity of light coming from an object (the number of photons striking the eye). If we place a filter over a projector or gradually (with a rheostat) lower its intensity, the brightness decreases.

15. **What are complementary colors?**
When equal quantities of complements are added, the result is white. Blue-green and red are complements, as are green and magenta. (This applies only to colored lights, not paints.)

16. **What is the color wheel?**
The color wheel is made up of all hues arranged in a circle so that each hue lies between those hues it most closely resembles and complementary hues lie opposite each other. Using the color wheel, we can predict the color that will result when two different lights are mixed. When noncomplements are mixed, the resultant color lies between the two original colors. The exact color seen depends on the quantity of each color used. For example, equal quantities of red and green result in yellow, whereas a large quantity of red and a relatively small quantity of green result in orange.

17. **How does the eye differ from the ear?**
Unlike the ear, which can distinguish several musical instruments playing at once, our eye and brain cannot determine the composition of a color we see. For example, if we present the eye with a light composed purely of 589 nm photons, the eye sees yellow. However, if we mix green and red lights in the proper proportions, the eye also sees yellow and cannot differentiate this from the other. Similarly, when two complements are mixed, we see white and cannot distinguish this white from the white seen when equal quantities of all wavelengths are present. Further, if we add white light to our original 589 nm yellow, the eye still sees yellow. Similarly, a light composed only of 490 nm photons is seen as blue-green and cannot be distinguished from an appropriate mixture of blue and green.

18. **What are the primary colors?**
When speaking of colored lights, the primary hues (also called the additive primaries) are red, green, and blue. Any color, including white, can be produced by overlapping red, green, and blue lights on a screen in the proper proportions. The reflecting screen can be regarded as a composite of an infinite number of tiny projectors. The eye, bombarded by all these photons, "adds up" their relative contributions. The color we see is determined by how many quanta of each wavelength reach the eye. Color television relies on this ability of the eye to add up tiny adjacent points of light. If one looks at a cathode ray tube color television from 6 inches away, one sees tiny dots of only three colors: red, green, and blue. If one then backs away, the full range of colors becomes apparent and the eye can no longer distinguish the tiny dots. It synthesizes (adds up) the adjacent colors (e.g., tiny dots of red and blue = purple; red and green = yellow; red and green and blue = white; and so forth).

19. **Where is the final determination of color made?**
The hue center, localized in the cortex, synthesizes information it receives from two "intermediate centers": the R–G center and the B–Y center. The information sent to the hue center from the R–G center depends on the relative stimulation of the R and G cones. For example, when light of 540 nm strikes the retina, it will stimulate both R and G cones. However, because the G cones are stimulated much more than the R cones, the message received by the hue center is predominantly "green." On the other hand, if light of 590 nm strikes the retina, the R cones are stimulated more than the G cones and we see yellow. When light of 630 nm strikes the retina, the G cones are not stimulated at all and we see red. The B cones send information to the B–Y center. The Y information does not come from Y cones because there are no Y cones. Information from the R and G cones combine to indicate yellow in the B–Y center.

20. **Why is brown, which is definitely a color, not on the color wheel?**
Because brown is a yellow or orange of low luminance.

21. **Describe the Bezold-Brucke phenomenon.**
As brightness increases, most hues appear to change. At low intensities, blue-green, green, and yellow-green appear greener than they do at high intensities, when they appear bluer. At low intensities, reds and oranges

appear redder and at high intensities, yellower. The exceptions are a blue of about 478 nm, a green of about 503 nm, and a yellow of about 578 nm. These are the wavelengths of invariant hue.

22. **What is the Abney effect?**
As white is added to any hue (desaturating it), the hue appears to change slightly in color. All colors except a yellow of 570 nm appear yellower.

23. **What are the relative luminosity curves?**
The relative luminosity curves illustrate the eye's sensitivity to different wavelengths of light. They are constructed by asking an observer to increase the luminance of lights of various wavelengths until they appear to be equal in apparent brightness to a yellow light, whose luminance is fixed. When the eye is light-adapted, yellow, yellow-green, and orange appear brighter than do blues, greens, and reds. The cones' peak sensitivity is to light of 555 nm.
A relative luminosity curve can also be constructed for the rods in a dark-adapted eye, even though the observer cannot name the various wavelengths used. The rods' peak sensitivity is to light of 505 nm (blue).

24. **Define lateral inhibition.**
As mentioned earlier, as cones of one kind (e.g., R cones) are stimulated, they may send an inhibitory message by way of horizontal and amacrine cells to adjacent cones of the same kind (e.g., other R cones). Therefore, when a purple circle is surrounded by a red background, the R cones in the purple area are inhibited, making the purple (a combination of red and blue) appear bluer than it really is. If the purple is surrounded by blue, it appears redder.

25. **What are afterimages?**
If one stares at a color for 20 seconds, it begins to fade (desaturate). Then, if one gazes at a white background, the complement of the original color (afterimage) appears (Fig. 4.3). These two phenomena depend on the fact that even when cones are not being stimulated, they spontaneously send baseline signals toward the brain. For example, when red light is projected onto the retina, the eye sees red because the R cones are stimulated much more than the G cones and B cones. The G and B contribution to the hue center is far outweighed by the R. After several seconds, the red color fades (becomes desaturated) because the red cones, being more strongly stimulated, cannot regenerate their pigment fast enough to continue to send such a large number of signals (fatigue). Now the G and B cone contribution to the hue center increases relative to that of the R cones and the brain "sees" a desaturated or paler red. It is as if we added blue-green light to the red. (Recall that blue-green is the complement of red and that mixing complements yields white.) When the red light is turned off, the frequency of the spontaneous messages sent to the brain by the fatigued R cones is far less than that sent by the G and B cones, so the brain sees blue-green, or cyan, the complement of red (Fig. 4.4).

26. **Why are white flowers white?**
The color of any object that is not white or black depends on the relative number of photons of each wavelength that it absorbs and reflects. Our ambient light, derived from the sun, contains approximately equal numbers of all the photons that make up the light spectrum. White paint reflects all photons equally well, and white flowers appear white.

Fig. 4.3 Stare at the black dot for 30 seconds and then look at a blank white area. The afterimage seen is the complement of each color.

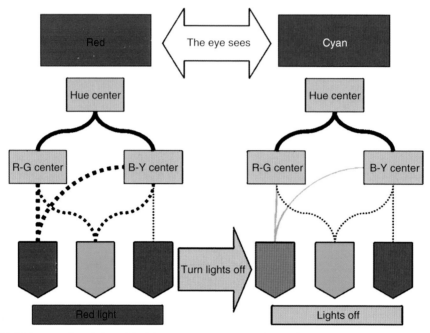

Fig. 4.4 Afterimages are formed when certain photoreceptors cannot regenerate pigment quickly enough, allowing other photoreceptors to appear relatively more stimulated.

27. Why is charcoal black?
    Charcoal absorbs most of the light that strikes it. Because very few photons are reflected toward the eye, the photoreceptors are not stimulated and no color is seen.

28. Why are blue flowers blue?
    The pigments in blue flowers absorb red and yellow photons best, green next best, and blue least of all; therefore, more blue photons are reflected than others, and the eye sees blue. A green leaf is green because chlorophyll strongly absorbs blue and red and reflects green.

29. Why does mixing red and blue-green *lights* result in white, but mixing red and green *paint* results in brown?
    Oil paints are made by mixing (suspending) tiny clumps of pigment in an opaque medium (the binder). Pigments reflect and absorb some wavelengths of light better than others. The dominant wavelength reflected is the color of the paint. When two lights are mixed, we speak of an "additive" mixture. But when two paints are mixed, each pigment subtracts some of the light the other would reflect. The resultant mixture is darker than either of the two originals. Red paint mixed with green paint results in brown because enough light is subtracted that the eye sees a yellow of low luminance.

30. Why does mixing paints yield unpredictable results?
    An artist or home decorator never knows the exact absorption spectrum of the originals. Two greens may appear to be the same, but because their pigments are not identical they do not yield the same color when mixed with the same yellow.

31. Why do colors appear different under fluorescent light as opposed to incandescent light?
    Tungsten (incandescent) light bulbs emit relatively more photons of the longer (red) wavelengths than of the shorter (blue) wavelengths, whereas fluorescent light bulbs emit relatively more light in the blue and green wavelengths. A shopper who picks out material for drapes in a store that has fluorescent lighting may be surprised to find out that the material looks quite different at home. A purple dress appears redder under incandescent light than it does under fluorescent light.

32. Why is the sky blue?
    The sun emits light of all of the spectral colors. If an astronaut in space looks at the sun, it appears white. If the astronaut looks away from the sun, he sees that the outer space is black, because the photons not coming

directly at him pass through space unhindered and are not reflected toward him. On Earth, the atmosphere, which contains ozone, dust, water droplets, and many other reflecting molecules and substances, is interposed between the sun and our eyes. The atmosphere scatters blue light more than it does green, yellow, or red. Therefore, if during the daytime we look away from the sun, we see the blue photons that are being bent toward us and the sky appears to be blue.

33. Why is the sunset red?
At dusk, to reach us, the light from the sun has to pass through much more of the earth's atmosphere than it does during the daytime. Therefore, even more of the blue and green photons are bent away from the atmosphere. The red and yellow photons penetrate better. If some of these are eventually reflected toward us by clouds or dust, we see a red sky. Similarly, the sun appears red.

34. Define trichromats.
Trichromats are the 92% of the population who have "normal" color vision. They have three different kinds of cones, normal concentration of the cone pigments, and normal retinal wiring.

35. What is congenital dichromatism?
In dichromats, the cones themselves are normal, but one of the three contains the wrong pigment. For example, in deuteranopes, the G cones are normal in every way except that they contain erythrolabe (red pigment) instead of chlorolabe (green pigment). In protanopes, the R cones are normal in every way except that they contain chlorolabe (green pigment) instead of erythrolabe (red pigment). Tritanopia is a defect of the B cones.

36. Why do deuteranopes have difficulty in distinguishing red from green?
In deuteranopia, because both R and G cones contain the same pigment, when red light strikes the retina, the R and G cones are stimulated equally and send an equal number of messages to the R–G center. Similarly, there is an increased R input to the B–Y center, where the R input now equals the G input. In other words, the hue center thinks that equal quantities of red and green light are striking the retina. When green or blue-green light strikes the retina, the R and G cones are again stimulated equally. An accurate analysis of the mechanics of color vision abnormalities is far more complicated, but it should be apparent that because both red and green light stimulate the R and G cones equally, the information the hue center receives from the R–G center is not useful in differentiating between the two colors and the deuteranope would have difficulty distinguishing red from green. Similarly, protanopes also have difficulty distinguishing red from green.

37. What is anomalous trichromatism?
In anomalous trichromatism, two of the three cone pigments are normal, but the third functions suboptimally. Depending on which pigment is abnormal, the affected persons are termed *protanomalous*, *deuteranomalous*, or *tritanomalous*. Anomalous trichromats can distinguish between fully saturated colors but have difficulty distinguishing colors of low saturation (pastels) or low luminance (dark colors), or both. Deuteranomaly is present in approximately 5% of the population; deuteranopia, protanopia, and protanomaly in 1% each; and tritanopia or tritanomaly in only 0.002%.

38. How is abnormal color vision inherited?
All red-green disorders are inherited in a sex-linked recessive pattern. This means that men almost exclusively manifest the disorder. Women are carriers. In other words, the women have perfectly normal color vision, but approximately 50% of their sons are affected by abnormal color vision. Both men and women can have the tritan disorders, which are inherited in an autosomal dominant fashion (Table 4.1).

39. What is Kollner's rule?
As a very general rule, the errors made by persons with optic nerve disease tend to resemble those made by protans and deutans, whereas those made by persons with retinal disease resemble those made by tritans.

Table 4.1 Inherited Color Vision Defects		
DEFECT	**INCIDENCE**	**INHERITANCE**
Deuteranomaly	5% (of males)	XR
Deuteranopia	1% (of males)	XR
Protanomaly	1% (of males)	XR
Protanopia	1% (of males)	XR
Tritanomaly and tritanopia	0.002%	AD

AD, Autosomal dominant; *XR*, X-linked recessive.

KEY POINTS: COLOR VISION

1. Rods function best in the dark-adapted state and cones function best in the light-adapted state.
2. Any color can be produced by overlapping red, green, and blue lights in the proper proportions.
3. Afterimages appear as the complement of the original color.
4. Protanopes and deuteranopes have difficulty distinguishing red from green.
5. All red-green disorders are inherited in an X-linked recessive pattern.

BIBLIOGRAPHY

Boynton RM: Color, hue and wavelength. In Carterette EC, Friedman MP, editors: Handbook of perception, vol V, New York, 1975, Academic Press, pp 301–350.

Gerritsen F: Theory and practice of color, New York, 1974, Van Nostrand.

Krill AE: Hereditary retinal and choroidal diseases. In Krill AE, editor: Evaluation of color vision, Hagerstown, MD, 1972, Harper & Row, pp 309–340.

Linksz A: Reflections, old and new, concerning acquired defects of color vision, Surv Ophthalmol 17;229–240, 1973.

Rubin ML, Walls GL: Fundamentals of visual science, Springfield, IL, 1969, Charles C. Thomas.

Smith VC: Color vision of normal observers. In Potts AM, editor: The assessment of visual function, St. Louis, 1972, Mosby, pp 105–135.

CHAPTER 5

OPHTHALMIC AND ORBITAL TESTING

Kendra A. Klein and Caroline R. Baumal

1. What is clinical electrophysiological testing?

   Electrophysiological testing refers to a variety of noninvasive tests that provide objective information about the function of the visual system. Standard electrophysiologic tests include the full-field electroretinogram (ffERG), pattern electroretinogram (PERG), multifocal electroretinogram (mfERG), electrooculogram (EOG), and visual evoked potential (VEP).

2. How are electrophysiologic tests performed?

   Electrophysiologic tests record electrical potentials evoked by visual stimuli. Light is delivered uniformly to the retina and the light-induced electrical discharges are recorded using electrodes placed on the surface or the eye, periocular area, or scalp. This response is secondary to transretinal movement of ions induced by the light stimulus.

KEY POINTS: COMPONENTS OF THE FULL-FIELD ELECTRORETINOGRAM

1. The **a-wave** is the initial negative electroretinogram (ERG) waveform arising from photoreceptor cells.
2. The positive **b-wave** follows the a-wave and is generated by the Müller cells and bipolar cells in the outer retina.
3. **Oscillatory potentials** are small wavelets that may be superimposed on the b wave and arise from cells in the midretinal layers (Fig. 5.1).
4. Under certain recording conditions, additional waveforms may be noted, such as the **c-wave** following the b-wave. This reflects electrical activity at the level of the retinal pigment epithelium (RPE) and is recorded in the dark-adapted eye.
5. The **early receptor potential** is a rapid transient waveform that occurs immediately after a light stimulus. This response originates from the bleaching of photopigments at the level of the photoreceptor outer segments.

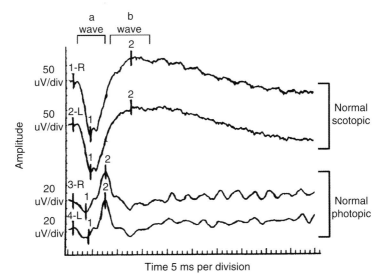

Fig. 5.1 Nocturnal scotopic (dark-adapted) and photopic electroretinogram responses to a high-intensity (0 dB) light flash demonstrating the a-wave and b-wave. Oscillatory potentials are present on the ascending limb of the b wave. The implicit time is measured from the stimulus onset to the peak of the a-wave *(1)* or b-wave *(2)*. The a-wave amplitude is measured from the baseline to the trough of the a-wave, and the b-wave amplitude is measured from the trough of the a-wave to the peak of the b-wave.

3. What does the full-field electroretinogram measure?
   The ffERG measures the global response of the retina under both light- and dark-adapted conditions. The ffERG allows distinction between outer and inner retinal dysfunction and primarily rod or cone dysfunction.

4. How is the full-field electroretinogram obtained?
   Light is delivered uniformly to the entire retinal. Ganzfeld or full-field stimulation is achieved with a bowl perimeter. The responses are recorded with electrodes in contact with cornea, conjunctiva, or periocular skin. The pupils are dilated to elicit maximal retinal response.

5. Describe different stimulus conditions in the full-field electroretinogram and the associated photoreceptor response.
   By utilizing dark- or light-adaptation protocols and particular light stimuli, isolation of either the cone or the rod responses is possible, allowing independent evaluation of distinct photoreceptors (Table 5.1 and Fig. 5.2).
   Following 20 minutes of dark adaptation (known as **scotopic** conditions) and stimulation with a weak flash of light, selective rod responses are obtained. Under scotopic conditions and stimulation with a standard or strong flash, both rod and cone responses are obtained. Following 10 minutes of light adaptation (known as **photopic** conditions) and stimulation with a 30 Hz flash or single flash, the rods are sufficiently dampened, and the response is primarily from cones.

6. What five responses are evaluated during a standard full-field electroretinogram?
   - Rod response (dark-adapted)
   - Maximal combined rod–cone response (dark-adapted)
   - Oscillatory potentials (dark-adapted)
   - Single-flash cone response (light-adapted)
   - 30-Hz flicker cone response (light-adapted)

Table 5.1 Photoreceptor Response Associated With Various Stimulus Conditions

STATE OF ADAPTATION	LIGHT STIMULUS	PHOTORECEPTOR RESPONSE
Scotopic	Dim white (24 dB)	Rod
Scotopic	Dim blue (10 dB)	Rod
Scotopic	Bright white (0 dB)	Mixed response: maximal rod and cone
Scotopic	Red (0 dB)	Mixed response: early cone, late rod
Scotopic	Bright white (0 dB)	Cone oscillatory potentials
Photopic	Bright white (0 dB)	Cone
Photopic	White flicker at 30 Hz	Pure cone

dB, Decibels; *Hz*, hertz.

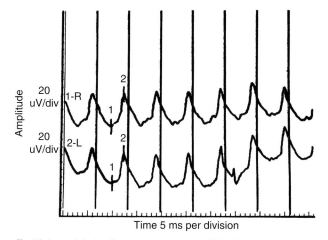

Fig. 5.2 A normal electroretinogram cone response to a flicker light stimulus at 30 Hz.

7. **What parameters are measured during evaluation of an electroretinogram?**
Two major ERG parameters, **amplitude** and **implicit time**, are measured. The amplitude (microvolts) of the a-wave is measured from baseline to the trough of the a-wave. The b-wave amplitude is measured from the trough of the a-wave to peak of the b-wave. The implicit time (milliseconds) is the time from the stimulus onset to peak of the response.

8. **How is the full-field electroretinogram amplitude affected in retinal disorders?**
The ffERG is a mass response reflecting activity from the entire retina. The amplitude of the ERG is proportional to the area of functioning retina stimulated and is abnormal only when large areas of the retina are functionally impaired.

9. **How is the full-field electroretinogram affected in age-related macular degeneration (AMD)?**
When AMD is characterized by localized perimacular lesions, the ffERG is normal. Because the ffERG measures global retinal response, it is not affected when small areas of the retina are damaged.

10. **What does the full-field electroretinogram demonstrate in retinal ganglion cell disease?**
The ganglion cells do *not* play a role in generation of the ffERG. Thus, disorders primarily affecting ganglion cells, such as glaucoma, do not alter the ffERG. On occasion, the b-wave may be reduced in optic atrophy or central retinal artery occlusion. This is postulated to result from transsynaptic degeneration from ganglion to the bipolar cell layer.

11. **Describe the clinical situations in which a full-field electroretinogram is utilized.**
    - To diagnose a generalized degeneration of the retina
    - To evaluate family members for a known hereditary retinal degeneration
    - To assess decreased vision and nystagmus present at birth
    - To assess retinal function in the presence of opaque ocular media or vascular occlusion
    - To evaluate functional visual loss

12. **List some retinal degenerations in which a full-field electroretinogram can help clarify the diagnosis.**
    - Retinitis pigmentosa (RP) and related hereditary retinal degenerations
    - RP sine pigmento
    - Retinitis punctata albescens
    - Retinal conditions simulating RP
    - Leber congenital amaurosis
    - Choroideremia
    - Gyrate atrophy of the retina and choroid
    - Goldman-Favre syndrome
    - Congenital stationary night blindness
    - X-linked juvenile retinoschisis
    - Achromatopsia
    - Cone dystrophies

13. **What are the clinical and full-field electroretinogram features of retinitis pigmentosa?**
RP is an inherited retinal disorder of the photoreceptors and other retina cell layers. Inheritance may be autosomal dominant, autosomal recessive, or X-linked. Both the rods and, to a lesser extent, the cones are abnormal in RP. Clinical features include decreased night vision (nyctalopia), visual field loss, and abnormal ERG (Fig. 5.3). Ocular features include waxy pallor of the optic nerve, attenuated retinal vessels, mottled RPE with bone-spicule pigmentation, cellophane maculopathy, cystic macular edema, pigment cells in the vitreous, and cataracts.
The ffERG shows reduced amplitude (usually b-wave) and prolonged photopic implicit time in early RP. Over time, the ERG becomes extinguished with no detectable rod or cone responses.

14. **What does the ffERG demonstrate in female carriers of X-linked retinitis pigmentosa?**
ERG abnormalities are noted in the majority of female carriers, including prolonged photopic b-wave implicit time and/or a reduction in the amplitude of the scotopic b-wave in the dark-adapted eye. Retinal examination in this group may be normal or demonstrate mild retinal abnormalities without subjective complaints.

15. **What does the full-field electroretinogram reveal in congenital rubella syndrome?**
Diffuse pigmentary retinal changes in congenital rubella syndrome may be confused with RP. However, the ERG is normal in congenital rubella. Other ocular signs of rubella include deafness and congenital cataracts.

16. **Describe the full-field electroretinogram in X-linked retinoschisis.**
ffERG reveals reduced scotopic and photopic b-wave amplitude, reflecting widespread midretinal anatomic changes induced by the schisis of the retina. Clinical findings include peripheral retinoschisis cavities in 50% of cases and foveal cystic changes in almost all cases.

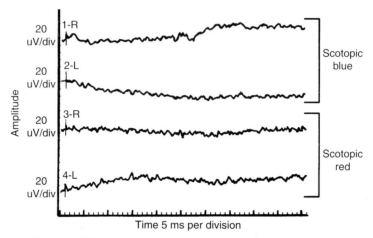

Fig. 5.3 The electroretinogram in retinitis pigmentosa reveals an extinguished response to scotopic blue and scotopic red-light stimuli.

17. **What does the full-field electroretinogram demonstrate in progressive cone dystrophy?**
The ffERG shows markedly reduced photopic flicker response and a normal rod scotopic response. This disorder initially affects peripheral cones, progressing to involve central cones. When the central cones are intact, the visual acuity and color vision are preserved; however, the acuity eventually decreases to the 20/200 range.

18. **Why is the full-field electroretinogram useful in patients with congenitally decreased vision?**
Three disorders characterized by nystagmus, congenitally reduced vision, and normal retinal examination can be diagnosed with an ERG:
- **Achromatopsia** (also known as rod monochromatism) is nonprogressive, has autosomal recessive inheritance, and involves near absence of cones. The ffERG demonstrates absent cone function and normal rod function.
- **Leber congenital amaurosis** is a group of hereditary (typically autosomal recessive), congenital retinal dystrophies that results in vision loss in infancy. It is characterized by decreased visual response, nystagmus, abnormal or poor pupillary response, and eye rubbing. The ffERG is markedly reduced or extinguished.
- **Congenital stationary night blindness** is an inherited retinal disorder (autosomal dominant, X-linked recessive, or autosomal recessive) that primarily affects rods. The ffERG reveals normal photoreceptors with a normal a wave, but an abnormal bipolar cell region as demonstrated by the absent b-wave (**negative ERG**).

19. **How can the full-field electroretinogram measure retinal function in the presence of opaque ocular media?**
The ffERG can be used to assess retinal function when the retina cannot be visualized, owing to cataracts or corneal or vitreous opacities. A normal ffERG provides information regarding the overall retinal function but does not indicate whether central vision is normal because macular degeneration and optic atrophy typically do not affect the ffERG amplitude. A cataract or corneal opacity may act as a diffuser of light, on occasion producing a "supernormal" ffERG.

20. **List the disorders that may demonstrate an extinguished electroretinogram.**
- RP and related disorders
- Ophthalmic artery occlusion
- Diffuse unilateral subacute neuroretinitis (DUSN)
- Metallosis
- Total retinal detachment
- Drugs such as phenothiazines or chloroquine
- Cancer-associated retinopathy (CAR)

21. **What is a negative electroretinogram?**
An ERG with selective reduction in amplitude of the b-wave, such that it does not exceed the a-wave.

22. **List the disorders that may demonstrate normal a-wave and reduced b-wave amplitude (negative electroretinogram).**
- Congenital stationary night blindness
- X-linked juvenile retinoschisis
- Central retinal vein or artery occlusion
- Myotonic dystrophy

- Oguchi's disease
- Quinine intoxication
- Transsynaptic degeneration from the ganglion to the bipolar cell layer (i.e., secondary to optic atrophy or central retinal artery occlusion)

23. List two disorders characterized by an abnormal photopic electroretinogram and a normal scotopic electroretinogram.
    - Achromatopsia (also known as rod monochromatism)
    - Cone dystrophy

24. The full-field electroretinogram is largely generated by which area of the retina?
    The retinal periphery (rod system).

25. Which electrophysiological tests are used to study macular function?
    The mfERG and the PERG.

26. What is a pattern electroretinogram?
    The PERG measures the electrical response to an alternating pattern stimulus that has a constant overall retinal luminance. The response appears to be localized to retinal ganglion cells. The PERG is extinguished after transection of the optic nerve, whereas the ffERG is not altered. The PERG may be used to diagnose or monitor disorders such as glaucoma, ocular hypertension, optic neuritis, optic atrophy, and amblyopia.

27. What is a multifocal electroretinogram?
    The mfERG provides a measure of the cone system function within the central macula. The spatial resolution of the mfERG is superior to the PERG and ffERG and objectively assesses the retinal electrical response at multiple locations. The resultant local responses contain components from all levels of the retina. The mfERG may be abnormal in Stargardt's disease, occult macular dystrophy, white dot syndromes, and hydroxychloroquine toxicity.

28. What is an electro-oculogram?
    The EOG is an indirect measure of the standing potential of the eyes (Fig. 5.4). This standing potential exists because of a voltage difference between the inner and the outer retina. The EOG is measured by placing electrodes near the medial and lateral canthi of each eye. The patient then moves his or her eyes back and forth over a specific distance.
    The clinical measurement of the EOG relies on the fact that the amplitude of the response changes when the luminance conditions are varied. After dark adaptation, the response progressively decreases, reaching a trough in 8 to 12 minutes. With light adaptation, there is a progressive rise in amplitude, reaching a peak in 6 to 9 minutes. The greatest EOG amplitude achieved in light (light peak) is divided by the lowest amplitude in the dark (dark trough). This calculated ratio is the **Arden ratio**. Normal subjects have an **Arden ratio** value of 1.80 or greater, whereas a ratio of less than 1.65 is distinctly abnormal.

29. Where is the electro-oculogram response generated?
    The electrical response in the EOG is generated by the RPE, with the light peak being produced by a depolarization of the basal portion of the RPE. To generate the EOG potential, it is necessary to have intact photoreceptors in physical contact with the RPE.

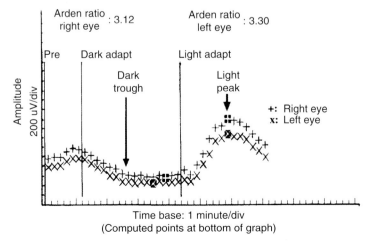

Fig. 5.4 Normal electrooculogram demonstrating the dark trough and the light peak.

30. **What are the clinical uses for the electro-oculogram?**
    The most important clinical use for the EOG is the diagnosis of Best's disease (also known as vitelliform dystrophy). Best's disease is inherited autosomal dominantly with phenotypic variability. Individuals with Best's disease usually have an EOG Arden ratio less than 1.5, but the ERG is normal. The EOG light rise is almost completely dependent on rod function, so it is normal in disorders of cone dysfunction. The EOG is abnormal in most other retinal disorders when the ERG is abnormal; thus, it has limited clinical utility aside from diagnosing Best's disease.

31. **What does the electro-oculogram demonstrate in pattern dystrophies?**
    The EOG light-peak to dark-trough Arden ratio in pattern dystrophy is usually either normal or minimally subnormal. This finding may help distinguish pattern dystrophy from Best's disease, in which the Arden ratio is always abnormal.

32. **How are the electroretinogram and electro-oculogram affected by chloroquine and hydroxychloroquine use?**
    Abnormal findings in the ERG and EOG have been reported in patients receiving these antimalarial drugs, which are frequently used for immune-mediated arthritides and other autoimmune disorders.

33. **What are the characteristics of dark adaptation?**
    Dark adaptometry measures the absolute threshold of cone and rod sensitivity and is tested with the Goldmann-Weekers adaptometer. Initially, the subject is adapted to a bright background light, which is then extinguished. In the dark, the patient is presented with a series of dim lights. The threshold at which the light is just perceived is plotted against time. The normal dark-adaptation curve (Fig. 5.5) is biphasic. The first curve represents the cone threshold and is reached in 5 to 10 minutes. The second curve represents the rod threshold and is reached after 30 minutes. The rod–cone break is a well-defined point between these two curves. Dark adaptometry is useful to evaluate retinal disorders with night blindness and some conditions with cone dysfunction.

34. **What are the indications for ophthalmic ultrasonography?**
    - Evaluation of the anterior or posterior segment in eyes with opaque ocular media
    - Assessment of ocular tumor dimensions as well as their tissue characteristics, such as calcium in retinoblastoma or choroidal osteoma
    - Evaluation of orbital disorders such as thyroid ophthalmopathy and orbital pseudotumor
    - Evaluation of optic nerve head fullness—optic nerve head drusen show calcific deposits vs. papilledema
    - Detection and localization of intraocular foreign bodies
    - Measurement of distances within the eye and orbit (also known as biometry)

35. **What frequency is used for standard ophthalmic ultrasonography?**
    Ultrasound is an acoustic wave that consists of an oscillation of particles within a medium. In standard ophthalmic ultrasound, frequencies are in the range of 8 to 10 MHz. This high frequency produces short wavelengths, which allow precise resolution of small ocular structures.

36. **What are the principles of ultrasonography?**
    Ultrasound is based on physical principles of tissue–acoustic impedance mismatch and pulse–echo technology. As the acoustic wave is propagated through tissues, part of the wave may be reflected toward the source of the emitted wave (i.e., the probe). This reflected wave is referred to as an echo. Echoes are generated at adjoining tissue interfaces that have differential acoustic impedance. The greater the difference in acoustic impedance, the stronger the echo. For example, strong reflections occur at the interface between retinal tissue and vitreous fluid.

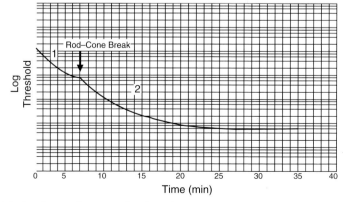

Fig. 5.5 Normal dark adaptation curve demonstrates the rod-cone break at 7 minutes, separating the cone threshold *(1)* and the rod threshold *(2)*.

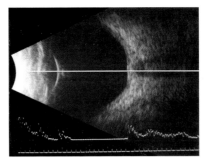

Fig. 5.6 A-scan *(bottom)* and B-scan *(top)* of a normal globe. A cross-sectional anterior–posterior view is presented in the B-scan. The lens capsule is seen toward the left of the display, and the optic nerve is seen toward the right. A vector line through the B-scan demonstrates the position of the A-scan information.

37. How is the clinical ophthalmic ultrasound displayed?
    The reflected echoes are received, amplified, electronically processed, and displayed in visual format as an A-scan or a B-scan (Fig. 5.6):
    - **A-scan ultrasonography**, or the A mode, is a one-dimensional, time–amplitude display. The horizontal base-line represents the distance and depends on the time required for the sound beam to reach a given interface and for its echo to return to the probe. In the vertical dimension, the height of the displayed spike indicates the amplitude or strength of the echo.
    - **B-scan ultrasonography**, or the B mode, produces a two-dimensional, cross-sectional display of the globe and orbit. The image is displayed in variable shades of gray, and the shade depends on the echo strength. Strong echoes appear white, and weaker reflections are gray.
    The A-scan is used predominantly for tissue characterization, whereas the B-scan is used to obtain architectural information. A-scans are used to determine axial lengths for intraocular lens power calculations for cataract surgery.

38. What lesion features are evaluated during the ultrasound examination?
    - The **topography** (location, configuration, and extension) of a lesion is evaluated by the two-dimensional B-scan.
    - The **quantitative features** include the reflectivity, internal structure, and sound attenuation of a lesion.
        - The **reflectivity** is evaluated by observing the height of the spike on an A-scan and the signal brightness on a B-scan. The internal reflectivity refers to the amplitude of echoes within a lesion and correlates with histologic architecture.
        - The **internal structure** refers to the degree of variation in histologic architecture within a lesion. Regular internal structure indicates a homogeneous architecture and is noted by minimal or no variation in the height of spikes on the A-scan and a uniform appearance of echoes on the B-scan. In contrast, an irregular internal structure is characterized by a heterogeneous architecture and variations in the echo appearance.
        - **Sound attenuation** occurs when the acoustic wave is scattered, reflected, or absorbed by a tissue and is noted by a decrease in the strength of echoes either within or posterior to a lesion. It is indicated by a decrease in spike height on the A-scan or a decrease in the brightness of echoes on the B-scan. Sound attenuation may produce shadowing seen as a void posterior to the lesion. Substances such as bone, calcium, and foreign bodies typically produce sound attenuation (Fig. 5.7).

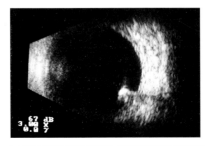

Fig. 5.7 B-scan showing a metallic foreign body on the retina surface. A bright echo is produced by the foreign body with shadowing of the structures posteriorly.

39. How is ultrasound used in preoperative cataract evaluation?

The A-scan is used to measure the axial length of the globe, which is required in the formulas used to calculate the intraocular lens power placed into the eye at the time of cataract surgery. The B-scan is useful if the ocular media are opaque to assess for a retinal disorder that may affect visual outcome after cataract surgery.

40. How is ultrasound used to assess intraocular tumors?

Ultrasound may be used for diagnosis, to plan treatment, and to evaluate tumor response to therapy. Specifically, the tumor shape, dimensions (such as thickness and basal diameter), and tissue characteristics are evaluated, along with the presence of extraocular extension.

41. What are the characteristic features of a choroidal melanoma on ultrasound?
    - Collar button or mushroom shape on B-scan (Fig. 5.8)
    - Low-to-medium internal reflectivity on A-scan (Fig. 5.8)
    - Regular internal structure
    - Internal blood flow (vascularity)

42. Describe the ultrasound patterns in the differential diagnosis of choroidal melanoma.

Ultrasound is often used in the evaluation of choroidal melanoma, choroidal hemangioma, metastatic choroidal carcinoma, choroidal nevus, choroidal hemorrhage, and a disciform lesion. It should be combined with clinical information because there are more tumor types than differentiating ultrasound patterns (Table 5.2).

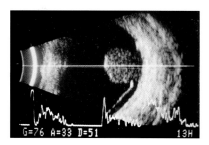

Fig. 5.8 A-scan and B-scan of choroidal melanoma. The B-scan reveals a collar-button-shaped mass with regular internal structure. A serous retinal detachment extends from the margin of the tumor. The A-scan reveals a strong initial echo from the retinal tissue overlying the tumor followed by a rapid decline in the A-scan echo amplitude (low internal reflectivity) within the tumor tissue. High reflectivity is noted again at the level of the sclera and orbital fat.

Table 5.2 Ultrasound Patterns in the Differential Diagnosis of Choroidal Melanoma

LESION	LOCATION	SHAPE	INTERNAL REFLECTIVITY	INTERNAL STRUCTURE	VASCULARITY
Melanoma	Choroid and/or ciliary body	Dome or collar button	Low to medium	Regular	Yes
Choroidal hemangioma	Choroid, posterior pole	Dome	High	Regular	No
Metastatic carcinoma	Choroid, posterior pole	Diffuse, irregular	Medium to high	Irregular	No
Choroidal nevus	Choroid	Flat or mild thickening (usually <2 mm)	High	Regular	No
Choroidal hemorrhage	Choroid	Dome	Variable	Variable	No
Disciform lesion	Macula	Dome, irregular	High	Variable	No

43. Describe the ultrasound features of a choroidal hemangioma.

Within a choroidal hemangioma, the adjoining cell and tissue layers have marked differences in acoustic impedance (acoustic heterogeneity). This creates large echo amplitudes at each interface. The A-scan reveals high internal reflections within the tumor, and lesions appear solid white on the B-scan.

44. Describe the ultrasound features of a retinal detachment.

A detached retina produces a bright, continuous, folded appearance on B-scan (Fig. 5.9). When detachment is total or extensive, the retina inserts into both the optic nerve and the ora serrata. The A-scan reveals a 100% high spike. There is motion of the detached retina with voluntary eye movement. Chronic retinal detachment may show intraretinal cysts, calcification, or cholesterol debris in the subretinal space.

45. Describe the ultrasound features that differentiate retinal detachment, posterior vitreous detachment, and choroidal detachment.

See Table 5.3.

46. What ocular conditions may demonstrate calcification on ultrasound?

- Tumors (retinoblastoma, choroidal osteoma, optic nerve sheath meningioma, choroidal hemangioma, choroidal melanoma)
- Toxocara granuloma
- Chronic retinal detachment
- Optic nerve head drusen
- Disciform retinal lesion
- Vascular occlusive disease of the optic nerve
- Phthisis bulbi
- Intumescent cataractous lens[1]

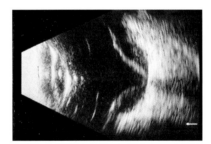

Fig. 5.9 B-scan of total retinal detachment. The anteroposterior view reveals the characteristic V-shaped appearance with attachment to the optic nerve. A cataract is also present.

Table 5.3 Ultrasound Features That Differentiate Retinal Detachment, Posterior Vitreous Detachment, and Choroidal Detachment

ULTRASOUND FEATURES	RETINAL DETACHMENT	POSTERIOR VITREOUS DETACHMENT	CHOROIDAL DETACHMENT
Topographic (B-scan)	Smooth or folded surface	Smooth surface	Smooth, dome, or flat surface
	Open or closed funnel with insertion at optic nerve	Open funnel with or without optic disc or fundus insertion	No optic nerve insertion
	Inserts at ora serrata	Inserts at ora serrata or ciliary body	
	With or without intraretinal cysts	Inserts at ora serrata or ciliary body	
Quantitative (A-scan)	Steep 100% high spike	Variable spike height that is <100%	Steeply rising, thick, double-peaked 100% high spike
Mobility after eye movement	Moderate to none	Marked to moderate	Mild to none

47. When is ultrasound used to evaluate ocular trauma?

Ultrasound may be used to evaluate the position of the lens and the status of the retina if visualization is impeded by an opaque cornea, hyphema, or vitreous hemorrhage resulting from trauma. It also may diagnose a posterior rupture site in the globe and assess for an intraocular foreign body.

The globe should be evaluated visually by the slit lamp technique before ultrasonography to determine whether ocular integrity has been severely disrupted and whether ultrasound examination is indicated. Given that the ultrasound probe contacts the eyelid and may apply pressure on the eye, ultrasound should be used cautiously if there is any evidence of a ruptured globe.

48. What are the ultrasound findings with an intraocular foreign body?

Foreign bodies have high reflectivity when the ultrasound probe beam is perpendicular to a reflective surface of the foreign body (see Fig. 5.7). On the B-scan, a metallic foreign body produces a bright echo that persists when the gain of the ultrasound output is decreased. Shadowing is often present behind a foreign body because of nearly complete reflection of the examining probe beam. Ultrasound is particularly useful with a nonmetallic intraocular foreign body that may not be visible on x-ray or computed tomography (CT) scan.

49. What is ultrasound biomicroscopy?

Ultrasound biomicroscopy (UBM) is a B-scan method that uses high frequencies in the range of 50 to 100 MHz. The depth of penetration is 5 to 7 mm. This technique produces high-resolution images of anterior segment structures (Fig. 5.10) and has been used to characterize the mechanism of secondary glaucoma.

50. How is color-Doppler ultrasonography used in ophthalmologic evaluation?

Color-Doppler ultrasonography is a noninvasive approach to evaluate ocular blood flow. It is useful for assessing morphologic and velocimetric data from the ophthalmic artery, central retinal artery, central retinal vein, and posterior ciliary vessels. This technique has been used to evaluate many ocular disorders, including glaucoma, optic nerve disorders, diabetes, hypertension, ocular ischemia, and the presence of arterial emboli.

51. What is required when you order orbital magnetic resonance imaging studies?

- Surface coil (orbital or head coil) for better visualization of structures of the orbit
- Precontrast axial, coronal, and sagittal T1-weighted images
- Axial, coronal T2-weighted images (fast spin-echo sequences)
- Postcontrast axial coronal T1-weighted images with fat-suppression techniques
- Sedation in children

52. What are paramagnetic agents?

Paramagnetic agents produce proton relaxation enhancement by shortening the intrinsic T1 and T2 relaxation times of the tissues in which they are present. Therefore, tissues containing paramagnetic agents will present with increased signal intensity, best seen on T1-weighted images. Melanin, methemoglobin, protein, and gadolinium are the most common paramagnetic agents. For example, a dermatoid cyst with a high proteinaceous content shows a higher signal intensity on T1- and T2-weighted images than a clear inclusion cyst does.

53. Which ocular and orbital tissues *do not* normally enhance on postcontrast magnetic resonance imaging studies?

- Lens
- Vitreous
- Retina
- Sclera
- Orbital fat
- Optic nerve sheath complex
- Peripheral nerve

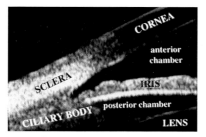

Fig. 5.10 Ultrasound biomicroscopic image of the anterior-segment angle structures.

- Tendon
- High-flow blood vessels

54. Which ocular and orbital tissues *do* normally enhance on postcontrast magnetic resonance imaging studies?
    - Choroid
    - Ciliary body
    - Extraocular muscles
    - Lacrimal gland
    - Nasal: sinus mucosa
    - Cavernous sinus
    - Low-flow blood vessels

55. What is the strategy for ordering imaging studies in a child with leukocoria and total retinal detachment?
    First, perform B-scan ultrasonography. It is cheap and easy to perform in the office without sedation. The goal is to identify calcification, which favors the diagnosis of retinoblastoma. If calcification is documented by ultrasonography, magnetic resonance imaging (MRI) is the second imaging step, to assess the optic nerve and orbital structures and to rule out extraocular retinoblastoma. MRI is also helpful in evaluating the pineal gland and parasellar region, particularly in patients with bilateral and/or familial retinoblastoma. If calcification is not visualized by ultrasonography, orbital CT should be the second imaging step because MRI cannot easily detect minor calcification.

56. What is the strategy for ordering imaging studies in an adult with the diagnosis of intraocular neoplasm?
    A- and B-scan ultrasonography is the first imaging step in evaluating an adult presenting with an intraocular tumor. If ultrasonography, fluorescein angiography, and indocyanine green (ICG) angiography do not help in the differential diagnosis, precontrast- and postcontrast-enhanced MRI studies with fat-suppression techniques are most helpful in detecting and diagnosing intraocular lesions.

57. In what clinical situation are contrast-enhanced magnetic resonance imaging studies most helpful in the evaluation of a child with leukocoria?
    Contrast-enhanced MRI distinguishes between retinoblastoma and Coats' disease.

58. What are the indications for ordering computed tomography orbital studies as a first choice?
    - Ocular trauma to rule out foreign body, especially metal
    - Orbital trauma to evaluate suspected fractures
    - Detection of calcification (i.e., retinoblastoma)
    - Lacrimal gland lesions
    - Infectious or noninfectious orbital inflammation
    - Bone lesions (i.e., osteoma, fibrous dysplasia, etc.) or to evaluate for bony erosion
    - Cases with contraindication for MRI

59. What size computed tomography scan slices should be ordered to evaluate for suspected foreign body or traumatic optic neuropathy?
    CT scan slices of 1.0 mm should be ordered.

60. What are the indications for ordering magnetic resonance imaging orbital studies as a first choice?
    - Optic neuritis (obtain MRI of the brain)
    - CN-III palsy—if pupil involving, obtain urgent MRI and magnetic resonance angiography (MRA) of the head
    - Central nervous system pathology (pituitary lesions, occipital lobe lesions, aneurysms)
    - Cavernous sinus or orbital apex pathology
    - Suspected papilledema (obtain urgent MRI and MRV of the brain)
    - To differentiate cystic and/or hemorrhagic lesions from solid tumors. *Note:* Imaging should not delay the prompt clinical diagnosis and management of an orbital compartment syndrome
    - Optic disc swelling or atrophy (to differentiate optic nerve from optic nerve sheath lesions)
    - Intraocular tumor with extraocular extension
    - Detection of wooden foreign body
    - Cases with contraindication for CT scan

61. What features of ocular and orbital structures on magnetic resonance imaging differentiate between T1- and T2-weighted images?
    - Vitreous is dark in T1 and bright in T2
    - Orbital fat is bright in T1 and dark in T2
    - With fat suppression (T1), vitreous and orbital fat will appear dark but extraocular muscles will appear bright
    - The majority of orbital tumors will be dark in T1 and bright postcontrast

62. What ocular and orbital lesions appear bright in T1 (without contrast)?
    - Lesions containing fat (e.g., dermoid)
    - Subacute hemorrhage (3 to 10 days); acute blood (<3 days) is dark in T1
    - Lesions containing mucus (e.g., mucocele)
    - Tumors containing melanin (e.g., melanoma)

KEY POINTS: SUMMARY OF MODALITIES FOR OPHTHALMIC IMAGING

1. Evaluation of ocular structure
   - Ultrasound—A-scan, B-scan, UBM
   - Optical coherence tomography (OCT)
   - Optical coherence tomography angiography (OCTA)
   - CT scan
   - MRI
   - Corneal topography
2. Evaluation of function
   - Angiography (fluorescein, ICG, OCTA)
   - Doppler blood flow

63. In which clinical situations are contrast-enhanced magnetic resonance imaging studies most helpful in the evaluation of a patient with proptosis?
    Precontrast and postcontrast MRI studies are very helpful in patients diagnosed with a well-circumscribed lesion because they can differentiate a solid (enhancing) tumor from a cystic (nonenhancing) tumor. In a young patient with acute proptosis, MRI studies can differentiate a hemorrhagic lymphangioma from a growing rhabdomyosarcoma. In suspected orbital inflammation, MRI characteristics of the ill-defined inflammatory tissues may predict the therapeutic response to steroids. Lesions showing high signal on T2-weighted images and marked contrast enhancement respond better to steroids than lesions presenting with lower signal intensity on T2-weighted images and/or with minimal or no contrast enhancement.

64. What are the indications for orbital ultrasonography in imaging orbital lesions?
    Orbital ultrasonography is of little help because of its poor histologic specificity and the rapid sound attenuation in the retro-ocular structures. It may be useful to evaluate extraocular extension of an intraocular tumor, the proximal portion of the optic nerve, and extraocular muscles adjacent to the sclera.

65. How can you differentiate optic nerve lesions from optic nerve sheath lesions with computed tomography and magnetic resonance imaging studies?
    Differentiation is almost impossible with CT except that optic nerve sheath meningioma may sometimes show linear calcifications best seen on CT. On MRI, the localization of the enhancement (best seen on T1-weighted images with fat-suppression techniques) helps to differentiate a true optic nerve lesion (neoplastic or inflammatory) from an optic nerve sheath process. An optic nerve tumor or inflammation demonstrates enhancement with the core of the optic nerve, whereas an optic nerve sheath neoplasm or inflammation demonstrates peripheral and/or eccentric enhancement. A cystic or hemorrhagic lesion does not enhance.

66. Summarize the magnetic resonance imaging features of normal ocular and orbital tissues.
    See Table 5.4.

67. What does OCT stand for?
    OCT stands for optical coherence tomography.

68. Explain the basic principles of optical coherence tomography.
    OCT is a noninvasive, noncontact imaging technique that measures variations in optical reflectivity across different tissue interfaces. It is analogous to ultrasound, which measures the reflectivity of sound waves. OCT provides high-resolution, micrometer-range, cross-sectional images of the retinal layers, choroid, and optic nerve. It is a vital tool for the management of a variety of retinal disorders.[1]

69. What is the difference between time-domain and spectral (or Fourier)-domain optical coherence tomography?
    Time-domain OCT uses a moving reference mirror, whereas spectral-domain OCT uses a fixed reference mirror. Spectral-domain technology allows for faster image acquisition, better resolution, and fewer movement artifacts.

70. Describe the retinal layers as seen on optical coherence tomography.[2]
    See Fig. 5.11.

Table 5.4 MRI Features of Normal Ocular and Orbital Tissues

LOCATION	SIGNAL INTENSITY T1-WEIGHTED IMAGES	SIGNAL INTENSITY T2-WEIGHTED IMAGES	ENHANCEMENT AFTER GADOLINIUM–DTPA INJECTION
Lens	High	Low	–
Vitreous	Low	High	–
Choroid	High	High	+++
Retina	Not detected	Not detected	–
Sclera	Low	Low	–
Optic nerve	Low	Low	–
Orbital fat	High	Low	–
Extraocular muscle	Low	Low	+++
Lacrimal gland	Low	Low	+++
Cortical bone	Low	Low	–

+++, Significant enhancement with gadolinium; –, no enhancement with gadolinium.
DTPA, Diethylenetriamine penta-acetic acid; *MRI*, magnetic resonance imaging.

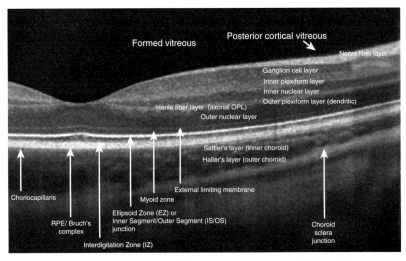

Fig. 5.11 Spectral-domain optical coherence tomography (OCT). The macular spectral-domain OCT image is labeled according to the international consensus definition. *OPL*, Outer plexiform layer.

71. Name common indications for optical coherence tomography.[3]

    OCT can be useful for diagnosis, monitoring response to therapy, and determining the pathogenesis of a variety of macular and optic nerve disorders, including the following:
    - Vitreoretinal interface disease such as vitreomacular traction (Fig. 5.12A) and epiretinal membrane (Fig. 5.12B).
    - Diagnosis of macular hole and differentiation of full-thickness macular hole (Fig. 5.12C) from lamellar hole and pseudohole.
    - Surgical planning for macular hole or epiretinal membrane surgery.
    - Assessment for the presence, location (intraretinal, subretinal, or subretinal pigment epithelium), and amount of fluid in diseases such as AMD (Fig. 5.12D), retinal vein occlusion, and diabetic macular edema.
    - Evaluate for the presence and stability of nerve fiber layer defects in glaucoma.
    - Monitor treatment response. For example, OCT imaging is used to evaluate response to anti-VEGF (vascular endothelial growth factor) agents (Fig. 5.13A and B).

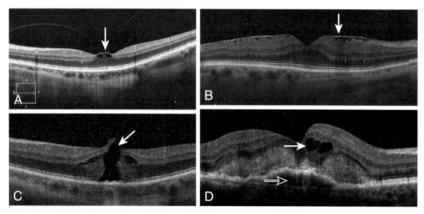

Fig. 5.12 Spectrum of retinal pathology demonstrated on optical coherence tomography. **A,** Vitreomacular traction with distortion of the foveal architecture *(arrow)* and an intraretinal cyst. **B,** Epiretinal membrane *(arrow)* with minimal distortion of the foveal contour. **C,** Full-thickness macular hole *(arrow)*. **D,** Intraretinal fluid *(solid arrow)*, subfoveal pigment epithelial detachment *(hollow arrow)*, and subretinal fibrosis in a patient with age-related macular degeneration.

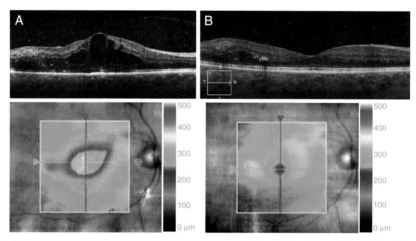

Fig. 5.13 Optical coherence tomography demonstrating reduction of diabetic macular edema in response to intravitreal ranibizumab. **A,** Macular optical coherence tomography (OCT) and thickness map demonstrating macular edema secondary to diabetic retinopathy prior to treatment. **B,** Macular OCT and thickness map with marked reduction in macular edema 4 weeks after intravitreal ranibizumab. The assessment of macular fluid and response to therapy is one of the most important uses of OCT.

72. What structure does enhanced-depth imaging optical coherence tomography help visualize?
    The choroid is external to both the retina and the RPE. Enhanced depth imaging OCT improves visualization of the choroid and may play a role in diagnosing certain disorders, including central serous chorioretinopathy, idiopathic polypoidal vasculopathy, and choroidal melanoma.[3]

73. Describe the technique of fluorescein angiography.
    Commercially available sodium fluorescein dye is injected intravenously at a dose of either 2.5 mL of a 25% concentration or 5 mL of a 10% concentration. Although most of the fluorescein is protein bound, approximately 20% of this dye circulates freely in the vasculature, including the vessels of the retina and choroid. Fluorescein dye fluoresces at a wavelength of 520 to 535 nm (green) after excitation by a light of 485 to 500 nm (blue). White light from a camera flash is passed through a blue filter, exciting unbound fluorescein molecules in the retinal and choroidal circulation and any that have leaked from the vasculature owing to ocular pathology. The blue light stimulates the fluorescein molecule to emit longer-wavelength yellow-green light. The emitted fluorescence and reflected blue light return to the camera, where a yellow-green filter blocks the reflected blue light and allows only the yellow-green fluorescence to enter the camera, by which it is captured onto film or a digital surface.

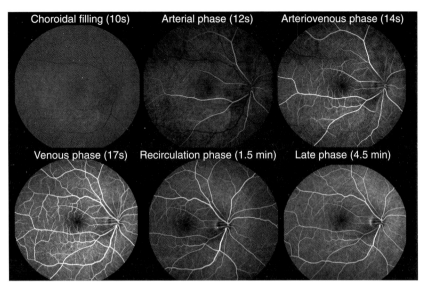

Fig. 5.14 Fluorescein angiography. The phases of a normal fluorescein angiogram are labeled, with the times after injection of fluorescein dye into a peripheral vein of the patient noted.

74. What are the normal phases of a fluorescein angiogram?
    1. Choroidal filling: This commences 10 to 20 seconds after intravenous fluorescein dye injection. The choroid fills within 5 seconds of dye appearance.
    2. Arterial phase: This begins 1 to 2 seconds after choroidal filling.
    3. Arteriovenous phase: Laminar venous flow is present.
    4. Venous phase: The retinal veins are completely filled with fluorescein dye.
    5. Recirculation phase: This begins 45 to 60 seconds after the arterial phase.
    6. Late phase: 3 minutes after the recirculation phase.

75. Describe fluorescence patterns visible with fluorescein angiography.
    Fluorescein angiograms are interpreted based on the pattern, timing, and location of the fluorescence (Fig. 5.14).

KEY POINTS: PATTERNS OF FLUORESCENCE ON FLUORESCEIN ANGIOGRAPHY

1. Hypofluorescence occurs when the fluorescence signal is blocked by overlying pigment, blood, or fibrous tissue or if the blood vessels do not fill properly, resulting in a vascular filling defect.
2. Hyperfluorescence can be seen in several major patterns, including leakage, staining, pooling, and transmission or window defects.
3. Leakage describes the gradual, marked increase in fluorescence throughout the angiogram as the fluorescein molecules diffuse through the RPE into the subretinal space, out of blood vessels, or from retinal neovascularization into the vitreous.
4. Staining denotes a pattern of fluorescence when fluorescein enters a solid tissue such as a scar or drusen. The fluorescence pattern of staining demonstrates a gradual increase in intensity into the late views with fixed borders that do not expand.
5. Pooling describes the accumulation of fluorescein in a fluid-filled space in the retina or choroid as in a detachment of the RPE.
6. Transmission or window defect refers to a view of the normal choroidal fluorescence through a defect in the pigment or loss of the RPE.

76. What structures are permeable to fluorescein?
    The choriocapillaris and Bruch's membrane are freely permeable to fluorescein. In contrast, the RPE and the retinal capillaries are impermeable to fluorescein.

77. Why is the fovea dark on a fluorescein angiogram?
    The fovea is dark for two reasons. First, the xanthophyll pigment in the outer plexiform layer blocks. Second, the retinal pigment epithelial cells in the fovea are taller and contain an increased concentration of melanin and lipofuscin.

78. What is the gold standard for the diagnosis of neovascularization?
    The gold standard is fluorescein angiography. This study demonstrates progressive leakage of dye in areas of neovascularization. This is useful for imaging retinal neovascularization as in diabetic retinopathy (Fig. 5.15A and B) and choroidal neovascularization as in AMD (Fig. 5.15C and D).

79. What are typical fluorescein angiographic findings in central serous chorioretinopathy?
    The classic pattern of central serous chorioretinopathy is a focal, expanding area of hyperfluorescence due to leakage of fluorescein dye from the choroid through the RPE with late pooling in the subretinal space. Some patients may demonstrate a "smokestack" pattern with an expanding area of hyperfluorescence that rises like smoke from a chimney. In more than 75% of patients, the leakage of fluorescein occurs within one disc diameter of the fovea.

80. What is indocyanine green dye?
    ICG is a water-soluble, high-molecular-weight dye that fluoresces with a peak absorption of 805 nm and peak emission of 835 nm. The dye is almost completely protein bound, which limits its diffusion through the small fenestrations of the choriocapillaris. Thus, it remains in the choroidal circulation.

81. What is the theoretical advantage of indocyanine green dye compared with fluorescein dye for retinal angiography?
    ICG dye excitation and emission occur at longer infrared wavelengths compared with fluorescein dye. ICG fluoresces through opacities such as pigment, fluid, lipid, and blood, which may produce hypofluorescence on fluorescein angiography.

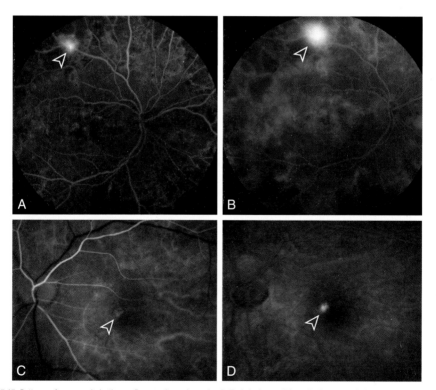

Fig. 5.15 Patterns of neovascularization on fluorescein angiography. **A,** Early leakage of the retinal neovascularization is demonstrated *(arrow)*, with hyperfluorescence with ill-defined borders, in this patient with proliferative diabetic retinopathy. **B,** The area of hyperfluorescence expands in the late-phase angiogram, indicating leakage. **C,** The arterial-phase angiogram demonstrates early parafoveal hyperfluorescence *(arrow)* indicative of a classic choroidal neovascular membrane in a patient with age-related macular degeneration. **D,** The late-phase angiogram demonstrates a small but expanding area of hyperfluorescence indicative of leakage from a CNVM *(arrow)*.

82. What are clinical uses of indocyanine green angiography?

ICG is most useful to demonstrate vascular polyps in idiopathic polypoidal choroidal vasculopathy (Fig. 5.16) and to differentiate this entity from AMD. ICG angiography may assist in the diagnosis of choroidal neovascularization, central serous chorioretinopathy, and choroidal inflammatory disorders.

83. What are the indications for obtaining an ICG in a patient with suspected age-related macular degeneration to differentiate from idiopathic polypoidal choroidal vasculopathy?

- Racially pigmented patients
- Serosanguineous macular detachment in the peripapillary area
- Serosanguineous macular detachment in the absence of drusen
- A large vascularized pigment epithelial detachment, particularly with extensive blood or lipid or minimal cystoid macular edema
- A vascularized pigment epithelial detachment that has proven resistant or minimally responsive to multiple anti-VEGF injections[4]

84. What cell layer does fundus autofluorescence evaluate?

Fundus autofluorescence (AF) assesses the RPE (Fig. 5.17). AF is the intrinsic fluorescence emitted by a substance after stimulation with excitation energy. The clinical use of fundus AF is based on the AF of lipofuscin, which accumulates as an oxidative by-product within RPE cells. RPE that is dead or atrophic is hypoautofluorescent, whereas RPE that is metabolically active, but sick, is hyperautofluorescent. Fundus AF is used to evaluate the area of geographic atrophy in AMD and to assess inflammatory diseases of the RPE. It is also used to evaluate for Plaquenil toxicity.

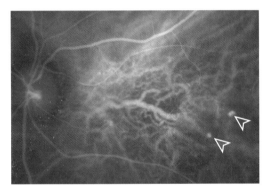

Fig. 5.16 Indocyanine green angiography demonstrating the discrete hyperfluorescence of vascular polyps (*arrows*) in a patient with polypoidal choroidal vasculopathy.

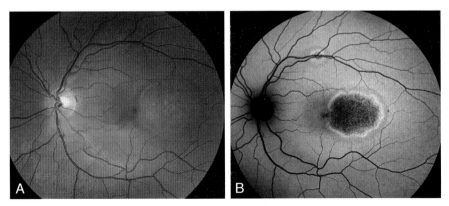

Fig. 5.17 A, Color fundus photography and **B,** fundus autofluorescence demonstrating a central area of hypoautofluorescence with a surrounding border of hyperautofluorescence in a patient with a presumed hereditary macular dystrophy of unknown etiology (other eye with similar findings).

KEY POINTS: SUMMARY OF KEY MODALITIES FOR RETINAL IMAGING

1. OCT: provides high-resolution cross-sectional images of the retina, RPE, and choroid and is vital for management of many retinal disorders.
2. Fluorescein angiography: provides an assessment of the retinal vasculature using an intravenous dye and is the gold standard for evaluating for the presence of neovascularization in conditions such as diabetic retinopathy, vein occlusion, and AMD.
3. OCTA: provides noninvasive, depth encoded images of flow in the retinal and choroidal circulation.
4. ICG angiography: dynamically images the choroidal vasculature and is helpful in evaluating disorders of the choroid, including central serous chorioretinopathy and polypoidal choroidal vasculopathy.
5. Fundus AF: allows for an assessment of the health of the RPE by imaging the intrinsic AF of the retina.

85. What is OCTA?
    Optical coherence tomography angiography is a noninvasive modality that produces detailed, depth-encoded, segmented images of the retinal and choroidal microvasculature (Fig. 5.18).

86. What are the principles behind optical coherence tomography angiography?
    OCTA uses motion contrast imaging to obtain volumetric blood flow information. OCTA compares the decorrelation signal between rapidly acquired, sequential, OCT B-scans. Sites of motion between the repeated OCT B-scans represents erythrocyte motion within the retinal vasculature.

87. What are the potential advantages of optical coherence tomography angiography over traditional fluorescein angiography?
    • Noninvasive
    • No systemic dye use, so no risk of allergic reaction
    • Higher image resolution
    • Three-dimensional image with volumetric data
    • Visualization of superficial and deep retinal and choroidal circulations
    • Faster image acquisition and repeatable

88. What are the disadvantages of optical coherence tomography angiography compared to traditional fluorescein angiography?
    • Smaller field of view
    • Affected by various artifacts (motion artifact, blink artifact)
    • Does not reveal dynamic leakage (static blood flow information)

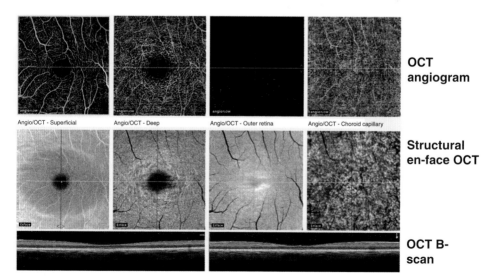

Fig. 5.18 Optical coherence tomography angiography readout of a normal OCT angiogram demonstrating segmentation of the retinal microvasculature.

89. What are some of the clinical disorders imaged with optical coherence tomography angiography?
    - Choroidal neovascularization (in AMD, myopia, macular telangiectasia, central serous chorioretinopathy) (Fig. 5.19)
    - Diabetic retinopathy
    - Retinal vascular occlusion
    - Inflammatory and inherited retinal conditions

90. What can optical coherence tomography angiography show in high-risk diabetic retinopathy?
    - Enlarged foveal avascular zone
    - Microaneurysms (seen as dilated capillary segments, focal dilations, or vascular loops)
    - Capillary remodeling
    - Intraretinal microvascular abnormalities (IRMAs)
    - Retinal and optic disc neovascularization (Fig. 5.20)

Angiography analysis: Angiography 6x6 mm

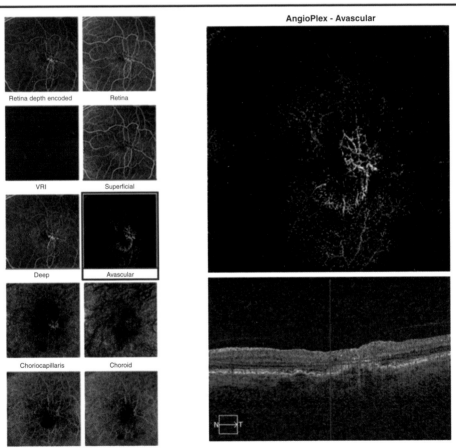

Fig. 5.19 Optical coherence tomography angiography demonstrating choroidal neovascularization in a patient with exudative macular degeneration.

Angiography analysis: Angio (12mmx12mm)

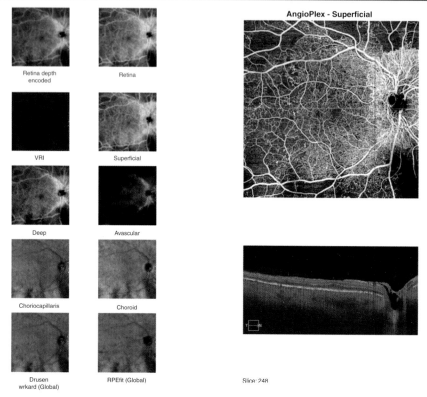

Retina depth encoded

Retina

AngioPlex - Superficial

VRI

Superficial

Deep

Avascular

Choriocapillaris

Choroid

Drusen wrkard (Global)

RPEfit (Global)

Slice: 248

Fig. 5.20 Optical coherence tomography angiography demonstrating retinal neovascularization, microaneurysms, and capillary dropout in a patient with proliferative diabetic retinopathy.

REFERENCES

1. Baumal CR: Clinical applications of optical coherence tomography, Curr Opin Ophthalmol 10:182–188, 1999.
2. Berson EL: Retinitis pigmentosa and allied diseases: Applications of electroretinographic testing, Int Ophthalmol 4:7–22, 1981.
3. Carr RE, Siegel IM: Electrodiagnostic Testing of the Visual System: A Clinical Guide. Philadelphia, 1990, F.A. Davis.
4. De Potter P, Flanders AE, Shields JA, et al.: The role of fat-suppression technique and gadopentetate dimeglumine in magnetic resonance imaging evaluation of intraocular tumors and simulating lesions, Arch Ophthalmol 112:340–348, 1994.
5. De Potter P, Shields JA, Shields CL: Computed tomography and magnetic resonance imaging of intraocular lesions, Ophthalmol Clin North Am 7:333–346, 1994.

BIBLIOGRAPHY

Berson EL: Retinitis pigmentosa and allied diseases: applications of electroretinographic testing, Int Ophthalmol 4:7–22, 1981.
Bilyk JR, Sergott RC, Savino PJ: Quick reference guide for CT and MRI of the eye and orbit, Wills Ophthalmology Review Course 2012.
Carr RE, Siegel IM: Electrodiagnostic testing of the visual system: a clinical guide, Philadelphia, 1990, F.A. Davis.
De Potter P, Flanders AE, Shields JA, et al.: The role of fat-suppression technique and gadopentetate dimeglumine in magnetic resonance imaging evaluation of intraocular tumors and simulating lesions, Arch Ophthalmol 112:340–348, 1994.
De Potter P, Shields JA, Shields CL: Computed tomography and magnetic resonance imaging of intraocular lesions, Ophthalmol Clin North Am 7:333–346, 1994.
De Potter P, Shields JA, Shields CL: MRI of the eye and orbit, Philadelphia, 1995, J.B. Lippincott.
De Potter P, Shields CL, Shields JA, Flanders AE: The role of magnetic resonance imaging in children with intraocular tumors and simulating lesions, Ophthalmology 103:1774–1783, 1996.
Deramo VA, Shah GK, Baumal CR, et al.: Ultrasound biomicroscopy as a tool for detecting and localizing occult foreign bodies after ocular trauma, Ophthalmology 106:301–305, 1999.
Fishman GA, Birch DG, Holder GE, Brigell MG: Electrophysiologic testing in disorders of the retina, optic nerve, and visual pathway, ed 2, San Francisco, 2001, American Academy of Ophthalmology.
Galuzzi P, Hadjistilianou T, Cerase A, De Francesco S, Toti P, Venturi C: Is CT still useful in the study protocol of retinoblastoma? AJNR Am J Neuroradiol 30:1760–1765, 2009.

Marmor MF, Arden GB, Nilsson SEG, Zrenner E: International Standardization Committee: standard for clinical electroretinography, Arch Ophthalmol 107:816–819, 1989.

Newton TH, Bilaniuk LT: Radiology of the eye and orbit, New York, 1990, Raven.

Robson AG, Nilsson J, Li S, et al.: ISCEV guide to visual electrodiagnostic procedures, Doc Ophthalmol 136:1–26, 2018.

Staurenghi G, Sadda S, Chakravarthy U, Spaide RF: International Nomenclature for Optical Coherence Tomography Panel: Proposed lexicon for anatomic landmarks in normal posterior segment spectral-domain optical coherence tomography: the IN•OCT consensus, Ophthalmology April 19, 2014.

Trope GE, Pavlin CJ, Bau A, et al.: Malignant glaucoma: clinical and ultrasound biomicroscopic features, Ophthalmology 101(6):1030–1035, 1994.

Yannuzzi LA: Indocyanine green angiography: a perspective on use in the clinical setting, Am J Ophthalmol 151(5):745–751, 2011.

Wong IY, Koizumi H, Lai WW: Enhanced depth imaging optical coherence tomography, Ophthalmic Surg Lasers Imaging 42(4):S75–S84, 2011.

CHAPTER 6

VISUAL FIELDS

Janice A. Gault

1. **What are the main types of visual-field tests?**
   - Confrontation visual fields
   - Kinetic perimetry
   - Static perimetry
   - Amsler grids

2. **How are confrontation fields used in practice?**
   Confrontation fields are used as a screening tool because they are a simple, quick, qualitative method for finding gross defects in the peripheral field. The test is performed with the examiner facing the patient and asking if the patient can see fingers in all four quadrants while looking directly at the examiner, testing one eye at a time. In clinical practice, this is more of a screening test. A defect picked up by confrontation fields can be described more definitively with formal field testing.

3. **What is the normal field of vision?**
   From the fixation point, the visual field is 60 degrees nasally, 110 degrees temporally, 75 degrees inferiorly, and 60 degrees superiorly.

4. **What is the difference between kinetic and static perimetry?**
   With kinetic perimetry, a stimulus of a particular size and intensity is moved throughout the visual field. The area within which a given target is perceived is known as that target's isopter. These are marked with different colors to easily differentiate the multiple stimuli used. Central vision is mapped with dimmer, smaller stimuli. Larger, more intense stimuli are used for peripheral vision. The Goldmann perimeter and tangent screen are examples of kinetic techniques. With static perimetry, a test site is chosen and the stimulus intensity or size is changed until it is large enough or bright enough for the patient to see it. The Humphrey and Octopus machines are examples of static perimetry.

5. **When is kinetic perimetry used?**
   The test can be helpful in patients who require significant supervision to complete visual-field testing, i.e., children, stroke victims, and patients with dementia and other mental challenges. Patients with low vision due to central vision loss are another indication.
   Highly trained personnel are needed to administer these tests.

6. **What is full-threshold testing?**
   Full-threshold testing refers to static visual-field testing in which the exact threshold of the eye is measured at every point tested. This technique differs from suprathreshold testing, in which test objects are presented at a fixed intensity. Suprathreshold testing is used mainly in screening programs and may miss early defects. Also, a shallow defect will appear the same as an extremely deep defect.

7. **You order a Goldmann visual field, and the isopters are labeled with notations such as I2e and V4e. What do these notations mean?**
   The target size and intensity are indicated by a Roman numeral (I to V), an Arabic numeral (1 to 4), and a lowercase letter (a to e). The Roman numeral represents the size of the target in square millimeters. Each successive number is an increase by a factor of 4. The Arabic numeral represents the relative intensity of the light presented. Each successive number is 3.15 times brighter than the previous one. The lowercase letter indicates a minor filter. The "a" is the darkest, and each progressive letter is an increase of 0.1 log unit.

8. **How is an Amsler grid used to test visual field?**
   The grids can be used to detect central and paracentral scotomas. If held at one-third of a meter, each square subtends 1 degree of visual field.

9. **Where is the physiologic blind spot located?**
   It is in the temporal visual field. The fovea is the center of the visual field. The blind spot is 15 degrees temporal and just below the horizontal plane. On the Humphrey visual field, it is marked by a triangle.

10. **When looking at a visual field, how do you differentiate the right eye from the left eye?**
    The right and left eyes are differentiated by noting where the blind spot is located. The right eye has the blind spot on the right side in its temporal field, and the left eye has the blind spot on the left in its temporal field. If the field loss is so great that the blind spot cannot be identified, the top of the printout should say which eye was tested.

11. What are causes of fixation errors? What can be done to decrease them?
    - Poor patient fixation
    - "Trigger-happy" patient
    - Mistake in locating the blind spot
        Fixation is tested by mapping the blind spot initially and then retesting throughout the test. A fixation loss is counted when the patient clicks the button when the blind spot is retested. Try replotting the blind spot, reinstructing the patient, or changing the fixation diamond to one that does not require central vision in patients with macular disease or central scotoma. Sometimes, giving the patient a break or having a technician remind the patient to stay alert can help. If the fixation loss is greater than 20%, the test is not reliable. Small defects may be missed and the depth of large defects can be underestimated. A kinetic field may be more helpful clinically.

12. What are false-negative errors?
    False negatives occur when a stimulus brighter than threshold is presented in an area where sensitivity has already been determined and the patient does not respond. The patient is usually inattentive and the field will appear worse than it actually is. They may also occur in patients with extremely dense defects.

13. What are false-positive errors?
    Most projection perimeters are fairly noisy, and there is an audible click or whirring while the machine moves from one position to another in the field. False positives occur when the projector moves as if to present a stimulus but does not and the patient responds. The patient is "trigger-happy," and the field will look better than it actually is.

14. On a Humphrey visual field, what is the difference between total deviation and pattern deviation?
    The total deviation is the point-by-point difference from expected values for normal patients who are in the same age range. It cannot confirm a scotoma but shows only generalized depression. The pattern deviation adjusts for the generalized depression or elevation and confirms the presence of a scotoma.

15. What is a scotoma?
    A scotoma is an area of lost or depressed vision within the visual field surrounded by an area of less depressed or normal visual field. On the pattern deviation plot, three or more nonedge points, clustered in an arcuate area, are suspicious for a scotoma.

16. On a Humphrey printout, what do MD, PSD, SF, and CPSD mean? Are they important?
    Mean deviation (MD) is similar to the total deviation plot, i.e., generalized depression. Pattern standard deviation (PSD) is a measure of the degree to which the numbers are different from each other, i.e., local irregularity. This shows more information regarding potential scotomas. Short-term fluctuation (SF) is a measure of intratest error in determining thresholds. Ten predetermined points are each tested twice. Corrected pattern standard deviation (CPSD) is the PSD corrected for the SF. If the SF shows unreliability, the CPSD is better. If the SF is due to true pathology, the PSD is better. If the CPSD or PSD is depressed with $p <5\%$, it is likely the patient has scotoma.

17. What are false field defects? What are some of their causes?
    False field defects occur when the interpreter overlooks physical factors and interprets them as true field defects:
    - Ptosis and dermatochalasis can cause loss in the upper parts of the field. Taping the lid up will clear these defects.
    - A tilted optic disc can cause local variations in retinal topography, giving the impression of a field defect for refractive reasons alone. When a patient has bilateral tilted discs, the effect can mimic a bitemporal visual field loss.
    - A small pupil may give a false impression of true field loss. Dilation of the pupil will clear these defects. This is especially important in patients on miotic therapy (Fig. 6.1).
    - The rim of the trial lens will give a defect in the periphery of the central visual field. This will be noted if the patient pulls the head back from the machine while taking the test or with a strong hyperopic corrective lens (Fig. 6.2).
    - Media opacities: cornea, lens, and vitreous opacities may cause routine test objects to be invisible. Using larger, brighter test objects may help clarify this problem. This generalized decreased sensitivity can be noted on the total deviation on a Humphrey visual field, but the pattern deviation may show no defects.

18. What is SWAP?
    Short-wavelength automated perimetry. A blue stimulus is projected on a yellow background. It may identity early glaucomatous damage by up to 5 years earlier than standard automated perimetry (SAP). It does have higher test-retest variability and media opacities can influence the results. The prolonged testing time makes is less accepted by patients and less efficient in practice. However, the SITA (Swedish interactive threshold algorithm) has lowered testing times without significantly decreasing diagnostic sensitivity in both SWAP and SAP.

19. What is frequency doubling technology (FDT)?
    Low spatial frequency and high temporal frequency preferentially target ganglion cells of the magnocellular pathway. This test selectively uncovers functional deficits in these ganglion cells and thus has high sensitivity and specificity for early glaucoma detection. It has lower test-retest variability compared to SAP, so it may be more advantageous in monitoring progressive visual field loss. A threshold screening test with FDT takes 5 minutes per eye.

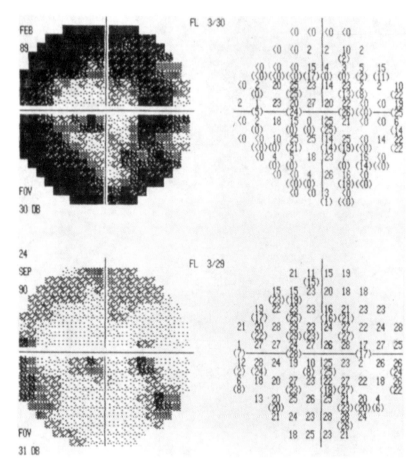

Fig. 6.1 A small pupil can create a false impression of visual-field defects. Note that a majority of the defects disappear or lessen when the pupil is dilated from 2 to 8 mm. (From Gross R: Clinical glaucoma management, Philadelphia, 2001, W.B. Saunders.)

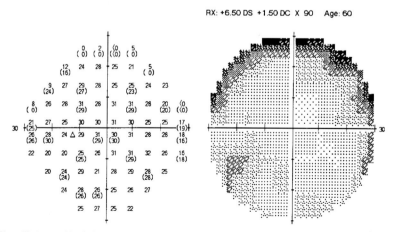

Fig. 6.2 Rim artifact caused by the lens and lens carrier. This is most commonly seen in patients on whom a hyperopic correction is being used. A clue to the presence of a rim artifact is the abrupt change from a fairly normal reading to a sensitivity of 0 dB. (From Alward WLM: Glaucoma: the requisites in ophthalmology, St. Louis, 2000, Mosby.)

20. Are visual field tests always done monocularly?
No. Although most visual field tests check one at a time, a binocular Esterman field tests both eyes at the same time; 120 points are presented at a suprathreshold level. The points are not evenly spaced as more points are displayed near the horizontal midline. They are useful in determining horizontal field of vision for driver's license requirements. Monocular Esterman visual fields are helpful in determining percentage of loss in visual field in each eye as 100 points are presented; 38 points not seen = 38% loss of visual field. Both of these fields are available on the Humphrey Field Analyzer.

KEY POINTS: CAUSES OF FALSE-POSITIVE FIELD DEFECTS

1. Ptosis
2. Tilted optic disc
3. Small pupil
4. Rim defect
5. Media opacities

21. What is hemianopia?
Hemianopia is defective vision or blindness in half of the visual field of one or both eyes.

22. Define the terms *homonymous* and *congruous* in relation to visual-field defects.
   • Homonymous: Pertaining to the corresponding vertical halves of the visual field of both eyes. In plain language, the term is used for defects that occur after neurologic insults that cause loss of a portion of the visual field subsumed by both eyes.
   • Congruous: Matched visual-field defects. The more congruous the defect, the more posterior the lesion.

23. How do you describe a visual-field defect?
   1. **Position:** Central (defined as the central 30 degrees), peripheral, or a combination of both. Note if the defects are unilateral or bilateral.
   2. **Shape:** Very helpful diagnostically. Visual-field defects can be monocular or binocular. The most common form of monocular sector defect is found in glaucoma. The shape is determined by physiologic interruption of nerve fiber bundles. The typical binocular sector defect is a hemianopia.
   3. **Intensity:** This refers to the depth of the defect.
   4. **Uniformity:** This refers to the depth of the defect throughout the defect.
   5. **Onset and course:** This is determined by serial visual fields.

24. What are the different types of hemianopia?
   • **Homonymous, total:** Loss of temporal field in one eye and nasal field of the other eye. The vertical midline is respected. The fixation point may be included or spared. This defect implies total destruction of the visual pathway beyond the chiasm unilaterally, anywhere from the optic tract to the occipital lobe. A complete homonymous hemianopia is nonlocalizing.
   • **Homonymous, partial:** The most common visual-field defect. It may be caused by injury to postchiasmal pathways. Again, it can result from damage at any point from the optic tract to the occipital lobe (Fig. 6.3).
   • **Homonymous quadrantanopia:** This is a form of partial homonymous hemianopia.
   • **Bitemporal:** May vary from a loss of a small amount of the temporal field to complete temporal hemifield loss. This defect signifies damage in the optic chiasm.
   • **Binasal:** This defect signifies an interruption of the uncrossed fibers in both lateral aspects of the chiasm, both optic nerves, or both retinas.
   • **Crossed quadrantanopia:** A rare defect in which the upper quadrant of one field is lost along with the lower quadrant of the opposite visual field. It can occur as part of the chiasmal compression syndrome in which the chiasm is compressed from beneath against a contiguous arterial structure. This produces pressure simultaneously from above and below.
   • **Altitudinal:** This defect can be unilateral or bilateral. A unilateral defect is prechiasmal such as that found in an ischemic optic neuropathy. Bilateral lesions may be produced by lesions that press the chiasm up, wedging the optic nerve, such as an olfactory groove meningioma (Fig. 6.4).
   • **Double homonymous hemianopia:** A result of lesions of the occipital area. There is a loss of all peripheral vision with a remaining small area of central vision representing the spared macula of both eyes. Most are vascular in origin, but they can result from trauma, anoxia, carbon monoxide poisoning, cardiac arrest, and exsanguination (Fig. 6.5).
   • **Macula sparing:** This is the rule in occipital damage. The central visual acuity can remain normal.
   • **Macula splitting:** Uncommon and difficult to detect because the patient will refixate often during the test. This defect occurs with homonymous hemianopia, caused by lesions in the anterior portion of the postchiasmal pathway.

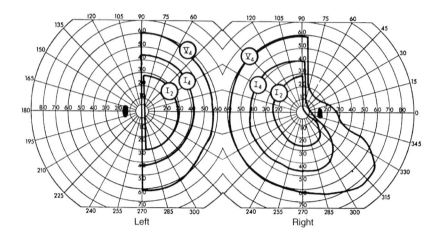

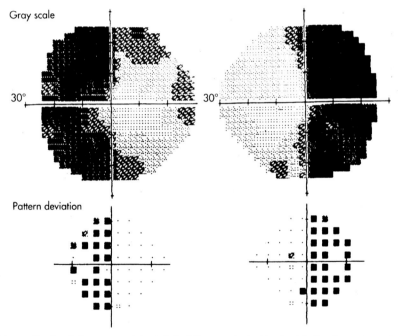

Fig. 6.3 Bitemporal hemianopia: incongruous noted on both the Goldmann perimeter *(above)* and the Humphrey perimeter *(below)*. (From Burde RM, Savino PJ, Trobe JD: *Clinical decisions in neuro-ophthalmology*, ed 2, St. Louis, 1992, Mosby.)

25. Describe the visual pathway.

The first-order neuron is the photoreceptor, a rod or a cone. They synapse with the second-order neurons, the bipolar cells. These synapse with the third-order neurons, the ganglion cells. Axons from these cells cross the retina as the nerve-fiber layer and become the optic nerve. The arrangement of these fibers determines the visual-field defects seen in glaucoma and other optic nerve lesions.

At the chiasm, the temporal fibers are uncrossed, but the nasal fibers cross. The optic tracts begin posterior to the chiasm and connect to the lateral geniculate body on the posterior of the thalamus. Crossed fibers go to laminae 1, 4, and 6. Uncrossed fibers terminate in laminae 2, 3, and 5. The retinal ganglion cell fibers synapse to cells that then connect to the occipital cortex (area 17) via optic radiations in the temporal and parietal lobes.

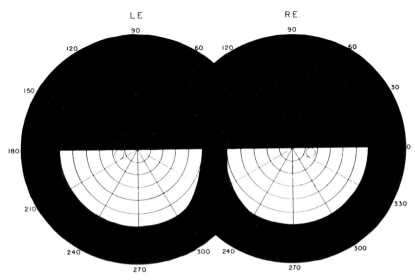

Fig. 6.4 Bilateral altitudinal hemianopia. (From Harrington DO, Drake MV: *The visual fields: text and atlas of clinical perimetry,* ed 6, St. Louis, 1990, Mosby.)

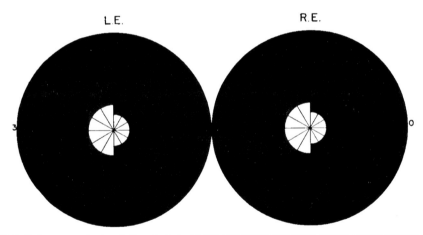

Fig. 6.5 Double homonymous hemianopia. (From Harrington DO, Drake MV: *The visual fields: text and atlas of clinical perimetry,* ed 6, St. Louis, 1990, Mosby.)

26. **What visual-field defects are characteristically seen in neuro-ophthalmologic disorders?**
    The pattern of visual-field loss in these patients can often be used to locate very precisely the area of the visual system involved (Fig. 6.6 and Table 6.1).

27. **Describe the visual-field defect in Fig. 6.7. What are its major causes?**
    This is a bitemporal hemianopia. Lesions of the chiasm cause bitemporal hemianopia because they damage the crossing nasal nerve fibers. Masses in this area include pituitary tumors, pituitary apoplexy, meningiomas, aneurysms, infection, craniopharyngiomas, gliomas, and other less common tumors. In addition, the chiasm may be damaged by trauma (typically causing a complete bitemporal hemianopia), demyelinating disease, and inflammatory diseases such as sarcoidosis and, rarely, ischemia.

28. **What causes binasal hemianopia?**
    Most nasal field defects are due to bilateral arcuate scotomas from glaucoma. True binasal hemianopias are rare, but they are never a result of chiasmal compression. They may be due to pressure upon the temporal aspect of

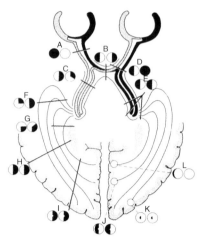

Fig. 6.6 Diagram of the visual pathway with sites of nerve fiber damage and corresponding visual fields produced by this damage. **A,** Optic nerve: blindness on involved side with normal contralateral field. **B,** Chiasm: bitemporal hemianopia. **C,** Optic tract: contralateral incongruous homonymous hemianopia. **D,** Optic nerve–chiasm junction: junctional scotoma. **E,** Posterior optic tract, external geniculate ganglion, posterior limb of internal capsule: contralateral homonymous hemianopia, complete or incomplete incongruous. **F,** Optic radiation, anterior loop in temporal lobe: incongruous contralateral homonymous hemianopia or superior quadrantanopia. **G,** Medial fibers of optic radiation: contralateral incongruous inferior homonymous quadrantanopia. **H,** Optic radiation in parietal lobe: contralateral homonymous hemianopia, may be mildly incongruous, minimal macular sparing. **I,** Optic radiation in posterior parietal lobe and occipital lobe: contralateral congruous homonymous hemianopia with macular sparing. **J,** Midportion of calcarine cortex: contralateral congruous homonymous hemianopia with wide macular sparing and sparing of contralateral temporal crescent. **K,** Tip of occipital lobe: contralateral congruous homonymous hemianoptic scotomas. **L,** Anterior tip of calcarine fissure: contralateral loss of temporal crescent with otherwise normal visual fields. (Adapted from Harrington DO, Drake MV: *The visual fields: text and atlas of clinical perimetry,* ed 6, St. Louis, 1990, Mosby.)

Table 6.1 Summary of Neuro-Ophthalmologic Visual-Field Defects

LESION	VISUAL FIELD
Optic nerve	Central and cecocentral scotomas (i.e., optic neuritis, compressive lesions) Altitudinal defects (i.e., optic nerve drusen, chronic papilledema, ischemic optic neuropathy, optic nerve colobomas)
Optic chiasm	Anterior chiasm or posterior optic nerve: junctional scotoma Body and posterior chiasm: bitemporal hemianopia
Optic tract	Incongruous homonymous hemianopia with or without central scotoma
Optic radiations	Internal capsule: congruous homonymous hemianopia Temporal lobe: superior quadrantanopia Parietal lobe: inferior quadrantanopia
Occipital lobe	Posterior: highly congruous homonymous hemianopia Anterior: monocular contralateral temporal defect Macular or extreme temporal fields may be spared

the optic nerve and the anterior angle of the chiasm or near the optic canal. Causes include aneurysm, tumors such as pituitary adenomas, and vascular infarction.

29. **Where would you expect the lesion causing a homonymous hemianopia without optic atrophy to be located?**
   It should be posterior to the lateral geniculate body. Any lesion anterior to the lateral geniculate body would cause the ganglion axon cells to degenerate.

30. **Does visual acuity help to locate the cause of a visual-field defect?**
   Patients with isolated retrochiasmatic lesions do not have decreased visual acuity unless the lesions are bilateral; then the visual acuity color plates are abnormal and the patient would have a relative afferent pupillary defect. Always examine the patient for optic disc abnormalities such as pallor, cupping, and drusen.

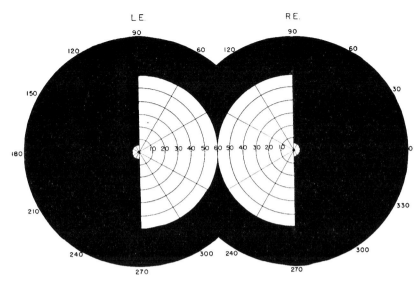

L.E.

R.E.

Fig. 6.7 Bitemporal hemianopia. (From Harrington DO, Drake MV: *The visual fields: text and atlas of clinical perimetry,* ed 6, St. Louis, 1990, Mosby.)

31. Describe the visual-field defect in Fig. 6.8. What causes this?

This is a cecocentral lesion defined as a lesion involving both the blind spot and the macular area (to the 25-degree circle). Four primary causes are typically cited: dominant optic atrophy, Leber's optic atrophy, toxic/nutritional optic neuropathy (i.e., tobacco, alcohol, lead, multiple medications), and congenital pit of the optic nerve with a serous retinal detachment. Optic neuritis also may cause cecocentral lesions.

32. Describe the visual-field defect in Fig. 6.9. Where is the lesion? Are there any coexistent symptoms?

A "pie-in-the-sky" lesion is a homonymous quadrantanopia involving the superior quadrant. The term indicates a lesion in the optic radiations through the temporal lobe, but similar defects can be seen with occipital lobe lesions as well. These patients often have coexistent seizures and visual hallucinations.

33. Describe the visual-field defect in Fig. 6.10. Where is the lesion? Are there any coexistent symptoms?

A "pie-on-the-floor" lesion is a homonymous quadrantanopia involving the inferior quadrant. The term indicates a lesion in the parietal lobe. These patients often have coexistent spasticity of conjugate gaze (tonic deviation of eyes opposite to the side of the lesion when attempting the Bell's phenomenon) and optokinetic asymmetry (diminished or absent response with rotation of optokinetic objects toward the side of the lesion).

34. Describe the visual-field defect seen in Fig. 6.11.

A junctional scotoma is a unilateral central scotoma associated with a contralateral superior temporal field defect. Thus, in a patient that comes in with poor vision in one eye, it is very important to check the contralateral visual field for superior temporal field loss.

35. What is the anatomic explanation for a junctional scotoma?

Inferonasal retina fibers cross in the chiasm, passing into the contralateral optic nerve (Willebrand's knee). The contralateral optic nerve is compressed near the chiasm. These patients have decreased visual acuity and a relative afferent visual defect.

36. What is an optic-tract syndrome?

Mass lesions of the optic tract are usually large enough to compromise the optic nerve and chiasm as well. Patients have an incongruous homonymous hemianopia (Fig. 6.12), bilateral optic disc atrophy, often in a "bow-tie" pattern, and a relative afferent defect on the side opposite the lesion (i.e., the eye with temporal field loss).

37. What are the most common visual-field findings in glaucoma?

Glaucoma is a disease of loss of retinal ganglion cells with characteristic optic nerve findings. The classic defects are determined by the anatomy of retinal ganglion cells as they travel to the optic nerve. The axons circle around the fovea in an arc. With damage to the nerve bundles, the classic findings include a nasal step, an arcuate

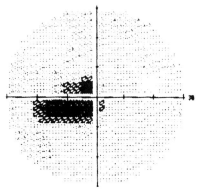

Fig. 6.8 Cecocentral scotoma. (From Burde RM, Savino PJ, Trobe JD: Unexplained visual loss. In Burde RM, Savino PJ, Trobe JD, editors: *Clinical decisions in neuro-ophthalmology,* ed 3, St. Louis, 2002, Mosby, pp 1–26.)

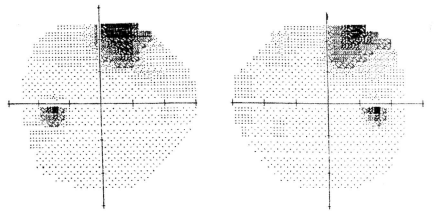

Fig. 6.9 Congruous right superior homonymous quadrantanopia following left temporal lobectomy for epilepsy. (From Burde RM, Savino PJ, Trobe JD: *Clinical decisions in neuro-ophthalmology,* ed 3, St. Louis, 2002, Mosby.)

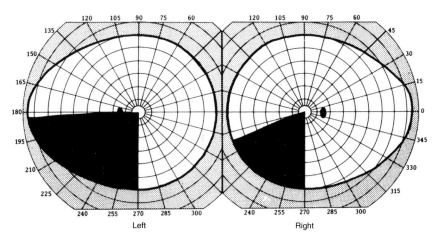

Fig. 6.10 Left inferior quadrantanopia in a patient with a right parietal lobe lesion. (From Kline LB, Bajandas FJ: *Neuro-ophthalmology review manual,* ed 4, Thorofare, NJ, 1996, Slack.)

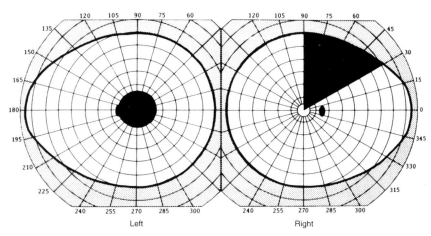

Fig. 6.11 Junctional scotoma from a lesion at the left optic nerve and anterior chiasm. (From Kline LB, Bajandas FJ: *Neuro-ophthalmology review manual,* ed 4, Thorofare, NJ, 1996, Slack.)

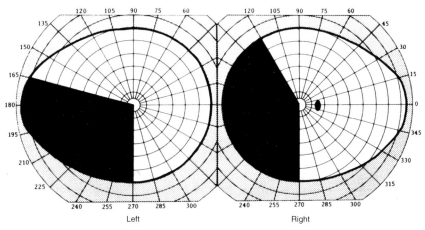

Fig. 6.12 Incongruous left homonymous hemianopia from a right optic-tract lesion. (From Kline LB, Bajandas FJ: *Neuro-ophthalmology review manual,* ed 4, Thorofare, NJ, 1996, Slack.)

defect within 15 degrees of fixation (also known as a Bjerrum defect), or a Siedel scotoma (a comma-shaped extension of the blind spot; Fig. 6.13). The defect obeys the horizontal midline (in contrast to neurologic field defects, which obey the vertical midline). An exam of the optic nerve is helpful in making the diagnosis in less clear cases. Defects in the optic nerve will predict the visual field loss (e.g., a superior notch of the nerve will be manifested by an inferior arcuate field defect). Usually, the central field is retained until a late stage of the disease. When the central field is lost, a small temporal island may remain.

38. When has the visual field of a person with glaucoma progressed?
   The answer remains controversial. First, do not base a diagnosis of glaucoma on one field. If the patient has clear optic nerve damage and corresponding visual field defects, one can make the diagnosis, but the baseline field needs to be repeated because patient performance will improve with practice. A first field with significant defects not corresponding to the clinical optic nerve exam may be full on a second attempt. Improved fixation can also cause field defects to appear more clearly. Persons with glaucoma tend to have more variable visual fields than normal subjects; thus, a single visual field showing worsening should be confirmed with a repeat field. One study concluded that to be certain of progression, one needs a minimum of 5 years of annual visual fields. However, use of clinical correlation can help (Fig. 6.14). Ongoing research is trying to improve our ability to determine which patients are progressing. Newer imaging with ocular

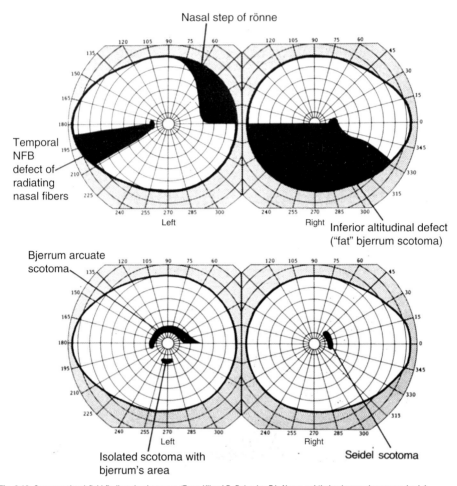

Nasal step of rönne

Temporal
NFB
defect of
radiating
nasal fibers

Left

Right

Inferior altitudinal defect
("fat" bjerrum scotoma)

Bjerrum arcuate
scotoma

Left

Right

Isolated scotoma with
bjerrum's area

Seidel scotoma

Fig. 6.13 Common visual-field findings in glaucoma. (From Kline LB, Bajandas FJ: *Neuro-ophthalmology review manual*, ed 4, Thorofare, NJ, 1996, Slack.)

coherence tomography, Heidelberg retinal tomography, and scanning laser polarimetry can help determine clinical correlation on visual field testing.

39. Describe the visual field in Fig. 6.15. What is your differential diagnosis?

This is a ring scotoma. Severe glaucoma, retinitis pigmentosa, panretinal photocoagulation, vitamin A deficiency, and other retinal and/or choroidal diseases affect the peripheral retina selectively. Aphakic patients may have a prominent ring scotoma from lens-induced magnification of the central field. A clinical exam should easily make the diagnosis from this differential. However, functional vision loss from hysteria or malingering may reveal a ring scotoma on visual-field testing. A Goldmann visual field may be helpful in this situation, as spiraling where an isopter of greater luminance overlaps one that is dimmer can rule out organic disease (Fig. 6.16).

40. What is the differential diagnosis of general depression of the field without localized field defects?

This is a general sign without diagnostic value, but can be an indication of glaucoma, media opacities, small pupils, refractive error, and/or an inexperienced or inattentive patient.

41. What clinical findings might mimic a neurologic defect?

An altitudinal defect can be seen with a hemibranch artery or vein occlusion. Peripapillary atrophy will reveal an enlarged blind spot. A disciform macular scar will show a central scotoma (Fig. 6.17). Retinal detachment will show a correlating visual-field defect, even after it has been repaired.

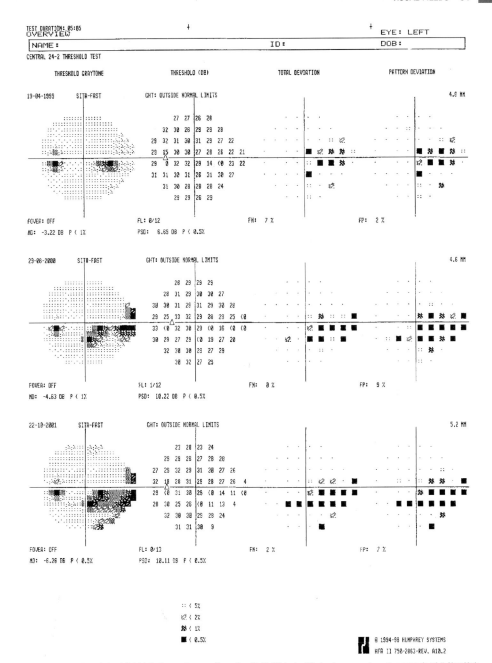

Fig. 6.14 Progression of visual-field defects over 3 years. (From Kanski JJ: *Clinical ophthalmology: a systematic approach,* ed 5, New York, 2003, Butterworth-Heinemann.)

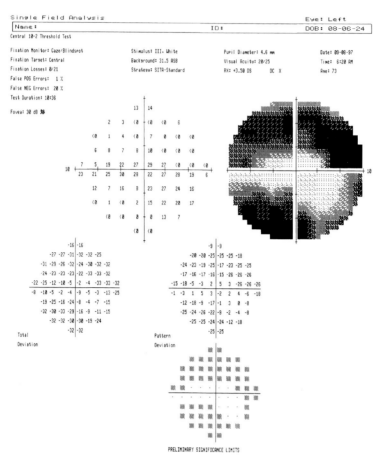

Fig. 6.15 Ring scotoma. (From Gross R: *Clinical glaucoma management,* Philadelphia, 2001, W.B. Saunders.)

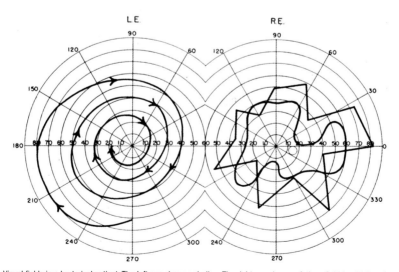

Fig. 6.16 Visual fields in a hysterical patient. The left eye shows spiraling. The right eye shows a fatigue field in which a star-shaped interlacing field results from testing opposite ends of the various meridians. (From Harrington DO, Drake MV: *The visual fields: text and atlas of clinical perimetry,* ed 6, St. Louis, 1990, Mosby.)

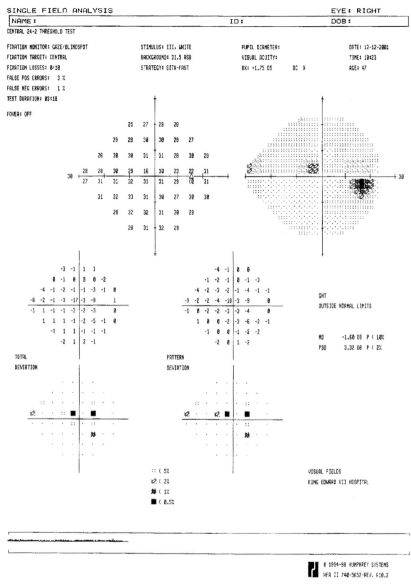

Fig. 6.17 Paracentral scotoma. (From Kanski JJ: *Clinical ophthalmology: a systematic approach*, ed 5, New York, 2003, Butterworth-Heinemann.)

KEY POINTS: USING VISUAL FIELDS TO DETERMINE CAUSE

1. Monocular defects are prechiasmal except that the far temporal visual field is seen only by one eye. Watch this in an anterior occipital infarct, which can produce a monocular temporal defect.
2. Lesions posterior to the chiasm do not cross the vertical meridian by more than 15 degrees.
3. Patients with postchiasmal defects typically have normal visual acuity, normal pupils, and a normal exam of the ocular fundus. Papilledema, however, may be seen in patients with space-occupying lesions.
4. Use clinical correlation to interpret fields.

42. What is the difference among 10-2, 24-2, and 30-2 visual fields?

10-2 tests only the central 10 degrees of visual field with 68 points. The other two test the central 24 degrees with 54 points and the central 30 degrees with 74 points, respectively. In the latter two tests, each point of the is six degrees apart, with only 12 points in the central 10 degrees. Only four of these points are in the macular area, the central 8 degrees. This area has 30% of the retinal ganglion cells in the eye as well as covering 60% of the visual cortex.

The 10-2 tests more than five times as many points as the other two tests in the central 10 degrees. These points are two degrees apart and thus have greater sensitivity. This is very helpful in paracentral scotomas that are often missed on the other two tests. This test is recommended in patients who have defects on visual fields within the central 12 degrees. It is possible that this test is underutilized in all glaucoma patients. That remains to be determined.

This test is also used in screening for plaquenil toxicity as it is associated with damage to the retinal pigment epithelium and a bull's-eye maculopathy. The subtle changes on an Humphrey visual field (HVF) 10-2 can alert the physician to an early case and stop the medication before the patient loses vision. It is important to detect it early as the drug clears slowly from the body and can cause ongoing damage even after the patient discontinues the medication.

43. What does the future hold for visual-field testing?

The most visual field testing done today is SAP. The most important advances in visual-field testing are faster algorithms that decrease test time. The new algorithm uses previous patient responses to help choose the testing threshold and thus takes less time. Test times are approximately 5 minutes per eye, as opposed to 15 minutes with the older algorithms.

BIBLIOGRAPHY

Anderson DA: Automated static perimetry, ed 2, St. Louis, 1998, Mosby.
Anderson DA, Johnson CA: Frequency-doubling technology perimetry, Ophthalmol Clin N Am 16:213-225, 2003.
Burde RM, Savino PJ, Trobe JD: Clinical decisions in neuro-ophthalmology, ed 3, St. Louis, 2002, Mosby.
Haley MJ, editor: The field analyzer primer, ed 2, San Leandro, CA, 1987, Allergan Humphrey.
Harrington DO, Drake MV: The visual fields: text and Atlas of clinical perimetry, ed 6, St. Louis, 1990, Mosby.
Johnson CA, Adams AJ, Casson EJ, et al.: Progression of early glaucomatous visual field loss for blue-on-yellow and standard white-on-white automated perimetry, Arch Ophthalmol 111:651–656, 1993.
Johnson CA, Brandt JD, Khong AM, Adams AJ: Short-wavelength automated perimetry in low-, medium-, and high-risk ocular hypertensive eyes, Arch Ophthalmol 113:70–76, 1995.
Johnson CA, Samuels SJ: Screening for glaucomatous visual field loss with frequency-doubling perimetry, Invest Ophthalmol Vis Sci 38:413–425, 1997.
Katz J, Tielsch JM, Quigley HA, Sommer A: Automated perimetry detects field loss before manual Goldmann perimetry, Ophthalmology 102:21–26, 1995.
Kline LB, Foroozan R: Neuro-ophthalmology review manual, ed 7, Thorofare, NJ, Slack.
Miller NR, Newman NJ: Walsh and Hoyt's clinical neuro-ophthalmology, vol 1, Baltimore, 1998, Williams & Wilkins.
Smith SD, Katz J, Quigley HA: Analysis of progressive changes in automated visual fields in glaucoma, Invest Ophthalmol Vis Sci 37:1419–1428, 1996.

CHAPTER 7

THE RED EYE

Janice A. Gault

CORNEA AND EXTERNAL DISEASES

1. Name the main causes of a red eye.
   - Conjunctivitis
   - Episcleritis
   - Subconjunctival hemorrhage
   - Scleritis
   - Corneal disease and trauma
   - Dry eye
   - Anterior uveitis
   - Acute glaucoma
   - Blepharitis

2. A 40-year-old woman complains of watery, itchy eyes with swollen lids. How should you proceed?

   In the differential diagnosis of a red eye, the history is often helpful. By asking more questions, you find that she has been mowing the grass; subsequently, her hay fever worsened and her eyes flared. Examination reveals red, edematous lids, chemosis, conjunctival papillae, and mucous strands in the cul-de-sac. A preauricular node is not palpable. She is on loratadine (Claritin), but despite improvement in her rhinitis, her eyes are still uncomfortable. Systemic antiallergy medications rarely affect ocular symptoms. Topical treatment is much more effective. Options for topical medications include:

   - Mast cell inhibitors
     - Lodoxamide (Alomide)
     - Nedocromil sodium (Alocril)
     - Cromolyn sodium (Crolom, Opticrom, generic)
     - Pemirolast (Alamast)
   - H_1 receptor antagonists
     - Direct: Epinastine (Elestat)
     - Selective: Emedastine (Emadine)
   - Combination H_1 antagonists/mast cell inhibitors
     - Ketotifen (Zaditor, Alaway, Claritin, generics) now over the counter (OTC)
     - Olopatadine (Patanol, Pataday, Pazeo)
     - Azelastine hydrochloride (Optivar, generics)
     - Nedocromil (Alocril)
     - Bepotastine (Bepreve)
     - Alcaftadine (Lastacaft)
   - Nonsteroidal anti-inflammatory drugs (NSAIDs)
     - Diclofenac (Voltaren)
     - Ketorolac (Acular)
     - Nepafenac (Nevanac, Ilevro)
     - Bromfenac (Prolensa)
   - Low-dose steroid (only for short-term use or under close supervision)
     - Loteprednol (Alrex, Lotemax)
   - Antihistamines/decongestants—OTC
     - Naphazoline/pheniramine (Opcon-A, Naphcon A, Visine A)
     - Naphazoline/antazoline (Vasocon A)

3. The next patient has a similar clinical exam but was seen by her primary care doctor with "pink eye." Since she started her gentamicin drops, she feels her eyes have gotten worse. Her eyelid skin is erythematous and scaly.

   A patient who is allergic to a medication used in or around the eyes presents in a fashion similar to other allergy sufferers, although the lid changes may be more severe. Typical offenders include aminoglycosides, sulfa medications, atropine, epinephrine agents, apraclonidine, trifluridine (Viroptic), pilocarpine, and any ophthalmic medication with preservatives. Immediate cessation of the offending agent, as well as cool compresses and preservative-free artificial tears or a topical antiallergy medication, is appropriate. Impress on the patient that lid rubbing will worsen the condition. If the lid reaction is severe, an ophthalmic steroid cream may be prescribed. Some patients are affected severely enough to develop an ectropion of their lower lids.

4. The next patient has no seasonal allergies and is not on any topical medications around her eye, but again, the clinical picture looks the same, with lots of itching.
Ask about exposures to items such as creams, lotions, detergents, fabric softener, hair dyes, cosmetics, nail lacquer, and glues. It can also be an old product, with new formulations or fragrances. A new cat or dog can cause a similar picture. The possibilities are nearly endless. Referral to an allergist for patch testing to determine the cause may be helpful. Cool compresses, preservative-free artificial tears, and topical antiallergy medicines can give symptomatic relief.

5. What might you expect to see in a patient with epidemic keratoconjunctivitis, or pink eye?
Examination may reveal tarsal conjunctival follicles as well as a preauricular node. In more severe cases, the patient may have membranes or pseudomembranes. Often, the condition begins in one eye and spreads to the other. Viral conjunctivitis may precede, accompany, or follow an upper respiratory infection. This condition is contagious, and patients need to be warned not to leave any contaminated material in a place where others may touch it. Frequent hand washing is crucial. The physician's exam room needs to be washed down thoroughly with an appropriate disinfectant, because an epidemic may occur among other patients as well as staff. Patients should not return to work or school until the eyes stop weeping, often as long as 2 weeks. The condition typically worsens in the first week before improving over the course of 2 to 3 weeks. Adults may have systemic symptoms of an upper respiratory infection with fevers and muscle pain. Children are less systemically affected. Ophthalmic treatment is supportive, with artificial tears and cool compresses. Steroids should be used only in select cases such as those with subepithelial infiltrates that reduce vision and membranes or pseudomembranes. Steroids decrease symptoms in the short-term but often increase the duration of the disease. Topical NSAIDs and antiallergy medications may alleviate discomfort without prolonging the disease course. Rapid immunoassay test strips are available to detect adenoviral antigens in the diagnosis of a viral conjunctivitis.

6. A 25-year-old man states that his eyes have been dripping with discharge over the past 8 hours. You notice significant purulent discharge, a preauricular node, and marked chemosis. What is the next step?
This condition is an emergency. The most likely diagnosis is gonococcal conjunctivitis. An immediate Gram stain and conjunctival scrapings for culture and sensitivities are imperative. Cultures should be done on blood agar, on chocolate agar at 37° C and 10% CO_2, and a Thayer–Martin plate. If they cannot be done at your office, send the patient to an emergency room that can perform and interpret them urgently.

7. What are you looking for on the Gram stain?
A positive Gram stain would show gram-negative intracellular diplococci.

8. How should the patient be treated?
   1. Ceftriaxone, 1 gm intramuscularly in a single dose. However, if corneal involvement exists or you are unable to visualize the cornea because of chemosis and lid swelling, the patient should be hospitalized and treated with ceftriaxone, 1 gm intravenously every 12 to 24 hours. *Neisseria gonorrhoeae* can perforate an intact cornea quickly. Penicillin-allergic patients can be treated orally with 500 mg of ciprofloxacin or 400 mg of ofloxacin, both as single doses. However, there is increasing fluoroquinolone resistance in certain areas. Consider an infectious disease consult.
   2. Topical bacitracin or erythromycin ointment four times a day or ciprofloxacin drops every 2 hours. Consider fluoroquinolones every hour if the cornea is involved.
   3. Eye irrigation with saline four times a day until the discharge is gone.
   4. Doxycycline, 100 mg twice a day for 7 days, or azithromycin, 1 gm orally as a single dose for chlamydial infection, which often coexists. Use erythromycin or clarithromycin in a patient who is pregnant or breast-feeding because of the risk of teeth staining in children.
   5. Referral of the patient and sexual partners to family doctors for evaluation of other sexually transmitted diseases.

9. A 35-year-old man complains of pain in his left eye for several days, watery discharge, and blurred vision. He thinks he has had the same symptoms before. He admits to stress on the job as well as a recent cold sore. What do you expect to see?
Herpes simplex virus (HSV) would be expected. With fluorescein staining of the eye, you can see a dendritic ulcer with terminal bulbs (Fig. 7.1). It is placed centrally, accounting for the decrease in vision. The patient may also have some anterior chamber cell and flare. He needs a topical antiviral such as ganciclovir (Zirgan), trifluridine (Viroptic), or vidarabine (Vira-A). Debridement of infected epithelium can speed recovery. Add a cycloplegic drop if photophobia and anterior chamber reaction are significant. Topical steroids should be tapered. Oral antivirals such as acyclovir (400 mg five times a day for 7 to 10 days) may be used if topical toxicity or compliance with the drops is a problem. However, they have not been shown to prevent stromal disease or iritis in HSV infection,

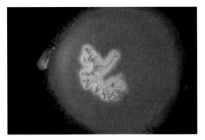

Fig. 7.1 A dendrite typical of herpes simplex keratitis with epithelial ulceration, raised edges, and terminal bulbs. (From Kanski JJ: *Clinical ophthalmology: a synopsis*, New York, 2004, Butterworth-Heinemann.)

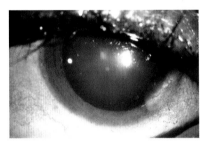

Fig. 7.2 Dry eye syndrome with rose bengal staining. (From Tu EY, Rheinstrom S: Dry eye. In Yanoff M, Duker JS, editors: *Ophthalmology*, ed 2, St. Louis, 2004, Mosby, pp 520–524.)

but they are beneficial if iritis is already present. Once the patient has healed from the acute episode, long-term, oral antiviral prophylaxis such as acyclovir 400 mg twice a day may be indicated if the patient has had multiple episodes of herpetic epithelial or stromal disease.

10. An 80-year-old woman complains of red eyes that constantly tear and burn. They worsen as the day goes on. She also feels foreign-body sensation and reports that her vision is not as clear as before. The vision varies with tear blink. She has noticed this condition over the past several years. What may you find?

    On exam, you may find a poor tear film filled with debris, a low tear meniscus, superficial punctate keratopathy (SPK) inferiorly or throughout the cornea, and, if severe, mucous filaments adherent to the cornea. A normal meniscus is 1 mm in height in a convex shape. A Schirmer's test can quantify her tear production. Fig. 7.2 shows the areas of rose bengal interpalpebral staining. Lissamine green staining would show a similar pattern. Both stains show devitalized cells in the conjunctiva and the cornea. Fluorescein only highlights areas of dead cells and can delay the diagnosis. Make sure that she can close her eyes completely, because lagophthalmos may cause similar symptoms. The condition may be due to an eyelid deformity from scarring, tumor, or Bell's palsy. Patients may have trouble closing their eyes completely after ptosis surgery.

11. What may cause superficial punctate keratopathy?

    Blepharitis, dry eye, Sjogren's syndrome, trauma from eye rubbing, exposure, topical drug toxicity, ultraviolet burns (welder's flash, snow blindness), foreign body under the upper lid, mild chemical injury, trichiasis, floppy-lid syndrome, entropion, and ectropion may cause bilateral SPK. Treatment consists of increasing lubrication and eliminating the cause.

12. What is Thygeson's superficial punctate keratopathy?

    Thygeson's SPK consists of bilateral stellate, whitish-gray corneal opacities that are slightly elevated with minimal to no staining. Tears are usually the only required treatment, with occasional topical steroids for severe cases. Thygeson's SPK has a chronic course with remissions and exacerbations.

13. An 83-year-old man has crusty lids and red eyes and complains of "sand in my eyes." What is your diagnosis?

    This is a common scenario indeed. Blepharitis may present with crusty, red, thickened eyelid margins with prominent blood vessels (Fig. 7.3). Inspissated oil glands at the lid margins cause meibomianitis. Patients often have both and complain of red, tearing eyes. The lids may be significantly swollen. Patients often have trouble

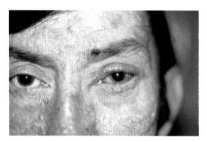

Fig. 7.3 Blepharitis. (From Kanski JJ: *Clinical ophthalmology: a test yourself atlas,* ed 2, New York, 2002, Butterworth-Heinemann.)

opening their eyes in the morning because of the amount of crusting. SPK is common. If severe and untreated, cornea scarring can develop.

Blepharitis can be divided into anterior and posterior blepharitis. Anterior blepharitis affects the eyelid follicles, base of the eyelash, and eyelid skin. Anterior blepharitis is staphylococcal, seborrheic, or a combination or both. Staphylococcal blepharitis has scaling, crusting, and redness of the lid margin with collarettes at the base of the eyelashes. *Staphylococcus aureus* is more common in these patients. Some think the antigens or toxins from these bacteria may be a factor in the pathophysiology of the disease. Dandruff-like material is seen in patients with seborrheic blepharitis; they may have seborrheic dermatitis of the eyebrows and scalp.

Posterior blepharitis affects the meibomian gland and its orifices. Some have proposed calling this meibomian gland dysfunction (MGD) instead. Foam at the eyelid margin and plugged, swollen meibomian glands and a decreased tear film breakup time are noted in slit lamp exam. Expression of the meibomian glands produces thick toothpaste-like meibomian gland secretions. Eventually, the glands atrophy and cicatrize. Acne rosacea frequently coexists.

14. **How do you treat blepharitis?**
    This chronic condition may require treatment indefinitely or only during flares. Warm compresses two times a day for 5 minutes at a time, baby shampoo on a washcloth or commercial lid scrubs to scrub the eyelid margins twice a day, and artificial tears as needed will help. It may take a week or two of compliance before improvement. Once the condition is under better control, the regimen can be reduced to once a day or as needed. However, when the condition flares, the regimen needs to be increased. Add bacitracin or erythromycin ointment at night. In severe cases, a topical antibiotic/steroid combination may be helpful in the short-term, but make sure that the patient understands the risks of long-term use of steroids (e.g., cataracts, glaucoma, increased risk of infection). Topical azithromycin (Azasite) scrubbed into the lashes at night and topical cyclosporine (Restasis) or lifitegrast (Xiidra) may be helpful for some patients, especially those with MGD. If the patient does not respond, epilating a lash and looking at it under the microscope may reveal *Demodex.* Infestation has been reported in patients with MGD and collarettes. Treatment with diluted tea tree oil or oral ivermectin has been reported to be of some benefit. MGD has been treated in the office with meibomian gland probing or devices using thermal pulsation (i.e., LipiFlow) to open the blocked orifices. There are no randomized clinical trials on the effectiveness of these procedures yet.

15. **If a patient with chronic blepharoconjunctivitis does not improve with multiple therapies, what should be in your differential?**
    The patient may have sebaceous cell carcinoma. It can be multicentric. Do a biopsy and stain with oil red O. Other tumors such as basal cell, squamous cell, and melanoma are less likely.

16. **What other ocular issues are commonly seen in patients with blepharitis?**
    Patients may have trichiasis or misdirected lashes that scratch the cornea and conjunctiva. If so, the lashes should be epilated. If they are a recurring problem, electrolysis or cryotherapy may provide a more permanent solution. Hordeolum and chalazion are frequently seen in patients with MGD.

KEY POINTS: RED EYE PATIENTS

1. History is important in diagnosis.
2. Itching usually points to allergy. Be suspicious of a diagnosis of allergy without itching.
3. Dry eye symptoms worsen as the day goes on.
4. Blepharitis symptoms may be worse from the beginning of the day.
5. Watery discharge points to a viral cause.
6. Purulent discharge points to a bacterial cause.

17. A 45-year-old man with red, weepy eyes complains of foreign-body sensation for several months. You note he has a bulbous nose and telangiectasias on both cheeks. What is your diagnosis? How do you treat?

Acne rosacea is a disease of the eyes and the skin. Pustules, papules, telangiectasias, and erythema develop on the nose, cheeks, and forehead. Rhinophyma occurs in the later stages of the disease. Telangiectasias of the eyelid margin and chalazia are common, as are blepharitis and meibomianitis. Dry eye, SPK, phlyctenules, and staphylococcal hypersensitivity may occur. In severe cases, the cornea may develop opacification, vascularization, and even perforation.

Treatment for blepharitis and meibomianitis with warm compresses and lid scrubs may be all that is necessary. If the patient does not respond, thinning of the abnormally thick meibomian gland secretions with tetracycline or doxycycline for several weeks may relieve the symptoms, but some patients require a low dose indefinitely. Erythromycin should be substituted in pregnant or nursing women and children because of the risk of teeth staining. A low-dose antibiotic/steroid combination may be useful if SPK or staphylococcal hypersensitivity is a problem; staphylococcal exotoxins may be the cause. Patients can develop infected corneal ulcers; thus, scrapings for smears and cultures may be necessary in patients with "sterile" corneal ulcers before steroids are used.

18. An 18-year-old contact lens wearer presents with her hand over her right eye. She noticed that her eye was somewhat red and irritated 2 days ago but believes that it has gotten worse even though she took out her lens at that time. What are you concerned about?

Whenever a contact lens wearer complains of a red, irritated eye that does not improve over a few hours, a corneal ulcer is high on the differential. After a corneal anesthetic such as proparacaine is instilled, the patient feels some relief and can tolerate examination. You notice a corneal infiltrate with an overlying epithelial defect and anterior chamber cell and flare. See the chapter on corneal infections for the necessary workup and treatment.

19. What else is in the differential diagnosis of a red eye in a contact lens wearer?

- Hypersensitivity reactions to preservatives in solution. The patient may develop an allergy or may not be rinsing the enzyme off completely before placing the lens in the eye. This is usually bilateral.
- Giant papillary conjunctivitis (Fig. 7.4). Patients have large conjunctival papillae on upper lid eversion. Patients may need to discontinue lens wear for several weeks, change their disposable lenses more frequently (even daily), and/or use topical medications such as nonsteroidal anti-inflammatory medications, mast cell inhibitors, or antihistamines. Increased enzyme use and discontinuation of overnight wear also help. This is usually bilateral.
- Contact lens deposits. Old lenses should be replaced. This can be unilateral or bilateral.
- Tight lens syndrome. Lenses shrink with age. On exam, the patient may have significant chemosis around the lens, and the lens will not move with a blink. In severe cases, a sterile hypopyon can develop. This can be unilateral or bilateral.
- Corneal abrasion. This is usually unilateral.

20. A young mother enters with her infant child. Her left eye is tearing profusely, and she has trouble keeping it open. She states that she was changing the child's diaper when he scratched her eye with his fingernail. What treatment do you recommend?

At the slit lamp, you see a fairly large, central corneal abrasion with no sign of an infiltrate. The upper lid is everted, and no foreign body is seen. The abrasion will heal fairly quickly regardless of treatment; the goals are comfort and prevention of infection. Some patients desire a pressure patch for comfort, but it should not be used in patients who wear contact lenses or who have had trauma from a fingernail or vegetable matter (e.g., a dirty nail or tree branch). Such injuries have a higher chance of contamination and need to be observed for the development of a corneal ulcer. Patching may increase the rate of infection in these patients. A cycloplegic drop, such as cyclopentolate 2%, may relieve the discomfort of ciliary spasm. Prophylactic antibiotics are controversial as they may increase the risk of resistant bacteria if an infected ulcer does develop. If the infection is considered "dirty," tobramycin or ciprofloxacin is a good choice for *Pseudomonas* sp. prophylaxis. A topical anti-inflammatory decreases pain, and some evidence

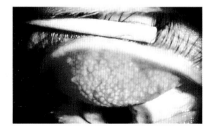

Fig. 7.4 A typical case of giant papillary conjunctivitis in a contact lens wearer. (From Rubenstein JB, Jick SL: Disorders of the conjunctiva and limbus. In Yanoff M, Duker JS, editors: *Ophthalmology*, ed 2, St. Louis, 2004, Mosby, pp 397–412.)

suggests that it may promote healing. However, long-term use of NSAIDs has been associated with corneal melts. The best choice is frequent lubrication with tears and/or ointments to promote healing.

21. **Does it make a difference where the abrasion is located?**
If the abrasion is large, central, or in a contact lens wearer, the patient should return the next day to make sure that no infection is developing and that the lesion is healing. A bandage contact lens can help with pain and reepithelialization in large defects. A contact lens wearer can resume his or her usual lenses after the defect has healed and the eye feels normal for 3 or 4 days. After the abrasion is healed, examine the patient while he or she is wearing the lenses to ensure that they fit well. Make sure that the lens does not have a tear or significant deposits, which may have contributed to the abrasion.

KEY POINTS: CAUSES OF RED EYE IN A CONTACT LENS WEARER

1. Corneal ulcer
2. Allergy to contact lens solutions
3. Giant papillary conjunctivitis
4. Old lenses
5. Corneal abrasion

---

22. **The same woman as in question 20 returns 3 months later complaining that she awoke in the morning with severe pain, redness, and tearing in the left eye. It feels like the original scratch. She denies rubbing her eye or any other trauma. What may have happened?**
Patients who have had a corneal abrasion from a sharp edge such as a paper edge or a fingernail may develop recurrent corneal erosions. Recurrent erosions also may be seen in patients who have corneal dystrophy, such as Meesmann's, map-dot-fingerprint, Reis-Bucklers', lattice, macular, or granular corneal dystrophy. Typically, patients awaken with severe pain and tearing, or symptoms develop after eye rubbing. On examination, an abrasion may be seen in the area of previous injury, or the epithelium may have healed the defect but appear irregular. Sometimes, no abnormalities can be seen, and the diagnosis must be made from the history. Look carefully for any signs of dystrophy, especially in the other eye. Treat with frequent lubrication to heal the epithelial defect. If the corneal epithelium is loose and heaped upon itself, debridement of the loose edges may be necessary first to allow the epithelial defect to heal.

23. **Do you treat if the exam is normal in this patient?**
After healing, lubrication is crucial. If the eye is dry and the lid becomes stuck to the abnormal epithelium, the cycle will begin again. Artificial tears during the day and lubricating ointment at night will help. A hypertonic solution of 5% sodium chloride theoretically draws out the water from the cornea and promotes epithelial adhesion to its basement membrane. If such treatment does not prevent further erosions, an extended-wear bandage soft contact lens or a self-retained amniotic membrane (ProKera) may help. Some patients require anterior stromal puncture or phototherapeutic keratectomy with an excimer laser, which causes small permanent corneal scars that prevent further erosions.

24. **A car mechanic complains of a painful red eye. He was fixing a muffler at the time of the onset of pain. What are your concerns?**
Most likely, he has a foreign body in his cornea or conjunctiva. It is important to find out what he was doing at the time of the injury. He states that he was hammering metal without safety glasses. This report increases your concern that he may have a ruptured globe. A metal piece that breaks off would travel at a high rate of speed.

On exam, he has 20/20 vision in both eyes. You see no foreign bodies in the conjunctiva or the cornea. You evert the upper lid and find nothing. The intraocular pressure is 2 mm Hg. The other eye has a pressure of 15 mm Hg. Slit lamp exam reveals a conjunctival defect with subconjunctival hemorrhage. It is impossible to determine whether a scleral laceration is present because of the blood blocking the view.

25. **What do you do now?**
First, put a shield over the eye to prevent further damage to the globe. It is best to examine and treat in the controlled setting of the operating room. The pupil should be dilated to determine whether the foreign body can be seen with the indirect ophthalmoscope. The patient should have nothing else by mouth. A computed tomography scan of the orbits and brain (axial and coronal) is necessary to screen for foreign bodies in the eye, orbit, and brain. Always evaluate the patient systemically to make sure no other injuries are missed. Begin intravenous antibiotics such as cefazolin and ciprofloxacin. Give a tetanus toxoid booster.

26. **How do you proceed if, instead of a potential ruptured globe, you find a superficial metallic foreign body at four o'clock on the cornea?**
Document visual acuity. Sometimes an infiltrate may be found around the foreign body, especially if it is over 24 hours old. Usually, the infiltrate is sterile. Apply a topical anesthetic (proparacaine), and remove the foreign

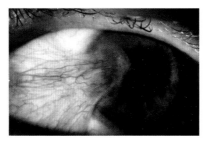

Fig. 7.5 An early pterygium with triangular, fibrovascular growth from the conjunctiva (tail) onto the cornea (head). A deposit of iron in the corneal epithelium (Stocker line) may be seen anterior to the head. (From Kanski JJ: *Clinical ophthalmology: a synopsis,* ed 5, New York, 2004, Butterworth-Heinemann.)

body with a 25-gauge needle or a foreign-body spud at the slit lamp. A rust ring may have formed, depending on how long the metal has been present. Often, it can be removed with the same instruments. It is sometimes safer to leave a rust ring if it is deep or in the center of the visual axis. The rust ring will eventually migrate to the corneal surface, where it is easier and safer to remove. Dilate the pupil, and make sure that the vitreous and retina are normal. The history of hammering makes a dilated exam imperative.

Treat with an antibiotic ointment or drop and a cycloplegic if the patient is severely photophobic and in pain. Large or central defects need to be followed up to make sure that healing occurs without infection. An antibiotic such as erythromycin, trimethoprim/polymyxin, or a fluoroquinolone is appropriate.

27. A lifeguard states that his eye has been red for a long time. He has a wing-shaped fold of fibrovascular tissue nasally in both eyes that extends onto the cornea. Should he be worried?
The lesion is a pterygium (Fig. 7.5). A similar lesion called a pinguecula involves the conjunctiva but not the cornea. Both are usually bilateral. They are thought to result from damage due to chronic ultraviolet exposure or chronic irritation from wind and dust. They may be associated with dellen, an area of corneal thinning secondary to drying because the area adjacent to raised areas may not receive adequate lubrication during blinks. It is necessary to rule out conjunctival intraepithelial neoplasia, which is unilateral, often elevated, and not in a wing-shaped configuration.

Counsel the lifeguard to wear ultraviolet blocking sunglasses and to use artificial tears frequently, especially on sunny, windy days. Surgical removal of a pterygium is indicated if it interferes with contact lens wear, causes significant irritation, or involves the visual axis. Newer surgical techniques and the use of antimetabolites such as mitomycin C are decreasing recurrences.

28. An unfortunate victim of domestic abuse had lye thrown in his face. What should you do?
Even before you check vision, quickly check pH and then begin copious irrigation with saline or Ringer's lactated solution for at least 30 minutes. An eyelid speculum and a topical anesthetic will help. Make sure to irrigate the fornices. Stop irrigation only when pH of 7.0 is reached. If it is not reached after a significant time, check for particulate matter that may be trapping the chemical.

29. What is his prognosis?
Acids tend to have a better outcome than alkalis. Acids precipitate proteins, which limit penetration. Alkalis (lye, cement, plaster) penetrate more deeply. A mild burn may have only SPK or sloughing of part or all of the epithelium. No perilimbal ischemia is seen. Patients need a cycloplegic, antibiotic ointment and rarely pressure patching. Check intraocular pressure, which may be elevated by damage to the trabecular meshwork.

A moderate to severe burn has perilimbal blanching and corneal edema or opacification with a poor view of the anterior chamber. A significant anterior chamber reaction may be seen. The intraocular pressure may be elevated and the retina may be necrotic at the point where the alkali penetrated the sclera. The patient may need hospital admission to monitor intraocular pressure and corneal status. A topical antibiotic, cycloplegic, and pressure patching are used. Steroids may be used if the anterior chamber reaction or corneal inflammation is severe. However, they cannot be used for more than 7 days because they promote corneal melting. Collagenase inhibitors such as acetylcysteine (Mucomyst) may help in a melt. Cyanoacrylate tissue adhesive and an emergency patch graft or transplant may be necessary if perforation occurs. Patients require long-term care.

30. A young boy presents with purulent discharge over the past few days. His mother thinks that he needs antibiotics. Do you agree?
Yes. Purulent discharge signals bacterial conjunctivitis as opposed to the watery discharge of viral conjunctivitis. Patients usually have a conjunctival papillary reaction and no preauricular node. Gram stain and conjunctival swab for culture and sensitivities should be done if the conjunctivitis is severe.

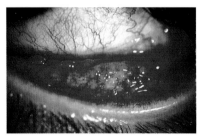

Fig. 7.6 Chronic follicular conjunctivitis with large conjunctival follicles, most prominent in the inferior forniceal conjunctiva, and scant mucopurulent discharge. Lymphadenopathy is also present. (From Kanski JJ: *Clinical ophthalmology: a synopsis*, ed 5, New York, 2004, Butterworth Heinemann.)

31. **What are the common organisms responsible for bacterial conjunctivitis in children? How should you treat?**
    S. aureus, Staphylococcus epidermidis, Streptococcus pneumoniae, and *Haemophilus influenzae* are common; *H. influenzae* is especially common in children. Topical antibiotics such as trimethoprim/polymyxin (Polytrim), ciprofloxacin, or erythromycin four times a day for 5 to 7 days is appropriate. *H. influenzae* should be treated with oral amoxicillin/clavulanate because of the possibility of systemic involvement, such as otitis media, pneumonia, or meningitis. Associated dacryocystitis also warrants oral antibiotics.

32. **A 27-year-old woman complains of red, irritated eyes with watery discharge over the past 6 weeks. A follicular conjunctivitis and palpable preauricular node are present. What is the differential diagnosis?**
    Conjunctivitis lasting longer than 4 weeks is considered chronic (Fig. 7.6). The differential for chronic conjunctivitis includes chlamydial inclusion conjunctivitis, ocular toxicity, Parinaud's oculoglandular conjunctivitis, trachoma, molluscum contagiosum, and silent dacryocystitis.

33. **How do you proceed?**
    History is important. On questioning, the patient reports a recent vaginal discharge. Chlamydial infection becomes high on the list. Such patients also may have white peripheral subepithelial infiltrates and a superior corneal pannus. Stringy, mucous discharge is common. Obtain a chlamydial immunofluorescence test and/or a chlamydial culture of the conjunctiva. Giemsa stain will show basophilic intracytoplasmic inclusion bodies in epithelial cells as well as polymorphonuclear leukocytes. Tetracycline, doxycycline, or erythromycin should be taken orally for 3 weeks by the patient and her sexual partners. Topical ocular erythromycin, tetracycline, or sulfacetamide ointment is used at the same time. Counseling and evaluation for other sexually transmitted diseases should be done by the family physician.

34. **How do you diagnose the other causes of chronic conjunctivitis?**
    1. **Toxic conjunctivitis** is common with many drops (see question 2 for offending agents). These patients may also have allergic dermatitis around the eyes. Treat with preservative-free artificial tears.
    2. **Parinaud's oculoglandular conjunctivitis** presents with a mucopurulent discharge and foreign-body sensation. Granulomatous nodules on the palpebral conjunctiva and swollen lymph nodes are necessary for the diagnosis. Fever and rash also may occur. The etiology includes cat-scratch disease (most common), tularemia (contact with rabbits or ticks), tuberculosis, and syphilis.
    3. **Trachoma** is seen in underprivileged countries with poor sanitation. It is also caused by chlamydial infection. Patients develop superior tarsal follicles and severe corneal pannus, which, if untreated, lead to significant dry eye, trichiasis, and scarring. Patients may become functionally blind. Diagnosis and treatment are the same as for chlamydial inclusion conjunctivitis.
    4. **Molluscum contagiosum** develops a chronic follicular conjunctivitis from a reaction to toxic viral products. On the lid or lid margin, multiple dome-shaped, umbilicated nodules are present. These lesions must be removed by excision, incision and curettage, or cryosurgery to resolve the conjunctivitis.
    5. **Dacryocystitis** is an inflammation of the lacrimal sac. Patients usually present with pain, erythema, and swelling over the inner aspect of the lower lid. They also may have a fever. However, a red eye may be the only sign. Pressure over the lacrimal sac may elicit discharge and a complaint of tenderness. Treatment is systemic antibiotics, warm compresses with massage over the inner canthus, and topical antibiotics. Watch patients closely because cellulitis can occasionally develop.

35. **A 40-year-old woman presents with a bright red eye that she noticed on awakening in the morning. On examination, she has a subconjunctival hemorrhage. What questions are important to ask?**
    You need to know whether this is her first episode. Does she have a history of easy bruising or poor clotting? Is she taking any medications or supplements that may increase bleeding time, such as warfarin, aspirin, vitamin E,

or garlic? Has she been rubbing her eye or had any injury to her eye? Has she done any heavy lifting or straining? Has she been sneezing or vomiting—anything that may cause a Valsalva maneuver?

36. **She answers no to the above questions and states that this is her first episode. Should she be worried?**
    No. Reassure her that the symptoms will resolve within 2 weeks. Artificial tears will make her more comfortable. Tell her to return if she has further episodes.

37. **With further thought, she remembers two other hemorrhages in her left eye and reports that her menses have been much heavier recently. What now?**
    At this point, referral to an internist for a complete blood count with differential, blood pressure check, prothrombin time, partial thromboplastin time, and bleeding time is appropriate.

38. **A 60-year-old woman complains that her eyes have been red and burning over the past several weeks. She also has some tearing and photophobia. On exam, you notice mild conjunctival injection and a slightly low tear meniscus. Should you think of anything else?**
    Make sure to elevate the upper eyelid. Superior limbic keratoconjunctivitis (Fig. 7.7) is a thickening and inflammation of the superior bulbar conjunctiva. Sometimes, a superior corneal micropannus, superior palpebral papillae, and corneal filaments can be found. Fifty percent of patients have associated dysthyroid disease. Artificial tears and ointments are all that are necessary for mild disease. Silver nitrate solution (*not* cautery sticks) may be applied to the superior tarsal and bulbar conjunctiva; mechanical scraping, cryotherapy, cautery, or surgical resection or recession of the superior bulbar conjunctiva may be necessary for more severe disease.

39. **A 22-year-old woman presents with mild redness in the temporal quadrant of her left eye for about 1 week. She notices no discomfort. On exam, she has normal vision. Large episcleral vessels beneath the conjunctiva are engorged in the area. They can be easily moved with a cotton swab, and no tenderness is present. The cornea and anterior chamber are clear. The sclera appears to be uninvolved. What is the diagnosis?**
    You must distinguish between episcleritis (Fig. 7.8) and scleritis. A drop of 2.5% phenylephrine blanches the episcleral vessels but leaves any injected vessels of the sclera untouched. Look for any discharge or conjunctival follicles and papillae to rule out conjunctivitis.

    Episcleritis is usually idiopathic. It may be diffuse or sectoral, unilateral or bilateral. Sometimes, a nodule may be seen. Rarely, it is associated with collagen-vascular disease, gout, herpes zoster or simplex, syphilis,

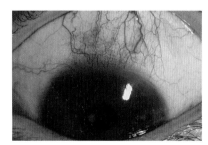

Fig. 7.7 Superior limbic keratoconjunctivitis. Slit lamp appearance of focal superior bulbar conjunctival injection is shown with rose bengal staining. (From Bouchard CS: Noninfectious keratitis. In Yanoff M, Duker JS, editors: *Ophthalmology*, ed 2, St. Louis, 2004, Mosby.)

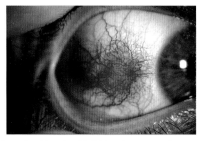

Fig. 7.8 A slightly tender and mobile elevated nodule with epithelial injection is typical for nodular episcleritis. (From Kanski JJ: *Clinical ophthalmology: a synopsis,* ed 5, New York, 2004, Butterworth-Heinemann.)

Lyme disease, rosacea, or atopy. Usually, artificial tears and/or a topical vasoconstrictor/antihistamine drop, such as naphazoline/pheniramine, will suffice. If the patient is unresponsive, a mild steroid drop should help. Rarely, oral NSAIDs are necessary. Warn the patient that episcleritis may recur.

40. The same patient returns 2 months later. Her left eye is still red, but it is now diffuse. She denies arthritis, rash, venereal disease, tick exposure, or other medical problems. She has been using a vasoconstrictor/antihistamine drop since her last visit. She began using it four times a day, then increased the frequency because her eye continued to be red unless she used it. She now applies drops every 1 to 2 hours. Does this make a difference?

Counsel patients not to use a vasoconstrictor for longer than 2 weeks and no more than four times a day. Just as patients can remain congested if using a vasoconstrictor nose spray frequently, vasoconstrictor eye drops can cause the eyes to stay red. She should stop the drop immediately. Her left eye will be very red for a time until the dependence resolves. Brimonidine tartrate 0.025% (Lumify) is now sold OTC as a topical drop for ocular redness and does not seem to have the same problems with rebound hyperemia. This would be a better choice for the patient once the source of the redness is diagnosed.

41. A 65-year-old woman with rheumatoid arthritis states that her left eye has been red and painful for a couple of weeks. The pain is severe and radiates to her forehead and jaw and has awakened her at night. It has worsened slowly. Her vision is decreasing. She thinks that she has had a similar condition before. On exam, the conjunctival, episcleral, and scleral vessels are injected temporally. The scleral vessels do not move, and the area is very tender. A scleral nodule is present. The sclera appears bluish in this area, adjacent to which is a peripheral keratitis with a mild anterior chamber reaction. The intraocular pressure is 24 mm Hg in the affected eye and 16 mm Hg in the unaffected eye. What may she have?

She may have nodular anterior scleritis (Fig. 7.9). The inflamed blood vessels are much deeper than those seen in conjunctivitis or episcleritis and do not blanch with 2.5% phenylephrine. In addition, the cornea and anterior chamber are involved. The deep, boring pain is typical with scleritis.

42. How else may scleritis present?
- Diffuse anterior scleritis.
- Necrotizing anterior scleritis with inflammation. The pain is severe, and the choroid is visible through the transparent sclera. The mortality rate is high owing to systemic disease.
- Necrotizing anterior scleritis without inflammation (scleromalacia perforans; Fig. 7.10). Such patients have almost a complete lack of symptoms, and most have rheumatoid arthritis.

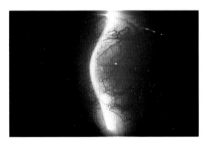

Fig. 7.9 Nodular scleritis is painful with a nonmobile nodule associated with swelling of the episclera and sclera. (From Kanski JJ: *Clinical ophthalmology: a synopsis*, ed 5, New York, 2004, Butterworth-Heinemann.)

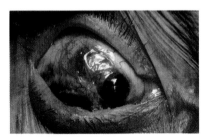

Fig. 7.10 Scleromalacia perforans is a noninflammatory form of necrotizing scleritis. (From Kanski JJ: *Clinical ophthalmology: a test yourself atlas*, ed 2, New York, 2002, Butterworth-Heinemann.)

- Posterior scleritis. It may mimic an amelanotic choroidal mass. An exudative retinal detachment, retinal hemorrhages, choroidal folds, and/or choroidal detachments may be seen. Restricted extraocular movements, proptosis, pain, and tenderness may also occur. Rarely is it related to a systemic disease.

43. **What percentage of patients with scleritis have systemic disease? What diseases are associated with scleritis?**
Fifty percent of patients with scleritis have systemic disease. The connective tissue diseases, such as rheumatoid arthritis, ankylosing spondylitis, systemic lupus erythematosus, polyarteritis nodosa, and Wegener's granulomatosis, are common associations. Herpes zoster ophthalmicus, Lyme disease, syphilis, and gout also may cause scleritis. Less frequently, scleritis may be associated with tuberculosis, sarcoidosis, or a foreign body.

44. **What workup is appropriate for a patient with scleritis?**
Any avascular areas of the scleritis must be identified. The red-free filter on the slit lamp is helpful for this purpose. The thinner the sclera, the more severe the disease. The risk of a melt is much higher. A dilated exam is necessary to check for posterior segment involvement. Patients should be referred to an internist or a rheumatologist for a complete physical exam; complete blood count; erythrocyte sedimentation rate; uric acid level; rapid plasma reagin test; fluorescent treponemal antibody, absorbed test; Lyme titer; rheumatoid factor; antinuclear antibody tests; fasting blood sugar; angiotensin-converting enzyme; CH50; C3; C4; and serum antineutrophilic cytoplasmic antibody. If history or symptoms warrant, a purified protein derivative test with anergy panel, a chest radiograph, sacroiliac radiograph, and/or B-scan ultrasonography to detect posterior scleritis should be ordered.

45. **How should you treat the patient?**
An oral NSAID, such as ibuprofen, 400 to 600 mg four times a day, or indomethacin, 25 mg three times a day, coupled with an antacid or H_2 blocker such as ranitidine is a good initial choice. If the patient is nonresponsive, oral steroids are the next step. In diseases such as systemic vasculitis, polyarteritis nodosa, and Wegener's granulomatosis, an immunosuppressive agent such as cyclophosphamide, methotrexate, cyclosporine, or azathioprine may be necessary. They may be used in combination. Biologics such as the antitumor necrosis factor agents infliximab (Remicade) and adalimumab (Humira) are showing promise in some patients. Decreased pain is an indication of successful treatment, although the clinical picture may not show a significant difference for a while.
Scleromalacia perforans does not have an ocular treatment except for lubrication. Patch grafts are used if perforation is a significant risk. Immunosuppression for the underlying systemic disease may be needed. A rheumatologic consult is appropriate to help with treatment with systemic biologics.

46. **What about topical steroids or a subconjunctival steroid injection?**
Topical steroids are not usually effective. Subconjunctival steroids are contraindicated because they may lead to scleral thinning and perforation.

47. **A 35-year-old man presents with severe photophobia, pain, and decreased vision in his right eye for 2 days. This condition has occurred several times before. He says that drops have helped. On examination, his vision is 20/50 in the right eye and 20/20 in the left eye. His pupil is poorly reactive on the right and miotic. The left eye is normal, and no afferent pupillary defect is present. The right eye is diffusely injected, especially around the limbus. The anterior chamber is deep, but 2+ cell and flare are present with a few fine keratic precipitates. The left eye is clear. The right eye has an intraocular pressure of 5 mm Hg; the left is 15 mm Hg. Dilated exam is normal. What are the diagnosis and treatment?**
The diagnosis is acute, nongranulomatous anterior uveitis. A cycloplegic drop such as cyclopentolate, 1% to 2% three times a day, for mild inflammation, and scopolamine 0.25% or atropine 1% three times a day for more severe inflammation will relax the ciliary spasm, making the patient more comfortable as well as preventing formation of synechiae in the angle and on the pupillary margin. Formation of synechiae increases the long-term risk of angle-closure glaucoma. A steroid drop every 1 to 6 hours, depending on the severity of the anterior chamber inflammation, is started. If no response occurs, a sub-Tenon's injection or oral steroids may be necessary. Rarely, systemic immunosuppressive agents are necessary.

48. **A 68-year-old Asian American woman presents with an acutely painful red left eye that developed after a recent anxiety attack. She has blurred vision and sees halos around lights. She has vomited twice. On exam, she has a fixed, middilated pupil and conjunctival injection. The cornea is cloudy. What are you concerned about?**
She may have acute angle-closure glaucoma. When the pressure rises quickly in the eye, severe pain and nausea with decreased vision develop. Asian Americans are at increased risk because of their shallow anterior chambers. Examination of the angle of the affected eye may be facilitated by glycerin to clear the corneal edema. If the shallow angle cannot be visualized, the other eye may reveal a narrow angle. For further information about diagnosis and treatment, see Chapter 16.

KEY POINTS: DISEASES THAT MAY MIMIC UVEITIS

1. Rhegmatogenous retinal detachment
2. Posterior segment tumors and lymphoma
3. Intraocular foreign body
4. Endophthalmitis

BIBLIOGRAPHY

American Academy of Ophthalmology: http://one.aao.org/preferred-practice-pattern/blepharitis-ppp-2013.

Foulks GN, Nichols KK, Bron AJ, et al.: Improving awareness, identification, and management of meibomian gland dysfunction, Ophthalmology 119(10):S1–S12, 2012.

Gerstenblith AT, Rabinowitz MP: Wills eye manual: office and emergency room diagnosis and treatment of eye disease, ed 6, Philadelphia, 2012, Lippincott Williams & Wilkins.

Herpetic Eye Disease Study Group: Acyclovir for prevention of recurrent herpes simplex virus eye disease, N Engl J Med 339:300–306, 1998.

Herpetic Eyes Disease Study Group: Oral acyclovir for herpes simplex virus eye disease: effect on prevention of epithelial keratitis and stromal keratitis, Arch Ophthalmol 118:1030–1036, 2000.

Langston DP: Oral acyclovir suppresses recurrent epithelial and stromal herpes simplex, Arch Ophthalmol 117:391–392, 1999.

Lin JC, Rapuano CJ, Laibson PR, et al.: Corneal melting associated with use of topical nonsteroidal anti-inflammatory drugs after ocular surgery, Arch Ophthalmol 118:1129–1132, 2000.

Lin JC, Sheha H, Tseng SCG: Pathogenic role of demodex mites in blepharitis, Curr Opin Allergy Clin Immunol 10(5):505–510, 2010.

PDR for ophthalmic medicines, ed 40, 2012, PDR Network.

Riordan-Eva P, Cunningham ET: Vaughn & Asbury's general ophthalmology, ed 18, New York, NY, 2011, McGraw Hill.

Tasman W, Jaeger EA: Wills Eye Hospital atlas of clinical ophthalmology, ed 2, Philadelphia, 2001, Lippincott Williams & Wilkins.

CHAPTER 8

CORNEAL INFECTIONS

Paramjit Bhullar, Nandini Venkateswaran, Alan N. Carlson, and Terry Kim

CORNEAL ULCERS

1. What is a corneal ulcer?
   The term *corneal ulcer* is used to describe an epithelial defect, stromal loss, stromal infiltrate, or any combination of these changes.

2. What clinical features distinguish an infectious corneal ulcer from a sterile corneal ulcer?
   Infectious corneal ulcers are caused by microorganisms such as bacteria, viruses, fungi, or parasites. Sterile corneal ulcers are not caused by microorganisms and can be due to several disease states such as severe dry eye disease, exposure keratopathy (e.g., from a prior cerebral stroke, facial nerve palsy or eyelid surgery), neurotrophic keratopathy (e.g., from previous corneal herpetic infections), autoimmune disorders (e.g., rheumatoid arthritis or Sjogren's syndrome), and secondary immunologic responses elicited by staphylococcal hypersensitivity or from corneal hypoxia (e.g., from extended contact lens wear).

   When evaluating symptomatology, infectious corneal ulcers are typically associated with rapid onset of pain accompanied by conjunctival injection, photophobia, and decreased vision, whereas sterile corneal ulcers are typically associated with a slow decline in vision but often with less significant pain, injection, or photophobia.

   On exam, infectious corneal ulcers typically have a visible corneal infiltrate with surrounding corneal edema. If the corneal inflammation is severe, there may also be associated anterior chamber cell and flare, keratic precipitates, and/or a hypopyon (Fig. 8.1). Bacterial corneal ulcers may also be associated with mucopurulent discharge. Some infectious causes of corneal ulcers may be caused by slow-growing organisms, such as anaerobes or mycobacteria; such infectious corneal ulcers may present with a nonsuppurative infiltrate and intact epithelium. In contrast, sterile corneal ulcers often present with mild conjunctival injection and anterior chamber reaction, minimal or absent corneal infiltrates, and/or an epithelial defect (Fig. 8.2).

3. What conditions predispose to corneal infections?
   Any condition that disrupts the corneal epithelial integrity can increase the likelihood of developing a corneal infection, including:
   - Contact lens wear (number one risk factor, associated with at least 30% of microbial keratitis cases seen in the emergency department setting and responsible for 19%–42% of cases overall). Sleeping while wearing soft contact lenses (extended wear) on a regular or even intermittent pattern of wear can increase the risk of developing microbial keratitis by 8–15-fold.
   - Trauma (e.g., corneal abrasions, exposure to a foreign body)
   - Structural eyelid abnormalities (e.g., ectropion/entropion, trichiasis, lagophthalmos)
   - Dry eye disease
   - Chronic epithelial disease (e.g., recurrent erosions, bullous keratopathy)
   - Topical medication toxicity (e.g., topical glaucoma medications, any eye drops with preservatives)
   - Local or systemic immunosuppression (e.g., oral steroid use, diabetes mellitus, human immunodeficiency virus)
   - Contaminated ocular medications

4. How can a contact lens wearer reduce the risk of infection?
   Contact lens wearers are at 10 times higher risk of developing a corneal ulcer as compared to their non–contact lens wearing counterparts. Contact lens wearers can reduce their risk of infection by practicing good contact lens hygiene. This includes never sleeping in contacts (including those that are approved for "extended wear"), changing contact lenses according to the manufacturers' instructions (the risk of infection is positively correlated with the number of consecutive days a contact lens is worn), properly disinfecting contact lenses prior to reinsertion, using fresh contact lens solution daily, and thoroughly cleaning contact lens cases. Patients should be aware that disposable contact lenses are no safer than conventional contact lenses and that lenses with higher oxygen permeability ("high DK" lenses) also increase the risk of developing a corneal infection.[1–3]

5. Describe the classic presentations and associations of various types of corneal infections (e.g., bacterial, viral, fungal).
   - History of trauma with any vegetable matter: Fungal keratitis
   - Oral and eyelid vesicles or repeated problems in only one eye: Herpetic keratitis
   - Contact lens wear: *Pseudomonas* or *Acanthamoeba* infections
   - Gram-positive organisms: Focal, discrete infiltrate

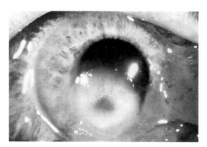

Fig. 8.1 Central pseudomonal corneal ulcer.

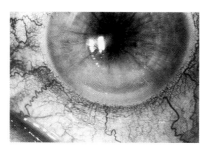

Fig. 8.2 Sterile corneal ulcer caused by rheumatoid arthritis.

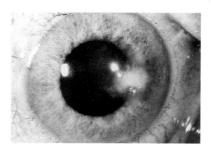

Fig. 8.3 Infectious ulcer caused by filamentous fungus. Note the indistinct, feathery borders.

- Gram-negative organisms: Spreading, diffuse infiltrate
- *Pseudomonas* infections: Suppurative infection, stromal necrosis, anterior chamber reaction with hypopyon
- Herpes simplex keratitis: Epithelial dendrite, stromal keratitis
- *Acanthamoeba* keratitis: pain out of proportion to exam, radial perineuritis, ring infiltrate late in the clinical course
- Infectious crystalline keratopathy: dense white, branching infiltrate with minimal inflammatory response (due to α-hemolytic *Streptococcus* species), particularly in a corneal graft or neurotrophic cornea
- Fungal keratitis: Feathery, irregular borders with satellite lesions (Fig. 8.3)

6. **When should corneal smears and cultures be performed?**
   Corneal smears and cultures should be obtained for most corneal ulcers suspected to be infectious, as studies show that clinical appearance alone is unreliable in determining the causative pathogen. Small, peripheral corneal infiltrates (less than 1 mm in diameter) do not have to undergo a smear and culture prior to the initiation of intensive empiric broad-spectrum topical antibiotic therapy. However, the American Academy of Ophthalmology practice guidelines recommend that initial cultures be obtained for infiltrates extending to the apex of the cornea, into the deep stroma, or across a large area (>2 mm), as well as for patients whose history or exam suggests a fungal, amoebic, mycobacterial, or drug-resistant etiology.

Table 8.1 Smears and Cultures for Infectious Keratitis	
Routine Tests	**Tests For**
Gram stain (smear)	Bacteria
KOH or Giemsa stain (smear)	Fungi/yeasts
Sabaroud's dextrose agar culture plate (without cycloheximide)	Fungi
Chocolate agar culture plate	*Hemophilus* and *Neisseria* species
Thioglycolate culture broth	Aerobic and anaerobic bacteria
Optional Tests (As Needed Based On Clinical Suspicion)	**Tests For**
Gomori methenamine silver stain (smear)	*Acanthamoeba*, fungi
Acid fast stain (smear)	Mycobacteria
Calcoflour white stain (smear)	*Acanthamoeba*, fungi
Löwenstein-Jensen agar culture plate	Mycobacteria, *Nocardia* spp.
Nonnutrient agar culture plate with *Escherichia coli* overlay	*Acanthamoeba*
HSV PCR	HSV

HSV, Herpes simplex virus; *PCR*, polymerase chain reaction.

Repeat smears and cultures should be obtained for ulcers that are unresponsive to first-line antimicrobial therapy; in these cases, it is helpful to provide the laboratory with documentation of the therapies attempted thus far. In addition, a 48-hour drug holiday can be conducted prior to obtaining repeat cultures to increase the chance of isolating a causative organism.[4]

7. What smears and cultures should be obtained? What culture plates should be used?
   See Table 8.1.

8. How should corneal smears and cultures be performed?
   Corneal smears and cultures should be performed at the slit lamp after the patient has been given topical anesthetic drops. Corneal scrapings should be obtained using a sterile Kimura spatula that is resterilized over a flame between each scraping or with sterile calcium alginate swabs, using a new swab for each scraping. A sterile needle or surgical blade can also be used. Separate slides should be used for each smear (e.g., Gram stain and potassium hydroxide [KOH] stain). Separate plates should be used for each culture and for Giemsa or calcfluor white stains.
   For viral cultures, Dacron swabs can be used to obtain viral-infected cells from the cornea or conjunctiva. Calcium alginate and cotton swabs should be avoided when obtaining viral cultures, as both can inhibit viral growth.
   Scrapings should be obtained from the margins of the ulcer, as that is the most active region and most likely to provide a good yield of microorganisms.

9. What is the diagnostic yield for smears and cultures performed prior to the initiation of therapy?
   Although Gram stain smears may provide early insight into the causative organism, they may be negative (with a highly variable positivity range of 0%–57%). Cultures grow organisms in approximately 50%–75% of suspected infectious ulcers. The yield for corneal smears and cultures is significantly higher prior to the initiation of antibiotic treatment.

10. How should the smear and culture results be used to modify treatment?
    Smears may provide a quick means of telling the clinician the general type of infection (e.g., bacterial, fungal, *Acanthamoeba*); however, smears have a poor correlation with culture results, often due to contamination. Begin broad-spectrum topical antibiotics should and continue until culture results are available, though the results of smears may help clinicians weigh therapy toward particular medications (e.g., in cases of a suspected fungal keratitis).
    Culture results identify the organism, help to target therapy, and eliminate extraneous medication, which can foster drug resistance. Sensitivities can be useful for guiding treatment but must be interpreted with caution as they are based on drug levels attainable in the serum and not on drug concentrations in the cornea. Corneal drug concentrations are much higher due to the direct topical administration; thus, antibiotics considered "resistant" can still be clinically effective in the cornea.

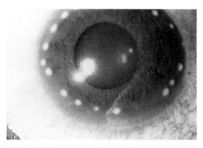

Fig. 8.4 Small peripheral infiltrates caused by a sterile reaction to contact lens solution.

11. **What is the recommended initial therapy for suspected infectious ulcers? How does one determine whether single-agent, broad-spectrum antibiotics, or combination fortified antibiotics should be used?**

    In general, initial therapy for corneal ulcers must cover a broad range of gram-positive and gram-negative bacteria and must be administered frequently (every 15–30 minutes). Previous multicenter studies have provided evidence that topical monotherapy with fluoroquinolones may be as effective as polytherapy with fortified antibiotics in many cases. It is our practice to treat small, peripheral ulcers with a single, fourth-generation fluoroquinolone antibiotic, such as gatifloxacin, moxifloxacin, or besifloxacin, which has shown improved coverage of gram-positive organisms like streptococcal and staphylococcal species. We reserve combination fortified antibiotics for more severe, sight-threatening infections. For ulcers that are >1 mm or sight-threatening, it is recommended to start initial broad-spectrum therapy with combination fortified antibiotics. Once culture results are available, therapy should be tailored to the offending microorganism.[5,6]

12. **What is the appropriate therapy for small peripheral infiltrates in a contact lens wearer?**

    Patients with infiltrates should immediately discontinue all contact lens wear and throw out the lens and contact lens case. Small infiltrates in a contact lens wearer may be sterile or infectious. Sterile infiltrates are usually peripheral and subepithelial in location, with an intact overlying epithelium. Patients often have minimal pain (Fig. 8.4). When in doubt of the etiology, however, it is best to presume infection.

    One can forego scraping and treat presumed infectious infiltrates frequently with a loading dose of a single broad-spectrum antibiotic (i.e., gatifloxacin, moxifloxacin, or besifloxacin every 30–60 minutes) and then an antibiotic ointment (i.e., ciprofloxacin) at bedtime. Patients should be followed closely and undergo scraping if the epithelial defect and infiltrate do not improve with treatment.

13. **Other than antibiotics, what adjunctive therapy may be necessary in the treatment of corneal ulcers?**

    Topical cycloplegic agents help relieve photophobia and pain from ciliary spasm and prevent the formation of posterior synechiae.

    Severe anterior chamber inflammation may cause the intraocular pressure to increase, often necessitating the use of ocular antihypertensive medications. Pilocarpine should be avoided as it can cause breakdown of the blood–aqueous barrier and lead to a subsequent increase in anterior chamber inflammation. In the case of impending or frank perforated corneal ulcer, cyanoacrylate tissue glue can be useful to temporarily, and sometimes permanently, seal the open wound. Cyanoacrylate is also thought to have bactericidal properties, which can aid in the treatment of infection in these cases.

    The role of topical corticosteroids in the management of bacterial keratitis is controversial, but these may be used as well (see later).

14. **What is the role of topical corticosteroids in the treatment of corneal ulcers?**

    The role of topical corticosteroids as an adjunctive therapy for corneal ulcers is controversial. In the Steroids for Corneal Ulcers Trial (SCUT), no significant benefit was seen with the use of corticosteroids as an adjunct to antimicrobial therapy for bacterial ulcers, as measured by 3-month best corrected visual acuity, infiltrate or scar size, time to reepithelialization, or corneal perforation, when compared to placebo. However, prespecified subanalyses suggested that patients with more severe ulcers (characterized as baseline best corrected visual acuity of counting fingers or worse, central ulcers covering the 4 mm pupil, or deep infiltrates) benefitted from the addition of corticosteroids, with significant improvements in logMAR visual acuity. In addition, ulcers caused by *Nocardia* species showed worse clinical outcomes with adjunctive corticosteroid use than ulcers caused by other bacterial organisms.

    Some clinicians advocate that corticosteroids help to reduce inflammation and decrease corneal scarring, whereas others fear that corticosteroids predispose to poor epithelialization, recurrent infection, progressive thinning and ultimately corneal perforation. As such, corticosteroids should not be used in the initial treatment of

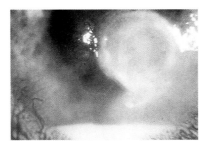

Fig. 8.5 Hypopyon associated with infectious corneal ulcer.

corneal ulcers but can be used in conjunction with antibiotics with caution only after a bacterial etiology has been confirmed and clinical improvement has been demonstrated with appropriate antibiotics.[7,8]

15. How does the presence of a hypopyon affect the management of infectious keratitis?
The presence of a hypopyon (Fig. 8.5) is indicative of corneal inflammation severe enough to cause a marked anterior chamber response. Therefore, the treatment should be aggressive, including administration of combined fortified antibiotics in most cases. For the most part, hypopyons associated with infectious corneal ulcers are sterile and do not require evaluation and treatment for endophthalmitis.

16. When should an anterior chamber and/or vitreous tap be performed?
Whenever endophthalmitis is suspected. Endophthalmitis must be considered when there is severe inflammation after intraocular surgery or perforating trauma, especially when vitreous inflammatory cells are present. Once diagnosed, topical antibiotics are inadequate and oral/intravenous antibiotics are unnecessary; antibiotics must be injected directly into the vitreous cavity after taking samples for culture (with vitrectomy indicated in severe cases). Endophthalmitis secondary to infectious keratitis in the absence of perforation is uncommon, and a sterile inflammatory response in the vitreous may be present that resolves with the clearing of the corneal infection. Fungal keratitis has a greater propensity to penetrate Descemet's membrane and gain access to the anterior chamber.

17. When should patients with corneal ulcers be hospitalized?
- If the patient lacks the ability or support to administer drops as frequently as every 30 minutes around-the-clock
- If the patient lives too far away to be followed on a daily and consistent basis
- Any condition requiring intravenous antibiotics or possible surgery (e.g., *Neisseria* infections involving the cornea and perforated corneal ulcers)

18. When are systemic medications indicated?
Systemic antibiotics are seldom indicated in bacterial corneal ulcers. However, oral and/or intravenous antibiotics are used with impending or progressive scleral involvement. Parenteral antibiotics play an important role in the treatment of aggressive infections from *Neisseria* and *Hemophilus* species with corneal involvement and imminent perforation.
Systemic antifungal agents are used in some cases of fungal keratitis where the infiltrate involves the deep corneal stroma or in cases that worsen on topical therapy alone.
Oral acyclovir is the primary mode of therapy for patients with ocular herpes zoster and is also used by some physicians to treat primary herpes simplex infection.

19. How should impending and frank corneal perforations be managed?
Corneal infections can be associated with corneal perforation, and the thinning of the cornea can be secondary to both active infection as well as robust associated inflammation. One study showed that having an outdoor occupation, exposure to vegetative matter with trauma, a central location of corneal ulcer, monotherapy with fluoroquinolones, lack of corneal neovascularization, as well as delay in starting management with antimicrobial therapy in infectious keratitis can lead to an increased risk of corneal perforation. In this study, *Staphylococcus epidermidis* was the most commonly isolated organism in cases of perforated corneal ulcers.
Any corneal infection associated with marked thinning or perforation (Fig. 8.6) should be protected with an eye shield without a patch. When the cornea becomes thinned to the point of imminent or existent corneal perforation, certain steps need to be taken. If the affected area is small, cyanoacrylate glue can be used to help seal the defect. However, most cases of perforation will eventually need a corneal patch graft and/or corneal transplantation to seal the eye, prevent intraocular spread of the infection, and attempt to salvage visual potential.[9]

20. What steps should be taken when a corneal ulcer does not respond to empirical therapy?
First, assess compliance with therapy. If compliance is suboptimal, consider hospitalization. If compliance is good, reevaluate the antimicrobial agent being used. Scrutinize the antimicrobial choice against the results of the corneal culture; perform an initial culture and repeat the corneal culture if needed. If the patient is being treated

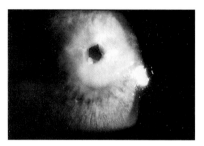

Fig. 8.6 Perforated corneal ulcer.

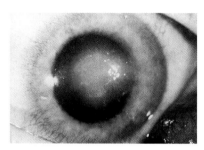

Fig. 8.7 Central *Acanthamoeba* ulcer.

empirically with a fluoroquinolone, escalate therapy to fortified antibiotics. If broad-spectrum antibiotics were used but unsuccessful, consider the possibility of atypical bacteria, viruses, or fungi. Antibiotics themselves may cause toxicity, impairing corneal healing and should be tapered in frequency or used in combination with other medications to help rehabilitate the ocular surface. Consider topical anesthetic abuse. Finally, consider the utility of topical corticosteroids in confirmed cases of bacterial keratitis (with the exception of *Nocardia* species), as they may be associated with improved clinical outcomes in more severe ulcers, as suggested by the SCUT trial.

21. **When should a corneal biopsy be considered?**
Whenever an ulcer is failing intensive antibiotic therapy and multiple cultures have been negative. *Acanthamoeba* (Fig. 8.7) is particularly difficult to grow in culture, and the infection may extend deep in the cornea. If this organism is suspected, a corneal biopsy is the best opportunity to identify cysts (more commonly) or trophozoites in the affected tissue. A single-use, sterile, dermatologic punch of a prespecified diameter (typically 2 or 3 mm) can be used to partially dissect the cornea in the location of the infiltrate; the section of corneal material can be carefully dissected with a sterile blade. The biopsy can be sectioned and subsequently plated on culture media. In rare circumstances, a femtosecond laser can also be used to safely obtain a corneal biopsy.

In cases with an intact epithelium, such as a deep fungal keratitis, where the infiltrate is not accessible by scraping, a 6-0, 7-0, or 8-0 silk suture can be passed through the cornea at the level of the infiltrate. The suture can then be removed, cut into pieces, and placed directly on culture media.

Corneal biopsies can significantly contribute to the diagnosis and management of infectious keratitis due to unknown etiology. In one study, a microorganism was successfully isolated in 82% of corneal biopsies conducted for infectious keratitis; these biopsies ultimately led to a change in antimicrobial therapy in 89% of patients.[10]

22. **What are the important immediate and delayed sequelae of corneal ulcers?**
The immediate concern with corneal ulcers is progressive thinning and perforation. Management and prognosis change considerably with perforation, and the concern for intraocular infection (i.e., endophthalmitis) rises dramatically. Perforated corneal ulcers can result in the loss of the eye. The delayed sequelae of corneal ulcers deal mainly with corneal scarring, which can severely limit visual acuity and function.

KEY POINTS: CORNEAL ULCERS

1. A corneal ulcer should be considered infectious until proven otherwise.
2. It is never wrong to culture an ulcer.
3. Some small, peripheral ulcers can be treated empirically and closely followed.
4. Any ulcer not responding to therapy should be recultured or biopsied and therapy should be escalated. Reconsider the differential.

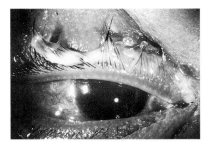

Fig. 8.8 Gonococcal conjunctivitis with marked conjunctival injection and copious mucopurulent discharge on the eyelid margins.

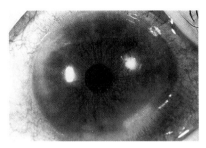

Fig. 8.9 Staphylococcal hypersensitivity infiltrate located in the inferior peripheral cornea. Note its marginal location and clear separation from the limbus.

BACTERIAL KERATITIS

23. What are the most common organisms that cause bacterial keratitis?

Staphylococcus aureus, Staphylococcus epidermidis, Streptococcus pneumonia and other Streptococcus spp., Pseudomonas aeruginosa (most common organism in soft contact lens wearers), and Enterobacteriaceae (Proteus spp., Enterobacter spp., and Serratia spp.).

24. When should a gonococcal infection be suspected? What additional workup and treatment should be initiated?

A gonococcal infection should be suspected when an acute onset of marked conjunctival injection is associated with severe mucopurulent discharge, marked chemosis, and preauricular adenopathy (Fig. 8.8). Corneal infiltrates can progress rapidly and perforate within 48 hours. Workup should include conjunctival scrapings for immediate Gram stain and culture using chocolate agar media. Treatment should include frequent irrigation with saline, a 1 g intramuscular dose of ceftriaxone, and frequent topical fluoroquinolone drops. If the cornea is involved or if compliance is problematic, the patient should be hospitalized for parenteral ceftriaxone therapy and be followed closely. Infants should be hospitalized for evaluation of disseminated Neisseria gonorrhea infection.

In patients with gonococcal keratitis, urethral symptoms most often precede ocular symptoms by several weeks. It is important to advise these patients be screened for other sexually transmitted diseases, especially Chlamydia.[11]

25. How are staphylococcal hypersensitivity infiltrates diagnosed and managed?

Staphylococcal marginal keratitis is usually a bilateral condition that involves the peripheral, inferior cornea adjacent to the limbus. Corneal infiltrates are separated from the limbus by a clear area (Fig. 8.9), may be observed in multiples, stain minimally or not at all with fluorescein, and are not associated with anterior chamber inflammation. They accompany staphylococcal blepharitis and meibomitis and represent an immunologic reaction to staphylococcal antigens. Some patients with staphylococcal marginal keratitis may also have comorbid acne rosacea. Mild cases of staphylococcal hypersensitivity should be treated with lid hygiene and antibiotic ointments. In more severe cases, combined antibiotic-steroid drops or ointments can be added. If concerned about an infectious etiology, treat the infiltrate(s) initially with intensive antibiotics. Contact lenses should be discontinued until the eye is fully cleared.[12]

HERPETIC KERATITIS

26. Why do herpetic infections occur?

Herpes simplex virus (HSV) keratitis is usually caused by the type 1 virus, often spread by physical contact with an oral "cold sore." The type 2 virus can cause a neonatal ocular infection after a newborn passes through an

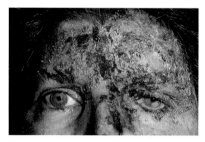

Fig. 8.10 Herpes zoster ophthalmicus with crusting and ulceration of skin innervated by the first division of the trigeminal nerve. (From Kanski JJ: Clinical ophthalmology: a synopsis, New York, 2004, Butterworth-Heinemann.)

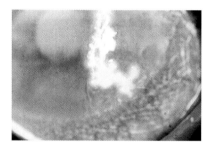

Fig. 8.11 Classic herpes simplex dendrite staining brightly with fluorescein.

infected birth canal. HSV is often associated with follicular conjunctivitis, corneal dendritic ulcers, cutaneous vesicles, and preauricular adenopathy. HSV keratitis frequently occurs without a history of oral involvement. Immunoglobulin G (IgG) for HSV is commonly positive in adults, so serologic investigation is seldom helpful, except when negative, ruling out the infection.

Herpes zoster ophthalmicus (shingles of the eye) represents reactivation of the varicella zoster virus (VZV) in the first division of cranial nerve V (Fig. 8.10). Nerve damage in a dermatomal distribution may lead to severe and chronic pain. Associated keratitis, uveitis, and glaucoma may be severe, chronic, and difficult to treat.

27. **Why is herpes a recurrent disease?**
    After primary contact with the herpes virus (HSV or VZV), the virus gains access to the central nervous system. The virus becomes latent in the trigeminal ganglia (HSV type 1 or VZV) or in the spinal ganglia (HSV type 2). Recurrent attacks occur when the virus travels peripherally via sensory nerves to infect target tissues such as the eye. These attacks may be triggered by any of the following stressors: fever, ultraviolet light exposure, trauma, stress, menses, and immunosuppression. The most impressive example of this pathway of recrudescence is the dermatomal involvement of the zoster virus.

28. **List some nonocular signs suggestive of a herpetic corneal infection.**
    Some nonspecific signs of primary herpetic corneal infection include fever, malaise, and lymphadenopathy (especially preauricular adenopathy on the involved side). The vesicular skin rash of herpes zoster infections characteristically involves the dermatome of the first division of cranial nerve (CN) V on one side, does not cross the midline, and progresses to scarring. The presence of this rash on the tip of the nose (referred to as Hutchinson's sign) suggests a greater likelihood for ocular involvement, because both areas are innervated by the nasociliary nerve, a branch of CN V_1. A lack of Hutchinson's sign should not be used to exclude ocular involvement. Patients with herpes simplex can present with vesicular lesions in the perioral and periocular region that resolve without scarring.

29. **Are there differences between corneal infections caused by herpes simplex and herpes zoster viruses?**
    Although corneal infections from herpes simplex and herpes zoster can present in a similar clinical fashion, there are subtle features that can help differentiate between the two. Herpes simplex keratitis is an episodic condition, whereas herpes zoster ophthalmicus results in chronic disease. Both conditions are associated with corneal dendrites. However, the dendrites due to HSV stain brightly with vital dye and fluorescein and have terminal bulbs (Fig. 8.11), while dendrites due to VZV display negative staining (due to the lesions being deep in the cornea and causing epithelial elevation) and lack terminal bulbs.

Herpetic infections can also produce iris atrophy, and the pattern of iris atrophy can often distinguish herpes simplex from herpes zoster infection. With HSV, the iris displays patchy atrophy, whereas with VZV, the iris displays sectoral atrophy.

30. What are the noninfectious manifestations of a herpetic keratitis?

Some ophthalmic findings of herpetic keratitis are not directly caused by the viral infection itself but instead relate to the immunologic response to the infection. Examples of this phenomenon include chronic keratouveitis (where large keratic precipitates are associated with corneal edema), as well as disciform and necrotizing keratitis (in which stromal infiltration with leukocytes and neovascularization can occur with an intact epithelium).

Corneal scarring and neurotrophic ulcers are signs of previous herpetic keratitis that can be visually debilitating and potentially necessitate surgical intervention with penetrating keratoplasty or tarsorrhaphy.

31. How should herpetic infections be treated?

Based on safety, efficacy, and tolerability, ganciclovir 0.15% (Zirgan) gel is considered a frontline topical drug in the treatment of dendritic HSV epithelial keratitis. The recommended dosing is one drop five times per day (i.e., approximately every 3 hours while awake) until the corneal ulcer heals, then one drop three times a day for an additional 7 days. The medication appears most effective when used early in the course of the infection. An alternative treatment is topical trifluridine 1% (Viroptic) drops, which is administered every 2 hours while awake until the corneal ulcer has completely reepithelialized. Ganciciclovir gel poses less toxicity and requires a simpler dosing regimen than trifluridine. Zovirax ointment can also be added for skin involvement but cannot be used in or near the eye. Disciform stromal keratitis should be managed with topical corticosteroids and prophylactic antiviral agents.

All VZV infections, regardless of ocular involvement, are treated primarily with oral acyclovir (800 mg PO five times/day for 7–10 days) or with oral valacyclovir (1 gm PO three times a day for 7–10 days). Skin lesions should receive antibiotic ointment and warm compresses. Topical medications should be added as needed according to other ocular involvement (e.g., conjunctivitis, uveitis, glaucoma).[13]

32. What is the role of topical corticosteroids in herpes simplex keratitis?

Although topical corticosteroids are contraindicated in the presence of active epithelial disease, such as in dendritic keratitis, they are useful in treating herpes simplex stromal keratitis with an intact epithelium. Prophylactic antivirals are necessary when patients with a history of herpes simplex keratitis are given topical steroids to prevent an outbreak. The Herpetic Eye Disease Study showed that topical steroids and prophylactic antivirals are safe and effective in the treatment of stromal keratitis.[14]

33. When should oral acyclovir be used in herpes simplex keratitis?

The Herpetic Eye Disease Study reported:

- Oral acyclovir (400 mg orally twice daily for 1 year) reduced the recurrence of ocular HSV in patients who had one or more recurrent episodes.
- Oral acyclovir (400 mg orally five times a day for 10 weeks) may be helpful for treating HSV iridocyclitis, but the results did not reach statistical significance.
- Oral acyclovir did not benefit patients with active stromal keratitis and did not prevent the development of stromal keratitis or uveitis in patients with active epithelial disease.
- Acyclovir is contraindicated during pregnancy and in patients with renal disease.[15]

KEY POINTS: HERPETIC KERATITIS

1. HSV typically causes episodic epithelial keratitis.
2. VZV causes a dermatomal rash and chronic ulcers and pain.
3. Polymerase chain reaction (PCR) is preferred over culture for HSV and HZV diagnosis.
4. Topical ganciclovir gel or trifluridine should be used for epithelial HSV keratitis.
5. Topical corticosteroids can be useful in the treatment of HSV stromal keratitis but are contraindicated in the setting of acute epithelial disease.
6. All patients with VZV eye disease should receive oral acyclovir.
7. Oral acyclovir is beneficial only in certain types of HSV eye disease, notably recurrent HSV epithelial keratitis.

REFRACTIVE SURGERY–ASSOCIATED KERATITIS

34. Are corneal infections common after refractive surgical procedures such as laser in situ keratomileusis and photorefractive keratectomy?

Corneal infection is a potentially vision-threatening complication after refractive surgery. The incidence of infectious keratitis after refractive surgery has varied widely in studies, from approximately 1 in 1000 to 1 in 5000. In January 2008, the ASCRS Cornea Clinical Committee sent a survey to 9121 international ASCRS members and determined an incidence of one infection in every 1102 procedures. Forty-two percent involved

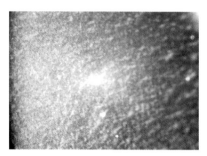

Fig. 8.12 Advanced case of diffuse lamellar keratitis.

laser in situ keratomileusis (LASIK) performed with a microkeratome, 10.5% involved LASIK performed with a femtosecond laser, and 42% involved surface ablation. The time of presentation ranged from 1 week to more than 1 month. The most common organisms cultured were methicillin-resistant staphylococci (MRSA) (28%) and non-methicillin-resistant staphylococci.[16]

35. **What other conditions can be mistaken for a corneal infection after LASIK?**
Although a microbial infection should always be considered, the more common condition that manifests with an infiltrate under the LASIK flap is diffuse lamellar keratitis (DLK) (Fig. 8.12). DLK is an inflammatory condition of unclear etiology that usually presents within 1–3 days after LASIK and has the appearance of sandy debris in the stromal interface (hence the term "sands of the Sahara syndrome").[17]

36. **Which clinical features help to distinguish diffuse lamellar keratitis from an infectious process after LASIK?**
DLK initially presents with a diffuse sandy infiltrate located in the periphery of the stromal interface. Patients are typically asymptomatic, with a quiet eye. As the condition progresses, the infiltrate moves toward the center of the cornea and may begin to aggregate in clumps. Advanced cases of DLK can cause decreased vision and melting of the flap. Early treatment consists of frequent topical corticosteroids. Advanced cases may require systemic corticosteroids, lifting of the flap, and irrigation of the stromal interface. The lack of a distinct corneal infiltrate, conjunctival injection, cell and flare, and keratic precipitates favors the presence of DLK rather than infection.

37. **How should corneal infections after LASIK be prevented and managed?**
Blepharitis should be treated preoperatively. Sterile technique, including proper hand hygiene, sterile gloves, prepping solution (i.e., povidone iodine 10%), and draping of eyelashes, should be used. Postoperative treatment with a single-agent, broad-spectrum topical antibiotic also helps to reduce the incidence of infectious keratitis.
Whenever an infection is suspected, the patient should be taken to an operating room where the flap can be lifted under a microscope for diagnostic smears and cultures. The patient should be treated with topical gatifloxacin 0.3% or moxifloxacin 0.5% every 30 minutes. These agents should alternate with either topical cefazolin 50 mg/mL or topical vancomycin 50 mg/mL in lieu of cefazolin for those exposed to a hospital environment if the infection presents within 2 weeks or with topical amikacin 35 mg/mL if the infection presents after 2 weeks. Additionally, patients should be started on oral doxycycline 100 mg twice a day and should discontinue topical corticosteroid use. As always, therapy should be tailored to the results of corneal cultures and scrapings, as some microorganisms (e.g. fungi) will not be responsive to the aforementioned treatment regimen.[18]

KEY POINTS: LASIK INFECTIONS

1. Infections after LASIK are uncommon.
2. Common organisms causing LASIK-associated keratitis include MRSA and non-methicillin-resistant staphylococci; late-onset infections are often caused by atypical mycobacteria.
3. A suspicious infiltrate after LASIK should always be cultured.
4. DLK is an inflammatory, and not an infectious, condition that occurs in the early postoperative period.

FUNGAL KERATITIS

38. **What are the common organisms that can cause fungal keratitis and what are the associated risk factors?**
Fungal keratitis can be caused by filamentous fungi with septae (such as *Fusarium* spp., *Aspergillus* spp., and *Curvularia* spp.), filamentous fungi without septae (such as *Rhizopus* spp.), and yeast-like fungi (such as *Candida* spp.). Prominent risk factors for fungal keratitis include a history of trauma, exposure to vegetable or plant matter,

prolonged topical corticosteroid use, living in warmer climates, and ocular surface disease. Rarely, fungal infections can occur after a lamellar or penetrating keratoplasty, in the setting of a positive donor rim culture.

39. **What other considerations are important when diagnosing fungal keratitis?**
These infections can often be indolent and be initially mistaken for bacterial, viral, or parasitic infections. A high index of suspicion for fungal infections is needed in cases with atypical risk factors, abnormal appearance, and minimal response to broad-spectrum initial antimicrobial therapy. Repeat cultures and corneal biopsy may be needed. If cultures return inconclusive, in vivo confocal microscopy may be used to identify fungal hyphae in early stages of fungal keratitis. In addition, for rapidly progressive fungal infections, frequent dilated exams and/or ultrasonography should be employed to monitor development of potential fungal endophthalmitis.

40. **How can fungal infections be treated?**
Fungal keratitis is a challenging condition to treat, often due to delayed diagnosis and recalcitrant disease. The mainstay of treatment is the use of topical antifungal medications, which need to be manufactured at compounding pharmacies. These medications include natamycin 5%, amphotericin 0.15%, and voriconazole 1%.
  According to the Mycotic Ulcer Treatment Trial 1 (MUTT), cases of filamentous fungal infections, notably *Fusarium* spp., were associated with better clinical and microbiological outcomes when treated with topical natamycin 5% as compared with topical voriconazole 1%. In the MUTT 2, no therapeutic benefit was noted with the addition of oral voriconazole to topical natamycin or voriconazole in advanced mycotic keratitis cases.[19]
  In clinical practice, topical antifungal therapy is frequently used in conjunction with oral voriconazole or fluconazole. Intrastromal and/or intracameral injections of injections can also be used as adjunctive therapies.[20] Oral, intrastromal, and intracameral agents are employed for larger and deeper infiltrates.
  Polyhexamethylene biguanide may also be considered as a treatment option for fungal keratitis, as it has been shown to be an effective inhibitor of Aspergillus growth.[21]
  Many times, in cases of deeply penetrating or diffuse fungal keratitis, a therapeutic keratoplasty may be needed to eradicate infection and prevent endophthalmitis. However, if the infection can successfully be treated medically and eventually form a corneal scar, the patient may become a candidate for rigid gas permeable lens use or a deep anterior lamellar keratoplasty, both of which can afford better postinfection visual acuity.

KEY POINTS: FUNGAL INFECTIONS

1. Fungal keratitis can be an extremely challenging condition to diagnose and treat.
2. Common organisms causing fungal keratitis include *Fusarium* spp., *Aspergillus* spp., *Curvularia* spp., and *Candida* spp.
3. Topical antifungal agents are the mainstay of therapy for cases of fungal keratitis; evidence is limited on the efficacy of oral and intrastromal/intracameral agents, although they are sometimes employed as adjunctive therapies.

ACANTHAMOEBA KERATITIS

41. **What are the risk factors for *Acanthamoeba* keratitis?**
Acanthamoeba are parasites that can be found in tap water, hot tubs, pools, and contact lens solutions. The main risk factor to develop an ocular infection with this organism is contact lens wear and concomitant exposure to the organism, often through contaminated water.

42. **List the clinical features of *Acanthamoeba* keratitis.**
Early signs of *Acanthamoeba* keratitis can be nonspecific, including epithelial defects, epithelial or subepithelial infiltrates, or pseudodendrites. In later stages, ring-shaped or disciform stromal infiltrates can develop along with radial keratoneuritis. Advanced disease can present with extreme corneal thinning and/or perforation. The hallmark symptom of *Acanthamoeba* keratitis is pain out of proportion to clinical findings.

43. **What additional imaging modalities can be used to diagnose *Acanthamoeba* keratitis?**
In addition to corneal cultures and biopsies, confocal microscopy can be used to detect *Acanthamoeba* cysts and has been shown to have high sensitivity and specificity.[22]

44. **How can *Acanthamoeba* keratitis be treated?**
Topical therapies typically include a biguanide (polyhexamethylene biguanide 0.02% or chlorhexidine 0.02%) in combination with a diamidine (propamidine isethanoate 0.1% or hexamidine 0.1%). These medications are started at high frequencies and slowly tapered, often continuing for up to 6 months or more as the double walled cyst stage can stay dormant for long periods of time. If not eradicated, they can cause late recurrences. The use of corticosteroids is controversial, with some advocating for their use to decrease the inflammatory response, while others argue that these agents may prolong the life cycle of the parasite. Case reports also suggest the use of triazoles, such as topical or oral voriconazole, in addition to standard therapy. A deep anterior lamellar or penetrating keratoplasty may be required in cases of recalcitrant disease or visually debilitating corneal scarring.[23]

KEY POINTS: *ACANTHAMOEBA* INFECTIONS

1. Contact lenses exposed to contaminated water remain a leading risk factor for *Acanthamoeba* keratitis.
2. Corneal scrapings, biopsies, and confocal microscopy all play a role in the diagnosis of these infections.
3. Treatment of these infections requires months of topical biguanide and diamidine therapy; the use of steroids is controversial.

NEW TREATMENTS FOR INFECTIOUS KERATITIS

45. What is the role of corneal collagen crosslinking in the treatment of infectious keratitis that is not responding to conventional therapy?

    Corneal collagen crosslinking has been used by some practitioners, predominately internationally, for the treatment of refractory infectious keratitis. Corneal collagen crosslinking is believed to play a role in infectious keratitis due to its ability to strengthen the cornea, protecting it from corneal melt, and its ability to kill infectious organisms by causing irreversible damage to their DNA/RNA.

    A 2016 systematic review and meta-analysis of 25 studies, including two randomized control trials, 13 case series, and 10 case reports, showed that 87% of eyes treated with corneal crosslinking (some with antibiotic therapy and some without) healed. Corneal crosslinking was helpful in infections due to bacteria, fungi, and *Acanthamoeba*; however, it was associated with corneal melting with the need for tectonic keratoplasty in viral infections. Given the small number of studies for different etiologies of infectious keratitis in this systematic review and meta-analysis, more randomized controlled trials are required to assess for the efficacy of corneal crosslinking in the treatment of infectious keratitis. However, corneal crosslinking does appear to be a promising procedure in the treatment of select cases of infectious keratitis refractory to conventional therapy.[24]

REFERENCES

1. Cohen EJ, Fulton JC, Hoffman CJ, et al.: Trends in contact lens-associated corneal ulcers, Cornea 24:51–58, 2005.
2. Robertson DM: The effects of silicone hydrogel lens wear on the corneal epithelium and risk for microbial keratitis, Eye Contact Lens 39(1):67–72, 2013.
3. Holden BA, Sweeney DF, Sankaridurg PR, et al.: Microbial keratitis and vision loss with contact lenses, Eye Contact Lens 29(1) S131–S134, 2003.
4. McLeod SD, Kolahdouz-Isfahani A, Rostamian K, et al.: The role of smears, cultures, and antibiotic sensitivity testing in the management of suspected infectious keratitis, Ophthalmology 103:23–38, 1996.
5. Kowalski RR, Dhaliwal DK, Karenchak LM, et al.: Gatifloxacin and moxifloxacin: An in vitro susceptibility comparison to levofloxacin, ciprofloxacin, and ofloxacin using bacterial keratitis isolates, Am J Ophthalmol 136:500–505, 2003.
6. O'Brien TP, Maguire MG, Fink NE, et al.: Efficacy of ofloxacin vs. cefazolin and tobramycin in the therapy of bacterial keratitis: report from the Bacterial Keratitis Research Group, Arch Ophthalmol 113:1257–1265, 1995.
7. Srinivasan M, Mascarenhas J, Rajaraman R, et al.: Corticosteroids for bacterial keratitis: the steroids for Corneal Ulcers Trial (SCUT), Arch Ophthalmol 130:143–150, 2012.
8. Srinivasan M, Mascarenhas J, Rajaraman R, et al.: The steroids for corneal ulcers trial (SCUT): secondary 12-month clinical outcomes of a randomized controlled trial, AJO 157:327–333, 2014.
9. Jhanji V, Young AL, Mehta JS, et al.: Management of corneal perforation, Surv Ophthalmol 56(5):522–538, 2011.
10. Alexandrakis G, Haimovici R, Miler D, et al.: Corneal biopsy in the management of progressive microbial keratitis, Am J Ophthalmol 129(5):571–576, 2000.
11. Kumar P: Gonorrhoea presenting as red eye: rare case, Indian J Sex Transm Dis 33(1):47–48, 2012.
12. Srinivasan M, Mascarenhas J, Prashanth CN: Distinguishing infective versus noninfective keratitis, Indian J Ophthalmol May-Jun 56(3):203–207, 2008.
13. Chou TY and Hong BY: Ganciclovir ophthalmic gel 0.15% for the treatment of acute herpetic keratitis: background, effectiveness, tolerability, safety, and future applications, Ther Clin Risk Manag 10:665–681, 2014.
14. Wilhelmus KR, Gee L, Hauck WW, et al.: Herpetic Eye Disease Study: a controlled trial of topical corticosteroids for herpes simplex stromal keratitis, Ophthalmology 101:1883–1895, 1994.
15. Herpetic Eye Disease Study Group: Oral acyclovir for herpes simplex virus eye disease: effect on prevention of epithelial keratitis and stromal keratitis, Arch Ophthalmol 118:1030–1036, 2000.
16. Solomon R, Donnenfeld ED, Holland EJ, et al.: Microbial keratitis trends following refractive surgery: results of the ASCRS Infectious Keratitis Survey and comparisons with prior ASCRS Surveys of Infectious Keratitis Following Keratorefractive Procedures, J Cataract Refract Surg 37(7):1343–1350, 2011.
17. Smith RJ, Maloney RK: Diffuse lamellar keratitis: a new syndrome in lamellar refractive surgery, Ophthalmology 105:1721–1726, 1998.
18. Donnenfeld ED, Kim T, Holland EJ, et al.: Management of infectious keratitis following laser in situ keratomileusis—American Society of Cataract and Refractive Surgery White Paper, J Cataract Refract Surg 31(10):2008–2011, 2005.
19. Prajna NV, Krishnan T, Rajaraman R, et al.: Effect of oral voriconazole on fungal keratitis in the mycotic ulcer treatment trial II (MUTT II): a randomized clinical trial, JAMA Ophthalmol 134:1365–1372, 2016.
20. Kalaiselvi G, Narayana S, Krishnan T, et al.: Intrastromal voriconazole for deep recalcitrant fungal keratitis: a case series, Br J Ophthalmol 99:195–198, 2015.

21. Rebong RA, Santaella RM, Goldhagen BE, et al.: Polyhexamethylene biguanide and calcineurin inhibitors as novel antifungal treatments for Aspergillus keratitis, Invest Ophthalmol Vis Sci 52:7309–7915, 2011.
22. Tu EY, Joslin CE, Sugar J, Booton GC, Shoff ME, Fuerst PA. The relative value of confocal microscopy and superficial corneal scrapings in the diagnosis of Acanthamoeba keratitis, Cornea 27:764–772, 2008.
23. Clarke B, Sinha A, Parmar DN, Sykakis E.: Advances in the diagnosis and treatment of Acanthamoeba keratitis, J Ophthalmol 2012; 2012: 484892.
24. Papaioannou L, Miligkos M, Papathanassiou M: Corneal collagen cross-linking for infectious keratitis, Cornea 35(1):62–71, 2016.

CHAPTER 9

OPHTHALMIA NEONATORUM

Janine G. Tabas and Kristin M. DiDomenico

1. **How does ophthalmia neonatorum typically present?**
   Inflammation of the conjunctiva within the first month of life is classified as ophthalmia neonatorum (neonatal conjunctivitis). One or both eyes may have a purulent or mucoid discharge along with conjunctival injection. The eyelids may be edematous and red.

2. **What is the usual means of transmission for neonatal conjunctivitis?**
   Conjunctivitis is usually transmitted to the newborn by passage through the mother's infected cervix at the time of delivery and reflects the sexually transmitted infections prevalent in the community. The organisms can ascend into the uterus as well and may cause conjunctivitis even in the setting of cesarean section. It may also be spread by people handling the baby soon after birth.

3. **What is the most common cause of neonatal conjunctivitis in the United States?**
   Neonatal conjunctivitis is the most common ocular disease of newborns. The most common infectious cause in the United States is *Chlamydia trachomatis*. *Neisseria gonorrhoeae,* previously the leading cause of blindness in infants, now causes less than 1% of cases of neonatal conjunctivitis. This is because of improved prenatal screening and ocular prophylaxis.

4. **List the common causes of ophthalmia neonatorum, their usual clinical presentations, and their approximate times of onset after birth.**
   See Table 9.1.

5. **What type of neonatal conjunctivitis is associated with the most severe complications to the eye?**
   N. gonorrhoeae has the ability to penetrate intact epithelial cells and divide within them. Its onset is rapid and can quickly lead to corneal perforation and endophthalmitis.

KEY POINTS: MOST COMMON CAUSES OF NEONATAL CONJUNCTIVITIS

1. Chemical
2. Chlamydial
3. Gonococcal
4. Bacterial (including *Staphylococcal* sp., *Streptococcal* sp., *Pseudomonas* sp.)
5. Herpetic

---

6. **What other diagnostic tool is used to differentiate the various causes of neonatal conjunctivitis?**
   In most cases, one cannot rely solely on clinical characteristics and time of onset for accurate diagnosis; therefore, initial therapy is also based on the results of Gram and Giemsa stains performed immediately on conjunctival swabs and scrapings. Their classic characteristics are listed in Table 9.2. Not all cases have classic findings. Specimens should be sent for culture and sensitivity testing and antigen detection tests. Once the results are known and the clinical response is observed, adjust treatment regimens accordingly. Polymerase chain reaction is playing an increasing role in the identification of pathogens causing conjunctivitis because of its high sensitivity and specificity.

7. **In a neonate, is a follicular reaction in the conjunctiva more indicative of a chlamydial or a gonococcal infection?**
   Neither. Follicular reactions are not seen in the neonate because of the immaturity of the immune system.

8. **Why is Crede prophylaxis (2% silver nitrate drops) no longer the standard agent of choice for routine neonatal conjunctivitis prevention?**
   Crede prophylaxis is no longer the favored agent because of its high incidence of associated chemical conjunctivitis.

9. **What is currently used for neonatal prophylaxis?**
   The best means of preventing ophthalmia neonatorum, specifically by *N. gonorrhoeae* and *C. trachomatis*, is screening all pregnant women and treatment with follow-up when appropriate. The American Academy of

Table 9.1 Common Causes of Ophthalmia Neonatorum With Time of Onset and Typical Characteristics

TYPE	TIME OF ONSET	TYPICAL CHARACTERISTICS
Chemical (e.g., silver nitrate drops)	Within hours of instillation	Self-limiting, mild, serous discharge (occasionally purulent) Lasts 24–36 hours
Chlamydia trachomatis	5–14 days	Mild to moderate, thick, purulent discharge (severity is variable) Erythematous conjunctiva, with palpebral more than bulbar involvement
Neisseria gonorrhoeae	24–48 hours	Hyperacute, copious, purulent discharge Lid swelling and chemosis common
Bacterial (nongonococcal)[a]	After 5 days	Variable presentation, depending on organism
Herpetic	Within 2 weeks	Conjunctiva only mildly injected Serosanguineous discharge Vesicular rash on lids sometimes seen Most have concomitant systemic herpetic disease

[a]Staphylococcus aureus, Staphylococcus epidermidis, Streptococcus pneumoniae, Streptococcus viridans, Haemophilus influenzae, Escherichia coli, Pseudomonas aeruginosa.

Table 9.2 Gram and Giemsa Stain Findings With Various Causes of Neonatal Conjunctivitis

CAUSE	STAIN	FINDINGS
Chemical	Gram	Polymorphonuclear neutrophils (PMNs)
Chlamydial	Giemsa	Basophilic intracytoplasmic inclusion bodies in conjunctival epithelial cells
Gonococcal	Gram	Gram-negative intracellular diplococci in PMNs
Bacteria	Gram	Gram-positive or gram-negative organisms
Herpes simplex	Giemsa	Multinucleated giant cells, lymphocytes, plasma cells

Pediatrics, the US Preventative Task Force, and the Centers for Disease Control and Prevention endorse the use of 0.5% erythromycin ointment for neonatal prophylaxis. This is aimed primarily at preventing gonococcal conjunctivitis, which can have devastating ocular consequences. Povidone-iodine 2.5% is under investigation for prophylaxis and may be more effective against chlamydial conjunctivitis. Topical azithromycin is also under investigation for prevention.

10. What is the differential diagnosis of neonatal conjunctivitis?
   - **Birth trauma:** Usually evident by history.
   - **Foreign body/corneal abrasion:** Usually diagnosed by a combination of history and exam with fluorescein.
   - **Congenital glaucoma:** Accompanying early signs are tearing, photophobia, blepharospasm, and fussiness. Later signs include corneal edema and corneal enlargement. Intraocular pressure is elevated.
   - **Nasolacrimal duct obstruction:** Occurs in 6% of neonates and is usually associated with edema of the inner canthus and matting of the eyelids. Tearing is common, and the conjunctiva is usually not affected.
   - **Dacryocystitis:** Infection of the lacrimal sac, with erythema and swelling of the inner canthus and nasal conjunctival injection. Purulent drainage can often be expressed from the punctum.

11. When is systemic treatment indicated for neonatal conjunctivitis? Why?
   Systemic treatment is necessary for all cases of chlamydial, gonococcal, and herpetic conjunctivitis because of the potential for serious disseminated disease. A complete systemic examination must be performed at the time of diagnosis to determine the extent of disease.

12. List the potential ocular and systemic sequelae of untreated neonatal conjunctivitis.
   See Table 9.3.

13. What is the treatment for chlamydial conjunctivitis?
   Oral erythromycin syrup is given for 2 to 3 weeks (50 mg/kg/day in four divided doses). Topical erythromycin or sulfa ointment may be used four times a day, although there is no clear evidence that this is effective. The mother

Table 9.3 Ocular and Systemic Sequelae of Untreated Neonatal Conjunctivitis

TYPE	OCULAR	SYSTEMIC
Chemical	None (a self-limited entity).	None
Chlamydial	Chronic infection may cause corneal scarring and symblepharon (adhesion of eyelid to eye).	Pneumonitis and otitis media
Gonococcal	Corneal ulceration, perforation, and endophthalmitis (may occur within 24 hours of onset).	Meningitis, arthritis, sepsis, and death
Bacterial	*Pseudomonas* sp. may cause corneal ulcer, perforation, and endophthalmitis.	Usually none
Herpetic	Recurrences throughout life may cause corneal scarring and profound amblyopia. Chorioretinitis and cataracts also may develop.	Meningitis and disseminated CNS disease (mortality rate can be as high as 85%)

CNS, Central nervous system.

and her sexual partner also are treated with oral tetracycline, 250 to 500 mg four times a day, or doxycycline, 100 mg two times a day, for 7 days for presumed systemic disease, even if asymptomatic. Tetracycline cannot be used in children, pregnant women, or breast-feeding mothers because of permanent yellow-gray-brown discoloration of developing teeth as well as enamel hypoplasia.

KEY POINTS: POTENTIAL SYSTEMIC COMPLICATIONS OF NEONATAL CONJUNCTIVITIS

1. Pneumonitis
2. Meningitis
3. Otitis
4. Arthritis
5. Sepsis/death

14. What is the treatment for gonococcal conjunctivitis?

As a result of the high incidence of penicillin-resistant organisms, the Centers for Disease Control and Prevention recommend treatment with penicillinase-resistant antibiotics. Start intravenous ceftriaxone (a third-generation cephalosporin) immediately for 7 to 14 days at a dose of 25 to 50 mg/kg/day. After significant clinical improvement is seen, change to an oral equivalent to complete a 7-day course. A single 125-mg intramuscular dose of ceftriaxone or a 100 mg/kg intramuscular dose of cefotaxime given immediately after diagnosis is an accepted alternative treatment. This single parenteral dosing is also indicated for infants born to mothers with known gonococcal infections, even without the diagnosis of conjunctivitis.

Administer topical bacitracin ointment every 2 to 4 hours, and perform saline lavage hourly until the discharge is eliminated. Patients are generally hospitalized and evaluated for evidence of dissemination.

Because of the high incidence of concomitant chlamydial infection in women who contract gonorrhea, the infant, the mother, and her sexual partner are also treated systemically for *Chlamydia* as outlined previously. It is reasonable to test for other sexually transmitted diseases, i.e., HIV, syphilis, etc.

15. What is the treatment for bacterial conjunctivitis?

Treat bacterial conjunctivitis with bacitracin or gentamicin ointment applied four times per day for 2 weeks for gram-positive or gram-negative conjunctival swab results, respectively. The antibiotic choice may be altered later once culture and sensitivity results are known. Use fortified topical antibiotics in cases of corneal involvement, especially as seen with virulent organisms such as *Pseudomonas* sp. Supplementation with systemic treatment may be recommended.

KEY POINTS: POTENTIAL OCULAR COMPLICATIONS OF NEONATAL CONJUNCTIVITIS

1. Corneal scarring
2. Symblepharon
3. Corneal perforation
4. Endophthalmitis

16. What is the treatment for herpes simplex viral conjunctivitis?

   Intravenous acyclovir, 45 mg/kg/day, every 8 hours for 14 to 21 days, along with vidarabine 3% ointment (Vira-A) five times per day, or trifluorothymidine 1% (Viroptic) every 2 hours for 10 to 21 days.

17. How can the incidence of ophthalmia neonatorum be reduced in future generations?

   The population most at risk for contracting neonatal conjunctivitis is infants born to mothers without adequate prenatal care or mothers with substance abuse. Because of its high association with serious systemic disease, neonatal conjunctivitis is still an important public health issue worldwide. Although not universally accepted, some countries (e.g., Sweden and England) have abandoned the use of routine prophylaxis after birth in favor of careful screening for sexually transmitted diseases and better prenatal care.

BIBLIOGRAPHY

Albert DM, Jakobiec FA: Principles and practice of ophthalmology, Philadelphia, 1994, W.B. Saunders.
Chandler JW: Controversies in ocular prophylaxis of newborns, Arch Ophthalmol 107:814–815, 1989.
Gerstenblith AT, Rabinowitz MP: The Wills eye manual, ed 6, Philadelphia, 2012, Lippincott Williams & Wilkins.
Elnifro E, Storey C, Morris D, Rullo A: Polymerase chain reaction for detection of *Chlamydia trachomatis* in conjunctival swabs, Br J Ophthalmol 81(6):497–500, 1997.
Hammerschlag M: Neonatal conjunctivitis, Pediatr Ann 22:346–351, 1993.
Laga M, Naamara W, Brunham R, et al.: Single-dose therapy of gonococcal ophthalmia neonatorum with ceftriaxone, N Engl J Med 315:1382–1385, 1986.
Matejcek A, Goldman R: Treatment and prevention of ophthalmia neonatorum, Can Fam Physician 59(11):1187–1190, 2013.
O'Hara M: Ophthalmia neonatorum, Pediatr Clin North Am 40:715–725, 1993.
Skuta G, Cantor L, Weiss J: Basic and clinical sciences course, Am Acad Ophthalmol 6:187–189, 2012.
Weiss A: Chronic conjunctivitis in infants and children, Pediatr Ann 22:366–374, 1993.
https://emedicine.medscape.com/article/1192190-overview
Neonatal Conjunctivitis (Ophthalmia Neonatorum) Puente, Jr, MA. updated Mar 3, 2021; accessed 09/09/2021.

CHAPTER 10

TOPICAL ANTIBIOTICS AND STEROIDS

Christopher J. Rapuano and Richard E. Sutton

1. **You are an antibiotic or steroid eyedrop just placed in the conjunctival fornix. Discuss the barriers to your journey into the eye.**

   Many eyedrop dispensers deliver a 50-μL eyedrop. However, only 20% of this is retained by the conjunctival cul-de-sac, and the excess immediately flows over the eyelids. Of the portion that remains, approximately 80% drains through the lacrimal system. In addition, because of the 15%/min tear turnover rate, almost all of the topically applied medication disappears from the conjunctival cul-de-sac in about 5 minutes. Irritating drugs can produce reflex tearing and may be cleared even more quickly.

   During this critical 5 minutes, the topically applied drug faces numerous tissue obstacles. Conjunctival absorption quickly disperses the medication systemically via the conjunctival vasculature. The small portion of drug that penetrates the episclera faces the relative impermeability of the sclera and the tight junctions of the retinal pigment epithelium. The cornea poses three different barriers to entry. The corneal epithelium and the endothelium possess tight junctions that force the drugs to pass through the cellular membranes and limit passage of hydrophilic drugs. The corneal stroma is water-rich and limits movement of lipophilic drugs. Even after entry into the anterior chamber, the lens effectively blocks most drug penetration, and very little enters the posterior segment of the eye through topical administration. While such formidable barriers seem insurmountable, inflammation and infection render these barriers less effective, and modifications of the drug and/or its vehicle can facilitate entry into the eye. In addition, the desired site of action may be the ocular surface and not inside the eye.

2. **Given the earlier barriers, how would you increase delivery of topical antibiotics or steroids to the desired site of action?**

   Punctal occlusion decreases the amount of drainage through the lacrimal system by 65% and leaves more drug for intraocular absorption. "Digital" punctal occlusion involves applying a finger to the medial canthal area to temporarily block the tear drainage system for 30–60 seconds. Silicone punctal plugs can also be placed in the tear drainage ducts to slow down the exit of tears (and eyedrops) from the eye. Of course, frequent instillation also increases drug absorption, but the practical limit is probably every 5 minutes because the subsequent eyedrop can wash out the previous eyedrop before intraocular absorption.

   Changing the characteristics of the drug and/or its vehicle can also improve delivery. Increasing the concentration of the drug may be limited by the solubility of the drug in the vehicle, and the high tonicity of higher concentrations triggers reflex tearing that quickly clears the drug from the ocular surface. Also, increasing the lipid solubility of the drug appears to promote corneal passage despite the dual barrier characteristic of the cornea. In addition, adding surfactants that disturb the corneal epithelium can dramatically increase drug entry.

3. **Name the four different formulations of topical medications and the advantages and the disadvantages of each.**

   - **Solutions** are easily instilled, but contact time is minimal, requiring frequent administration. In addition, the "pulse" nature of absorption invites transient overdose and toxicity.
   - **Suspensions** allow a longer contact time, but the particulate nature of the preparation may be irritating and trigger reflex tearing. Suspensions settle to the bottom of the bottle and the bottle needs to be shaken before eyedrop instillation. Patients also may complain of accumulation of the precipitates or forget to shake the bottle before administering the eyedrops.
   - **Gels** are more viscous than solutions and suspensions and they are retained on the eye longer, allowing for better penetration of the active ingredients. In contrast to the suspensions, in which the active ingredient may precipitate, the gels allow for a more uniform distribution. Gels tend to blur the vision temporarily more than solutions or suspensions.
   - **Ointments** increase the contact time further, requiring the least frequent instillation, but leave a film over the eye that blurs vision even more than gels and for a much longer time. They are not practical to use bilaterally or for any length of time unless there is no other choice as they make the patient functionally blind in that eye. In addition, water-soluble drugs do not dissolve in the ointment vehicle and are present as crystals. Crystals are trapped in the ointment vehicle until the ointment melts with exposure to body temperature at the ocular surface, freeing the crystals to be absorbed. This type of absorption allows entry of constant but low amounts of the drug.

   Other methods of delivery include soft contact lenses, soluble ocular inserts, or implantable devices. Medications inserted into punctal plugs are becoming more available.

KEY POINTS: STRATEGIES TO INCREASE THE PENETRATION OF TOPICAL MEDICATIONS

1. Punctal occlusion.
2. Increase the frequency.
3. Increase the concentration of drug in the drop.
4. Increase the lipid solubility of the drug.
5. Use surfactants to disrupt the corneal epithelium.

4. What are some of the indications for using topical antibiotics?

Topical antibiotics are used to treat infections of the conjunctiva (conjunctivitis, conjunctival ulceration), cornea (keratitis, corneal ulceration), and lacrimal drainage system (canaliculitis). They are also used as prophylaxes against infection before and after ocular surgeries such as cataract, glaucoma, retina, corneal transplant, refractive, and ocular surface surgeries. Topical antibiotics are also used as prophylaxis in patients with corneal epithelial defects (e.g., after trauma, foreign body or suture removal) and in some cases eyes with therapeutic contact lenses. Prophylaxis with antibiotics is somewhat controversial as it may select for more resistant bacteria should an infection occur.

5. A 60-year-old man complains of crusting of the eyelids in the morning and chronic foreign-body sensation. Examination reveals moderate blepharitis with numerous collarettes around the eyelashes. What would you recommend?

Blepharitis responds well to warm compresses and eyelid scrubs in many cases, but supplemental antibiotic gels or ointments applied to the eyelash base or conjunctiva may be helpful, especially when numerous collarettes are seen around the eyelashes. Frequently used antibiotic ointments include erythromycin, bacitracin, and polymyxin-bacitracin (e.g., Polysporin). Azithromycin comes as an ophthalmic gel drop. Erythromycin and azithromycin are macrolide antibiotics that inhibit bacterial protein synthesis by binding to the 50S ribosomal unit. They have a broad spectrum of coverage but suffer from relatively poor intraocular absorption. They are most appropriate for blepharitis and conjunctivitis. Bacitracin is composed of numerous cyclic polypeptides that inhibit gram-positive bacterial cell wall synthesis. Polysporin combines bacitracin and polymyxin B, the latter of which is also a cyclic peptide that acts like a detergent to lyse bacterial cell membranes, and offers better coverage of gram-negative bacteria.

6. A 30-year-old woman with "cold" symptoms presents with redness and mucous discharge in both eyes. The ocular symptoms began in the right eye several days ago but now involve both eyes despite treatment of the right eye with sulfacetamide drops four times a day, as prescribed by her family physician. Examination reveals bilateral follicular conjunctivitis with preauricular adenopathy. What would you recommend?

History and examination are consistent with viral conjunctivitis. Artificial tears and cool compresses may provide comfort. Follow-up in 1 to 2 weeks is advisable to look for potential membranous conjunctivitis that may require treatment with topical steroids. Sulfacetamide is a bacteriostatic structural analog of *p*-aminobenzoic acid and inhibits synthesis of folic acid. It has a broad spectrum of coverage of bacteria and good corneal penetration and becomes more effective when combined with trimethoprim, which blocks a successive step in bacterial folate metabolism. It is used often by nonophthalmologists for initial treatment of red eyes; it is effective for mild bacterial conjunctivitis but is not helpful for viral conjunctivitis and should be discontinued in this patient. Viral conjunctivitis is very contagious, typically until the eye is no longer red and weeping. This patient should avoid close contact with others, perform frequent hand washing, and avoid sharing items such as towels or handkerchiefs.

7. A 55-year-old woman complains of discharge and redness of her right eye for 4 weeks. Her family physician told her that she had "pink eye" and prescribed erythromycin ointment, then sulfacetamide, and then ciprofloxacin, but the symptoms have not improved. Examination reveals diffuse papillary conjunctivitis with purulent discharge. There is no preauricular adenopathy or previous history of "cold" symptoms. What should you do?

The patient has chronic conjunctivitis, possibly bacterial. Topical therapy usually brings prompt relief, and you should make sure that she is using the medications properly. Assuming that she is getting the medications into the eye in a proper dosing regimen, conjunctival cultures can be performed to look for resistant or unusual bacteria. Testing for ocular *Chlamydia* may also be helpful. Chronic dacryocystitis should be investigated by applying firm pressure below the medial canthal tendon in an attempt to produce a diagnostic purulent discharge through the lacrimal punctum. An abscess in the nasolacrimal sac may provide a source of bacteria resistant to topical antibiotics.

8. A 25-year-old man holding a towel over his right eye complains of copious discharge that began in the morning. Examination reveals diffuse conjunctival hyperemia and chemosis

with thick, purulent discharge. A prominent preauricular adenopathy is also present. What should you do?

Prompt urgent conjunctival smears and cultures to look for gonococcal conjunctivitis in sexually active patients with hyperactive bacterial conjunctivitis. Although rare, gonococcal conjunctivitis requires *immediate* systemic antibiotics (typically intramuscular or intravenous ceftriaxone plus oral azithromycin), with topical antibiotics as an adjunctive treatment only. Screen for other sexually transmitted diseases and notified the authorities according to directions from the local health department.

9. A 26-year-old physician in a general surgery residency with a doctorate in pharmacology presents with foreign-body sensation and photophobia in both eyes after sleeping with soft contact lenses during his call night. A midperipheral 2-mm corneal ulcer with surrounding corneal stromal edema is present with scant anterior chamber reaction. What should you do?

The chances of developing a corneal ulcer increase by a factor of 10 when the patient sleeps with contact lenses, even those approved for such by the Food and Drug Administration (FDA). Corneal cultures are often recommended, although many ophthalmologists manage small corneal ulcers without cultures.

Initial therapy should cover a broad spectrum of bacteria. Traditionally, fortified cephalosporin and aminoglycoside have been used, but frequent use of fluoroquinolones offers similar efficacy (especially for small ulcers) with less toxicity. In addition, fortified topical antibiotics are not universally available and need to be refrigerated.

Fluoroquinolones inhibit bacterial DNA synthesis by binding to DNA topoisomerases and gyrase, thus introducing lethal breaks in bacterial DNA. They offer a superb spectrum of coverage in in vitro studies, although there is increasing resistance to both gram-positive and gram-negative bacteria. Even so, they appear to be highly effective for most contact lens–induced corneal ulcers.

Aminoglycosides bind to bacterial ribosomal subunits and interfere with protein synthesis. They offer a broad spectrum of coverage but require transport into the bacteria, which may be reduced in anaerobic environments of an abscess. Coadministration of antibiotics that alter bacterial cell wall structure (e.g., penicillins) improves aminoglycoside penetration into bacteria and may result in a synergistic inhibitory effect.

Cephalosporins are β-lactam antibiotics synthesized or derived from compounds isolated from the fungus *Cephalosporium acremonium*. They inhibit various penicillin binding proteins that are critical for bacterial cell wall synthesis. In general, later generations provide broader coverage with better gram-negative but poorer gram-positive activity. Cefazolin is a first-generation cephalosporin that is traditionally combined with an aminoglycoside for the initial treatment of more severe or centrally located corneal ulcers. It covers gram-positive and some gram-negative organisms but misses *Pseudomonas* sp. and therefore requires the addition of an aminoglycoside or fluoroquinolone for initial broad-spectrum coverage.

10. After corneal cultures are done, the patient is instructed to take ciprofloxacin drops every hour around the clock. The next day, he is in worse pain, and the corneal ulcer has enlarged to 3 mm with tenacious purulent discharge. What is your next step?

Make sure the eyedrops are getting into the eye. Ask the patient to demonstrate eyedrop administration. Several eyedrops fall on the floor, then on his cheeks, and finally he announces success when the eyedrops fall on his closed eyelids. Often, antibiotic failure is due to improper administration. Patients should be observed taking their eyedrops. A friend or family member may need to administer the eyedrops to be sure that the medications are getting to the source of infection, especially when frequent instillation is required. Indeed, some patients require hospitalization to receive intensive eyedrop administration.

In addition, the patient should have taken the drug more often initially.

The manufacturer's recommended dose of ciprofloxacin for corneal ulcers:

- **First 6 hours:** Two drops every 15 minutes
- **Remainder of the first day:** Two drops every half-hour
- **Day 2:** Two drops every hour
- **Days 3 to 14:** Two drops every 4 hours

However, this regimen may be altered in response to clinical exam and culture results. Frequent dosing of ciprofloxacin may produce a white precipitate over the ulcer, but this precipitate does not appear to impede the bactericidal activity and usually resolves when the dose is tapered.

Ofloxacin is also used but has different manufacturer's recommendations:

- **Days 1 and 2:** One to two drops every 30 minutes while awake
- **Awaken at 4 and 6 hours after retiring:** Give one to two drops
- **Days 3 to 7 or 9:** One to two drops hourly while awake
- **Days 7–9 to completion:** One to two drops four times a day

Fourth-generation fluoroquinolones, gatifloxacin, moxifloxacin, and besifloxacin, are also available topically, with better gram-positive coverage and comparable gram-negative coverage. These medications have not been FDA approved for the treatment of corneal ulcers, but they are frequently used off-label for this condition.

11. The patient now prefers a "proven" treatment regimen with a long history and requests topical fortified antibiotics. However, he recalls that minimal bactericidal concentration for

most pathogenic bacteria is far below that provided by the fortified antibiotics and accuses you of wasting money and drugs. Is he right?

No. In vitro and in vivo results in other sites of the body are not directly applicable to the eye. Indeed, in the vitreous, the dose–response relationship has been demonstrated up to 100 times the in vitro minimal bactericidal concentration.

12. The patient reminds you that he is penicillin-allergic and is concerned about anaphylaxis. What antibiotics should you choose? How do you begin therapy?

Topical penicillin is not often used in ophthalmology because of poor penetration into the eye and active transport out of the eye by the organic acid transport system of the ciliary body. However, inflammation improves ocular penetration. Penicillin inhibits bacterial transpeptidase and prevents bacterial cell wall synthesis. Various modifications of the original compound have produced differing spectra of activity. Penicillin G and V are still highly effective for many gram-positive and gram-negative bacteria, but many strains of *Staphylococcus aureus* and *Staphylococcus epidermidis* are now resistant. Penicillinase-resistant penicillins such as methicillin, nafcillin, and oxacillin are useful for penicillinase-producing staphylococci. Broad-spectrum penicillins, ampicillin and amoxicillin, have better gram-negative coverage, and semisynthetic penicillins such as carbenicillin, piperacillin, and ticarcillin extend coverage to *Pseudomonas*, *Enterobacter*, and *Proteus* spp.

Immediate allergic response to penicillin, such as anaphylaxis, is a strong contraindication for its use, and there is 10% cross-reactivity with cephalosporins. Therefore, for patients with penicillin allergy, cefazolin is typically replaced with vancomycin. Vancomycin is a complex glycopeptide that inhibits bacterial cell wall synthesis with principally gram-positive coverage, including methicillin-resistant *S. aureus* and Enterococcal spp., of which *Enterococcus faecalis* is a frequent bacterial pathogen in infections of filtering blebs.

As mentioned earlier, aminoglycosides can be synergistic with cell wall–inhibiting antibiotics, and the patient should be started on fortified vancomycin and tobramycin. Give the patient four doses—an alternating dose every 5 minutes—followed by alternation every half-hour to 1 hour, usually starting around the clock. Actual dosing will vary in different institutions.

13. The next morning, the ulcer looks worse with 4-mm corneal infiltrate and purulent material overlying the ulcer but the patient feels better. The corneal culture confirms *Pseudomonas aeruginosa*. Why did the patient not improve?

This particular *Pseudomonas* organism could be resistant to the prescribed medications, but many cases of *Pseudomonas* corneal ulcers take a day or two to turn the corner, even when receiving appropriate treatment. Less eye pain is a good indication of improvement. *Pseudomonas* corneal ulcers sometimes require double coverage. Fortified amikacin, piperacillin-tazobactam or ticarcillin could be added in a non-penicillin-allergic patient. Frequent ciprofloxacin (or a newer generation fluoroquinolone) could also be resumed, especially in this case.

14. Two days later, the ulcer looks stable, but the patient complains of persistent and perhaps worsening pain. Examination reveals diffuse punctate corneal epithelial defects outside the area of ulceration, inferior conjunctival erythema with overlying conjunctival epithelial defect, and swollen lower eyelids. What should you do?

Overall toxicity is often less severe with topical compared to systemic administration; indeed, some common topical antibiotics such as neomycin and polymyxin cannot be given intravenously because of systemic toxicity. However, intensive regimens of potent topical antibiotics often produce surface toxicity with prominent involvement of lower more than upper conjunctiva. The toxicity is related to several factors, including the pH of the antibiotic drop and the presence of preservative in the solution. Fortified antibiotic drops, which are generally prepared by diluting intravenous antibiotics with preservative-free artificial tears and topical moxifloxacin, are preservative free. Occasionally, only analgesics and cool compresses can be offered if the infection is not under control. In this case, the fortified vancomycin should be decreased or discontinued because tobramycin and ciprofloxacin are more important for *Pseudomonas* ulcer, and the ulcer appears to be stabilizing.

15. One week later, the patient presents to you complaining of a dense white opacity in his cornea. Examination reveals superficial dense white material with gritty appearance in the area of the healing ulcer (Fig. 10.1). What is going on?

Prolonged use of ciprofloxacin drops/ointments causes characteristic macroscopic deposits in up to 20% of patients through a compromised corneal epithelium. These eventually disappear after discontinuation of the ciprofloxacin eye medication.

16. The patient slowly improves, but significant corneal opacity remains. He would like binocular vision for his surgical career and asks you to get rid of his corneal haze. How do you respond?

Read on to learn about topical steroids. Often, inflammatory opacities fade with time, but the effect may be enhanced with topical steroids. When, how much, and how long to use topical steroids are controversial, but a trial of topical steroids is often warranted before considering surgical options. The infection should be under control first before applying any topical steroids.

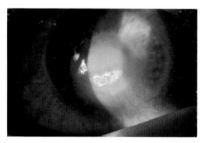

Fig. 10.1 Anterior segment of the right eye demonstrates refractile superficial crystalline deposits overlying an area of epithelial defect in a patient who was treated with a prolonged course of topical ciprofloxacin.

KEY POINTS: CORNEAL ULCERS

1. Small, noncentral ulcers can be managed without cultures.
2. Fluoroquinolones every half-hour to 1 hour initially may offer similar efficacy with less toxicity than fortified topical antibiotics.
3. *Pseudomonas* ulcers may require double antibiotic coverage.
4. The use of topical steroids after the infection is under control can decrease the size and density of the scar.

17. Review the currently available topical antibiotics in generic and brand names.
    See Table 10.1.

18. How do topical steroids work?
    The specific mechanisms of action of steroids are not completely understood. At a molecular level, the most important effect may be inhibition of arachidonic acid release from phospholipids. Arachidonic acid is converted to prostaglandins and related compounds that are potent mediators of inflammation. At a cellular level, steroids must be carried to the cytoplasm, where they bind to soluble receptors and then enter the nucleus to alter transcription of various proteins involved in immune regulation and inflammation. At the tissue level, steroids suppress the cardinal signs of inflammation such as edema, heat, pain, and redness through a variety of mechanisms. They cause vasoconstriction and decrease vascular permeability to inflammatory cells. Steroids stabilize cellular and intracellular membranes inhibiting release of inflammatory mediators such as histamine. They inhibit neutrophilic leukocytosis and decrease macrophage recruitment and migration. Overall, steroids are potent anti-inflammatory and immunosuppressive agents with wide-ranging ophthalmic applications, but their adverse effects as well as their benefits should be understood before use.

19. Because steroids are not cures, what general categories of disorders warrant ophthalmic use of topical steroids?
    There are three broad categories of disorders that warrant steroid use: postsurgical, immune hyperreactivity, and combined immune and infectious processes. Although their use in the postoperative setting is almost universal, some ophthalmologists report adequate control of postoperative inflammation with topical nonsteroidals for various ophthalmic procedures, most commonly cataract surgery. The second category includes various uveitides, allergic and vernal conjunctivitis, corneal graft rejections, and other processes in which the immune system activity is harmful to the host tissue. The last category includes viral and bacterial corneal ulcers, especially herpes simplex and varicella zoster, in which control of infectious processes must be balanced with control of inflammation that may scar delicate ocular tissue.

20. The physician with the residual corneal opacity wants to minimize his corneal opacity but is concerned about the potential side effects of topical steroids. How do you advise him?
    The most immediate concern is exacerbation of the existing infection with reactivation of dormant organisms or inhibition of wound healing. Other well-known adverse effects include glaucoma and cataracts, but numerous other side effects have been observed, including blepharoptosis, eyelid skin or scleral atrophy, and mydriasis.
    In a randomized, multicenter clinical trial, investigators compared the effects of topical prednisolone sodium phosphate 1% to placebo in culture-positive bacterial corneal ulcers that were treated with topical moxifloxacin for at least 48 hours prior to randomization. Improvement in the overall best spectacle-corrected visual acuity at 3 months was not observed in the group treated with corticosteroids compared to placebo. In addition, there were no differences in the scar/infiltrate size, time to reepithelialization, and rate of corneal perforation between the groups. However, subgroup analysis demonstrated that ulcers with central location and presenting vision of counting fingers (CFs) or worse did better in the steroid-treated group. At 1 year, a small

Table 10.1 Commonly Commercially Available Topical Antibiotics

GENERIC	BRAND NAME	CLASS	PREPARATION
Gentamicin	Genoptic S.O.P.	Aminoglycosides	0.3% ointment or solution
Tobramycin	Garamycin		0.3% ointment or solution
	Gentacidin		
	Gentak		
	Tobrex		
Besifloxacin	Besivance	Fluoroquinolones	0.6% suspension
Ciprofloxacin	Ciloxan		0.3% solution or ointment
Ofloxacin	Ocuflox		0.3% solution
Moxifloxacin	Vigamox		0.5% solution
Gatifloxacin	Zymar		0.3% solution
Levofloxacin	Zymaxid		0.5% solution
	Quixin		0.5% solution
Azithromycin	Azasite	Macrolides	1% gel drop solution
Erythromycin	AK-Mycin		0.5% ointment
	Ilotycin		
Sulfacetamide	Bleph-10	Sulfonamides	10% ointment or solution
	AK-Sulf		10% ointment or solution
	Sodium Sulamyd		10% ointment or solution
Polymyxin B	Neosporin Neocidin	Polymyxins	10,000 units, 1.75 mg,
	Polymycin		0.025 mg/mL solution
	AK-Spore (with		
	Neomycin		
	Gramicidin)		
Tetracycline	Achromycin	Tetracycline	1% solution or ointment
Bacitracin	AK-Tracin		500 units/g ointment
Chloramphenicol	Chloromycetin		0.5% ointment, 1.0%
	Ocu-Chlor		solution
	Chloroptic		
Polymyxin B/trimethoprim	Polytrim	Combination antibiotic	0.1%/10,000 units/mL
Polymyxin B/bacitracin	Polysporin	medications	solution
Polymyxin B/bacitracin/	Neosporin		10,000 units/g, 500 units/g
neomycin	Neosporin Neocidin		ointment
Polymyxin/neomycin/	Polymycin		10,000 units, 3.5 mg,
gramicidin	AK-Spore		400 units/g ointment
			10,000 units, 1.75 mg,
			0.025 mg solution

amount of visual improvement (one line) was noted in eyes treated with steroids whose ulcer was *not* caused by *Nocardia*, especially if the steroids were begun 2 to 3 days after the antibiotics were started, as opposed to 4 days or longer.

Systemic absorption may be significant with frequent use. Encourage punctal occlusion in these cases. A 6-week regimen of topical 0.1% dexamethasone sodium phosphate suppresses the adrenal cortex, and some patients with systemic hay fever improve with topical ocular steroids. Of course, all of these effects are more frequent with intensive and chronic use of steroids.

21. After a lengthy discussion, the patient agrees to try topical steroids. However, given his interest in pharmacology, he requests a brief discussion of the pharmacokinetics of a few of the available topical steroids.

Topical steroids may be prepared as solutions, suspensions, or ointments. Phosphate preparations may be prepared as solutions because they are highly water-soluble in the aqueous vehicles but penetrate less well into intact corneal epithelium than acetate or alcohol suspensions, which have biphasic solubility. Nevertheless, 1% prednisolone phosphate achieves a significant corneal level of 10 μg/g within 30 minutes of instillation, which improves to 235 μg/g when the corneal epithelium is removed. Dexamethasone phosphate enters the cornea and anterior chamber within 10 minutes, reaches a maximum in 30 to 60 minutes, and slowly disappears over the next few to 24 hours.

22. The patient also requests that a potent steroid be used with rapid taper so that the overall course may be shortened. Which steroid do you choose?

The anti-inflammatory effects of topical steroids differ depending on the clinical setting and method of measurement. However, certain generalizations can be made:

- Higher concentrations and more frequent instillations, up to every 5 minutes, increase concentrations of steroids in the cornea and aqueous.
- Potency with intact corneal epithelium is highest in prednisolone acetate suspension > dexamethasone alcohol solution > prednisolone sodium phosphate solution > dexamethasone phosphate ointment.
- Potency with corneal epithelial defects is highest in prednisolone sodium phosphate solution > dexamethasone phosphate solution > prednisolone acetate suspension.

23. The patient is started on 1% prednisolone acetate four times a day. His opacity is beginning to recede, but he returns 2 days later with complaints of a white precipitate that forms on his conjunctiva and insists on a change of medication to prevent this annoying buildup. Which steroid do you choose now?

Suspensions leave a milky precipitate that some patients find unpleasant. In addition, despite shaking the bottles before instillation, a variable amount of the suspension may be delivered if particles are not evenly distributed. Therefore, some ophthalmologists prefer phosphate solutions despite lower potency with intact epithelium. A change to 1% prednisolone phosphate is reasonable if it improves patient compliance.

24. On day 10 of steroid therapy, the corneal opacity is receding, but the patient complains of foreign-body sensation. Examination reveals large corneal epithelial dendrites. What should you do?

Steroids do not cause herpetic keratitis but may promote herpetic keratitis when viral shedding is timed with the presence of steroids on the ocular surface. Often, the dendrites are large and numerous in the presence of steroids, and steroids should be rapidly tapered or stopped. Of course, start full dosing of a topical antiviral (e.g., ganciclovir or trifluridine) or an oral antiviral (e.g., acyclovir, valacyclovir, or famciclovir).

25. Fortunately, the dendrite heals rapidly and the previous corneal opacity has faded significantly with return to 20/20 vision in that eye. Four years have passed, and the patient is now seeking employment. Opportunities are scarce, and his only job offer is from a large organized health company that hopes to use him as a pharmacist as well as a physician as a cost-saving measure. Understandably, he is stressed. Now he notices extreme photophobia and redness of his eye. Examination reveals corneal stromal edema and focal keratic precipitates consistent with herpes simplex keratouveitis. What should you do?

Many stimuli, including stress, may promote recurrence of herpetic keratitis. Other potential stimuli include menses, sun exposure, and fever. If the inflammation is severe or central vision is threatened, start topical steroids concurrent with antiviral coverage to decrease corneal scarring and intraocular inflammation. One regimen is acyclovir 400 mg two times a day and 1% prednisolone acetate four times a day. Other regimens are acceptable. Antiviral coverage is probably unnecessary below one drop a day of 1% prednisolone acetate. In patients with a history of multiple episodes of herpes simplex keratitis, prophylactic antivirals (e.g., acyclovir 400 mg two times a day) are successful in decreasing the chances of recurrences.

26. Two days later, only marginal improvement is noted, but intraocular pressure is 35 mm Hg. What happened?

Significant steroid-induced rises in intraocular pressure are seen in up to 6% of patients after 6 weeks of topical dexamethasone. Patients with glaucoma or a family history of glaucoma are particularly susceptible. The mechanism appears to be decreased aqueous outflow, perhaps as a result of deposition of mucopolysaccharides in the trabecular meshwork. The extent of intraocular pressure rise varies with type and dose of steroids. Usually, steroids with greater anti-inflammatory potency elicit greater elevation of intraocular pressure. For example, steroids with low intraocular bioavailability and potency, such as fluorometholone, cause lower rises in intraocular pressure after a greater duration of therapy than more potent steroids such as dexamethasone. Loteprednol appears to be an exception. It suppresses anterior chamber cell and flare similar to 1% prednisolone acetate, with intraocular pressure elevation similar to fluorometholone. Regardless, the elevated intraocular pressure subsides, usually within 2 weeks, by decreasing or discontinuing steroid therapy, but topical aqueous suppressants may be needed in some patients.

However, steroid-induced rises in intraocular pressure rarely occur in less than 2 weeks and certainly not after 2 days of steroid therapy. Patients with intraocular inflammations, especially in herpetic keratouveitis, may have increased intraocular pressure as a result of intraocular inflammation. Therefore, in the present patient, the topical steroids should be increased and not decreased.

27. The frequency of prednisolone acetate administration was increased to every 3 hours while awake, and timolol, two times a day, was added. One week later, the intraocular pressure is normal, and intraocular inflammation has subsided. Prednisolone acetate is decreased

to two times a day. The patient returns 2 days later with recurrence of pain and photophobia and return of intraocular inflammation. What happened?

You tapered the steroids too quickly. A useful rule is to decrease steroids by no more than half of the previous dose every week to many weeks, especially in herpetic keratouveitis, in which rebound inflammation is frequent. Make sure that the patient is still taking the eyedrops. Sometimes, patients abruptly stop the eyedrops when they feel better and then suffer rebound inflammation.

28. Review the commonly available topical steroids and their generic and brand names.
    See Table 10.2.

29. What are some of the topical antibiotic/steroid combinations and when is it appropriate to use them?
    There are many antibiotic/steroid combination drops and ointments available on the market. See Table 10.3.

Table 10.2 Commonly Commercially Available Topical Steroids

GENERIC NAME	BRAND NAME	PREPARATION
Difluprednate	Durezol	0.05% emulsion
Dexamethasone sodium phosphate	AK-Dex, Decadron	0.1% solution
Dexamethasone sodium phosphate	AK-Dex, Decadron	0.05% ointment
Fluorometholone	FML Forte	0.25% suspension
Fluorometholone	FML Liquifilm, Fluor-Op	0.1% suspension
Fluorometholone	FML	0.1% ointment
Fluorometholone acetate	Flarex	0.1% suspension
Prednisolone acetate	Pred Forte, Econopred Plus	1% suspension
	Pred Mild, Econopred	0.125% suspension
Prednisolone sodium phosphate	Inflamase Forte, AK-Pred 1%	1% solution
	Inflamase Mild, AK-Pred 0.125%	0.125% solution
Rimexolone	Vexol	1% suspension
Loteprednol	Alrex	0.2% suspension
	Lotemax	0.5% suspension, 0.5% geldrop
	Lotemax SM	0.38% geldrop
	Inveltys	1% suspension

Table 10.3 Commonly Commercially Available Topical Steroid/Antibiotic Combinations

GENERIC	BRAND NAME
Dexamethasone (0.1%)/neomycin(0.35%), polymyxin B (10,000 units)	Maxitrol suspension, Maxitrol ointment
Dexamethasone (0.1%)/tobramycin (0.3%)	Tobradex suspension, Tobradex ointment
Dexamethasone (0.05%)/tobramycin (0.3%)	Tobradex ST suspension
Hydrocortisone (1%)/neomycin (0.35%)/polymyxin B (10,000 units) ointment	—
Hydrocortisone (1%)/neomycin (0.35%)/bacitracin (400 units)/polymyxin B (10,000 units) ointment	—
Loteprednol (0.5%)/tobramycin (0.3%)	Zylet suspension
Prednisolone (1%)/gentamicin (0.3%)	Pred-G suspension
Prednisolone (0.6%)/gentamicin (0.3%)	Pred-G ointment
Prednisolone (0.5%)/neomycin (0.35%)/polymyxin B (10,000 units)	Poly-Pred solution
Prednisolone (0.2%)/sulfacetamide (10%)	Blephamide solution
Prednisolone (0.2%)/sulfacetamide (10%)	Blephamide ointment

These medications are often used in eyes with mild superficial infections associated with some inflammation, such as staphylococcal marginal hypersensitivity. Combination medications should be used cautiously as steroids can cause a rapid progression and worsening of corneal ulcer. Also, long-term use of these medications can lead to the formation of cataract and elevated intraocular pressure and/or glaucoma. Be careful to warn patients not to use steroids or combination medications that include them "as needed" for irritation, redness, or similar symptoms without close medical follow-up to prevent these side effects.

BIBLIOGRAPHY

Abelson MB, Butrus S: Corticosteroids in ophthalmic practice. In Jakobiec FA, Albert D, editors: Principles and practice of ophthalmology, vol. 6, Philadelphia, 1994, W.B. Saunders, pp 1013–1022.

Austin A, Lietman T, Rose-Nussbaumer J: Update on the management of infectious keratitis, Ophthalmology 124(11):1678–1689, 2017.

Awwad ST, Haddad W, Wang MX, Parmar D, Conger D, Cavanagh HD: Corneal instrastromal gatifloxacin crystal deposits after penetrating keratoplasty, Eye Contact Lens 30(3):169–172, 2004.

Axelrod J, Glew R, Barza M, et al.: Antibacterials. In Jakobiec FA, Albert D, editors: Principles and practice of ophthalmology (vol 6), Philadelphia, 1994, W.B. Saunders, pp 940–960.

Baum JL: Initial therapy of suspected microbial corneal ulcers. I: broad antibiotic therapy based on prevalence of organisms, Surv Ophthalmol 24:97–105, 1979.

Brar VS, et al.: Ocular pharmacotherapeutics. In Brar VS, Law SK, Lindsey JL, et al., editors: Basic and clinical science course, Fundamentals and principles of ophthalmology, section 2, San Francisco, 2019, American Academy of Ophthalmology, pp 399–411, 417–431.

Callegan MC, Engel LS, Hill JM, et al.: Ciprofloxacin versus tobramycin for the treatment of staphylococcal keratitis, Inv Ophthalmol Vis Sci 35:1033–1037, 1994.

Foster CS, Alter G, Debarge LR, et al.: Efficacy and safety of rimexolone 1% ophthalmic suspension vs. 1% prednisolone acetate in the treatment of uveitis, Am J Ophthalmol 122:171–182, 1996.

Henderer JD, Rapuano CJ: Ocular pharmacology. In Brunton LL, editor: Goodman & Gilman's the pharmacological basis of therapeutics, ed 13, New York, 2018, McGraw-Hill Education, chapter 69, pp 1251–1262.

Herretes S, Wang X, Reyes JM: Topical corticosteroids as adjunctive therapy for bacterial keratitis, Cochrane Database Syst Rev 10, 2014.

KhalafAllah MT, Basiony A, Salama A: Difluprednate versus prednisolone acetate after cataract surgery: a systematic review and meta-analysis, BMJ Open 9(11), 2019.

Leibowitz HM, Bartlett JD, Rich R, et al.: Intraocular pressure-raising potential of 1% rimexolone in patients responding to corticosteroids, Arch Ophthalmol 114:933–937, 1996.

McDonald EM, Ram FS, Patel DV, McGhee CN: Topical antibiotics for the management of bacterial keratitis: an evidence-based review of high quality randomised controlled trials, Br J Ophthalmol 98(11):1470-1477, 2014.

Poggio EC, Glynn RJ, Schein OD, et al.: The incidence of ulcerative keratitis among users of daily-wear and extended-wear soft contact lenses, N Engl J Med 321(12):779–783, 1989.

Prajna NV, Krishnan T, Mascarenhas J, et al.: The Mycotic Ulcer Treatment Trial: a randomized trial comparing natamycin vs voriconazole, JAMA Ophthalmol 131(4):422–429, 2013.

Ray KJ, Srinivasan M, Mascarenhas J, et al.: Early addition of topical corticosteroids in the treatment of bacterial keratitis, JAMA Ophthalmol 132(6):737–741, 2014.

Schein OD, Glynn RJ, Poggio EC, Seddon JM, Kenyon KR: The relative risk of ulcerative keratitis among users of daily-wear and extended-wear soft contact lenses. A case-control study. Microbial Keratitis Study Group, N Engl J Med 321(12):773–778, 1989.

Sharma A, Taniguchi J: Review: emerging strategies for antimicrobial drug delivery to the ocular surface: implications for infectious keratitis, Ocul Surf 15(4):670–679, 2017.

Srinivasan M, Mascarenhas J, Rajaraman R, et al.: Corticosteroids for bacterial keratitis: the Steroids for Corneal Ulcers Trials (SCUT), Arch Ophthalmol 130(2):143–150, 2012.

Srinivasan M, Mascarenhas J, Rajaraman R, et al.: Steroids for Corneal Ulcers Trial Group. The Steroids for Corneal Ulcers Trial (SCUT): secondary 12-month clinical outcomes of a randomized controlled trial, Am J Ophthalmol 157(2):327–333, 2014.

Stroman DW, Dajcs JJ, Cupp GA, et al.: In vitro and in vivo potency of moxifloxacin and moxifloxacin ophthalmic solution 0.5%, a new topical fluoroquinolone, Surv Ophthalmol 50:S16–S31, 2005.

Ueno N, Refojo MF, Abelson M: Pharmacokinetics. In Jakobiec FA, Albert D, editors: Principles and practice of ophthalmology, vol. 6, Philadelphia, 1994, W.B. Saunders, pp 916–928.

CHAPTER 11

DRY EYES

Janice A. Gault

1. **What is the definition of dry eye?**
   A dry eye, or keratoconjunctivitis sicca, is a condition in which the tear film is abnormal and cannot lubricate the anterior surface of the cornea adequately. The resulting changes in the ocular surface can cause ocular discomfort, scarring, and, in severe cases, loss of vision and perforation. It is a multifactorial disease with a loss of homeostasis of the tear film, causing ocular surface inflammation and subsequent damage.

2. **Describe the normal tear film.**
   The normal tear film is a 1.0-mm convex band with a regular upper margin.

3. **What are the components of the tear film?**
   The normal tear film is made of three components. The outer layer is a thin lipid layer produced by the Meibomian glands, which open along the upper and lower lid margins. The middle layer, the thickest, is composed of aqueous produced from the main and accessory lacrimal glands. The innermost layer is a mucin layer produced by conjunctival goblet cells.

4. **What is the function of the outer lipid layer?**
   It retards evaporation of the aqueous middle layer. If it is dysfunctional, evaporative dry eye will result.

5. **What causes dysfunction of the outer lipid layer?**
   It could be caused by oil deficiency, as in Meibomian gland dysfunction (i.e., blepharitis). Also, an abnormal lid contour, as in ectropion or lid tumor, or poor blinking, found in Bell's palsy, can cause outer lipid layer dysfunction.

6. **What is the function of the aqueous middle layer?**
   It supplies oxygen from the atmosphere to the corneal epithelium, washes away debris, and has antibacterial properties due to immunoglobulin A (IgA), lysozyme, and lactoferrin present. If deficient, hyposecretive dry eye results, as found in Sjögren's syndrome.

7. **What is the function of the inner mucin layer?**
   It covers the villus surface of the corneal epithelium, converting it from a hydrophobic surface to a hydrophilic one, thus allowing the aqueous layer to lubricate the cornea.

8. **What diseases of the conjunctiva can cause dry eye?**
   Conjunctival scarring can injure the goblet cells. Patients with cicatricial ocular pemphigoid, Stevens-Johnson syndrome, chemical burns (especially alkali), and graft-versus-host disease in bone marrow transplantation may have dry eye. Patients with other conjunctival disorders that accompany conditions such as aniridia may also have dry eyes. Vitamin A deficiency can result in the loss of goblet cells. This is becoming more common with the increase in gastric bypass procedures who do not take adequate vitamin supplements postoperatively.

9. **What is necessary for the normal resurfacing of the tear film?**
   A normal blink reflex, normal lid anatomy and contour, and a normal corneal epithelium. Of course, a normal tear film makeup is essential.

10. **What are the types of dry eye?**
    There are three main types:
    - **Aqueous deficient (i.e., Sjögren's or non-Sjögren's syndrome):** The aqueous component is low. Ten percent of severe dry eye patients have Sjögren's syndrome. Lacrimal deficiency/obstruction, systemic drugs, reflex block from contact lens wear or local anesthesia from previous ocular surgery, or herpetic disease are other causes.
    - **Evaporative**
      - Extrinsic causes are vitamin A deficiency, topical drugs and their preservatives, contact lens wear, and environmental factors such as low humidity or allergens.
      - Intrinsic factors are meibomian gland dysfunction, eyelid abnormalities (i.e., Bell's palsy, ectropion) or corneal surface changes such as dellen, and poor blink.
    - **Mixed:** This combines features of the other two. The majority of patients fit in this group—dry eye is a continuum.

11. **What are the symptoms of dry eye?**
    Burning, irritation, foreign body sensation, light sensitivity, and fluctuating blurred vision. Usually, the symptoms are worse in the afternoon and evening and better on awakening. A dry or dusty environment may cause more difficulties in patients with dry eye than in others. Cigarette smoke can be extremely irritating. Symptoms are

worse in low-humidity environments, such as those with central air and in an airplane, during prolonged reading, driving, or screen use with a decreased blink rate owing to increased concentration, and windy conditions.

12. What are the most common signs of dry eye?

In the early stages, ocular symptoms may be more impressive than what is found on the examination. Signs of dry eye include a decreased tear meniscus, debris in the tear film, conjunctival injection, and superficial punctate keratitis and conjunctivitis. Abnormal fluorescein or rose bengal staining of the corneal and conjunctival epithelium in the exposed interpalpebral fissure (at 3 and 9 o'clock) of the lower third of the cornea is often present. The upper half of the cornea is usually spared. In more severe disease, filamentary keratitis, as well as corneal scarring, can develop. Blepharitis with a frothy tear film may be seen in tandem with dry eye.

13. What is Sjögren's syndrome?

Sjögren's syndrome is a triad of dry eye, dry mouth (xerostomia), and a collagen vascular disease. Rheumatoid arthritis is the most common, but systemic lupus erythematosus, Wegener's granulomatosis, scleroderma, systemic sclerosis, and primary biliary cirrhosis may also be associated. The lacrimal gland acini and ducts are damaged in the autoimmune disease. Ten percent of severe dry eye patients have Sjögren's syndrome.

14. How do you determine if a patient has Sjögren's syndrome?

Order anti-Sjögren's syndrome A antibody (SSA or anti-Ro), anti-Sjögren's syndrome B antibody (SSB or anti-La), rheumatoid factor, and antinuclear antibody. A biopsy of the lacrimal gland may be necessary. Then, refer to a rheumatologist for systemic evaluation and treatment.

15. Who gets dry eye?

Women are more likely than men to develop this, probably in relation to changes in hormone levels. It is also associated with birth control use. Contact lens wearers frequently have problems with dry eye, especially with long histories of contact lens use. Other likely risk factors include diabetes, rosacea, and thyroid disease.

It may be seen in all age groups, but it is most common after 60 years of age. It can occur in patients in their 20s and 30s but may be overlooked unless patients are specifically questioned about symptoms. However, dry eye is becoming more frequent in all ages because of increased screen use and the subsequent decreased blink rate. LASIK and blepharoplasty can exacerbate underlying dry eye. Radiation treatments can also cause dry eye. Many systemic medications have a side effect of dry eye.

16. What medications may be a cause of dry eye?

Topical eye drops such as those used in glaucoma can cause or worsen dry eye. The medication or the preservative may cause toxicity to the epithelial cells. Aminoglycoside antibiotics (i.e., Neosporin and gentamicin), β-blockers, and pilocarpine are common offenders.

Systemic medications that can decrease tear production include antimuscarinics (scopolamine, Detrol, anti-Parkinson's medications), antihistamines, lithium, diuretics, antiandrogens and estrogens (including birth control pills), antihypertensives (β-blockers, α-agonists), antidepressants, chemotherapy agents, antipsychotics, marijuana, and morphine.

17. What stains are used in dry eye diagnosis?

Fluorescein stains corneal and conjunctival epithelial defects. Rose bengal stains mucin and epithelial cells that are dead or devitalized, but still in place, as well as breaks in the tear film on the cornea or conjunctiva. Thus, rose bengal will show earlier, more subtle abnormalities in comparison to fluorescein. Lissamine green stains damaged or devitalized cells but does not stain healthy cells in contrast to the other two dyes.

18. How do you measure a tear breakup time?

Instill fluorescein into the lower fornix. Ask the patient to blink several times and then stop. The tear breakup time (TBUT) is the time from the last blink to the development of a dry spot noted by black spots in the fluorescein film. Normal is 10 or more seconds. It decreases with age, but less than 5 seconds is good evidence for dry eye. Meibomian gland dysfunction may show a TBUT of zero.

19. What is Schirmer's test?

A Schirmer's test filter strip is placed with the notched edge over the lid margin. The tear film in the lacrimal lake is absorbed over 5 minutes and measured. A normal Schirmer's test wets the strip 10 mm. Usually, it is done with topical anesthesia so as to not cause reflex tearing.

20. What other tests are done in dry eye patients?

Tear film osmolarity is elevated in patients with dry eye disease as well as other disease states such as bacterial conjunctivitis and meibomitis. Tear lactoferrin levels are low in dry eye disease. Matrix metalloproteinase-9 (MMP-9) is a marker of inflammation and elevated in tears in dry eye disease. Quick and simple in-office tests are available for all of these. Dry spots or irregular mires in corneal topography is suggestive of corneal surface disease. Tear meniscus height can estimate tear volume. Anything less than 0.25 mm is suggestive of dry eye. Tear film interferometry of the lipid layer of the tear film is used to grade tear film quality and estimate lipid layer thickness. The LipiView interferometer is commercially available and a noninvasive in-office test. It remains to be seen if the community at large will adopt any of these. They all give evidence to make a diagnosis of dry eye disease as well as objective markers to observe treatment effectiveness or failure.

21. How should patients be screened for dry eye?

A positive symptom score on the Dry Eye Questionnaire-5 (DEQ-5) (Fig. 11.1), Standard Patient Evaluation of Eye Dryness (SPEED) (Fig. 11.2), or Ocular Surface Disease Index (OSDI) (Fig. 11.3), should alert the practitioner to look more closely for dry eye disease. These have all been validated in clinical practice and can be used to judge improvement with treatment. If a patient has a reduced noninvasive TBUT, a large interocular disparity in osmolarity or ocular surface staining, dry eye disease is confirmed.

DEQ 5

1. Questions about **EYE DISCOMFORT:**

   a. During a typical day in the past month, **how often** did your eyes feel discomfort?

0	Never
1	Rarely
2	Sometimes
3	Frequently
4	Constantly

   b. When your eyes felt discomfort, **how intense was this feeling of discomfort** at the end of the day, within two hours of going to bed?

Never have it	Not at all intense				Very intense
0	1	2	3	4	5

2. Questions about **EYE DRYNESS:**

   a. During a typical day in the past month, **how often** did your eyes feel dry?

0	Never
1	Rarely
2	Sometimes
3	Frequently
4	Constantly

   b. When your eyes felt dry, **how intense was this feeling of dryness** at the end of the day, within two hours of going to bed?

Never have it	Not at all intense				Very intense
0	1	2	3	4	5

3. Questions about **WATERY EYES:**

   During a typical day in the past month, **how often** did your eyes look or feel excessively watery?

0	Never
1	Rarely
2	Sometimes
3	Frequently
4	Constantly

   Score: 1a + 1b + 2a + 2b + 3 = Total

   _____ + _____ + _____ + _____ + _____ = _____

Fig. 11.1 Five-item dry eye questionnaire (DEQ 5). (Copyright© Begley & Chalmers 2018, all rights reserved.)

SPEED™ QUESTIONNAIRE

Name: _____ Date: ___/___/___ Sex: M F (Circle) Date: ___/___/___

For the standardized patient evaluation of eye dryness (SPEED) questionnaire, please answer the following questions by checking the box that best represents your answer. Select only one answer per question.

1. Report the type of <u>SYMPTOMS</u> you experience and when they occur:

Symptoms	At this visit		Within past 72 hours		Within past 3 months	
	Yes	No	Yes	No	Yes	No
Dryness, grittiness or scratchiness						
Soreness or Irritation						
Burning or watering						
Eye fatigue						

2. Report the <u>FREQUENCY</u> of your symptoms using the rating list below:

Symptoms	0	1	2	3
Dryness, grittiness or scratchiness				
Soreness or Irritation				
Burning or watering				
Eye fatigue				

0 = Never   **1** = Sometimes   **2** = Often   **3** = Constant

3. Report the <u>SEVERITY</u> of your symptoms using the rating list below:

Symptoms	0	1	2	3	4
Dryness, grittiness or scratchiness					
Soreness or irritation					
Burning or watering					
Eye fatigue					

0 = No Problems
1 = Tolerable - not perfect, but not uncomfortable
2 = Uncomfortable- irritating, but does not interfere with my day
3 = Bothersome- irritating and interferes with my day
4 = Intolerable- unable to perform my daily tasks

4. Do you use eyedrops for lubrication?   ☐ YES ☐ NO   If yes, how often? _____

Cornea. 2013 Sep;32(9):1204–10

For office use only
Total SPEED score (frequency + severity) = _____/ 28

Fig. 11.2 Standard patient evaluation of eye dryness (Speed questionnaire). (Copyright © 2011 TearScience, Inc. All rights reserved.)

Ocular Surface Disease Index© (OSDI©)[2]

Ask your patients the following 12 questions, and circle the number in the box that best represents each answer. Then, fill in boxes A, B, C, D, and E according to the instructions beside each.

Have you experienced any of the following *during the last week?*	All of the time	Most of the time	Half of the time	Some of the time	None of the time
1. Eyes that are sensitive to light? . .	4	3	2	1	0
2. Eyes that feel gritty?	4	3	2	1	0
3. Painful or sore eyes?	4	3	2	1	0
4. Blurred vision?	4	3	2	1	0
5. Poor vision?	4	3	2	1	0

Subtotal score for answers 1 to 5 (A)

Have problems with your eyes limited you in performing any of the following *during the last week?*	All of the time	Most of the time	Half of the time	Some of the time	None of the time	N/A
6. Reading?.	4	3	2	1	0	N/A
7. Driving at night?	4	3	2	1	0	N/A
8. Working with a computer or bank machine (ATM)?	4	3	2	1	0	N/A
9. Watching TV?	4	3	2	1	0	N/A

Subtotal score for answers 6 to 9 (B)

Have your eyes felt uncomfortable in any of the following situations *during the last week?*	All of the time	Most of the time	Half of the time	Some of the time	None of the time	N/A
10. Windy conditions?	4	3	2	1	0	N/A
11. Places or areas with low humidity (very dry)?	4	3	2	1	0	N/A
12. Areas that are air conditioned? . . .	4	3	2	1	0	N/A

Subtotal score for answers 10 to 12 (C)

Add subtotals A, B, and C to obtain D
(D = sum of scores for all questions answered) (D)

Total number of questions answered
(do not include questions answered N/A) (E)

Please turn over the questionnaire to calculate the patient's final OSDI© score.

Fig. 11.3 A, B, Ocular surface disease index (OSDI). (Copyright © 1995 Allergan.)

Continued

Evaluating the OSDI© Score[1]

The OSDI© is assessed on a scale of 0 to 100, with higher scores representing greater disability. The index demonstrates sensitivity and specificity in distinguishing between normal subjects and patients with dry eye disease. The OSDI© is a valid and reliable instrument for measuring dry eye disease (normal, mild to moderate, and severe) and effect on vision-related function.

Assessing Your Patient's Dry Eye Disease[1,2]

Use your answers D and E from side 1 to compare the sum of scores for all questions answered (D) and the number of questions answered (E) with the chart below.* Find where your patient's score would fall. Match the corresponding shade of red to the key below to determine whether your patient's score indicates normal, mild, moderate, or severe dry eye disease.

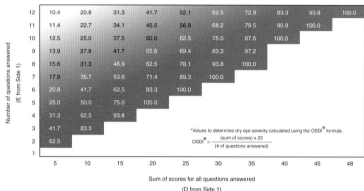

Patient 's Name: .... Date: ....

How long has the patient experienced dry eye disease? ....

Eye Care Professional 's Comments ....
....
....
....
....

1. Data on file, Allergan, Inc.
2. Schiffman RM, Christianson MD, Jacobsen G, Hirsch JD, Reis BL. Reliability and validity of the Ocular Surface Disease Index. *Arch Ophthalmol.* 2000; 118:615–621

Fig. 11.3, cont'd

22. What are the treatments for dry eye patients?

Dry eye is now recognized as a vicious cycle of tear film instability and hyperosmolarity causing ocular surface inflammation, damage, and sensory abnormalities. Hyperosmolarity is considered to be the trigger for a cascade of signaling effects in the corneal epithelial cells. This leads to a release of inflammatory mediators and proteases. The goal is to restore homeostasis.

The Tear Film and Ocular Surface Society (TFOS) Dry Eye Workshop (DEWS) II recommends a staged approach based on the presence or absence of symptoms with clinical signs (Box 11.1). Begin with patient education, environmental and dietary modifications, stopping any topical and/or systemic medications that might be worsening the symptoms, warm compresses, and blepharitis treatment. Start tear replacement therapy. They are used as needed depending on the patient's symptoms. Once or twice a day may be fine for some; others may need nearly

Box 11.1 DEWS II Staged Management and Treatment Recommendations

Step 1:

- Education regarding the condition, its management, treatment, and prognosis
- Modification of local environment
- Education regarding potential dietary modifications (including oral essential fatty acid supplementation)
- Identification and potential modification/elimination of offending systemic and topical medications
- Ocular lubricants of various types (if MGD is present, consider lipid-containing supplements)
- Lid hygiene and warm compresses of various types

Step 2:

If the previous options are inadequate, consider:

- Nonpreserved ocular lubricants to minimize preservative-induced toxicity
- Tea tree oil for *Demodex* (if present)
- Tear conservation
- Punctal occlusion
- Moisture chamber spectacles/goggles
- Overnight treatments (such as ointment or moisture chamber devices)
- In-office, physical heating and expression of the meibomian glands (including device-assisted therapies, such as LipiFlow, TearScience)
- In-office intense pulsed-light therapy for MGD
- Prescription drugs to manage DED
- Topical antibiotic or antibiotic/steroid combination applied to the lid margins for anterior blepharitis (if present)
- Topical corticosteroid (limited duration)
- Topical secretagogues
- Topical nonglucocorticoid immunomodulatory drugs (such as cyclosporine)
- Topical LFA-1 antagonist drugs (such as lifitegrast)
- Oral macrolide or tetracycline antibiotics

Step 3:

If previous options are inadequate, consider:

- Oral secretagogues
- Autologous/allogeneic serum eye drops
- Therapeutic contact lens options
- Soft bandage lenses
- Rigid scleral lenses

Step 4:

If previous options are inadequate, consider:

- Topical corticosteroid for longer duration
- Amniotic membrane grafts
- Surgical punctal occlusion
- Other surgical approaches (e.g., tarsorrhaphy, salivary gland transplantation)

DED, dry eye disease; *DEWS II*, Dry Eye Workshop II; *LFA*, lymphocyte function-associated antigen; *MGD*, Meibomian gland dysfunction.
Adapted and reprinted from Jones L, Downie LE, Korb D, et al.: TFOS DEWS II management and therapy report, *Ocular Surf* 580–634, 2017. Copyright © 2017, with permission from Elsevier.

every hour. Lacrisert is a solid form of artificial tear placed in the lower cul-de-sac that melts over a period of 12 hours. It is seldom used but can be very effective in a small number of patients. Patients should also be counseled to avoid conditions with low humidity such as central air heating, to prevent air from blowing into their eyes as from an air conditioner vent at home or in the car, and to use a humidifier while sleeping and at work if possible. Increased lubrication is often necessary during plane travel, as airplane cabins have very low humidity, and during periods of intense reading, driving, and screen use, as the blink reflex is decreased during concentration.

Dry eye patients may better tolerate newer contact lenses with a high-Dk and high water content. Daily disposable lenses are a good choice.

23. **What if the patient uses tears six to eight times a day and returns with red, painful eyes and more superficial punctate keratitis?**
The patient may be sensitive to the preservatives in the tears. In these patients, preservative-free tears may be necessary. Lubricating ointments can be used at night. It will blur vision but may be necessary during the day if exposure is a significant problem, as in Bell's palsy. If Meibomian gland disease is a factor, consider in-office heating and expression of the Meibomian gland (i.e., Lipiflow). Intense pulsed light therapy is showing promise for Meibomian gland disease in clinical use. Treatment of blepharitis with a steroid/antibiotic drop for short periods can help. Mild steroids can calm the inflammation of dry eye but should not be used for long periods because of the risk of cataract, infection, and a rise in intraocular pressure in some patients.

24. What if this is still not enough or the patient has a clinical exam that is worsening?

Punctal occlusion is an option. Patients who use tears every 2 hours or more may benefit from closing the lower puncta. Placement of a punctal plug can be easily done as an office procedure. Patients may notice local irritation for a short time, but this usually resolves. Occasionally, epiphora may result from overflow tearing and the plug can quickly be removed in the office. If the patient is comfortable with this, but the plug falls out, permanent closure can be done by using cautery. Between 10% and 20% of the tear film is drained through the upper puncta, and these may be closed subsequently if the lower lid punctal closure is not adequate to control symptoms. Of course, any lid contour abnormalities should be addressed as well (e.g., ectropion, lid laxity).

KEY POINTS: SEVERE DRY EYE

1. Frequent tear use may make symptoms worse if the patient is sensitive to the preservatives.
2. Occlude the lower lid puncta first and then proceed to upper lid punctal occlusion.
3. Cyclosporine may increase tear production, but it may take months to see results.
4. Lifitegrast may improve tear quality and decrease inflammation more quickly.
5. Dry eye must be treated prior to cataract surgery as an irregular tear film can dramatically change the measurements needed for intraocular lens determination as well as the quality of the vision.

25. A patient with punctal occlusion returns with more irritation and burning since the procedure was done. The tear film meniscus is greatly improved. What happened?

If a patient has significant blepharitis, the symptoms can worsen after punctal occlusion. The debris is trapped and not drained and now has a higher concentration than before. Make sure blepharitis is treated adequately before placing punctal plugs to prevent this.

26. Is there any treatment to increase tear production and improve tear quality?

Topical cyclosporine (Restasis) decreases cell-mediated inflammation of the lacrimal tissue and ultimately can increase tear production. Patients need to use it twice a day for 1 to 3 months to get a response and then continue for up to 6 months or more. Some practitioners are using a mild steroid four times a day for the first 2 weeks of Restasis to decrease inflammation and stinging until the cyclosporine begins to work.

Lifitegrast (Xiidra) is a topical lymphocyte function-associated antigen (LFA-1) antagonist that hinders T-cell activation and release of inflammatory mediators. It appears to inhibit the inflammatory pathways in dry eye disease. Some patients complain of a bad taste after instilling, it but punctal occlusion usually makes it tolerable. Patients may notice an improvement in symptoms faster with this medicine in comparison with cyclosporine.

27. What is the role of acetylcysteine?

Acetylcysteine is a mucolytic agent used to break up mucus in patients who have filamentary keratitis and mucous plaques.

28. What other agents are used in a patient severe of dry eye?

Other options are systemic cholinergic and anti-inflammatory agents, autologous serum tears, moisture chamber goggles, and a temporary or permanent lateral tarsorrhaphy. Rheumatologic evaluation may help elucidate the cause and coordinate systemic treatments. Many more treatments are on the horizon and in clinical testing.

29. What about patients who have symptoms but no clinical signs?

They may have preclinical ocular surface disease or neuropathic pain. Treat them initially as if they have dry eye, but if they do not respond, consider other strategies. Autologous serum tears may help with aberrant nerve regeneration. These patients often have peripheral neuropathic pain elsewhere and fibromyalgia; this can be part of a systemic complex pain syndrome. The intensity of the pain correlates with depression. Tricyclic antidepressants, nonsteroidal anti-inflammatory drugs (NSAIDs), dronabinol, tramadol, and gabapentin have been used with various measures of success. Botulinum toxin has been used in select cases for trigeminal neuralgia and may be applicable in these cases. Referral to a pain management specialist may be helpful.

BIBLIOGRAPHY

Abidi A, Shukla P, Ahman A: Lifitegrast: a novel drug for treatment of dry eye disease, J Pharmacol Pharmacother 7(4):194, 2016.

American Academy of Ophthalmology: Dry eye syndrome PPP—2018. https://www.aao.org/preferred-practice-pattern/dry-eye-syndrome-ppp-2018.

Chalmers RI, Begley CG, Caffery B: Validation of the 5-Item Dry Eye Questionnaire (DEQ-5): discrimination across self-assessed severity and aqueous tear deficient dry eye diagnosis, Cont Lens Anterior Eye 33:55-60, 2010.

Chow CYC, Gibard JP: Tear film. In Krachmer JG, Mannis MJ, Holland EJ, editors: Cornea, vol. 1, St. Louis, 1997, Mosby, pp 49–60.

Craig J, Nichols K, Akpek E, et al.: TFOS DEWS II definition and classification report, Ocul Surf 15:276, 2017.

Fox FI: Systemic diseases associated with dry eye, Int Ophthalmol Clin 34:71–87, 1994.

Goyal S, Hamrah P: Understanding neuropathic corneal pain—gaps and current therapeutic approaches, Semin Ophthalmol 31(1–2):50–70, 2016.

Jones L, Downie L, Korb D, et al.: TFOS DEWS II management and therapy report, Ocul Surf 15:575, 2017.

Kanski J: Clinical ophthalmology: a systematic approach, Edinburgh, 2003, Butterworth-Heinemann.

Lemp MA: Definition and Classification Subcommittee of the International Dry Eye Workshop, Ocul Surf 5:77, 2007.

Lemp MA: Report of the national eye institute/industry workshop on clinical trials in dry eyes, CLAO J 21:221–232, 1996.

Ngo W, Situ P, Kier N, Korb D, Blackie C, Simpson T: Psychometric properties and validation of the Standard Patient Evaluation of Eye Dryness Questionnaire, Cornea 32:1204, 2013.

Sall K, Stevenson OD, Mundorf TK, Reis BL: Two multicenter, randomized studies of the efficacy and safety of cyclosporine ophthalmic emulsion in moderate to severe dry eye disease. CsA phase 3 study group, Ophthalmology 107:1220, 2000.

Schiffman R, Christianson M, Jacobsen G, Hirsch J, Reis B: Reliability and validity of the Ocular Surface Disease Index, Arch Ophthalmol 118:614, 2000.

Stevenson D, Tauber J, Reis BL: Efficacy and safety of cyclosporine A ophthalmic emulsion in the treatment of moderate-to-severe dry eye disease: a dose-ranging, randomized trial. The Cyclosporine A Phase 2 Study Group, Ophthalmology 107:967–974, 2000.

Tu EY, Rheinstrom S: Dry eye. In Yanoff M, Duker JS, editors: Ophthalmology, ed 2, St. Louis, 2004, Mosby, pp 520–526.

CHAPTER 12

CORNEAL DYSTROPHIES

Sadeer B. Hannush and Lorena Riveroll-Hannush

1. **What are corneal dystrophies?**
Corneal dystrophies are bilateral, inherited, noninflammatory, commonly progressive alterations of the cornea that are usually not associated with any other systemic condition. Most corneal dystrophies are autosomal dominant disorders presenting after birth. Because each dystrophy may exhibit a spectrum of clinical manifestations, examining multiple family members frequently aids in establishing the diagnosis.

2. **How do degenerations differ from dystrophies?**
In contrast to dystrophies, degenerations are unilateral or bilateral aging changes that are not inherited. They are also not associated with systemic disease.

3. **Discuss the general anatomic classification of corneal dystrophies.**
   - **Anterior membrane dystrophies** include disorders affecting the corneal epithelium, epithelial basement membrane (Fig. 12.1), and Bowman's layer.
   - **Stromal dystrophies** occur anywhere in the stromal layer of the cornea between Bowman's layer and Descemet's membrane (DM).
   - **Posterior membrane dystrophies** are primarily abnormalities of the endothelium and DM.

KEY POINTS: DIFFERENCES BETWEEN CORNEAL DYSTROPHIES AND DEGENERATIONS

1. Corneal dystrophies are always bilateral.
2. They are inherited.
3. They may present shortly after birth.

4. **What is the International Committee for Classification of Corneal Dystrophies?**
The International Committee for Classification of Corneal Dystrophies (IC3D) was created in 2008 to study what genetic analyses had brought to light and the relations between genetic abnormalities and their phenotypic description available at the time. Members of The Cornea Society assigned a category number from 1 to 4 to each one of the known dystrophies, reflecting the "level of evidence" of its existence. All dystrophies were given names, alternative names, and eponyms; their Mendelian inheritance in humans, genetic locus, and gene; their onset, signs, symptoms, and course; their light microscopy, transmission electron microscopy, immunohistochemistry, and confocal microscopy findings; and a category.

  All anterior membrane dystrophies are autosomal dominant. Examples are Meesmann's juvenile epithelial dystrophy, epithelial basement membrane dystrophy, and corneal dystrophies of Bowman's layer.

5. **Which is the most common anterior membrane dystrophy? Which dystrophy is strictly epithelial?**
Epithelial basement membrane dystrophy is by far the most common anterior membrane dystrophy. In fact, it has the highest prevalence of all of the corneal dystrophies. Areas of extra basement membrane result in map-like and/or fingerprint changes as well as intraepithelial microcysts. Five percent of otherwise normal corneas have been observed to have such changes. Of interest, many cornea specialists no longer consider epithelial basement membrane disease (EBMD) a dystrophy, especially in view of its prevalence in patients with chronic blepharitis. EBMD behaves more like a degeneration.

  Second in prevalence are the corneal dystrophies of the Bowman's layer (CDBs): Reis-Bücklers (CDB-I) and Thiel-Behnke honeycomb-shaped dystrophy (CDB-II). These disorders consist of gray reticular opacities beneath the epithelium.

  Meesmann's dystrophy is the rarest of the three and is strictly epithelial. This disorder, noted in the first few years of life, presents as a bilaterally symmetric pattern of microcysts or vesicles seen strictly in the epithelial layer of the cornea, usually in the interpalpebral fissure.

6. **What are the most common presenting symptoms of anterior membrane dystrophies?**
First are the symptoms associated with corneal erosions—pain, foreign body sensation, photophobia, and tearing, especially with opening of the lids during sleep or upon awakening in the morning. Erosions are most common in the setting of epithelial basement membrane dystrophy. The second symptom is blurred vision secondary to

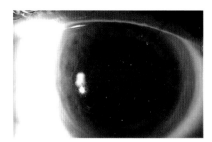

Fig. 12.1 Typical mare's tail sign in epithelial basement membrane dystrophy.

either irregularity of the surface, seen in epithelial basement membrane dystrophy, or corneal clouding, frequently seen in the dystrophies of Bowman's layer or Meesmann's dystrophy.

7. **Discuss treatment options for recurrent corneal erosions associated with anterior membrane dystrophies.**
   The conservative approach includes the generous use of lubricating eyedrops during the day and ointments at night. Some physicians advocate the use of topical steroids to stabilize the basement membrane, and others advocate hypertonic saline, especially in ointment form at night to dehydrate the epithelium and aid in its attachment to the underlying layers. Patching, either conventional or with collagen or bandage contact lenses, hypothetically decreases the mechanical effect of lid movement on the already weakened corneal epithelium. Again, some physicians have used amniotic membrane devices to aid with comfort and healing, but there is no evidence that these offer any advantage over a conventional bandage contact lens in a neuro-competent cornea. Recalcitrant cases may require surgical intervention.

KEY POINTS: RECURRENT CORNEAL EROSIONS

1. Recurrent corneal erosions may be associated with anterior membrane and stromal dystrophies.
2. They have common symptoms: pain, blurred vision, and photophobia.
3. Recurrent corneal erosions are frequently amenable to medical therapy with lubrication and hyperosmotic agents.
4. They can be treated surgically with mechanical or laser keratectomy or stromal puncture.

8. **Discuss the role of surgery in the treatment of anterior membrane dystrophies.**
   In the setting of recalcitrant corneal erosions, mechanical debridement of the loose epithelium and basement membrane or anterior stromal puncture, together with the use of a bandage lens, may aid in re-epithelialization of the surface and adherence of the epithelium to the underlying layers. Mechanical debridement also may be used to remove an irregular epithelial basement membrane if an associated visual decline is noted. Typically, these patients do not have symptoms of corneal erosion but complain of blurred vision. Topography reveals marked irregularity of the Placido rings. Removal of the abnormal epithelium and basement membrane can restore normal anterior corneal anatomy paralleled by improvement in vision. For Bowman's layer dystrophies, a more aggressive superficial or lamellar keratectomy may be required. This may be microkeratome assisted. Lamellar keratoplasty may also be considered.

9. **Do lasers have a role?**
   The yttrium–aluminum–garnet (YAG) laser has been used instead of a needle to accomplish anterior stromal puncture but does not offer a clear advantage. The excimer laser has been used for treatment of recurrent erosions associated with basement membrane dystrophies and for removal of deeper layers in conditions such as Reis-Bücklers' and Thiel-Behnke dystrophies (phototherapeutic keratectomy). Although in the first instance the excimer laser may not offer a clear advantage over mechanical debridement except in possibly allowing for better epithelial adherence, in the second, it has supplanted manual lamellar keratectomy as the treatment of choice. Microkeratome-assisted lamellar keratectomy may be equally effective.

10. **What controversy surrounds the dystrophies affecting the Bowman's layer?**
    Until recently, there has been some confusion over dystrophies affecting the Bowman's layer because they present with two different sets of characteristics, but historically they have been lumped under Reis-Bücklers' dystrophy. The first set was described by Reis in 1917 and later by Bücklers in 1949 and the second by Thiel and Behnke in 1967. Küchle et al. divided the Bowman's membrane dystrophies into two classifications: corneal dystrophy of the Bowman's layer type I and type II. Type I is synonymous with the original Reis-Bücklers' dystrophy and equivalent to what also has been described as superficial variant of granular dystrophy. Type II is

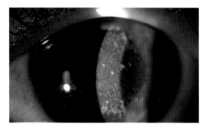

Fig. 12.2 Slit lamp appearance of granular dystrophy.

Table 12.1 Clinical Features of the Three Major Stromal Dystrophies

	Age of Onset		
FEATURE	**GRANULAR DYSTROPHY**	**LATTICE DYSTROPHY**	**MACULAR DYSTROPHY**
Deposits	First decade	First decade	First decade
Symptoms	Third decade or none	Second decade	First decade
Decreased vision	Fourth or fifth decade	Second or third decade	First or second decade
Erosions	Uncommon	Frequent	Common
Corneal thickness	Normal	Normal	Thinned
Opacities	Discrete with sharp borders and clear intervening stroma early but becoming hazy later, not extending to the limbus	Refractile lines and subepithelial spots, diffuse central haze, not extending to the limbus except in advanced cases	Indistinct margins with hazy stroma between, extending to the limbus; central lesions more anterior and peripheral lesions more posterior

honeycomb shaped and is also known as the Thiel-Behnke corneal dystrophy. The two dystrophies have slightly different characteristics on light microscopy. Transmission electron microscopy, on the other hand, differentiates them unequivocally.

11. Describe the inheritance patterns of the stromal dystrophies.
    - **Autosomal dominant:** Granular (Groenouw type I; Fig. 12.2), lattice, Avellino granular–lattice, Schnyder's crystalline, fleck, central cloudy dystrophy of François, pre-Descemet, congenital hereditary (stromal), and posterior amorphous dystrophies
    - **Autosomal recessive:** Macular (Groenouw type II) and possibly gelatinous drop-like dystrophies
      Note: these have been revised and altered with the publication and revision of IC3D in 2008 and 2015, respectively.

12. Match the stromal dystrophy with the histochemical stain for the accumulated substance.
    - **Granular:** Masson trichrome stains hyaline.
    - **Lattice:** Congo red stains amyloid (amyloid deposits exhibit polarized light birefringence and dichrois).
    - **Macular:** Alcian blue stains mucopolysaccharides (glycosaminoglycans).
    - Lattice and macular dystrophies also stain with periodic acid–Schiff stain.

13. Describe the clinical features of the three major stromal dystrophies.
    See Table 12.1.

14. Is lattice dystrophy associated with systemic amyloidosis?
    There are three types of lattice dystrophy. Only type II (Meretoja's syndrome or familial amyloid polyneuropathy type IV), which has less corneal involvement than type I or III, is associated with systemic findings, including blepharochalasis, bilateral facial nerve palsies, peripheral neuropathy, and systemic amyloidosis.

15. What is the differential diagnosis of corneal stromal crystals? What systemic findings are associated with Schnyder's crystalline dystrophy?
    The differential diagnosis of corneal stromal crystals includes Bietti's peripheral crystalline dystrophy, cystinosis, and dysproteinemias, such as multiple myeloma, Waldenstrom's macroglobulinemia, and benign monoclonal gammopathy.

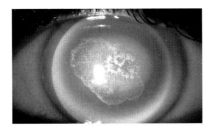

Fig. 12.3 Schnyder's crystalline stromal dystrophy.

Schnyder's dystrophy (Fig. 12.3) is strongly associated with hypercholesterolemia with or without hypertriglyceridemia. There is no direct association with primary hyperlipidemias, and serum lipid levels do not correlate with the density of the corneal opacities. The dystrophy more likely represents a localized defect in cholesterol metabolism. Of importance, not all patients with Schnyder's dystrophy have clinical evidence of corneal crystalline deposits.

16. How does central cloudy dystrophy of François differ from posterior crocodile shagreen?
    Although some physicians have argued that the location of the lesions differs in the two conditions, the lesions are clinically the same. It is generally accepted that the polygonal "cracked-ice" lesions of the central cloudy dystrophy of François are more central, deeper, and, by definition, bilateral with an inheritance pattern. On the other hand, posterior crocodile shagreen is more commonly peripheral and anterior stromal and is classified as degeneration. Of importance, both conditions are associated with normal corneal thickness and no recurrent erosions or significant visual compromise.

17. What characterizes Avellino dystrophy?
    Avellino dystrophy also has been called granular–lattice dystrophy. The granular deposits occur in the anterior stroma early in the progression of the condition, followed later by lattice-like lesions in the mid to posterior stroma and finally by anterior stromal haze. More patients with Avellino dystrophy experience recurrent erosions than patients with typical granular dystrophy. The disease-causing genes of lattice dystrophy type I, granular dystrophy, Avellino dystrophy, and Reis-Bücklers' dystrophy have been mapped to chromosome 5q, suggesting one of the following possibilities:
    • A corneal gene family exists in this region.
    • These corneal dystrophies represent allelic heterogeneity (i.e., different mutations within the same gene manifest as different phenotypes).
    • They are the same disease.

18. How are stromal dystrophies treated?
    To the extent that some dystrophies, such as lattice and Avellino, are associated with recurrent erosions, they are treated as discussed earlier. When the lesions obscure vision and are restricted to the anterior third of the stroma, they are usually amenable to manual lamellar, microkeratome-assisted lamellar, or phototherapeutic keratectomy with the excimer laser. If the lesions are deeper, lamellar or penetrating keratoplasty (PK) is necessary.

19. Is keratoplasty a definitive treatment?
    Deep anterior lamellar keratoplasty (DALK) offers the advantage of preserving the host DM and endothelium. PK may be considered as well, especially if the surgeon is not comfortable with the DALK technique. Both keratoplasty techniques are associated with recurrence of the pathology in the graft as early as 1 year after surgery. The recurrent pathology is sometimes milder than in the original cornea but may require regrafting not infrequently (Fig. 12.4).

KEY POINTS: KERATOPLASTY

1. DALK is the procedure of choice for stromal dystrophies with deep stromal involvement not amenable to surgical or phototherapeutic keratectomy.
2. Endothelial keratoplasty (Descemet stripping endothelial keratoplasty or Descemet membrane endothelial keratoplasty) is the procedure of choice for posterior membrane dystrophies.
3. PK may also be considered for stromal or posterior membrane dystrophies, especially when the surgeon is not familiar with the anterior and posterior keratoplasty techniques.
4. DALK and PK do not prevent recurrence of stromal dystrophies in the donor graft.

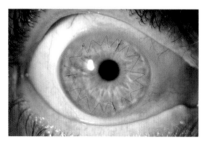

Fig. 12.4 Appearance of the eye after penetrating keratoplasty.

20. Name the three posterior membrane dystrophies.
    • Posterior polymorphous dystrophy (PPMD)
    • Fuchs' endothelial dystrophy
    • Congenital hereditary endothelial dystrophy (CHED)

21. What is their common clinical manifestation?
    All three essentially share the pathway of corneal edema and increased corneal thickness, resulting in visual compromise.

22. Describe the inheritance patterns of the three posterior membrane dystrophies.
    Posterior polymorphous and Fuchs' dystrophies have an autosomal dominant inheritance pattern. Two forms of CHED exist. The autosomal dominant form presents in early childhood and is slowly progressive and frequently symptomatic. The autosomal recessive form presents at birth and is nonprogressive, but it is associated with significant visual compromise and nystagmus due to marked corneal edema.

23. Describe the main clinical characteristics of the three posterior membrane dystrophies.
    See Table 12.2.

24. How does Fuchs' dystrophy differ from cornea guttata?
    Cornea guttata basically refers to a pattern of corneal guttae that are usually found on the central cornea. They sometimes coalesce, produce a beaten-metal appearance, and are associated with increased pigmentation. This condition does affect vision, although not significantly. In 1910, Fuchs described a more severe form of the condition associated with stromal thickening and epithelial edema with secondary marked visual compromise (Fig. 12.5). This represents an advanced stage of the same dystrophy.

Table 12.2 Main Clinical Characteristics of the Three Posterior Membrane Dystrophies

FEATURE	PPMD	FUCHS' DYSTROPHY	CHED
Onset	Second to third decade, rarely at birth	Fifth to sixth decade	Birth to first decade
Corneal findings	Vesicles, diffuse opacities, and corneal edema	Guttae, stromal thickening, epithelial edema, and subepithelial fibrosis	Endothelium rarely visible with marked corneal thickening and opacification
Other ocular abnormalities	Peripheral synechiae, iris atrophy/corectopia, and glaucoma	Narrow angles and glaucoma	None
Differential diagnosis	ICE syndrome, early-onset CHED	Pseudoguttae, Chandler's syndrome, herpes simplex keratitis, aphakic or pseudophakic bullous keratopathy, and other guttate conditions	Congenital glaucoma, metabolic opacification, Peters' anomaly, forceps injury, early-onset PPMD, and infectious etiologies

CHED, Congenital hereditary endothelial dystrophy; *ICE*, iridocorneal endothelial syndrome; *PPMD*, posterior polymorphous dystrophy.

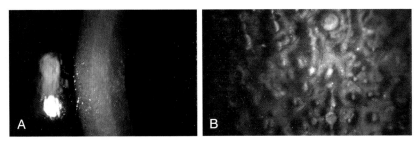

Fig. 12.5 A, Slit lamp photo of cornea with advanced Fuchs' dystrophy. **B,** Confocal microscopy of guttate changes in Fuchs' dystrophy.

25. Describe the workup of a patient with Fuchs' dystrophy.
    • History: Ask about previous intraocular surgery
    • Biomicroscopic examination: Guttae on the posterior corneal surface, increased stromal thickness, and epithelial edema with possible subepithelial bullae
    • Intraocular pressure measurement
    • Ultrasound, optical, or optical coherence tomography (OCT) pachymetry
    • Specular microscopy to evaluate number, size, and shape of endothelial cells
    • Anterior segment OCT to characterize the appearance of the cornea on a subclinical level. High-resolution and ultrahigh-resolution OCT is new technology that enables mapping of corneal morphology with an axial resolution of 2–3 microns.

26. What overlapping features are seen in posterior polymorphous dystrophy and iridocorneal endothelial syndromes?
    The overlapping features of PPMD and iridocorneal endothelial syndrome (ICE) are abnormal corneal endothelium, peripheral anterior synechiae, corectopia, and glaucoma.

27. What is unique about the congenital hereditary endothelial dystrophy cornea?
    The CHED cornea shows markedly increased corneal thickness, sometimes above 1,000 microns, unlike any other corneal dystrophy.

28. Discuss the management and prognosis of posterior membrane dystrophies.
    Conservative management has a role, especially in the earlier stages of Fuchs' dystrophy. Topical hypertonic saline solution, dehydration of the cornea with a blow dryer, and reduction of intraocular pressure may decrease corneal edema and improve vision. Bandage contact lenses may be used in the setting of recurrent erosions or subepithelial bullae. However, when vision is significantly compromised by Fuchs' or other posterior membrane dystrophies, the definitive solution is endothelial keratoplasty (Descemet stripping endothelial keratoplasty [DSEK] or Descemet membrane endothelial keratoplasty [DMEK]). DSEK involves transplantation of a layer of donor posterior stroma with DM and endothelium (Fig. 12.6A–C). DMEK is a pure anatomic replacement of the host DM and endothelium with healthy donor tissue. This is surgically challenging because of the very thin nature of the donor tissue (15 to 20 μm) (Fig. 12.6D–G). Keratoplasty, endothelial or penetrating, has the best prognosis in Fuchs' dystrophy, especially in the absence of glaucoma; a fairly good prognosis in PPMD in the absence of glaucoma; and a guarded prognosis in CHED, especially in the early pediatric age group. Recently, a procedure named Descemet stripping only (DSO) has gained popularity. In Fuchs' dystrophy, the visually significant corneal guttae are usually concentrated centrally, while the peripheral endothelium is healthy. The concept behind DSO is to denude the central 4 mm of the cornea's posterior surface of visually significant guttae, allowing the peripheral corneal endothelium to migrate centrally and clear the temporary corneal edema through their pump function (Fig. 12.7). Going forward, a significant amount of work is being done on the replacement of abnormal or deficient host endothelium with injected cultured cells together with the use of a rho kinase (ROCK) inhibitor... much to look forward to!

29. Can posterior polymorphous dystrophy recur in the graft?
    Recurrence of PPMD has been reported.

30. Discuss the considerations for combined cataract extraction and corneal transplantation in patients with Fuchs' dystrophy.
    • **First scenario: Visually significant cataract and borderline corneal function.** The decision whether to perform corneal transplantation at the time of cataract extraction (CE) may be based on a number of factors, including appearance of the corneal endothelium by specular microscopy, corneal thickness, vision variation throughout the day, and postoperative visual requirements of the patient. Patients with no evidence of frank stromal edema, including absence of morning blur and a stable central corneal thickness less than 620 μm, are likely to tolerate CE alone. The risk of corneal decompensation is outweighed by the advantage of rapid

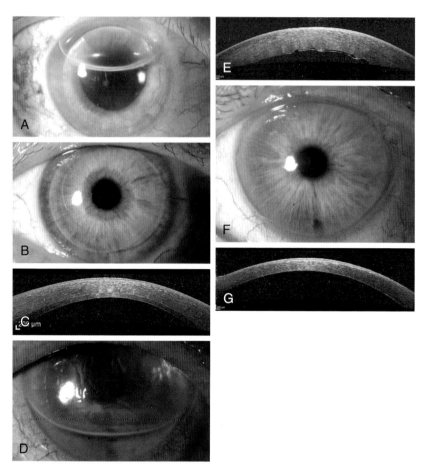

Fig. 12.6 A, One day after Descemet stripping endothelial keratoplasty (DSEK). Postoperative bubble allows one to check the border and adherence of the graft. **B,** 1 week after DSEK. The border of the graft is visible. **C,** Anterior segment optical coherence tomography (OCT) of the cornea after DSEK. **D,** One day after Descemet's membrane endothelial keratoplasty (DMEK). **E,** Anterior segment OCT 1 day after DMEK with Descemet's membrane almost indistinguishable, showing in complete adherence of the graft. **F,** One month after DMEK. **G,** Anterior segment OCT 1 month after DMEK.

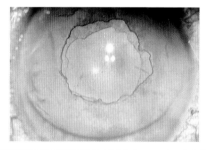

Fig. 12.7 Immediately after Descemet stripping only showing the central 4-mm area denuded of guttae compared to the surrounding cornea.

visual rehabilitation from cataract surgery alone. The patient understands the possibility of corneal decompensation after cataract surgery requiring endothelial keratoplasty secondarily. On the other hand, in patients with frank stromal edema, central corneal thickness greater than 650 μm, or an increase of more than 10% in corneal thickness in the morning compared with later in the day, the cornea is unlikely to tolerate routine CE. The patient will benefit from a triple procedure (i.e., CE with implant combined with keratoplasty, usually DSEK or DMEK). Having said that, most surgeons are opting to offer their patients with early, but visually significant Fuchs' dystrophy and cataract the modern triple procedure, which includes endothelial keratoplasty (DSEK or DMEK) combined with CE and intraocular lens (IOL) implantation, because of the high success of and the rapid visual rehabilitation after this combined procedure.

- **Second scenario: Corneal edema requiring corneal transplantation and mild to moderate cataract.** With the wide acceptance of DSEK and DMEK as the preferred procedures for the surgical management of visually significant Fuchs' dystrophy, together with the predictability of the refractive outcome when combined with CE and IOL implantation, more triple corneal procedures (DSEK or DMEK + CE/IOL) are being performed for corneal endothelial disease and even early cataract. Some surgeons, however, prefer to stage the procedures, starting with endothelial keratoplasty, followed a few months later, when the cornea is stable physiologically and refractively, with CE/IOL. Especially in the presence of corneal epithelial microcystic edema, this approach allows for clearing of the cornea and more accurate biometry before cataract surgery, giving the patient the best chance for good vision postoperatively and the opportunity to select a toric or presbyopia-correcting IOL implant. The incidence of graft decompensation after secondary CE/IOL is small.

31. List some interesting trivia about corneal dystrophy.
- The apostrophe in Fuchs' dystrophy is after the "s," not before.
- In cornea guttata, guttata is the adjective describing the cornea. The actual excrescences of DM between the endothelial cells are corneal guttae, not corneal guttata.
- Although keratoconus is usually bilateral and may have an inheritance pattern, it is considered an ectasia, not a dystrophy.
- Dua's layer (pre-Descemet layer [PDL]) is a structure in the posterior stroma, 5 to 8 collagen lamellae and 5 to 16 μm thick, devoid of keratocytes, and with a high bursting pressure reaching 750 mm Hg.
- When the DM is stripped off, the posterior stroma it always scrolls endothelial side out!

WEBSITES

1. www.corneasociety.org
2. www.nkcf.org
3. www.cornealdystrophyfoundation.org

BIBLIOGRAPHY

Adamis AP, Filatov V, Tripathi BJ, Tripathi RC: Fuchs' endothelial dystrophy of the cornea, Surv Ophthalmol 38:149–168, 1993.
Aldave AJ, Yellore VS, Self CA, Holsclaw D, Small K: The usefulness of buccal swabs for mutation screening in patients with suspected corneal dystrophies, Ophthalmology 111:1407–1409, 2004.
Aldave AJ, Han J, Frausto RF: Genetics of the corneal endothelial dystrophies: an evidence based review, Clin Genet 84(2):109–119, 2013.
Arffa RC: Grayson's diseases of the cornea, ed 4, St. Louis, Mosby.
Casey TA, Sharif KW: A color atlas of corneal dystrophies and degenerations, London, Wolfe Publishing.
Cheng JI, Qi X, Zhao J, Zhai H, Xie L: Comparison of penetrating keratoplasty and deep lamellar keratoplasty for macular corneal dystrophy and risk factors of recurrence, Ophthalmology 120(1):34–39, 2013.
Coleman CM, Hannush S, Covello SP, et al.: A novel mutation in the helix termination motif of keratin K12 in a U.S. family with Meesmann corneal dystrophy, Am J Ophthalmol 128:687–691, 1999.
Cullom RD, Chang B, editors: The wills eye manual: Wills Eye Hospital office and emergency room diagnosis and treatment of eye disease, ed 6, Philadelphia, J.B. Lippincott Williams & Wilkins.
Dinh R, Rapuano CJ, Cohen EJ, Laibson PR: Recurrence of corneal dystrophy after excimer laser phototherapeutic keratectomy, Ophthalmology 106:1490–1497, 1999.
Dua HS, Faraj LA, Said DG, et al.: Human corneal anatomy redefined, Ophthalmology 120:1778–1785, 2013.
Kim MJ, Frausto RF, Rosenwasser GOD, et al.: Posterior amorphous corneal dystrophy is associated with a deletion of small leucine-rich proteoglycans on chromosome 12, PLoS One 9(4):e95037, 2014.
Kinoshita S, Koizumi N, Ueno M: Cultured cells and ROCK inhibitor for bullous keratopathy, N Engl J Med 379(12):1185, 2018.
Klintworth GK: Advances in the molecular genetics of corneal dystrophies, Am J Ophthalmol 128:747–754, 1999.
Krachmer JH, Palay DA: Cornea color atlas, expert consult, ed 3, St. Louis, Mosby.
Krachmer JH, Mannis MJ, Holland EJ: Cornea, St. Louis, Mosby.
Kruse FE, Laaser K, Cursiefen C, et al.: A stepwise approach to donor preparation and insertion increases safety and outcome of Descemet membrane endothelial keratoplasty, Cornea 30(5):580–587, 2011.
Küchle M, Green WR, Volcker HE, Barraquer J: Reevaluation of corneal dystrophies of Bowman's layer and the anterior stroma (Reis-Bücklers and Thiel-Behnke types): a light and electron microscopic study of eight corneas and review of the literature, Cornea 14:333–354, 1995.

Moloney G, Iovieno A, Colby KA: Cornea 37(4):e21–e22, 2018.

Paparo LG, Rapuano CJ, Raber IM, et al.: Phototherapeutic keratectomy for Schnyder's crystalline corneal dystrophy, Cornea 19: 343–347, 2000.

Pineros OE, Cohen EJ, Rapuano CJ, Laibson PR: Triple versus nonsimultaneous procedures in Fuchs' dystrophy and cataract, Arch Ophthalmol 114:525–528, 1996.

Price MO, Gorovoy M, Price FW Jr, Benetz BA, Menegay HJ, Lass JH: Descemet's stripping automated endothelial keratoplasty: three-year graft and endothelial cell survival compared with penetrating keratoplasty, Ophthalmology 120(2):246–251, 2013.

Ridgway AE, Akhtar S, Munier FL, et al.: Ultrastructural and molecular analysis of Bowman's layer corneal dystrophies: an epithelial origin, Invest Ophthalmol Vis Sci 41:3286–3292, 2000.

Seitz B, Lisch W: Corneal dystrophies, developments in ophthalmology, vol 48, Karger.

Small KW, Mullen L, Barletta J, et al.: Mapping of Reis-Bucklers' corneal dystrophy to chromosome 5q, Am J Ophthalmol 121:384–390, 1996.

Stone EM: Three autosomal dominant corneal dystrophies mapped to chromosome 5q, Nat Genet 6:47–51, 1994.

Terry MA, Shamie N, Chen ES, et al.: Endothelial keratoplasty for Fuchs' dystrophy with cataract: complications and clinical results with the new triple procedure, Ophthalmology 116(4):631–639, April 2009.

von Marchtaler PV, Weller JM, Kruse FE, et al.: Air versus sulfur hexafluoride gas tamponade in Descemet membrane endothelial keratoplasty: a fellow eye comparison, Cornea 37(1):15–19, 2018.

Waring GO, Rodriguez MM, Laibson RR: Corneal dystrophies. I: dystrophies of epithelium, Bowman's layer and stroma, Surv Ophthalmol 23:71–122, 1978.

Waring GO, Rodriguez MM, Laibson RR: Corneal dystrophies. II: endothelial dystrophies, Surv Ophthalmol 23:147–168, 1978.

Weiss JS, Møller HU, Aldave A, et al.: IC3D classification of corneal dystrophies, edition 2, Cornea 34:117–159, 2015.

Weiss JS, Moller HU, Lisch W, et al.: The IC3D classification of the corneal dystrophies, Cornea 27(2):S1–S42, 2008.

Woo JH, Ang M, Htoon HM, et al.: Descemet membrane endothelial keratoplasty versus Descemet stripping automated endothelial keratoplasty and penetrating keratoplasty, Am J Ophthalmol 207:288–303, 2019.

CHAPTER 13

KERATOCONUS

Irving Raber

1. **What is keratoconus?**

   Keratoconus is a noninflammatory ectatic disorder of the cornea that leads to variable visual impairment. The cornea becomes steepened and thinned, thereby inducing myopia and irregular astigmatism. In advanced stages, the cornea assumes a conical shape, hence the term *keratoconus*. The condition is usually bilateral, although frequently asymmetric.

2. **Who gets keratoconus?**

   It is difficult to estimate the incidence of keratoconus because the diagnosis is easily overlooked, especially in the early stages. In a recent meta-analysis, the prevalence of keratoconus in the entire population was 1.38 per 1000 population. The highest reported prevalence, 47.9 per 1000, was reported in a Saudi population, while the lowest, 0.17 per 1000, was reported in an American population. Some studies report a female predominance, whereas other studies report a male predominance. There is no known racial predilection.

3. **What is the cause of keratoconus?**

   The cause of keratoconus is unknown. The etiology is multifactorial with both genetic and environmental factors playing a role. Various biochemical abnormalities have been documented in keratoconic corneas, including reduced collagen content, decreased or altered keratin sulfate molecules, reduced total protein and increased nonproteinaceous material, and increased collagenolytic and gelatinolytic activity associated with reduced matrix metalloproteinase inhibitor levels. Several studies have shown that the enzyme and proteinase inhibitor abnormalities are most prominent in the epithelial layer of the cornea. This suggests that the basic defect in keratoconus may reside in the epithelium and its interaction with the stroma. Additional studies implicate abnormal processing of free radicals and superoxide within keratoconus corneas leading to buildup of destructive aldehydes and/or peroxynitrites. Eye rubbing has been implicated as a cause of keratoconus. When asked, patients with keratoconus will frequently admit to excessive eye rubbing.

4. **What is the relationship between contact lens wear and keratoconus?**

   The relationship between contact lens wear and keratoconus is controversial. Circumstantial evidence suggests that contact lens wear may lead to the development of keratoconus, especially long-term use of rigid contact lenses. Such patients tend to present at an older age and have a flatter corneal curvature than typical patients with keratoconus. In addition, the so-called contact lens–induced cones tend to be more centrally located in the cornea than the more typical cones, which are characteristically decentered inferiorly.

   Contact lens warpage is diagnosed when contact lens wear induces irregular astigmatism without the slit lamp features of keratoconus. Discontinuing lens wear for weeks to months eliminates the irregular astigmatism and allows the cornea to resume its normal shape, whereas in the so-called contact lens–induced keratoconus, the changes are permanent and do not resolve when contact lens wear is discontinued.

   Some contact lens practitioners are of the opinion that contact lenses can be used to flatten the cornea and reverse or at least retard further progression of keratoconus. However, I believe that corneal flattening induced by contact lens wear in patients with keratoconus is temporary and that the cornea ultimately reverts to its pre–contact lens shape once lens wear is discontinued.

5. **Is keratoconus hereditary?**

   The role of heredity in keratoconus has not been clearly defined. The majority of cases occur sporadically with no familial history. However, some cases of keratoconus are transmitted within families. One study used corneal topography to diagnose subclinical cases of keratoconus. Familial transmission was documented in 7 of 12 families (58.3%) of patients with keratoconus and no known family history of corneal or ocular disease. The authors postulate autosomal dominant inheritance with incomplete penetrance as the mode of transmission. Other studies report that 6% to 25% of keratoconus patients have a positive family history, and there are numerous reports of concordance between monozygotic twins and discordance between dizygotic twins. Autosomal recessive inheritance has been suggested in a few studies with high consanguinity. Numerous genetic loci have been mapped in keratoconus families, but the roles of these gene loci are inconclusive, and as of 2021, no genetic mutations have been confirmed. It may be that there are multiple genes involved in the development of keratoconus. Genetic heterogeneity may also be involved in keratoconus, wherein different gene abnormalities manifest a similar phenotype.

6. **What systemic conditions are associated with keratoconus?**

   There is a definite relationship between atopy and keratoconus. The prevalence of atopic diseases, such as asthma, eczema, atopic keratoconjunctivitis, and hay fever, is higher in patients with keratoconus than in normal controls. Atopic patients are bothered by ocular itching, and excessive eye rubbing also may contribute to the development of keratoconus.

There is an association between Down's syndrome and keratoconus. Approximately 5% of patients with Down's syndrome manifest signs of keratoconus. The incidence of acute hydrops in keratoconus patients with Down's syndrome is definitely higher than in patients without Down's syndrome. As in atopic subjects, keratoconus patients with Down's syndrome tend to be vigorous eye rubbers. This may explain, at least in part, the relationship with keratoconus.

Keratoconus is also associated with various connective tissue disorders, such as Ehlers-Danlos syndrome, osteogenesis imperfecta, and Marfan's syndrome. There are conflicting reports of an association between keratoconus, mitral valve prolapse, and joint hypermobility. One study has reported an association between keratoconus and false chordae tendineae in the left ventricle. The relationship between various connective tissue diseases and keratoconus suggests a common defect in the synthesis of connective tissue.

7. What ocular conditions are associated with keratoconus?
Keratoconus has been described in association with various ocular diseases, including retinitis pigmentosa, Leber's congenital amaurosis, vernal conjunctivitis, floppy eyelid syndrome, corneal endothelial dystrophy, and posterior polymorphous corneal dystrophy.

8. What are the symptoms of keratoconus?
The characteristic onset of keratoconus is in the late teens or early 20s, although earlier and later onset has been reported. Symptoms usually begin as blurred vision with shadowing around images.

Vision becomes progressively more blurred and distorted with associated glare, halos around lights, light sensitivity, multiple images, and ocular irritation.

9. How is the diagnosis of keratoconus made?
During the early stages of keratoconus, the patient presents with myopic astigmatism, and a normal slit lamp examination. Corneal topography/tomography is helpful in documenting the presence of keratoconus even before keratometric or slit lamp findings become apparent. As the disease progresses, an irregular light reflex with scissoring on retinoscopy can be appreciated through the dilated pupil. The cornea steepens and thins with irregularity of the mires on keratometry. Obvious signs of keratoconus become apparent at the slit lamp later in the course of the disease.

KEY POINTS: DIAGNOSIS OF KERATOCONUS

1. Topographic mapping of the anterior corneal surface.
2. Elevation analysis of the anterior and posterior corneal surfaces.
3. Slit lamp examination of the cornea
4. Evaluation of the light reflex through a dilated pupil.

10. What are the topographic signs of keratoconus?
With conventional topography, the Placido rings of light are reflected off the cornea, and corneal curvature is derived from the distance between the rings and displayed as a color-coded map. Distortion of the rings is noted early on in the disease.
- The characteristic sign of keratoconus on topography is inferior midperipheral steepening (Fig. 13.1). Numerous studies have tried to develop quantitative topographic parameters to define keratoconus. In one study, central corneal power >47.20 diopters (D) combined with steepening of the inferior cornea compared with the superior cornea of >1.20 D detected 98% of patients with keratoconus. However, it may be difficult to make a definitive diagnosis of keratoconus based on topographic findings alone. This is of particular importance in patients seeking refractive surgery because the results of the surgery are poorly predictable in patients with keratoconus. Patients with apparently normal corneas may have inferior midperipheral steepening >1.20 D but normal central corneal powers in the range of 43 to 45 D. It is difficult to know whether such patients represent a forme fruste of keratoconus and, as such, should be dissuaded from considering refractive surgery, especially laser-assisted in situ keratomileusis (LASIK) because such surgery can result in cornea ectasia, thereby manifesting characteristic signs and symptoms of keratoconus. However, excimer laser photorefractive keratectomy can be a viable option in select patients with borderline findings. Each case must be analyzed on an individual basis.
- Corneal tomography units utilize scanning slit technology or a Scheimpflug-based imaging system to document corneal shape, corneal thickness measurements across the cornea, and elevation of the front and back corneal surfaces in relation to a computer-generated best-fit sphere. These instruments also present standard Placido disc color maps. The additional information, especially the corneal elevation and corneal thickness profile, is very helpful in differentiating between forme fruste or early keratoconus and nonkeratoconic corneas. Of particular note is when the thinnest area of the cornea corresponds with the area of maximal elevation. Some of the units provide specialized diagnostic software to help with making the diagnosis of keratoconus. In addition, some tomography units, as well as some high-frequency ultrasound biomicroscopy machines, provide corneal epithelial

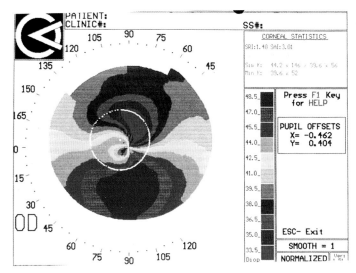

Fig. 13.1 Map showing symmetric inferior steeping.

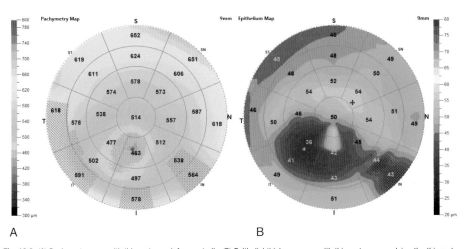

A   B

Fig. 13.2 (A) Pachymetry map with thinnest area inferocentrally. (B) Epithelial thickness map with thinnest area overlying the thinnest portion of the cornea. Courtesy of Dr Christopher Rapuano.

thickness profiles that add to our diagnostic armamentarium (Fig. 13.2). The corneal epithelium tends to be thinner over the area of corneal ectasia, which is usually decentered inferiorly with compensatory epithelial thickening centrally. However, no technology is 100% specific and 100% sensitive, requiring the surgeon's input, especially when evaluating patients presenting for refractive surgery.

11. **What are the slit lamp findings of keratoconus?**
The earliest slit lamp signs of keratoconus are apical thinning and steepening, usually located inferior to the center of the pupil. As the keratoconus progresses, the thinning and ectasia become more prominent with the development of apical scarring that begins in the anterior stroma and progresses into the deeper layers of the stroma (Figs. 13.3 to 13.6). Fine linear striae become apparent in the deep stroma just anterior to the Descemet's membrane, usually oriented vertically or obliquely. They are thought to represent stress lines in the posterior stroma and are known as Vogt's striae. They can be made to disappear when the intraocular pressure is transiently raised by applying external pressure to the globe. In some mild cases of keratoconus, the pressure from rigid

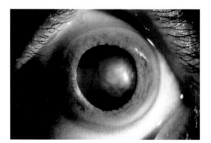

Fig. 13.3 Apical scarring.

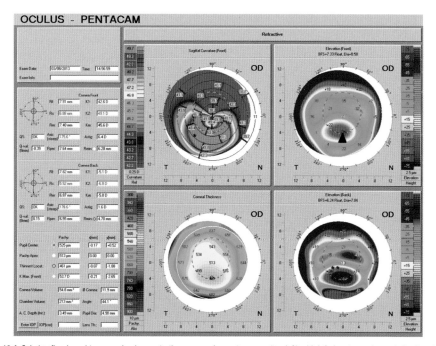

Fig. 13.4 Scheimpflug-based tomography demonstrating a corneal curvature map (top left) with inferior steepening, anterior (top right) and posterior (bottom right) with inferocentral elevation posterior greater than anterior, and corneal thickness (bottom left) with thinnest area corresponding to the area of maximal elevation.

gas-permeable contact lens wear can induce the formation of such striae, which disappear when the lens is removed. A Fleischer ring is commonly seen outlining the base of the cone. This is the result of hemosiderin pigment deposition within the deeper layers of the corneal epithelium. A Fleischer ring may only partially outline the cone but, as the ectasia progresses, tends to become a complete circle with more dense accumulation of pigmentation that is best appreciated while viewing with the cobalt blue filter on the slit lamp (Fig. 13.7). Subepithelial fibrillary lines in a concentric circular pattern have been described just inside the Fleischer ring. The source of these fibrils is unknown but has been postulated as epithelial nerve filaments. Anterior clear spaces thought to represent breaks in the Bowman's membrane are sometimes seen within the thin portion of the conical protrusion. Prominent corneal nerves are reportedly more common in keratoconic corneas. In the more advanced stages, when the eye is rotated downward, the corneal ectasia causes protrusion of the lower lid. This is known as Munson's sign.

12. How does keratoconus progress?

The onset of keratoconus characteristically occurs in the mid to late teens, progressing slowly for several years before stabilizing. However, delayed onset or late progression of keratoconus is not uncommon. As the disease progresses, the corneal thinning and epithelial ectasia become more prominent with increasing apical scarring.

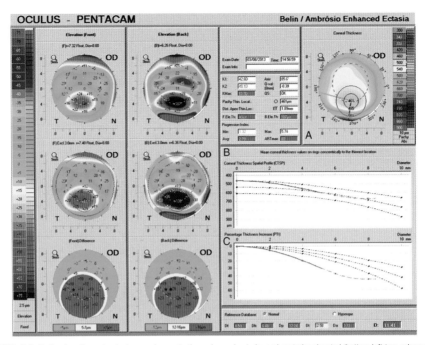

Fig. 13.5 Belin/Ambrosio enhanced ectasia map demonstrating enhanced anterior and posterior elevated (bottom left two columns) as well as various corneal thickness profiles (right images **A**, **B**, and **C**) that further support the diagnosis of keratoconus.

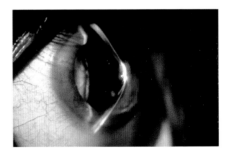

Fig. 13.6 Apical thinning and scarring demonstrated in slit beam.

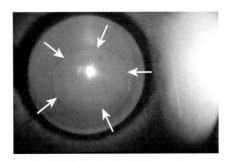

Fig. 13.7 Cobalt blue illumination demonstrating Fleischer ring outlining the extent of the cone. *Arrows* point to margins of the ring.

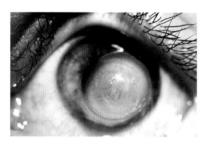

Fig. 13.8 Acute hydrops.

Two types of cones have been described: (1) a small round or nipple-shaped cone that tends to be more central in location and (2) an oval or sagging cone that is usually larger and displaced inferiorly, with the thinning extending close to the inferior limbus. Progression of keratoconus tends to manifest as increased thinning and protrusion, although enlargement of the cone also occurs with extension peripherally.

13. **What is acute hydrops?**
   Acute hydrops (Fig. 13.8) occurs in the more advanced cases of keratoconus. Ruptures in the Descemet's membrane allow aqueous to enter into the corneal stroma, resulting in marked thickening and opacification of the cornea that are usually restricted to the cone. The involved stroma becomes massively thickened with large, fluid-filled clefts, overlying epithelial edema, and bulla formation. Rarely, a fistulous tract may develop through the cornea, with resultant leakage of aqueous from the anterior chamber through the fluid-filled stroma and epithelium onto the corneal surface. The corneal edema gradually resolves over weeks to months as endothelial cells adjacent to the rupture in the Descemet's membrane enlarge and migrate across the defect, laying down new Descemet's membrane. With healing, scarring tends to flatten the cornea, thereby facilitating the possibility of subsequent contact lens fitting with significant usual improvement as long as the scarring spares the visual axis. Some corneas with acute hydrops tend to develop stromal neovascularization that increases the potential risk of graft rejection if corneal transplantation ultimately becomes necessary. Acute hydrops is more common in patients with Down's syndrome and vernal keratoconjunctivitis, presumably related to the repeated trauma of eye rubbing in these patients. Most cases of acute hydrops resolve spontaneously, requiring supportive treatment with topical hyperosmotic agents such as 5% sodium chloride drops and/or ointment to promote corneal deturgescence. Some patients with acute hydrops complain of severe photophobia and benefit from the use of topical steroids and/or cycloplegic agents. In addition, topical steroids should be instituted in patients with signs of corneal neovascularization. Studies have reported quicker resolution of acute hydrops with injection of air or nonexpansile concentrations of SF_6 and C_3F_8 into the anterior chamber to promote closure of the rupture in Descemet's membrane. However, several injections are sometimes required and many surgeons feel the benefits do not outweigh the risks, such as cataract and pupillary block glaucoma. Once the hydrops has resolved, the resultant scarring tends to result in corneal flattening. The patient can then try to resume contact lens wear if the central cornea has not become excessively scarred. Otherwise, the only alternative is a corneal transplant.

14. **What is the histopathology of keratoconus?**
   Most histopathologic studies of keratoconic corneas are performed on advanced cases that require lamellar or penetrating keratoplasty. In addition, most patients were previous long-term contact lens wearers, which also may affect the histopathologic findings, as contact lens wearers may induce more apical scarring. Changes have been described in every layer of the cornea. The stroma of the cone is thinner than the surrounding cornea. The apical epithelium tends to be flattened and thinned with scattered fragmentation and dehiscence of the epithelial basement membrane. Iron noted in the epithelial cells outlining the cone corresponds to the Fleischer ring.
   Among the most characteristic histologic changes of keratoconus are breaks in Bowman's membrane that are sometimes filled in with epithelium and/or stromal collagen. Ultimately, the anterior corneal stroma may become replaced with irregularly arranged connective tissue.
   The Descemet's membrane is normal unless acute hydrops has occurred. Depending on the stage of the reparative process, breaks in the Descemet's membrane with curled edges subsequently become covered by adjacent endothelial cells that slide over and lay down new membrane. The corneal endothelial cells tend to be normal, although they may exhibit increased pleomorphism and polymegathism.

15. **How is keratoconus treated?**
   Mild cases of keratoconus can be successfully managed with spectacles. However, as the keratoconus progresses and the amount of irregular astigmatism increases, patients are unable to obtain satisfactory vision with spectacle correction. Contact lenses can be used to neutralize the irregular astigmatism, thereby offering significant visual improvement over spectacles. As the cornea becomes more distorted, scarred, and ectatic, contact lens fitting becomes more difficult and vision deteriorates, ultimately necessitating surgical intervention.

16. **What types of contact lenses are used to treat keratoconus?**

Conventional spherical myopic soft contact lenses may be used successfully in mild cases of keratoconus with minimal manifest astigmatism. Toric soft contact lenses also may be used in some patients without excessive amounts of irregular astigmatism. The vast majority of patients with keratoconus are managed with rigid gas-permeable contact lenses. Fitting such lenses over a distorted ectatic cornea is difficult. Numerous lens designs are available for fitting patients with keratoconus, including varying diameters of spherical lenses, aspheric lenses, toric lenses, and lenses with multiple curvatures on the posterior surface that have a steeper central curve to vault the apex of the cone and a flatter peripheral curve to align with the more normal peripheral cornea. Computed topography/tomography can be helpful in fitting these challenging patients.

Large gas-permeable scleral contact lenses that vault the cornea and are filled with a fluid reservoir that bathes the corneal surface are now being used more frequently in managing patients with prominent ectatic cones who cannot be fit with more conventional gas-permeable lenses. A piggyback system is another option available for treating patients with keratoconus: A gas-permeable contact lens is fitted on top of a soft contact lens. This system is a little more expensive and time consuming for both practitioner and patient but can be helpful in managing select cases that have failed more conventional contact lens fitting. Another specialized lens design incorporates a rigid gas-permeable center with a soft peripheral skirt to reduce the edge awareness of conventional gas-permeable lenses. Such hybrid lenses may actually center better and offer a more stable fit by virtue of their large diameter, which extends beyond the limbus. However, they have a tendency to be tighter over time, sometimes causing corneal neovascularization and hypoxia.

17. **Can keratoconus be prevented?**

Developed in Germany, collagen crosslinking is a technique to prevent the progression of keratoconus. It involves saturating the corneal stroma with riboflavin drops and then applying ultraviolet light (UV-A) at a wavelength of 365 nm. The riboflavin serves as a photo-sensitizing agent that interacts with the UV-A, leading to crosslinking within collagen and the extracellular matrix of the corneal stroma, resulting in strengthening of the cornea. The riboflavin absorbs the UV-A in the anterior stroma sparing the endothelium of any adverse effects. The procedure is limited to corneas greater than 400 μm in thickness to avoid endothelial toxicity. Thinner corneas can be "thickened up" by using hypotonic riboflavin solution.

The procedure has been used all around the world for the past 15 years but was approved by the Food and Drug Administration (FDA) in the United States only in 2016. It has been shown to stabilize the cornea and prevent progression in 90% of cases. Moreover, in countries that have been using collagen crosslinking for many years, the incidence of corneal transplantation for keratoconus has been drastically diminished. Numerous studies demonstrate the long-term safety and efficacy of the procedure. Although it must be stressed that the crosslinking prevents progression rather than treating the disease, some patients have been shown to gain 1 to 2 D of corneal flattening, associated with a small improvement in visual acuity.

The traditional crosslinking technique requires removal of the corneal epithelium to allow the riboflavin better access to the corneal stroma. Removing the epithelium carries with it the risk of infection as well as stromal haze that usually resolves spontaneously. Several investigators have been studying "epi on" techniques by modifying the riboflavin solution and/or the corneal epithelium to promote transepithelial transport of the riboflavin, eliminating the need for epithelial debridement. To date, the "epi on" technique does not seem to be as efficacious as "epi off." Not only does the transepithelial absorption of riboflavin have to be worked out, there is also the issue of the corneal epithelium blocking UV-A from getting through into the stroma to exert its effect. However, "epi on" is certainly a much simpler procedure with little or no discomfort and little or no risk of infection.

Investigators are also studying the benefits of combining collagen crosslinking with intracorneal ring segments, topographic guided excimer laser surface ablation, and conductive keratoplasty.

18. **What are the surgical options for treating keratoconus?**

Surgical intervention is reserved for patients with keratoconus who cannot be successfully fit with contact lenses or who fail to obtain satisfactory vision with contact lenses. Atopic patients with keratoconus tend to require surgery much more frequently than nonallergic patients because the allergic diathesis tends to interfere with contact lens tolerance.

- **Penetrating keratoplasty (full-thickness corneal transplantation)** is the most common surgical technique used to rehabilitate patients with keratoconus. The surgical procedure requires excision of the entire cone, frequently determined by the outline of the Fleischer ring using a manual trephine or femtosecond laser. The donor tissue is cut the same size or slightly larger to obtain good wound apposition with sutures, most commonly 10-0 nylon, utilizing various interrupted running or combined suturing techniques. If the cone extends close to the limbus (usually inferiorly), a large corneal graft is needed. Usually, the grafted tissue is centered on the pupil, but when the cone is eccentric, an eccentric graft is used to encompass the entire cone, taking care to leave the optical zone free of sutures. Increasing graft size with proximity to the limbal blood vessel reduces the "immune privilege" of the usually avascular cornea, thereby increasing the risk of immunologic reaction.
- **Lamellar (partial-thickness) keratoplasty** has become increasingly popular for the treatment of keratoconus. A lamellar graft has the advantage of being an extraocular procedure that avoids the risk of intraoperative positive pressure, wherein intraocular contents can be expelled through the trephined opening in the cornea made during penetrating keratoplasty. It also eliminates the risk of endothelial rejection while

increasing the donor pool because it does not require a healthy corneal donor endothelium, which is discarded at the time of surgery.

A lamellar procedure is more demanding technically than a full-thickness procedure. It involves replacing as much of the corneal stroma as possible while leaving behind the patient's own endothelial layer and Descemet's membrane. The resultant visual acuity is similar to that from a penetrating keratoplasty when no stroma is left behind. This is best accomplished in deep anterior lamellar keratoplasty (DALK) with the Anwar "Big Bubble" technique. Air is used to cleanly separate Descemet's membrane from the overlying stroma. When some recipient stoma remains during manual lamellar dissection, the resultant interface usually causes some degradation of the usual image, which can limit the visual recovery.

- **Intracorneal rings** are polymethylmethacrylate ring segments of varying thickness and configuration inserted into the midperipheral corneal stroma. They are useful in treating mild keratoconus in patients who are contact lens intolerant. The therapeutic rationale is to support the ectatic area of the cornea, thereby reducing corneal steepening and regularizing the astigmatism associated with keratoconus, with improvement in both uncorrected and best spectacle-corrected visual acuity. However, they do not slow or prevent progression of corneal ectasia. In the United States, Intacs (Addition Technology) are the only ring segments that are FDA approved.
- **Epikeratophakia** is a type of onlay lamellar procedure using a freeze-dried donor cornea that is sewn on top of a deepithelialized host cornea. The purpose is to flatten the cornea with the hope of offering improved spectacle-corrected visual acuity and/or better contact lens fitting. After initial enthusiasm in the late 1980s, the procedure has been abandoned by most surgeons because of complications and poor visual results. However, in select cases in which a full-thickness corneal transplant is contraindicated, such as patients with Down's syndrome who may aggressively rub their eyes and dehisce a full-thickness wound or patients at high risk for immune rejection (e.g., multiple graft failures in the other eye), lamellar grafts, or epikeratophakia are worthy of consideration.
- **Thermokeratoplasty** is a technique in which heating the cornea from 90° C to 120° C causes shrinkage of corneal collagen fibers with resulting flattening of the cornea. This procedure has been abandoned for the most part because of unpredictable results, induced scarring, and the potential for recurrent corneal erosions because of damage to the epithelial basement membrane complex. However, when the apex of the cone spares the visual axis, thermokeratoplasty may be used to flatten the cornea, thereby allowing more favorable spectacle-corrected visual acuity and/or contact lens fitting. In addition, thermokeratoplasty may be helpful in promoting resolution of acute hydrops.

Additionally, some patients with keratoconus develop an elevated subepithelial scar at the apex of the cone as the result of chronic apical irritation from contact lens wear. Corneal epithelial breakdown may develop over the scar, thereby interfering with contact lens wear. These scars can be removed or smoothed out manually with a blade or with the excimer laser, thereby allowing resumption of contact lens wear and sparing the patient an otherwise needed corneal transplant.

19. What are the results of corneal transplant in patients with keratoconus?

As mentioned previously, most corneal transplantation surgery for keratoconus involves penetrating keratoplasty, although DALK is increasing in popularity. The results of such surgery are excellent, with clear grafts in approximately 90% of patients, most of whom obtain best corrected visual acuity of 20/40 or better. The most frequent problem arising in patients with keratoconus who undergo corneal transplantation is high postkeratoplasty astigmatism. However, the astigmatism following corneal transplant surgery tends to be much more regular than the irregular astigmatism of the original disorder. This difference allows most patients to achieve satisfactory visual results with spectacle correction, even if they have a large amount of astigmatism that most patients without keratoconus would not be able to tolerate in spectacles. If the astigmatism cannot be tolerated in spectacles, contact lens wear or refractive surgery (excimer laser ablation or incisional keratotomy) can be offered. Because keratoconus tends to be asymmetric, many patients undergoing corneal transplantation in one eye manage with a contact lens in the lesser involved eye and thus prefer to wear a contact lens in the operated eye as well. The contact lens tends to neutralize most of the astigmatism in the corneal transplant and frequently offers a little better vision than spectacles, especially if there is some degree of irregularity in the astigmatism.

It usually takes up to a full year or more for the corneal transplant wound to heal. If the patient is seeing well with the sutures in place, the sutures are left undisturbed and tend to disintegrate spontaneously over a few years. Sometimes, disintegrating sutures erode through the corneal epithelium and cause a foreign body sensation. If they are not removed from the surface of the cornea, they can cause secondary infection. After sutures disintegrate and/or are removed, a significant change in the refractive error may occur. All graft sutures should have disintegrated or have been removed before keratorefractive surgery is contemplated postcorneal transplantation.

Graft rejection occurs in approximately 20% of patients with keratoconus who undergo penetrating keratoplasty. Most immune rejections can be reversed with appropriate local steroid therapy if caught early. Irreversible rejection leads to permanent corneal clouding that requires repeat penetrating keratoplasty. A repeat graft has a reasonably good prognosis, although the success rate is lower than the primary graft and tends to diminish with each successive transplant. If multiple graft failures occur, an "artificial cornea," i.e., keratoprosthesis, can always be considered.

BIBLIOGRAPHY

Bran AJ: Keratoconus, Cornea 7:163–169, 1988.

Colin J, Cochener B, Savary G, Malet F: Correcting keratoconus with intracorneal rings, J Cataract Refract Surg 26:1117–1122, 2000.

Hashemi H, Heydarian S, Hooshmand E, et al.: The prevalence and risk factors for keratoconus: a systematic review and meta-analysis, Cornea 39(2):263–270, 2020.

Kenney MC, Brown DJ, Rajeev B: The elusive causes of keratoconus: a working hypothesis, CLAO J 26:10–13, 2000.

Krachmer JH, Feder RS, Belin MW: Keratoconus and related noninflammatory thinning disorders, Surv Ophthalmol 28:293–322, 1984.

Lawless M, Coster DJ, Phillips AJ, Loane M: Keratoconus: diagnosis and management, Aust NZ J Ophthalmol 17:33–60, 1989.

Loukovitis E, Sfakianakis K, Syrmakesi P, et al.: Genetic aspects of keratoconus: a literature review exploring potential genetic contributions and possible genetic relationships with comorbidities, Ophthalmol Ther 7(2):263–292, 2018.

Macsai MS, Valery GA, Krackmer JH: Development of keratoconus after contact lens wear: patient characteristics, Arch Ophthalmol 108:534–538, 1990.

Maeda N, Klyce SD, Smolek MD: Comparison of methods for detecting keratoconus using video keratography, Arch Ophthalmol 113:870–874, 1995.

Tuft SJ, Moodaley LC, Gregory WM, et al.: Prognostic factors for the progression of keratoconus, Ophthalmology 101:439–447, 1994.

Wollensak G, Spoerl E, Seifer T: Riboflavin/ultraviolet influenced collagen cross-linking for the treatment of keratoconus, Am J Ophthalmol 135(5):620–627, 2003.

Wheeler J, Hauser MA, Afshari NA, et al.: The genetics of keratoconus: a review, Reprod Syst Sex Disord 65:001, 2012.

CHAPTER 14

REFRACTIVE SURGERY

Neil Vadhar and Brandon D. Ayres

1. **What are the refractive components of the eye?**

   The cornea and the lens refract incident light so that it is focused on the fovea, the center of the retina. The cornea contributes approximately 44 diopters (D) compared with only 18 D from the lens. In addition, the anterior chamber depth and axial length of the eye contribute to the refractive status.

2. **What are the various types of refractive errors?**
   - **Myopia,** or nearsightedness, exists when the refractive elements of the eye place the image in front of the retina.
   - **Hyperopia,** or farsightedness, exists when the image is focused behind the retina.
   - **Astigmatism** usually refers to corneal irregularity that requires unequal power in different meridians to place a single image on the fovea. Lenticular astigmatism (due to the lens) is less common than corneal astigmatism.
   - **Presbyopia** is the natural impairment in accommodation often noted around age 40 years. The power of the corrective "add" or bifocal segment to combat presbyopia increases with age.

3. **How is myopia related to age?**

   Myopia is common among premature infants, less common in full-term infants, and uncommon at 6 months of age, when mild hyperopia is the rule. Myopia becomes most prevalent in adolescence (approximately 25%), peaking by 20 years of age and subsequently leveling off. This information is important for determining the appropriate age to consider refractive surgery.

4. **What are the goals of refractive surgery?**

   Goals vary for each patient. Certain patients desire refractive surgery because of professional or lifestyle issues; examples include athletes and police, fire, and military personnel, who may find glasses or contact lenses hindering or even dangerous. Other patients, such as high myopes, may find spectacle correction inadequate because of image minification or may be intolerant of contact lenses. In general, the goals of refractive surgery are to reduce or eliminate the need for glasses or contact lenses without altering the quality of vision or best-corrected vision.

5. **What features characterize a good candidate for retractive surgery? Are there any contraindications?**

   First, patients considering refractive surgery should be at least 18 to 21 years of age with a stable refraction. Patients with certain ocular conditions (such as severe dry eye or uveitis) or particular systemic diseases (such as autoimmune collagen vascular disease or uncontrolled diabetes) and patients taking medications that impair wound healing are poor candidates. Keratoconus, a condition in which the cornea is irregularly cone shaped, remains a contraindication for refractive surgery because results are unpredictable. Analysis of corneal curvature with computerized corneal topography should be performed on all patients before surgery because early keratoconus has a prevalence of up to 13% in this population and may be missed by other diagnostic methods.

   Second, patients' motivations and expectations should be explored thoroughly so that unrealistic hopes may be discovered preoperatively. For example, the patient who is constantly cleaning his or her glasses because of "excruciating glare" from dust on the lenses or who desires perfect uncorrected vision is not a good candidate for refractive surgery. A careful discussion of the risks and benefits of surgery is particularly important. Patients may want to try contact lenses before considering surgery. The concept of presbyopia must also be explained; many patients are prepresbyopic and have no understanding that achieving excellent uncorrected vision at distance will require correction for reading at near within a few years.

6. **How is corneal topography used in the evaluation of patients undergoing refractive surgery?**

   Corneal topography is extremely useful for evaluating patients undergoing refractive surgery because it generates precise images of corneal curvature that correspond to a large area of the cornea. This information aids in presurgical planning and postsurgical evaluation. Placido disc-based systems detect reflected images of rings projected onto the cornea. A computer generates a topographic "map" of corneal curvature based on the measured distance between the rings reflected from the cornea (Fig. 14.1A and B). Optical coherence tomography systems provide high-resolution cross-sectional images of the cornea and are based on the reflection of infrared wavelengths from biological tissues. Scheimpflug-based systems use slit beams and a rotating camera, which maps sections of the cornea (Fig. 14.2). These systems allow for anterior and posterior corneal topography measurement and can also estimate corneal thickness.

   Subtle corneal abnormalities, such as early keratoconus (forme fruste) or contact lens–induced corneal warpage, may be detected only by topography. The Oculus Pentacam Scheimpflug system provides the Belin/Ambrósio enhanced

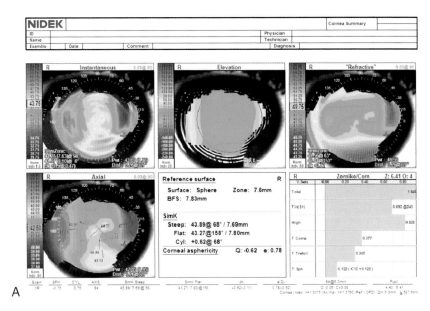

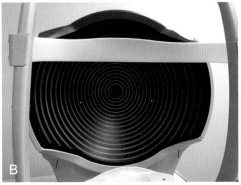

Fig. 14.1 A, Corneal diagnostic summary in a post-LASIK patient. **B,** The Nidek OPD Scan III Placido–based corneal analyzer.

ectasia display, which aides in screening of keratoconus and corneal ectasia (Fig. 14.3). In addition, postoperative and preoperative topographic maps may be analyzed to generate "difference" maps that isolate the procedure-induced changes. Computerized corneal topography is also extremely useful for determining the cause of imperfect vision after refractive surgery commonly due to irregular astigmatism.

7. What are the major options for the surgical treatment of myopia?
   - Radial keratotomy (RK)
   - Photorefractive keratectomy (PRK)
   - Laser-assisted in situ keratomileusis (LASIK)
   - Small incision lenticule extraction (SMILE)
   - Intracorneal ring segments (Intacs)
   - Phakic intraocular lens (IOL) implants
   - Clear lens extraction

8. How does radial keratotomy reduce myopia?
   RK is a historical method for the treatment of myopia and now has largely been replaced by excimer laser procedures. Deep radial incisions cause steepening of the cornea peripherally, which results in secondary flattening of the central cornea. The number, length, and depth of incisions and the size of the clear, central optical zone, along with the patient's age, determine the refractive effect. Typically, four incisions are used for low myopia (Fig. 14.4) and eight incisions for moderate myopia. However, some patients had as many as 32 incisions for high myopia.[1,2]

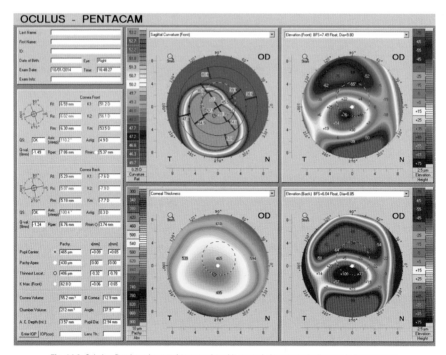

Fig. 14.2 Scheimpflug-based corneal topography with corneal changes typically seen in keratoconus.

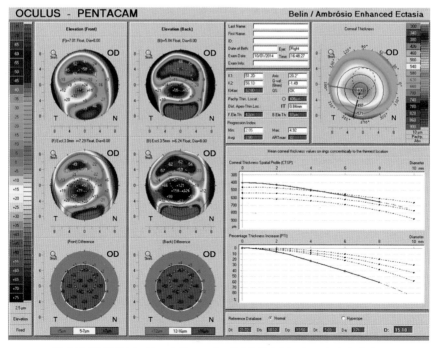

Fig. 14.3 Scheimpflug-based corneal topography with Belin/Ambrósio enhanced ectasia display.

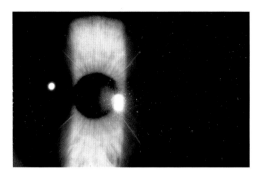

Fig. 14.4 Three weeks after four-incision radial keratotomy.

9. What are the various radial keratotomy techniques?
   - The "American" technique involves making centrifugal incisions (from the center toward the limbus) with an angled diamond knife blade.
   - The "Russian" technique uses centripetal incisions (from the limbus toward the center) with a straight vertical diamond knife blade. The Russian technique gives deeper incisions and a more refractive effect; however, there is a greater danger of entering the optical zone.

     Based on statistical analysis of previous cases, standardized nomograms are used to determine the number of incisions and optical zone size, depending on the patient's age and desired refractive change.

10. What results have been achieved with radial keratotomy? What about complications?
    Several major investigations have been performed, the most important of which is the Prospective Evaluation of Radial Keratotomy study. This study showed that 60% of treated eyes were within 1 D of emmetropia up to 10 years postoperatively. After 10 years, 53% had at least 20/20 uncorrected vision, and 85% had at least 20/40 vision. However, 43% of eyes had a progressive shift toward hyperopia of at least 1 D after 10 years. This shift was noted to be worse for eyes with the smaller optical zone of 3 mm. Only 3% of patients lost two or more lines of best-corrected visual acuity, and all had 20/30 vision or better. Three of more than 400 patients complained of severe glare or starburst that made night driving impossible. Corneal perforations occurred in 2% of cases; none required a suture for closure. Overall, the best results were achieved in the low-myopia group (−2.00 to −3.00 D). As with any invasive procedure, infection is a small but real risk (Fig. 14.5).[3]

11. How does photorefractive keratectomy reduce myopia?
    PRK involves direct laser treatment of the central corneal stroma. Specifically, the "excited dimer" (excimer) 193-nm UV laser causes flattening of the central cornea through a photoablative/photodecomposition process whereby more tissue is removed centrally than peripherally. Under topical anesthesia, the central corneal epithelium is removed either with a spatula or with the laser. The laser is then used to ablate a precise quantity of stromal tissue with submicrometer accuracy to achieve the desired refractive effect. PRK is preferred over LASIK in cases of irregular astigmatism, thin corneas, epithelial basement membrane disease, prior corneal surgery, or LASIK complications. In some cases, if the LASIK flap cannot be created safely, the procedure may be converted to PRK.

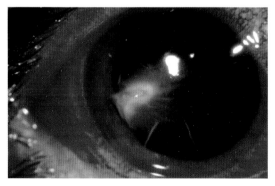

Fig. 14.5 Infection at radial keratotomy incision.

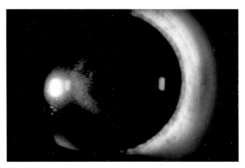

Fig. 14.6 Mild stromal haze, 3 months after photorefractive keratectomy.

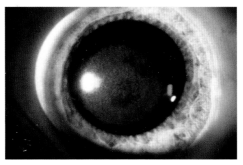

Fig. 14.7 Moderate to severe stromal haze, 6 months after photorefractive keratectomy.

12. **What results have been achieved with photorefractive keratectomy? What about complications?**
    A randomized 20-year prospective clinical trial of PRK found the following:
    - Slight but significant increase in myopia (0.54 D) after PRK between 1 and 20 years, particularly in those under 40 at the time of treatment and in female patients.
    - Corneal power remained unchanged, but axial length increased.
    - The procedure was safe, with no long-term sight-threatening complications and with improvements in corrected distance visual acuity and corneal transparency with time.
        Residual corneal haze is a known complication of PRK (Figs. 14.6 and 14.7).[4]

13. **What is LASIK?**
    LASIK stands for laser-assisted in situ keratomileusis. The procedure involves creating a corneal flap to ablate midstromal tissue directly with an excimer laser beam, ultimately flattening the cornea to treat myopia and steepening the cornea to treat hyperopia. Whereas earlier techniques of keratomileusis consisted of removing a corneal cap and resecting stromal tissue manually, technological advancements have revolutionized this procedure into a highly automated process. Contemporary techniques use a femtosecond laser for flap creation and an excimer laser for tissue ablation. After a lid speculum is placed and topical anesthetic is applied, the suction ring is centered on the cornea to stabilize the eye. Historically, a mechanical microkeratome blade was used to create the corneal flap, but currently, most surgeons have switched to femtosecond laser for creating the LASIK flap. After the flap is created, the vacuum on the ring is released, and the flap is then lifted, exposing the bare stromal bed. Next, the excimer laser is applied directly to the stromal tissue. Afterward, the corneal flap is replaced to its original position, typically without sutures, and allowed to heal.

14. **How has the use of the femtosecond laser in the LASIK procedure helped to improve results versus the microkeratome?**
    A meta-analysis of multiple studies found that:
    - No significant differences were identified between the two groups in regard to a loss of two or more lines of vision or to patients achieving 20/20 vision or better ($P = .24$).
    - The femtosecond group had more patients who were within ± 0.50 D of target refraction.
    - Flap thickness was more predictable in the femtosecond group.
    - The microkeratome group had more epithelial defects.
    - The femtosecond group had more cases of diffuse lamellar keratitis (DLK).[5]

15. **What is the range of myopia recommended for correction with LASIK?**

    LASIK is generally recommended for myopia as low as 1 D and as high as 10 to 12 D, although it is Food and Drug Administration (FDA) approved for myopia up to 14 D.

16. **What are the advantages and disadvantages of LASIK versus radial keratotomy and photorefractive keratectomy?**

    LASIK offers the advantage of minimal postoperative pain as well as earlier recovery of vision because the epithelium is left essentially intact. There is less chance of corneal scarring and haze than after RK and PRK. The disadvantages of LASIK include the brief intraoperative period of marked visual loss (due to high intraocular pressures generated by the suction ring); the risk of flap irregularities, subluxation, or dislocation (Fig. 14.5); and the expense of the procedure. Additional problems associated with LASIK include irregular astigmatism and the potential for epithelial ingrowth or infection under the flap.

    LASIK offers several advantages to the surgeon. Because the technique involves making a flap in the anterior corneal stroma, the risk of corneal perforation associated with RK is virtually nonexistent. The creation of a uniform smooth flap with preservation of the central Bowman's layer also reduces the subepithelial scarring seen with PRK. The use of the femtosecond laser allows little room for surgeon error. However, its automated aspect also poses disadvantages. The surgeon has limited intraoperative control over creation of the flap and ablation of the stroma. The vacuum ring can be difficult to place on a patient with narrow palpebral fissures or deep orbits. Femtosecond-created flaps can be difficult to lift and tears in the flap can be created. On occasion, gas could cause perforation in the flap (vertical gas breakthrough).

17. **How do the surgical results of LASIK compare with those of photorefractive keratectomy?**

    Several studies have compared the results of LASIK and PRK in both low-to-moderate and moderate-to-high myopia. Overall, the refractive and visual results are comparable after the first 1 to 3 months. LASIK allows faster visual recovery. Pop and Payette compared the results of LASIK and PRK for the treatment of myopia between −1 and −9 D. They concluded that visual and refractive outcomes were similar at follow-up visits between 1 and 12 months, but LASIK patients were more likely to experience halos. In general, when refractive subgroups are analyzed, less predictable results are achieved in the higher myopia groups for both procedures. Nevertheless, LASIK may be the best corneal technique available for treating higher degrees of myopia.[6]

18. **What is "wavefront?" Are wavefront ablations any better than standard LASIK?**

    In standard LASIK, the spherical and cylindrical aberrations are measured using computerized corneal topography and manifest and cycloplegic refraction. The excimer laser is then programmed based on these data. A wavefront measurement has the ability to measure many more aberrations than just sphere and cylinder. To measure a wavefront, an aberrometer shines low-intensity laser light through the pupil. The laser light is then reflected off the retina and through the lens, pupil, and cornea and is distorted by the refractive properties of the eye. This wavefront of light is then used to detect an infinite number of ocular aberrations (evaluated, for example, by Zernike polynomials or Fourier analysis).

    In a wavefront ablation, the data collected by the aberrometer are converted into a sphere and cylindrical equivalent (usually with room for physician adjustment) and the customized ablation is carried out. Although the hope for wavefront-guided LASIK and PRK is high, there is no significant clinical evidence that it is better than carefully planned standard LASIK. Some studies have shown a reduction in higher-order aberrations after wavefront-guided ablations, while others have shown an increase. As surgical techniques and technology improve, perhaps the clinical results of wavefront LASIK will begin to outshine standard LASIK.

19. **Name the important potential complications of LASIK.**

    Complications are uncommon and are not listed in order of frequency:
    - Premature release of suction ring
    - Intraoperative flap amputation (microkeratome)
    - Postoperative flap dislocation/subluxation (may require suturing of flap into place) (Fig. 14.8)
    - Epithelialization of the flap-bed interface (causes irregular astigmatism, light scattering, and possibly flap damage) (Fig. 14.9)
    - Irregular astigmatism
    - Infection
    - DLK
    - Progressive corneal ectasia[7]

KEY POINTS: COMMON POTENTIAL CONTRAINDICATIONS TO LASIK

1. Thin cornea.
2. Irregular astigmatism.
3. Keratoconus.
4. Anterior basement membrane dystrophy.
5. Herpes simplex or zoster keratitis.

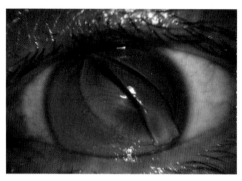

Fig. 14.8 Dislocated LASIK flap.

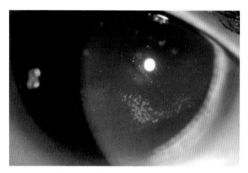

Fig. 14.9 Epithelial ingrowth under the LASIK flap.

20. What is SMILE?

    The SMILE procedure developed by Zeiss utilizes the VisuMax femtosecond laser to create a thin disc of tissue (lenticule) inside the corneal stroma, which is then extracted through a small incision. Unlike LASIK, this procedure does not require a flap. It is intended for treatment of myopia up to −8.00 D.

21. What is the range of myopia for correction of SMILE?

    SMILE is FDA approved for the treatment of myopia between −1.0 and −8.0 D with up to 3.0 D of astigmatism.

22. What are the advantages and disadvantages of SMILE?

    Advantages include:
    - Biomechanical stability
    - No risk of traumatic flap dislocation
    - Decreased dry eye
    - Better for larger pupils due to less induced higher order aberrations (HOAs)

    Disadvantages include:
    - More technically challenging than LASIK and PRK
    - Not indicated for hyperopia, high HOAs, or topographic irregularities
    - Contraindicated for epithelial basement membrane dystrophy (EBMD) or corneal opacities

23. How do the surgical results of SMILE compare to LASIK?

    The long-term efficacy and safety of SMILE is comparable to LASIK as demonstrated by numerous meta-analyses. 88% and 98% of eyes were within ±0.5 D and ±1.0 D, respectively, after 3 months. Compared to LASIK, SMILE has demonstrated reduced postoperative dry eye, fewer HOAs, and improved biomechanical stability.

24. Name the potential complications of SMILE.

    - Premature loss of suction
    - Formation of opaque bubble layer (OBL)
    - Subconjunctival hemorrhage
    - Incisional bleeding
    - Incisional tears
    - Lenticule remnant

- Lenticule adhesions
- Corneal abrasion
- Dry eye
- Infection

KEY POINTS: COMMON POTENTIAL CONTRAINDICATIONS TO SMILE

1. Thin cornea.
2. Irregular astigmatism.
3. Keratoconus.
4. Anterior basement membrane dystrophy.
5. Severe dry eye.
6. Corneal scarring.
7. Herpes simplex or zoster keratitis.
8. Uncontrolled glaucoma or uveitis.
9. Active eye infection or inflammation.
10. Women who are pregnant or breastfeeding.

25. **What is diffuse lamellar keratitis? How is it treated?**

DLK was originally termed "sands of the Sahara syndrome" because of the clinical appearance of a wavy inflammatory reaction in a LASIK flap interface. It generally appears 1 to 3 days after a primary LASIK procedure or an enhancement. The exact cause is unknown and is most likely multifactorial. Suspected etiologies include bacterial endotoxins, meibomian secretions, oils from the microkeratome, and excessive laser energy from the IntraLase femtosecond laser. Treatment involves high-dose topical steroids. In severe cases, lifting the flap and irrigating the interface may be helpful.[8]

26. **What is Epi-LASIK? What are the potential advantages?**

Epi-LASIK is a modified surface ablation, which uses a keratome and an epithelial separator that creates a plane between the epithelial basement membrane and the Bowman's membrane. As the "epitheliatome" passes over the eye, it creates an epithelial flap on a hinge, very similar to a LASIK flap. The epithelial flap is then reflected, exposing the surface of the Bowman's membrane. The excimer laser is then used to alter the shape of the cornea, after which the epithelial flap is repositioned. The advantage of Epi-LASIK is the safety of a surface procedure but with potentially faster visual recovery, less postoperative discomfort, and less haze than PRK. Epi-LASIK has largely been abandoned in favor of LASIK, or the flap is removed entirely as in PRK.

27. **What is the femtosecond laser? What are its potential advantages?**

Current femtosecond laser technology systems use neodymium:glass 1053-nm (near-infrared) wavelength light. Laser energy is converted into mechanical energy in a process known as photodisruption. The femtosecond laser uses ultrafast pulses of energy to ablate tissue with extreme precision. The ultrashort pulses prevent heat buildup, thus allowing minimal to no damage to surrounding tissues. In refractive surgery, this laser is used to cut a lamellar flap in the cornea. The potential advantages of using the femtosecond laser include greater safety, reproducibility of flap thickness, decreased flap complications, and decreased epithelial defects. Flap striae and interface deposits may also be reduced. Currently available femtosecond lasers for LASIK flap creation include the IntraLase FS and iFS laser systems from Abbott and Femto LDV systems from Ziemer.

In cataract surgery, the femtosecond laser creates a very precise capsulotomy and fragments the lens nucleus. These features may reduce surgical risks associated with traumatic cataracts, zonular instability, and pseudoexfoliation. Primary and secondary corneal cataract incisions can also be created more precisely by the laser. Arcuate incisions that reduce astigmatism can also be created during cataract surgery, taking into account surgically induced astigmatism from cataract incisions. Many of the femtosecond lasers that are used in cataract surgery can also be used to create LASIK flaps.[9–12]

28. **What is progressive corneal ectasia?**

Corneal ectasia is progressive corneal thinning and steepening with irregular astigmatism that causes poor vision. It is thought to result mainly in eyes with forme fruste keratoconus or from a stromal bed that is too thin after LASIK. Most surgeons believe that the stromal bed (calculated by taking the central corneal thickness minus the flap thickness minus the laser ablation) should be at least 250 μm to prevent corneal ectasia. However, other surgeons believe that the minimal stromal bed thickness should be greater. Long-term follow-up is required to determine the answer. Corneal collagen crosslinking is a treatment option for corneal ectasia, but it is not yet FDA approved.

29. **What are intracorneal ring segments?**

Intacs are an FDA-approved procedure for the correction of low myopia and mild to moderate keratoconus. This procedure involves the placement of two 150-degree arc segments of polymethylmethacrylate plastic at two-thirds depth in the peripheral cornea. This "tissue addition" results in flattening of the central cornea.[13]

30. How much myopia does Intacs treat?

    Intacs are FDA approved to treat between -1 and -3 D of nearsightedness in patients with no more than 1 D of astigmatism and who are at least 21 years of age.

31. What are the refractive results of Intacs for myopia?

    In US clinical trials at 1 year, 97% of patients had 20/40 vision or better, 74% had 20/20 vision or better, and 53% had 20/16 vision or better without correction.

32. List the potential complications of Intacs.

    Complications are not common and are not listed in order of frequency.
    - Induced astigmatism
    - Fluctuating vision
    - Anterior or posterior perforation of the cornea
    - Infection
    - White deposits along the ring segment
    - Extrusion of the ring segment

33. Is the Intacs procedure reversible?

    The Intacs can be removed, and most eyes return to their original refractions.

34. What are phakic intraocular lens implants?

    These lens implants are placed in the eye without the removal of the patient's own crystalline lens. There are currently three main types: an anterior chamber lens clipped to the iris, an angle-supported anterior chamber lens, and a posterior chamber lens in the ciliary sulcus (just in front of the crystalline lens). The Artisan or Verisyse iris-clip anterior chamber lens is currently FDA approved for -5 to -20 D of myopia with up to 2.5 D of astigmatism. The Visian implantable collamer lens (ICL) implant (Fig. 14.10) sits in the posterior chamber behind the pupil and is approved for -3 to -20 D of myopia. The toric version of this lens was approved in September 2018 and can be used to correct up to 4.0 D of astigmatism.[14,15] The EVO Visian ICL features a hole in the center of the lens, eliminating the need for an iridectomy, and is available outside the United States. The EVO+ version has an expanded optic for patients with larger pupils and is also available outside the United States.

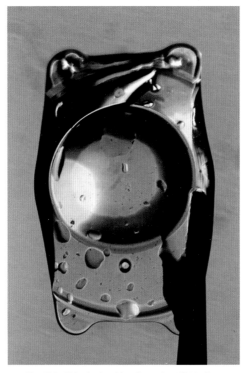

Fig. 14.10 Visian implantable collamer lens (ICL) implant.

35. What is the effect of the Verisyse phakic intraocular lens implant on endothelial cell count?
The FDA found no significant loss in endothelial cell counts with the Verisyse iris-claw phakic IOL at 2 years after implantation. In a worst-case scenario (by adjusting for measurement inaccuracy), 9% of eyes would have been at risk for 10% loss of endothelial cells at 12 months. Eyes at risk were found to have higher preoperative endothelial cell counts. Several authors have reported that the iris-claw lenses do accelerate endothelial cell loss.[16,17]

36. What are accommodative, multifocal, and extended depth of focus intraocular lenses?
As opposed to the more common single-vision IOLs implanted after cataract surgery, which leave the eye with very little ability to focus, the accommodative IOLs allow the eye to move the implant by various mechanisms to allow a greater range of focus. The only FDA-approved accommodative IOLs as of this writing are the Crystalens and Trulign Toric by Bausch + Lomb. The optic is on hinges and allows for vitreous pressure to move the IOL anteriorly and posteriorly. This movement changes the refractive power of the IOL and allows patients greater reading ability. In the FDA Crystalens 1-year trial, 98% of patients with bilateral implants were 20/25 at distance, 96% could read 20/20 at arm's length, and 73% could read at near without any assistance from glasses or contact lenses. The Trulign is similar to the Crystalens but provides astigmatic correction.
Multifocal IOLs simultaneously focus near and distance light. Refractive options include the Array (first generation) and ReZoom (second generation). Both IOLs consist of five concentric zones that create multiple focal points. Bifocal diffractive options include the ReSTOR and Tecnis. The ReSTOR lens has apodized diffractive changes on the lens surface. The Tecnis lens has its diffractive steps on the posterior surface. The PanOptix is a trifocal diffractive IOL with improved intermediate vision.
Extended depth of focus IOLs create a single elongated focal point to provide a range of vision. The Tecnis Symfony features a posterior diffractive surface with an echelette design.
Many patients complain of haloes, glare, and problems driving at night with multifocal, bifocal, and extended depth of focus lenses. Make sure these patients are consented appropriately prior to implant them in patients.
The Light Adjustable Lens uses UV light to alter the IOL shape and correct residual postoperative myopia, hyperopia, and astigmatism. It is not FDA approved in the United States at the time of printing.

37. Are there any other surgical options for the treatment of myopia or presbyopia?
Because the crystalline lens adds about 18 D of power to the optical system, clear lens extraction may be used in patients with a comparable level of myopia. However, performing intraocular surgery for a purely refractive goal is controversial. In addition, highly myopic eyes carry a moderate risk of retinal detachment, which is increased after lens extraction.
Kamra is a corneal inlay that offers a surgical option for presbyopia. The Kamra inlay (Fig. 14.11) works on the same principle as a camera aperture by increasing the depth of focus. The opening in the inlay allows only focused light into the eye, allowing one to see near, far, and everything in between. The Kamra received FDA approval April 2015 in the United States.

38. What are the treatment options for astigmatism?
The correction of astigmatism is slightly more forgiving than the correction of myopia. A patient with 3.00 D of astigmatism is usually quite pleased with a postoperative residual of 1.25 D of cylinder correction because of reasonably good vision results. Each of the procedures for myopia has adaptations to address astigmatism alone or simultaneously with myopia. Astigmatic keratotomy refers to making transverse (straight) or arcuate astigmatic cuts in the midperiphery of the steep corneal meridian. Crossing transverse and radial incisions is problematic. Epithelial ingrowth into the stroma, healing difficulties, and significant scarring may result. Excimer laser photo-astigmatic refractive keratotomy uses a cylindrical ablation pattern rather than spherical ablation to remove tissue in a chosen meridian (astigmatic correction). In patients with compound myopic astigmatism, a combination of

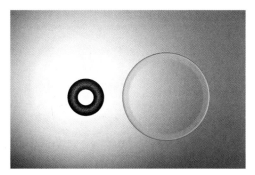

Fig. 14.11 Kamra corneal inlay.

spherical and cylindrical patterns corrects both myopia and astigmatism. Similar astigmatic corrections have been achieved with LASIK. Whichever procedure is employed, the axis of the astigmatism should be marked with the patient seated, because it may shift when the patient reclines. Corneal astigmatism can also be addressed during cataract surgery with a toric IOL implanted after crystalline lens extraction.

39. **What can be done about astigmatism after a corneal transplant?**
There are several options. First, selective removal of sutures in steep meridians may improve astigmatism. A rigid gas-permeable contact lens may be especially effective in alleviating irregular astigmatism. However, many patients do not tolerate or desire contact lenses after corneal transplant surgery. Once all sutures are out and the refraction is stable, arcuate relaxing incisions may be performed in the donor cornea along the steep meridian to reduce astigmatism. An alternative technique involves using a blade to open the wound partially and relax several clock hours of the graft–host junction as opposed to creating incisions in the donor tissue. The femtosecond laser can also be used to create arcuate keratotomy incisions. As described earlier, the excimer laser also has been used to correct post–corneal transplant astigmatism. Relaxing incisions combined with compression sutures (across the graft–host interface) have been used successfully to correct astigmatism of 5 to 10 D by causing steepening of the cornea in the sutured median (Fig. 14.12). For astigmatism greater than 10 D, a wedge resection (of corneal tissue followed by sutured closure of the wound) may be performed in the flat meridian.

40. **A 40-year-old Olympic ski coach desires refractive surgery so that he may see distance clearly. His refraction is −3.00 × −2.00 at 180 in both eyes. The surgeon performs radial incisions for 3.00 D of myopia and transverse incisions to flatten the steep meridian by 2.00 D at 90 degrees. Is the patient happy?**
The patient is unhappy because of residual myopia. He now knows more about the "coupling effect" than his surgeon. When one incision causes corneal flattening in one meridian, there is a compensatory steepening of the unincised corneal meridian 90 degrees away. In this case, the coupling effect of the incised and unincised meridians (90 degrees apart) should have been anticipated. Radial incisions must be used to correct the 3.00 D of spherical myopia as well as the approximate 1.00 D of steepening induced by the transverse incisions. In general, short incisions tend to cause less steepening of the unincised meridian than longer incisions do.

41. **What about procedures for hyperopia?**
Of the available options, none is as effective or reliable as the procedures for myopia.
　　For low levels of hyperopia, *holmium laser thermokeratoplasty* has been used with some success. This procedure is FDA approved for the "temporary reduction" of hyperopia in patients 40 years of age or older with between +0.75 and +2.50 D of manifest spherical equivalent with −0.75 D of astigmatism. Eight (or 16) peripheral laser spots are placed in a ring (or two), with each spot causing shrinkage of the stromal collagen and resulting in steepening of the central cornea. Problems to be resolved include regression of effect and induced astigmatism.
　　Conductive keratoplasty (CK) involves the use of low-energy radiofrequency energy delivered to the cornea with a guarded needle in a ring pattern around the midperiphery of the cornea. The heat generated causes collagen shrinkage, allowing the central cornea to steepen. CK was FDA approved in 2002 for the treatment of hyperopia in patients 40 years of age and older with a manifest refraction between +0.75 and +3.25 D. The procedure is effective for low to moderate hyperopia, but the trend is for regression over several years. CK has also recently been FDA approved to treat presbyopia in people over 40.
　　Hyperopic excimer laser PRK also has been approved by the FDA to treat hyperopia between +1 and +6 D. Treatment of hyperopic astigmatism also has been approved by the FDA in patients with +0.5 to +5.0 D of sphere with refractive astigmatism of +0.5 to +4.0 D and a maximal manifest refraction spherical equivalent of +6.0 D at the spectacle plane. The laser is used to create a large, donut-shaped ablation that requires a generous epithelial defect (often 9 mm or more).

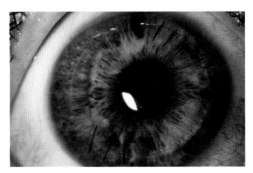

Fig. 14.12 Treatment for postcorneal transplant astigmatism. Compression sutures were placed in the flat meridians (1:00 to 3:00 and 6:30 to 8:00), and relaxing incisions were performed in the graft wound 90 degrees away.

Hyperopic LASIK treatments are currently FDA approved to treat up to 6 D of hyperopia with up to 6 D of astigmatism. Performing the laser ablation under a corneal flap has the theoretical advantage of decreased haze (ablation performed deep to the Bowman's layer) and faster healing response (no large epithelial defect).

Phakic IOLs can treat hyperopia as well as myopia; however, they are not currently FDA approved to do so.

Clear lens extraction is a technique already familiar to most surgeons. Phacoemulsification is performed with implantation of one or two IOLs as required by the degree of hyperopia. However, accommodation is completely eliminated by the procedure. Moreover, the risks of intraocular surgery, including endophthalmitis, are difficult to justify in eyes without organic disease.

42. What are the effects of refractive surgical procedures on corneal endothelial cells?

Although endothelial cell loss was an early concern in RK, studies using specular microscopy have demonstrated only a small, nonprogressive loss of endothelial cells. After excimer laser treatment of myopia, studies in animals and humans suggest a small, insignificant loss of endothelial cells that diminishes over time. Certainly, it is much more of a concern with intraocular surgery, especially phakic IOLs. Ongoing studies are important. As the treated population grows older, patients eventually will require cataract surgery. There are already case reports of a renewed hyperopic shift in post-RK patients undergoing cataract surgery. Is corneal decompensation in Fuchs' endothelial dystrophy accelerated by previous refractive surgery? Many questions remain unanswered. The effects of the laser itself, the inflammatory response, and the toxicity of topically applied drugs may contribute to endothelial cell loss and require further study.

43. What is the role of drugs in refractive surgery?

The first issue is pain, which is important in all treatment modalities but most significant for PRK. After PRK, increased levels of prostaglandin E-2 have been found, which sensitize the pain response of nerves. Topical nonsteroidal anti-inflammatory drugs (NSAIDs) such as ketorolac and diclofenac sodium have been shown to decrease pain by reducing prostaglandin E-2 levels. However, these agents also increase white blood cell response in the cornea and should be used concomitantly with a topical steroid. One study found increased sterile corneal infiltrates when topical NSAIDs were used alone.

Another issue is corneal haze after PRK. The cornea undergoes a wound-healing response to the excimer laser ablation. Activated keratocytes lay down new collagen and proteoglycan matrix (the haze). This is first apparent at 1 month postoperatively, peaks at 3 months, and then decreases as remodeling ensues. Several experimental and retrospective studies have shown that topical steroids reduce corneal haze after PRK. However, a prospective, double-masked study revealed no benefit from topical steroids versus placebo. Still, in a subgroup of patients, steroids may be beneficial, and they are typically used postoperatively.

Topical steroids also have been studied in the modulation of corneal curvature. Despite controversy in the literature, topical steroids apparently help to prevent regression of myopic effect after PRK. In fact, cessation of steroids has been associated with myopic regression, which may be reversed on reinstituting therapy in certain patients.

Mitomycin C (MMC) is a cell-cycle-nonspecific alkylating agent that targets rapidly dividing cells. MMC is being used by topical application during PRK for people with moderate to high myopia. The goal is to reduce the proliferation of keratocytes and fibroblasts, thus reducing the haze seen after moderate to deep ablations. MMC has shown great promise in refractive surgery and is felt to be safe for use on the cornea; however, the adverse reactions to MMC when used on the conjunctiva or sclera can be quite severe. Reported complications of MMC include corneal and scleral melts, cataract formation, and corneal edema.

REFERENCES

1. Sanders DR, Deitz MR, Gallagher D: Factors affecting predictability of radial keratotomy, Ophthalmology 92:1237–1243, 1985.
2. Waring GO III: Refractive keratectomy for myopia, St. Louis, Mosby.
3. Waring GO III, Lynn MJ, McDonnell PJ: Results of the prospective evaluation of radial keratotomy (PERK) study 10 years after surgery, Arch Ophthalmol 112:1298–1308, 1994.
4. O'Brart DP, Shalchi Z, McDonald RJ, et al.: Twenty-year follow-up of a randomized prospective clinical trial of excimer laser photorefractive keratectomy, Am J Ophthalmol 158(4):651.e1–663.e1, 2014.
5. Chen S, Feng Y, Stojanovic A, et al.: IntraLase femtosecond laser vs mechanical microkeratomes in LASIK for myopia: a systematic review and meta-analysis, J Refract Surg 28(1):15–24, 2012.
6. Pop M, Payette Y: Photorefractive keratectomy versus laser in situ keratomileusis: a control-matched study, Ophthalmology 107:251–257, 2000.
7. Tham VM, Maloney RK: Microkeratome complications of laser in situ keratomileusis, Ophthalmology 107:920–924, 2000.
8. Holland SP, Mathias RG, Morck DW, et al.: Diffuse lamellar keratitis related to endotoxins released from sterilizer reservoir biofilms, Ophthalmology 107:1227–1234, 2000.
9. Donaldson KE, Braga-Mele R, Cabot F, et al.: Femtosecond laser–assisted cataract surgery, J Cataract Refract Surg 39:1753–1763, 2013.
10. Binder PS: Flap dimensions created with the IntraLase FS laser, J Cataract Refract Surg 30:26–32, 2004.
11. Durrie DS, Kezirian GM: Femtosecond laser versus mechanical keratome flaps in wavefront-guided laser in situ keratomileusis: prospective contralateral eye study, J Cataract Refract Surg 31:120–126, 2005.

12. Touboul D, Salin F, Mortemousque B, et al.: Advantages and disadvantages of the femtosecond laser microkeratome, J Fr Ophthalmol 28:535–546, 2005.
13. Rapuano CJ, Sugar A, Koch DD, et al.: Intrastromal corneal ring segments for low myopia: a report by the American Academy of Ophthalmology, Ophthalmology 108:1922–1928, 2001.
14. Alio JL, de la Hoz F, Perez-Santonja JJ, et al.: Phakic anterior chamber lenses for the correction of myopia: a 7-year cumulative analysis of complications in 263 cases, Ophthalmology 106:458–466, 1999.
15. Nanavaty MA, Daya SM: Refractive lens exchange versus phakic intraocular lenses, Curr Opin Ophthalmol 23(1):54–61, 2012.
16. Benedetti S, Whomsley R, Baltes E, Tonner F: Correction of myopia of 7 to 24 diopters with the Artisan phakic intraocular lens: two-year follow-up, J Refract Surg 21:116–126, 2005.
17. Pop M, Payette Y: Initial results of endothelial cell counts after Artisan lens for phakic eyes: an evaluation of the United States Food and Drug Administration Ophtec Study, Ophthalmology 111:309–317, 2004.

CHAPTER 15

GLAUCOMA

Mary J. Cox and George L. Spaeth

GLAUCOMA

1. **What is glaucoma?**

   Glaucoma is a highly heterogeneous group of conditions in which tissues of the eye are damaged. Usually, the optic nerve is damaged, resulting in a characteristic optic neuropathy with associated visual-field loss. In conditions such as acute angle-closure glaucoma, the lens, cornea, and other structures may be affected as well. The etiology of glaucoma is multifactorial. Elevated intraocular pressure (IOP) is one of the factors responsible for the damage. The role of IOP in glaucoma damage is variable. Increased IOP is the sole cause for the damage in acute angle-closure glaucoma, whereas in low-tension glaucoma (LTG), IOP may play less of a role in the disease process.

2. **How is glaucoma classified?**

   The broad classifications of glaucoma are somewhat artificial; they tend to blur as we learn more about the disease and its pathogenesis. Traditionally, glaucoma has been classified as open angle or closed angle based on the gonioscopic angle appearance. This differentiation plays an important role in treatment. Open- and closed-angle glaucomas have been further classified as primary or secondary. Open-angle glaucoma is classified as primary when no identifiable contributing factor for the increased IOP can be identified. Secondary glaucoma identifies an abnormality to which the pathogenesis of glaucoma can be ascribed. Examples include pseudoexfoliative, uveitic, angle recession, and pigmentary glaucoma.

3. **How prevalent is glaucoma?**

   Glaucoma is the second leading cause of irreversible blindness in the United States and the third leading cause of blindness worldwide. Primary open-angle glaucoma (POAG) affects approximately 2.5 million Americans. Half are unaware that they have the disease. Population-based studies have shown prevalence among Whites 40 years of age and older ranging from 1.1% to 2.1%. The prevalence among Blacks is three to four times higher. Prevalence increases with age. People over 70 have a prevalence three to eight times higher than people in their 40s.[1]

4. **Name the risk factors for the development of primary open-angle glaucoma.**

   Known risk factors include elevated IOP, age, race, and a positive family history of glaucoma. Decreased central corneal thickness also has been shown to contribute to the risk of developing glaucoma. A newly described risk factor is corneal hysteresis. For every 1 mm Hg reduction in corneal hysteresis, the risk of glaucoma increases by 21%.[2,3]

   Presumed risk factors for which evidence exists but sometimes appears conflicting include myopia and diabetes mellitus. Potential risk factors for which some association has been found include hypertension, cardiovascular abnormalities, sleep apnea, and vasospastic conditions such as Raynaud's phenomenon or migraine. Disc hemorrhage, increased cup-to-disc ratio, and asymmetric cupping of the optic nerve may represent either risk factors or evidence of early disease.[4]

5. **Discuss the genetics of primary open-angle glaucoma.**

   POAG is most likely inherited as a multifactorial or complex trait. A combination of multiple genetic factors or of genetic and environmental factors is required to develop the disease. One specific gene, the TIGR/myocilin gene, has been found to confer susceptibility to POAG. Family history is an important risk factor for the development of glaucoma. The Baltimore Eye Survey found that the relative risk of having POAG is increased approximately 3.7 times for individuals having siblings with POAG.[5,6]

6. **What is the pathogenesis of glaucoma?**

   The pathogenesis of glaucoma has been only partially elucidated. In some cases, elevated IOP may cause optic nerve damage by mechanically deforming the optic nerve with posterior bowing of the lamina cribrosa. In other cases, a decrease in perfusion of the optic nerve may cause damage. This may happen from a sudden drop in blood pressure in response to blood loss or medications. Anemia can result in ischemia of the optic nerve. Focal vasospasm may contribute to a decreased perfusion and ischemia in patients with the low-tension forms of glaucoma. In most patients, several different pathogenetic mechanisms probably operate simultaneously.[7]

7. **What is the clinical presentation of primary open-angle glaucoma?**

   POAG is slowly progressive and painless. It is usually bilateral but often asymmetric. Central visual acuity is relatively unaffected until late in the disease; therefore patients are often asymptomatic. Advanced disease may be present before symptoms are noticed.

8. What is normal intraocular pressure?

The line between normal and abnormal IOP is not clear. Mean IOP is around 16 mm Hg, with a standard deviation of 3 mm Hg. It is a non-Gaussian distribution skewed toward higher pressures. Elevated IOP has been shown to be a risk factor for glaucoma; however, only 5% of people with pressures above 21 mm Hg eventually develop glaucoma. Conversely, patients with glaucoma damage may have IOPs consistently in the normal range.[8,9]

9. True or false: Loss of peripheral vision is a warning sign of early glaucoma.

False. Loss of temporal vision (side vision) is the last to be affected in most types of glaucoma. The first area to be damaged in most people with glaucoma is vision to the nasal side of central vision. This helps explain why patients do not notice loss of vision until the damage is marked. Both eyes provide vision to the nasal side so that a blind spot is not noted with both eyes open until vision is lost in both eyes.[1]

KEY POINTS: COMMON VISUAL-FIELD DEFECTS FOUND IN GLAUCOMA

1. Superior/inferior nasal step.
2. Superior/inferior arcuate defect.
3. Generalized depression.
4. Paracentral loss.
5. Temporal or central island in advanced disease.

---

10. Who is a glaucoma suspect?

A glaucoma suspect is an adult who has an open angle on gonioscopy and one of the following findings in at least one eye:
- Optic nerve appearance suspicious for glaucoma (see later)
- Visual-field defect consistent with glaucoma
- Elevated IOP consistently greater than 22 mm Hg

    If a patient has two or more of the earlier findings, then a diagnosis of glaucoma is likely. The decision to treat a glaucoma suspect takes into account the earlier findings as well as additional risk factors and the general health of the patient.[7]

11. In examination of the optic nerve, what findings could be consistent with a diagnosis of glaucoma or suspicion of glaucoma?

Diffuse narrowing of the optic nerve rim, focal narrowing or notching of the optic nerve rim, vertical elongation of the optic cup, nerve fiber layer defects, nerve fiber layer hemorrhages, and asymmetric cupping of the optic nerves are all signs of glaucoma or suspicion of glaucoma. An acquired pit of the optic nerve is a pathognomonic sign of glaucoma.[10]

KEY POINTS: COMMON OPTIC NERVE FINDINGS IN GLAUCOMA

1. Diffuse narrowing of the neuroretinal rim.
2. Focal narrowing or notching of the neuroretinal rim.
3. Nerve fiber layer defects.
4. Disc hemorrhages.
5. Asymmetry of optic nerve cupping.

---

12. A patient presents with optic nerve damage in one eye as shown in Fig. 15.1. The other eye has lower pressures and a healthier optic nerve with a normal visual field. What is the prognosis for the healthier optic nerve?

The optic nerve in Fig. 15.1 shows complete loss of the inferotemporal rim. Optic nerve damage in one eye has been associated with a significantly increased risk of future damage in the other eye. Twenty-nine percent of untreated fellow undamaged eyes will show visual-field loss in an average of 5 years.[11]

13. A 74-year-old Black female presents for a routine eye examination. She has not been to an ophthalmologist in 10 years. Her IOPs are 26 mm Hg in the right eye (OD) and 24 mm Hg in the left eye (OS). Her optic nerves are as shown in Fig. 15.2. What information is important to obtain from the patient?

The optic nerves in Fig. 15.2 show significant asymmetry with a narrower rim supertemporally in the right eye in comparison to the left eye. She has not been seen by an ophthalmologist for years. The history is a crucial part of the evaluation; it identifies possible secondary causes for glaucoma (e.g., trauma, steroid use) as well as risk

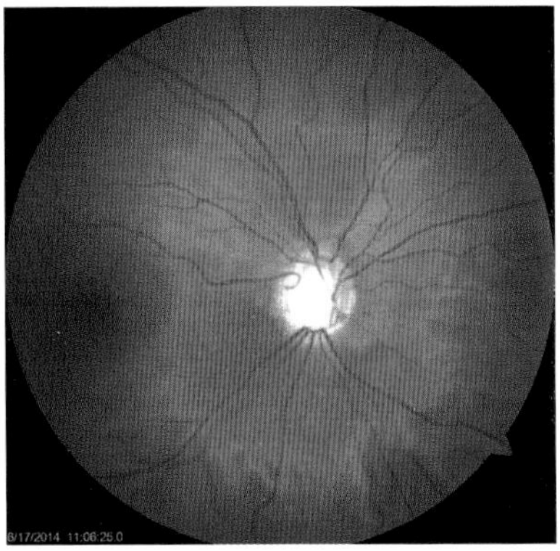

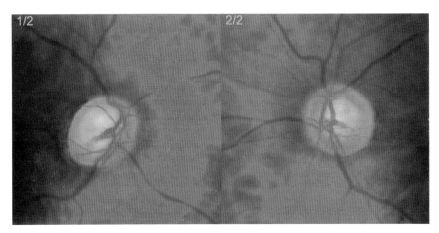

Fig. 15.1 Complete loss of the neuroretinal rim is a sign of advanced glaucoma.

Fig. 15.2 Asymmetry of the cup-to-disc ratio can be an early sign of glaucoma.

factors such as family history, helps determine the visual demands and support system of the patient, and can give an idea of the patient's general health and life expectancy. All of these components help formulate a treatment plan most likely to be agreeable to the patient, least likely to be damaging, and of an appropriate level of aggressiveness for each individual patient.

14. If the patient in question 13 had been to another ophthalmologist several times a year and was presenting for the first time in your office, what information would be important to obtain?
    Old records are valuable. Knowing about previous surgeries, lasers, and medicines (both those that worked and those that did not) helps formulate a current treatment plan. Previous IOP readings, former visual-field tests, and optic nerve evaluations can establish the rate of progression of the disease, a key piece of information in determining the level of aggressiveness needed in treatment.

15. True or false: If the patient in question 13 had a normal visual field, she would be unlikely to have glaucoma.
    False. Visual-field defects may not be apparent until as much as 50% of the optic nerve fiber layer has been lost.

16. True or false: If the patient in question 13 had intraocular pressures of 19 mm Hg OD and 18 mm Hg OS, then she would be unlikely to have glaucoma.
    False. A single IOP measurement in the normal range is not enough to eliminate the possibility of glaucoma. Several studies suggest that as many as 30% to 50% of individuals in the general population having glaucomatous optic nerve damage and visual-field defects have an initial IOP measurement of less than 22 mm Hg. Diurnal IOP

fluctuation and artificially low measurements due to decreased central corneal thickness or other factors may contribute to the normal IOP. In addition, patients with normal-tension glaucoma (NTG) or LTG have glaucomatous optic neuropathies without ever demonstrating elevated IOPs.[12,13]

17. **How does intraocular pressure fluctuate in glaucoma patients?**
    Individuals without glaucoma may have an IOP fluctuation of 2 to 6 mm Hg over a 24-hour period. IOP in glaucoma patients may vary widely. In untreated glaucoma patients it may vary by 15 mm Hg or more in 24 hours. The majority of patients demonstrate the highest pressures in the morning with a decrease throughout the day. Other patterns with peak pressures at night or midday as well as flat patterns without variation have been reported.[14]

18. **What role does central corneal thickness play in the evaluation of glaucoma?**
    Corneal thickness is important to consider for two reasons. First, corneal thickness affects the measurement of IOP so that the measured IOP may be inaccurate if the corneal thickness is not average. The actual average central corneal thickness is approximately 544 μm. IOP is about 5 mm Hg lower than measured for each 100 μm that the cornea is thicker than normal. The true IOP is actually higher than measured when the cornea is thinner than average. Second, a thin central cornea, in itself, is associated with more severe glaucoma. The Ocular Hypertension Treatment Study identified reduced central corneal thickness as a risk factor for glaucoma in patients with IOP between 24 and 32 mm Hg.[15,16]

19. **Name factors that affect the measurement of intraocular pressure.**
    IOP measurements can be overestimated and underestimated based on several factors (see Table 15.1).

20. **What role does imaging play in the evaluation and management of glaucoma?**
    Significant structural retinal nerve fiber layer (RNFL) loss occurs prior to functional visual-field loss. Periodic stereoscopic optic disc photography remains the gold standard for documentation of the optic nerve appearance and assessment of glaucoma progression over time. However, newer technologies such as optical coherence tomography (OCT) are now available to assess the RNFL, optic nerve head, and ganglion cell complex. This technology may assist in the detection of RNFL loss in situations in which the subtle signs of disease could be overlooked on clinical exam. It can also help confirm the diagnosis or progression of glaucoma in the setting of corresponding RNFL defects and visual-field defects.[17]

21. **What parameters on optical coherence tomography are useful in the diagnosis and management of glaucoma?**
    As shown in Fig. 15.3, OCT measures the RNFL thickness and then compares those data with a normative age-matched database. Green, yellow, and red colors signify the percentage chance that the thickness is within the

Table 15.1 Factors Influencing the Accurate Measurement of IOP
Overestimation of IOP
Pressing on the globe
Thick tear meniscus (too much fluorescein)
Thick central cornea
Valsalva (breath-holding or straining)
Thick neck/obese patients
Anxiety
Astigmatism
Orbital disease/restrictive ocular myopathy, as with Graves' disease
Corneal scarring and high corneal rigidity
Flat anterior chamber
Underestimation of IOP
Thin tear meniscus (too little fluorescein)
Thin central cornea
Corneal edema
Repeated IOP measurements/prolonged contact with cornea
Low corneal rigidity

IOP, Intraocular pressure.

Name:

	OD	OS
ID: 38536	Exam date:	8/8/2013	8/8/2013
DOB: 2/27/1948	Exam time:	8:06 AM	8:07AM
Gender: Male	Serial number:	4000–7549	4000–7549
Doctor:	Signal strength:	9/10	9/10

ONH and RNFL OU analysis: Optic disc cube 200×200   OD ○ | ○ OS

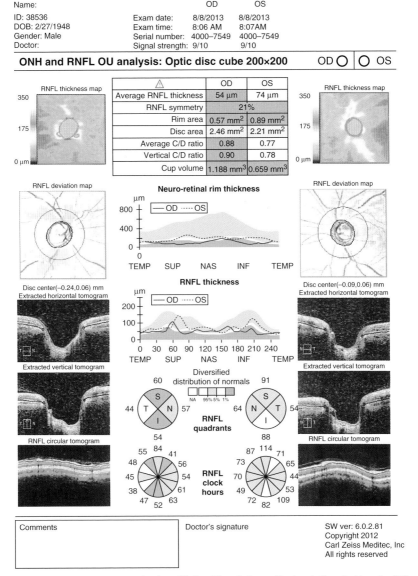

⚠	OD	OS
Average RNFL thickness	54 µm	74 µm
RNFL symmetry	21%	
Rim area	0.57 mm²	0.89 mm²
Disc area	2.46 mm²	2.21 mm²
Average C/D ratio	0.88	0.77
Vertical C/D ratio	0.90	0.78
Cup volume	1.188 mm³	0.659 mm³

Fig. 15.3 Optical coherence tomography shows thinning of the retinal nerve fiber layer in the patient from Fig. 15.2.

normal range for an age-matched population. OCT also documents optic nerve head parameters including optic rim area, optic disc area, average cup/disc ratio, vertical cup/disc ratio, and optic cup volume.[18] These are helpful to compare over time as well as a good way to show patients objectively their disease state and progression. Newer technology allows for techniques to measure blood flow and optic nerve head perfusion as well.[19] However, their clinical usefulness is not yet fully determined

22. True or false: If the OCT showed no evidence of RNFL thinning, then the patient does not have glaucoma.
    False. OCT technology may be limited by signal quality, image artifact, and confounding ocular disease. Serial imaging can be used as an adjunct to standard perimetry and optic disc photography. Clinical decisions should not be made on the basis of a single test or technology.

23. What is the primary goal of treatment of patients with glaucoma?

The primary goal in the treatment of glaucoma is enhancing the patient's health by improving or preserving his or her vision. One way of preserving vision is by lowering the IOP. It is important not to lose sight of the primary goal in treatment. All treatment options carry side effects and risks. The patient's general health and visual demands always need to be considered.

24. Name the initial treatment options for primary open-angle glaucoma.

Options include observation or lowering the IOP by using eyedrops, selective laser trabeculoplasty, or surgery.

25. What factors help determine which option to try?

When deciding on an initial treatment for a patient with glaucoma, several factors need to be considered. First, determine how aggressive the treatment needs to be. The level of aggressiveness takes into consideration the severity of the disease, the rapidity of progression, and the general health of the patient. Second, the toxicity and cost of the various treatment options need to be assessed. This will help predict compliance. For example, a 70-year-old healthy patient with advanced disease and an inability to tolerate medicines would most likely benefit from surgery. A healthy 45-year-old with mild to moderate disease may begin with medication or a laser trabeculoplasty. An elderly sick patient with mild to moderate disease may benefit from observation alone.

26. Are eyedrops safer than oral medications?

No. Eyedrops are directly absorbed into the blood through the nasal mucosa. This route bypasses the first-pass metabolism of drugs by the liver and can allow increased effects for a given amount of absorption.

27. Are some optic nerves more resistant to intraocular pressure damage than others?

Yes. Small nerves with no peripapillary atrophy but small central cups in which it is not possible to see laminar dots are less likely to become damaged than eyes with large optic nerves, large cups, peripapillary atrophy, and prominent laminar dots. A large cup does not necessarily correlate with glaucoma if the optic nerve head itself is large. It is important to determine the optic nerve size when evaluating neuroretinal rim.

28. A patient being treated for glaucoma presents for a follow-up examination with an optic nerve appearance as shown in Fig. 15.4. Discuss the findings.

Fig. 15.4 demonstrates an optic nerve with vertical elongation of the cup. Narrowing at the superior and inferior rim often occurs in glaucoma. A nerve fiber layer hemorrhage is present at the inferotemporal rim of the optic nerve. Disc hemorrhages are commonly found in glaucoma patients. They are important prognostic signs for the development or progression of visual-field loss.[20]

29. Name five potential causes of disc hemorrhages.
   • Glaucoma
   • Posterior vitreous detachments
   • Diabetes mellitus
   • Branch retinal vein occlusions
   • Anticoagulation

30. What is low-tension glaucoma?

LTG is one of the traditional labels for a glaucomatous optic neuropathy that occurs without evidence of elevated IOP. Because "low" is a relative word, and because many people with "low tension" have IOP above the mean, but in the normal range, the term *normal-tension glaucoma* is also used interchangeably with *low-tension glaucoma*. There is much controversy over whether NTG is part of a spectrum of POAG with IOP that is not elevated above the average range or its own disease entity. The optic nerve in patients with NTG is susceptible to damage at normal IOP. Ischemia may contribute significantly to the progression of the disease. Studies suggest

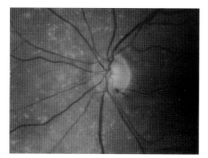

Fig. 15.4 Elongation of the optic nerve cup can be an early finding in glaucoma. Splinter disc hemorrhages can be a prognostic indicator for progressive disease.

Table 15.2 Differential Diagnosis of Glaucoma-Like Optic Discs and Visual Fields

1. Missed elevated IOP
   - Diurnal variability
   - Incorrect measurement
   - Thin central cornea (<500 μm)
2. Previous IOP elevation, no longer present
3. Shock-induced optic neuropathy
4. Compressive optic neuropathy
5. Ischemic optic neuropathy
6. Giant cell arteritis (temporal arteritis)
7. Optic nerve anomalies (pituitary tumors, etc.)
8. Macular degeneration
9. Juxtapapillary choroiditis
10. Myopia
11. Demyelinating disease

IOP, Intraocular pressure.

a higher prevalence of vasospastic disorders such as migraine or Raynaud's phenomenon, coagulopathies, cardiovascular disease, sleep apnea, and autoimmune disease in patients with LTG. Nocturnal hypotension and anemia may also result in decreased optic nerve perfusion in patients with LTG. Working with the primary care doctor to change systemic antihypertensive medications so that the lowest blood pressure is not during nocturnal hours can help in these patients.

31. **What disease entities can mimic low-tension glaucoma?**
Undetected "high-tension glaucoma" can mimic LTG. This could be the result of a missed elevation of IOP that occurs at times when the IOP was not measured, a thin central cornea, or an error in applanation. The patient could have suffered a previous episode of severe IOP elevation from a secondary glaucoma such as uveitic or steroid-induced glaucoma that had subsequently normalized. He or she could have suffered intermittent spikes from angle closure. The patient may have suffered an episode of optic nerve hypoperfusion due to blood loss from surgery or trauma. Compressive optic nerve lesions, ischemic optic neuropathy, congenital anomalies, and certain retinal disorders can also mimic NTG (Table 15.2).[21]

32. **What tests should be considered in the workup of a patient with glaucomatous-appearing optic nerves and visual fields without elevated intraocular pressure?**
Usually, the diagnosis is clear on the basis of the appearance of the optic nerve, the visual field, and the asymmetry of IOP with the higher pressure in the eye with more damage. When not clear, a diurnal curve and central corneal thickness should be checked to be certain that the condition is not a "high-tension" glaucoma with low IOP readings. A computed tomography or magnetic resonance imaging scan to evaluate for compressive lesions of the optic nerve or chiasm may be indicated. If history or symptoms suggest, rapid plasma reagin/Venereal Disease Research Laboratory, rheumatoid factor/antinuclear antibody, or erythrocytic sedimentation rate may be checked to look for syphilis, autoimmune diseases, or temporal arteritis (giant cell arteritis) as potential causes. If a patient is on blood pressure medicines or has a history of hypotension, a 24-hour Holter monitor to check for nocturnal hypotension may be indicated.

33. **How is normal-tension glaucoma treated?**
The Collaborative Normal-Tension Glaucoma Study found that by reducing the IOP by 30%, the rate of progression of visual-field loss was reduced from 35% to 12%. Lowering intraocular pressure is the mainstay of treatment for normal-tension glaucoma, as well as POAG.[22]

REFERENCES

1. Tielsch JM, Sommer A, Katz J, et al.: Racial variations in the prevalence of primary open-angle glaucoma. The Baltimore Eye Survey, JAMA 266:369–374, 1991.
2. Medeiros F, Meira-Freitas D, Lisboa R, et al.: Corneal hysteresis as a risk factor for glaucoma progression: a prospective longitudinal study, Ophthalmology 120:1533–1540, 2013.
3. Susanna C, Diniz-Filho A, Daga F, et al.: A prospective longitudinal study to investigate corneal hysteresis as a risk factor for predicting development of glaucoma, Am J Ophthal 187:148–152, 2018.

4. Caprioli J, Bateman J, Gaasterland D, et al.: Primary open-angle glaucoma: preferred practice pattern, San Francisco, 2003, American Academy of Ophthalmology.
5. Tielsch JM, Katz J, Sommer A, et al.: Family history and risk of primary open-angle glaucoma. The Baltimore Eye Survey, Arch Ophthalmol 112:69–73, 1994.
6. Wolfs R, Klaver C, Ramrattan R, et al.: Genetic risk of primary open-angle glaucoma: population-based familial aggregation study, Arch Ophthalmol 116:1640–1645, 1998.
7. American Academy of Ophthalmology: Basic and clinical science course, section 10, San Francisco, 2004, American Academy of Ophthalmology.
8. Colton T, Ederer F: The distribution of intraocular pressures in the general population, Surv Ophthalmol 25:123–129, 1980.
9. Dielemans I, Vingerling JR, Wolfs RC, et al.: The prevalence of primary open-angle glaucoma in a population-based study in the Netherlands. The Rotterdam study, Ophthalmology 101:1851–1855, 1994.
10. Coleman AL, Morrison JC, Callender O: Evaluation of the optic nerve head. In Higginbotham E, Lee D, editors: Clinical guide to glaucoma management, Boston, 2004, Elsevier, pp 183–191.
11. Kass MA, Kolker AE, Becker B: Prognostic factors in glaucomatous visual field loss, Arch Ophthalmol 94:1274–1276, 1976.
12. Mitchell P, Smith W, Attebo K, et al.: Prevalence of open-angle glaucoma in Australia. The Blue Mountains Study, Ophthalmology 103:1661–1669, 1996.
13. Sommer A, Tielsch JM, Katz J, et al.: Relationship between intraocular pressure and primary open angle glaucoma among white and black Americans. The Baltimore Eye Survey, Arch Ophthalmol 109:1090–1095, 1991.
14. Zeimer RC: Circadian variations in intraocular pressure. In Ritch R, Shields MB, Krupin T, editors: The glaucomas, ed 2, St. Louis, 1996, Mosby, pp 429–445.
15. Brandt JD, Beiser JA, Kass MA, et al.: Central corneal thickness in the ocular hypertension treatment study, Ophthalmology 108:1779–1788, 2001.
16. Ehlers N, Bramsen T, Sperling S: Applanation tonometry and central corneal thickness, Acta Ophthalmol 53:34–43, 1975.
17. Quigley HA, Dunkelberger GR, Green WR: Retinal ganglion cell atrophy correlated with automated perimetry in human eyes with glaucoma, Am J Ophthalmol 107(5):453–464, 1989.
18. Aref AA, Budenz DL: Spectral domain optical coherence tomography in the diagnosis and management of glaucoma. Ophthalmic surgery, Lasers Imaging 41(6):S15–S27, 2010.
19. Jia Y, Wei E, Wang X, et al.: Optical coherence tomography angiography of optic disc perfusion in glaucoma, Ophthalmology 121(7):1322–1332, 2014.
20. Diehl D, Quigley HA, Miller NR, et al.: Prevalence and significance of optic disc hemorrhage in a longitudinal study of glaucoma, Arch Ophthalmol 108:545–550, 1990.
21. Kent AR: Low-tension glaucoma. In Higginbotham E, Lee D, editors: Clinical guide to glaucoma management, Boston, 2004, Elsevier, pp 183–191.
22. Collaborative Normal-Tension Glaucoma Study Group: Comparison of glaucomatous progression between untreated patients with normal-tension glaucoma and patients with therapeutically reduced intraocular pressures, Am J Ophthalmol 126:487–497, 1998.

CHAPTER 16

ANGLE-CLOSURE GLAUCOMA

George L. Spaeth

1. **What landmarks are seen in the anterior chamber angle?**
   The structures noted in anterior-to-posterior sequence are as follows (numbered list corresponds to numbers in Fig. 16.1):
   1. **Schwalbe's line:** The peripheral or posterior termination of Descemet's membrane, seen clinically as the apex or termination of the corneal light wedge. This technique requires perfect focus in which the focal planes of the microscope oculars are the same as those of the examiner. Schwalbe's is often shiny and may bulge slightly into the anterior chamber (AC). With increasing age, dots of pigment deposit on its surface, most markedly at the 6 o'clock position, and lessening nasally and temporally. Such pigment is not present superior to the 4 or 8 o'clock positions.
   2. **Anterior, *nonpigmented,* trabecular meshwork (TM):** Clear whitish band, nonreflective.
   3. **Posterior, *pigmented,* TM:** Variably pigmented band of homogeneous width. It is best identified by noting it has texture, rather like fine-grain velvet. The pigment is located within the meshwork, not on its surface contrasting to the pigmentation on the surface of Schwalbe's line. It is usually more intensely pigmented at the 12 o'clock than the 6 o'clock position and less pigmented at 3 and 9 o'clock. In brown eyes, pseudoexfoliation syndrome, and following trauma, the pigmentation is greatest inferiorly (Fig. 16.2).
   4. **Schlemm's canal:** Elevated episcleral venous pressure or pressure from the edge of the goniolens may cause blood to reflux, making it appear as a faint red band.
   5. **Scleral spur:** Narrow, refractile white band of sclera invaginating between the TM and the ciliary body (CB). Marks the insertion site of the longitudinal muscle fibers of the CB to the sclera.
   6. **CB band:** Pigmented band marking the anterior face of the CB. Variably, iris processes may be seen as lacy projections crossing this band. By definition, iris processes do not extend anterior to the scleral spur. Projections that cross the scleral spur to the TM are usually peripheral anterior synechiae (PAS) and may occur in a variety of relatively diagnostic patterns associated with the various conditions causing them. They may be focal, pillar-like, or broad sheets.
   7. **Iris**

2. **Why is a goniolens necessary to visualize the anterior chamber angle?**
   Light from the AC angle undergoes total internal reflection at the cornea (tear)–air interface, preventing direct visualization. A goniolens changes the refractive index at the interface, enabling visualization.

3. **What are the different types of gonioscopy? How do they differ?**
   - A Koeppe contact lens is used for direct gonioscopy. This technique is cumbersome, requiring a separate illuminator, a handheld binocular microscope, and the patient to be supine. A clear liquid is used as a coupling medium. As the patient is supine, the angle usually appears deeper than when the patient is seated.
   - Indirect gonioscopy uses a mirrored contact lens. Several styles are available. The Goldmann, three-mirror lens allows examination of the angle, the posterior pole and peripheral retina. As the curvature of the lens is greater than that of the cornea, a coupling fluid such as methylcellulose is required. This has the disadvantage of blurring the patient's vision and making subsequent visualization of the ocular fundus suboptimal. There are also several styles of goniolenses that do not require a coupling fluid as they have a curvature similar to that of the cornea and a much smaller surface diameter. Thus they can be used for indentation gonioscopy. Lenses with a much wider anterior surface diameter are easier to use, but cannot be used for indentation gonioscopy that is essential for diagnosing narrow AC angles properly. Among the indentation-type lenses are the Zeiss (Fig. 16.3), Posner, and Sussman four- or six-mirror lenses. These directly contact the cornea and thus do not require a coupling agent, beyond the patient's normal tear film. All direct gonioscopic lenses are used at the slip lamp.

4. **Which goniolens is preferred by most glaucoma specialists and why?**
   The Zeiss, Posner, and Sussman lenses are preferred by a majority of glaucoma specialists for the following reasons:
   - Speed and ease of use (they do not require a viscous coupling liquid and, because of their four or six mirrors, they do not need to be rotated to see all 360 degrees of the angle).
   - The ability to perform indentation. The ability to indent the cornea in order to displace aqueous and deepen the peripheral AC is essential for differentiating appositional contact between the peripheral iris and the wall of the eye and from the anterior synechiae between these two surfaces. The suction effect of the Goldmann lens can sometimes artificially widen narrow angles. These two qualities can be critically important when evaluating eyes with narrow angles.
   - Elimination of the transient degradation of corneal clarity that is a consequence of the viscous liquid and Goldmann lens manipulation, which can make subsequent fundus examination difficult.

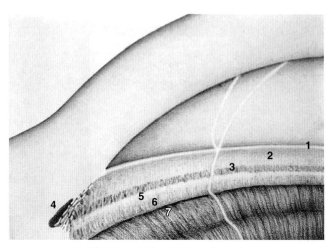

Fig. 16.1 Diagram of the anterior chamber anatomy.

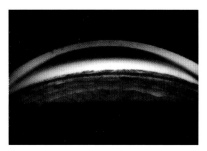

Fig. 16.2 Inferior quadrant of a heavily pigmented open angle.

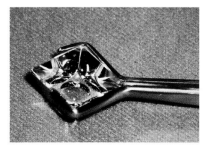

Fig. 16.3 Zeiss goniolens.

Warning: When first mastering gonioscopy, the Zeiss lens can be more difficult than the Goldmann lens. In inexperienced hands, excessive indentation can easily occur, which will (1) blur the view and (2) make the angle appear wider than it really is. Zeiss gonioscopy demands a light touch. If contact with the lens is light enough so that part of the contact meniscus is occasionally lost, pressure is not too excessive. If corneal striae are noted or the view is not crystal clear, the pressure is causing corneal indentation and much be lessened.

5. How is gonioscopy performed?
   This depends on the type of lens being used, the nature of the eye being examined, and the purpose of the examination. It must be clearly understood that gonioscopic skill cannot be adequate until one has gonioscoped approximately 1000 normal eyes. While it is easier to learn with a Goldmann-type lens, the novice should quickly

progress to an indentation type. Every patient should be examined at every visit until the examiner can examine and write the grading of the angle in 1 minute at the most (per eye). A major concern is causing corneal erosions. These can be avoided by being certain the cornea is moist and by not keeping the lens on the eye for more than a minute. After a minute, the lens should be removed, the person asked to blink in order to moisten the cornea or given a moistening drop if necessary before the gonioscopy is resumed. This is not usually a problem when employing a Goldmann-type lens. The problem can be avoided by having the patient blink immediately before the process of gonioscopy is started and, IMPORTANTLY, by having the patient keep both eyes closed when not being examined!! In almost all cases, the examining room must be dark enough, and the illuminating beam focused enough that the pupil is minimally constricted. A topical anesthetic is required, and the cornea must be kept moist in order to avoid causing corneal erosions. The slit lamp must be prepared for the particular examiner and the patient. The illuminating beam must always be 30 degrees temporal to the visual axis. Magnification should be as low as possible and can be increased later if necessary.

The patient must be told that they will feel the lens and will want to blink and also that the procedure will not be painful, even though it will be felt.

Goldmann-type examination: After the previous steps, a coupling substance is placed on the surface of the lens that will contact the eye. The patient places their head in the slit lamp and is told to blink and then to look slightly up, elevating the upper lid. When examining the right eye, the examiner holds the Goldmann lens with the thumb and third finger of the left hand and with the curved-most mirror at the 12 o'clock position. While looking around the temporal side (examiner's left side) of the slit lamp, when the patient is looking slightly up, the lens is placed firmly on the right eye and held there. The examiner tells the patient to keep their head in the slit lamp and to look straight ahead. The examiner then looks through the microscope into the superior mirror, moves the joy stick to get the view in meticulous focus, and attempts to identify the TM. It has texture, and usually a relatively homogeneous brown pigmentation, which may be minimal or even totally absent in the young or the blue-eyed. It is posterior to the shiny Schwalbe's line, which often has pigment spots on its surface at the 6 o'clock position. It is anterior to the Scleral Spur, a totally unpigmented line anterior to the gray or brown CB. In the abnormal angle, the pigmented trabecular meshwork (PTM) may not be visible. If not, the examiner should try to identify another structure, such Schwalbe's line. The gonioscopy does not continue until the examiner has identified one structure with relative certainty. Start at the inferior angle because that is where the angle usually deepens and the structures are most easily identified. The examiner notes the most posteriorly visible structure and documents such:

A. for anterior to Schwalbe's line—that is no angle structures are visible.
B. for behind Schwalbe's line; that is, nothing posterior to Schwalbe's line can be seen.
C. if the scleral spur is visible
D. for deep, so that the CB can be seen
E. if the angle is extremely deep so that more than 1 mm of the CB is visible.

Next, estimate the degrees of the angle between the anterior surface of the iris and the posterior surface of the cornea, the apex of the triangle being Schwalbe's line.

Then, determine whether the iris is flat (f) or bowed anteriorly (b) or curved convexly posteriorly (c) or rises steeply anterior from its insertion and then becomes flat, that is, has a plateau appearance (p). If the angle has a 10 degree or less angularity, or if the PTM is not visible, then indentation must be done. The indentation-type goniolens is pushed against the corneal dome, forcing the aqueous humor toward the periphery of the AC, near the root of the iris. This iris will be displaced posteriorly but only where it is not adherent to the wall of the glove or lying on the surface of the lens. This will displace the iris posteriorly, but only where it is not adherent to the wall of the globe or lying on the surface of the lens. Therefore it is possible to differentiate between inability to see the landmarks due to the iris obstructing the view—because it has either a bowed or a plateau configuration—or whether the iris is actually adherent to the inner wall of the eye. Thus the examiner describes the configuration.

Next, the qualitative characteristics are described: pigmentation, adhesions, other aspects such as blood in Schlemm's canal, or abnormal blood vessels.

At the slit lamp:
- Topical anesthesia is essential for patient comfort and cooperation.
- Rest your elbow on the slit lamp platform and your ring and/or small fingers on the side bar or on the patient's cheek to help stabilize your hand.
- Examination can be facilitated by asking the patient to stare straight ahead with the fellow eye without blinking.
- To facilitate viewing a particular quadrant of the angle with indirect gonioscopy, either tilt the mirror toward the quadrant or have the patient look toward that mirror. For example, when viewing the superior angle, either tilt the inferior mirror upward, toward the superior angle, or have the patient look down slightly, toward the inferior mirror.
- The superior–inferior relationships in the nasal and temporal mirrors and the nasal–temporal (right–left) relationships in the superior and inferior mirrors are preserved, not inverted as in indirect ophthalmoscopy. For example, when viewing the superior angle through the inferior mirror, an area of PAS seen at 5 o'clock in the mirror is actually at 1 o'clock, not 11 o'clock.

6. How can I determine which patients may have narrow angles and need gonioscopy?
The van Herick technique uses a thin slit beam focused at the limbus to approximate angle depth by comparing the peripheral AC depth to corneal thickness. Grade I has a peripheral AC depth less than one-quarter of the

corneal thickness; grade II is one-quarter of the corneal thickness; grade III is one-half of the thickness; and grade IV is one corneal thickness or more. Patients who are grade I or II certainly have narrow angles and should have gonioscopy. This technique, however, should never replace gonioscopy in eyes with clear media as part of a glaucoma evaluation. It falsely gives the appearance of an open angle in some eyes with plateau iris or anterior rotation of the CB (see classification later).

7. What are the different gonioscopic anterior chamber angle classification systems?
Table 16.1 summarizes the *Scheie* system, which is rarely used, and the *Schaffer* system, which is the one most commonly used.

The *Spaeth system*, however, is the most descriptive. The first element is a capital letter (A to E), for the level of iris insertion:
- **A** = Anterior to the TM
- **B** = Behind the Schwalbe's line, or at the TM
- **C** = At the scleral spur
- **D** = Deep angle, CB band visible
- **E** = Extremely deep
  If, during indentation gonioscopy, the true iris insertion is noted to be more posterior than originally apparent, then the original impression is put in parentheses, followed by the true iris insertion outside parentheses.
  The second element is a number that denotes the iridocorneal angle width in degrees at the level of the TM, usually from 5 to 45 degrees.
  The third element is a lower-case letter describing the peripheral iris configuration:
- **f** = Flat
- **b** = Bowed or convex
- **c** = Concave
- **p** = Plateau configuration
  In addition, the pigmentation of the posterior TM is graded on a scale of 0 (none) to 4 (maximal). For example, (A)C10b, 2+PTM refers to an appositionally closed 10-degree angle that, with indentation, opened to the scleral spur and revealed moderate pigmentation of the posterior TM.

8. How do I know if I can safely dilate a patient, with or without a slit lamp?
If no slit lamp is available, use a penlight and shine it from the temporal side perpendicular to the central visual axis. In an eye with a normal or "safe" AC depth, the entire nasal half of the iris will be illuminated as well as the temporal half. In an eye with a shallow or questionable AC depth, none or only part of the nasal half of the iris will be illuminated. This technique does not hold true in eyes with plateau iris.

If a slit lamp is available, angles that are less than or equal to 15 degrees are at risk for closure and probably should not be dilated. An eye with a 20-degree angle should be watched closely, as it may narrow further with time, and should be reevaluated with tonometry and gonioscopy after dilation. An exception to these general guidelines is plateau iris (discussed later), in which the angle may be wider than 20 degrees and still at risk for closure. Thus the peripheral iris configuration is also very important.

9. What are other methods of evaluating anterior chamber angles besides gonioscopy?
There are several imaging devices that can display the AC angles. Ultrasound biomicroscopy (UBM) uses ultrasound to visualize the angles. The ultrasound waves are not blocked (absorbed) by the iris pigmented epithelium. Therefore it has the advantage of visualizing the CB. UBM is particularly useful to identify a plateau iris configuration (PIC). Anterior-segment optical coherence tomography (OCT) uses a diode laser to obtain anterior segment imaging. Limbus-to-limbus images are possible in a single scan with the Visante OCT. OCTs designed for retinal imaging can perform anterior segment imaging if used with adaptive lenses. However, because the diode laser can be blocked by the iris pigmented epithelium (especially in dark irises), OCT cannot visualize the CB as clearly as UBM in individuals with dark irises. In addition to UBM and OCT, Scheimpflug cameras (Pentacam) use a specific optical principle to image angles. Classification of angles by UBM and OCT is different from that by gonioscopy. Gonioscopy is still the gold standard of angle classification. Gonioscopy also gives valuable information such as pigmentation or presence of abnormal vessels that cannot be demonstrated by imaging devices.

Table 16.1 The Scheie and Schaffer Classification Systems

	GRADE 0	GRADE I	GRADE II	GRADE III	GRADE IV
Scheie		Wide open	Scleral spur visible, CB band not seen	Can see only to anterior TM	Closed
Schaffer[a]	Closed	10 degrees	20 degrees	30 degrees	40 degrees

[a]The angle is graded as a slit when it is between grades 0 and I.
CB, Ciliary body; *TM*, trabecular meshwork.

10. How is angle closure classified?
   I. By clinical presentation
      A. Acute
      B. Subacute or intermittent
      C. Chronic
   II. By mechanism
      A. Posterior pushing mechanism
         1. Pupillary block (can occur in phakic, pseudophakic, or aphakic eyes)
            a. Relative idiopathic (i.e., primary angle closure [PAC]), miosis induced
            b. Absolute or true: By posterior synechiae from any inflammatory etiology
         2. Lens induced
            a. Phacomorphic (due to an intumescent cataractous lens or a swollen lens in a diabetic)
            b. Lens subluxation
               i. Trauma
               ii. Pseudoexfoliation syndrome
               iii. Hereditary/metabolic disorder (e.g., Marfan's syndrome, homocystinuria)
            c. Lens pushed forward
               i. Aqueous misdirection syndrome (malignant or ciliary-block glaucoma)
               ii. Mass (e.g., tumor, retinopathy of prematurity, persistent hyperplastic primary vitreous)
         3. Plateau iris
            a. True plateau iris
            b. Pseudoplateau—iris and CB cysts
         4. Swelling/anterior rotation of the CB (some overlap within this)
            a. Inflammatory (e.g., scleritis, uveitis, post–panretinal photocoagulation [PRP])
            b. Congestive (e.g., after scleral buckling surgery, nanophthalmos)
            c. Choroidal effusion—secondary to medications (e.g., topiramate), hypotony after trauma or surgery, uveal effusion, etc.
            d. Suprachoroidal hemorrhage (SCH)—intraoperative or postoperative. Risk factors for SCH include previous intraocular pressure (IOP) elevation followed by hypotony, high myopia, advanced age, aphakia, previous vitrectomy, systemic hypertension or atherosclerotic vascular disease, and postoperative Valsalva maneuver
      B. Anterior pulling mechanism—synechial angle closure
         1. Chronic appositional closure from any of the above
         2. Intraocular inflammation (uveitis)—forming synechial membrane
         3. Neovascular glaucoma (NVG)
            a. Central retinal vein occlusion (CRVO), accounts for one-third of cases
            b. Diabetes mellitus, accounts for another one-third of cases
            c. Carotid occlusive disease, comprises approximately 10% of cases
            d. Miscellaneous (e.g., central retinal artery occlusion [CRAO], tumors, chronic retinal detachment)
         4. Iridocorneal endothelial syndrome
            a. Progressive iris atrophy
            b. Chandler's syndrome
            c. Cogan-Reese syndrome

11. What do the terms PACS, PAC, APAC, and PACG signify? How are they related to acute, subacute, and intermittent angle closure?
PACS stands for primary angle closure suspect
PAC stands for primary angle closure
PACG stands for primary angle-closure glaucoma
APAC stands for acute primary angle closure

   The terms refer to a new classification system of angle closure currently used in most clinical and epidemiological studies. This system was developed by the International Society of Geographical and Epidemiological Ophthalmology between 1998 and 2005. PACS refers to patients with narrow angle on *gonioscopy* but without elevated IOP or presence of PAS. PAC refers to patients with narrow angle and elevated IOP or PAS. PACG refers to patients with narrow angle and glaucomatous optic neuropathy and/or visual field defects (Table 16.2).
   The purpose of this new classification system is to unify the definition of glaucoma. It reserves the term *glaucoma* for the presence of optic neuropathy. For example, a patient presenting with acute elevated IOP secondary to angle closure will be referred to as APAC instead of acute angle-closure glaucoma, as the patient may not have developed (yet) glaucoma optic neuropathy during the episode of acute angle closure.
   The new classification system relates to the traditional classification of angle-closure glaucoma to some degree. Acute angle-closure glaucoma is referred to as acute primary angle closure; chronic angle-closure glaucoma can be either PAC or PACG depending on the status of the optic nerve and visual field. Subacute or intermittent angle-closure glaucoma can be PACS, PAC, or PACG with self-limited symptoms. The status of the angle and optic

Table 16.2 The International Society of Geographic and Epidemiological Ophthalmology Classification of Angle Closure

	NARROW ANGLES	ELEVATED IOP OR PAS	GLAUCOMATOUS OPTIC NEUROPATHY
Primary angle closure suspect (PACS)	+	−	−
Primary angle closure (PAC)	+	+	−
Primary angle closure glaucoma (PACG)	+	+/−	+

IOP, Intraocular pressure; *PAS*, peripheral anterior synechiae.

nerve dictates the classification of angle closure instead of the patient's symptomatology and probably has better prognostic value than the previous system.

The new classification intends to describe the natural history of angle closure. Anatomically narrow angles (i.e., PACS) are common; about 4% to 10% of the population above the age of 40 have some degree of narrow angle. Angles narrow with age as the lens thickens throughout life. *Some* (not all) PACS will progress to PAC and eventually to PACG. Some PACS will develop APAC. We are still trying to identify which subgroup of PACS will progress to PACG and evaluating effective preventive treatments.

A study of almost 900 individuals considered angle-closure suspects at the Zongshan Ophthalmic Center in China who were followed for 72 months after treatment of one eye, the fellow being a control, found a low in incidence of development of angle closure in untreated eyes—specifically 36 eyes. Angle closure developed in 19 of the 889 eyes treated with laser iridotomy. The authors report that no cases had serious adverse effects. They recommend not routinely treating eyes considered to be at risk for angle closure.

It is important not to generalize these conclusions to other populations. The fact that 19 of the treated eyes developed angle closure indicates that either the iridotomy was not performed properly or that the patients did not have angle closure due to relative pupillary block, a mechanism responsible for PAC in individuals of European extraction. Furthermore, that there were no adverse effects from the angle closure reinforces the fact that the clinical condition being evaluated has different characteristics than acute primary angle closure in Europeans, many of whom develop excruciating pain and have permanent ocular damage following the attack. This Chinese study must not be considered to show that PAC in other populations is so benign that there is no need to prevent its occurrence.

PRIMARY ANGLE CLOSURE (RELATIVE PUPILLARY BLOCK AND OTHER MECHANISMS)

12. What is the epidemiology of primary angle-closure glaucoma?

Inuit or Eskimos have the highest incidence of APAC, followed by Asians and then Caucasians and those of African descent. It is more common in Northern European Caucasians than in Mediterranean Caucasians. The peak incidence is between the ages of 55 and 65. In both Asians and Caucasians, women are three to four times more likely to develop angle closure than men. In those of African descent, the incidence is equal between men and women. There is a greater incidence in hyperopes. The inheritance appears to be polygenic. However, the asymptomatic form of angle-closure glaucoma (PACG) is the most common form of angle-closure glaucoma across all ethnicities.

13. Which is more common: chronic angle-closure glaucoma or symptomatic acute angle closure?

The chronic, asymptomatic form of PACG is much more common across all ethnicities. Most of the angle-closure diseases are asymptomatic. This highlights the importance of gonioscopy in *every patient* presenting with elevated IOP and/or glaucoma optic neuropathy. In fact, patients with PACG are often misdiagnosed as having primary open-angle glaucoma (POAG) because gonioscopy is omitted during clinical examination. It is very important to differentiate PACG from POAG, as the treatments are different for the two. The treatment of PACG starts with addressing the mechanism of angle closure—performing laser peripheral iridotomy (PI) or removing the lens. The treatment of POAG starts with aqueous suppression or enhancing outflow by medication or laser.

14. What are the symptoms of acute primary angle closure?

Patients may complain of ocular pain, redness, blurred or foggy vision, halos around lights, nausea, and vomiting. The visual symptoms are partly caused by the corneal edema that occurs from the sudden severe rise in IOP. This, the most common presentation, is most often induced by stress, low ambient light levels, and, occasionally, various medications. If the IOP exceeds the pressure in the ophthalmic or central retinal artery, visual loss occurs as a result of ischemia of the optic nerve or retina. Most APACs progress into chronic angle closure with elevated IOP (i.e., PAC) and the development of glaucomatous optic neuropathy (i.e., PACG).

15. Describe the signs or exam findings seen in acute primary angle closure.
    - **IOP:** Typically greater than 45 mm Hg.
    - **Conjunctiva and episclera:** Dilated vessels.
    - **Cornea:** Epithelial and stromal edema.
    - **AC:** Shallow; cells or flare variably present.
    - **Iris:** Dilated vessels (as distinguished from neovascularization of the iris), middilated nonreactive or sluggish pupil, and sector atrophy from ischemia (only if previous episodes have occurred).
    - **Lens:** Glaukomflecken (not seen acutely, but if present initially, may indicate previous episodes of angle closure).
    - **Gonioscopy:** With narrow angle or closed angle, one may be unable to view structures owing to corneal edema (glycerin may be used to clear the cornea); superior angle is usually the narrowest and the first to develop PAS.
    - **Optic nerve:** Occasional swelling and hyperemia from vascular congestion; may mimic papilledema.
    - **Retina:** May be normal or may show signs of vascular occlusion.
    - **Fellow eye:** Examination of the fellow eye is *very important* in making the diagnosis. It usually also has a shallow AC and narrow angle. If the fellow eye has a normal AC depth and a normal angle width, the diagnosis of primary angle closure should be reevaluated and secondary causes need to be addressed.

KEY POINTS: COMMON SIGNS OF ACUTE PRIMARY ANGLE CLOSURE

1. Dilated conjunctival and episcleral vessels.
2. Corneal edema.
3. Shallow AC with or without cells or flare.
4. Middilated, sluggish, or unreactive pupil.
5. Lens glaukomflecken.
6. Shallow AC and narrow angle in fellow eye.

16. How does subacute or intermittent angle closure present clinically?
    The symptoms are similar to an acute attack but usually less severe, tend to recur over days to weeks, and may be confused for headaches. They resolve on their own, often when the individual goes to sleep or enters a well-lit area (both induce miosis). These episodes can result in chronic angle closure. Between episodes, the IOP is normal and the ocular exam is usually normal, except for the presence of narrow angles and, sometimes, glaukomflecken, cataracts, and PAS on gonioscopy.

17. How does chronic angle closure present clinically?
    It is usually asymptomatic, unless marked visual-field loss has occurred. Gradual closure of the angle, by simple apposition and/or PAS, leads to a more gradual rise in IOP. The IOP is more variable but can be as high as 60 mm Hg without any symptoms. The cornea is usually clear, because the IOP rises gradually, resulting in a lack of pain, redness, decreased vision, or other symptoms. This is the most dangerous form of angle closure. Because of the lack of symptoms and very high IOP, patients tend to present late with very advanced disease.

18. What are the anatomic characteristics of eyes with primary angle closure?
    Anatomically, the eyes have short axial length, hyperopia, anterior segment crowding, including a thicker lens, and/or peripheral iris.

19. What is the pathophysiologic mechanism of relative pupillary block?
    The crystalline lens grows thicker throughout life. In eyes that are predisposed, apposition between the posterior iris surface and the anterior lens capsule gradually increases. As the iridolenticular touch increases, the resistance to aqueous flow from the posterior to the AC increases, gradually increasing posterior chamber pressure. Under conditions in which the pupil is in a middilated position (e.g., from stress, low ambient light levels, sympathomimetic or anticholinergic medications), the elevated posterior chamber pressure causes the lax or floppy iris to bow anteriorly and occlude the TM. It is hypothesized that thinner or lighter-colored irises are more likely to cause an acute rise in IOP because they are thinner and floppier, causing acute angle closure. Less floppy, thicker irises are pushed anteriorly more gradually, especially peripherally. This leads to creeping chronic angle closure, with or without PAS, and a more gradual IOP rise (Fig. 16.4).

20. What nonmedical maneuver may help to lower intraocular pressure even before medicating the patient?
    Even before starting medical treatment, indentation gonioscopy can sometimes help lower IOP by pushing aqueous from the central AC peripherally, opening the angle if it is not sealed with PAS. This must be done carefully to avoid abrading the corneal epithelium, which is swollen and may abrade more easily than normal. An AC paracentesis with a blade or needle may more rapidly decompress the eye, and medications would further lower the IOP.

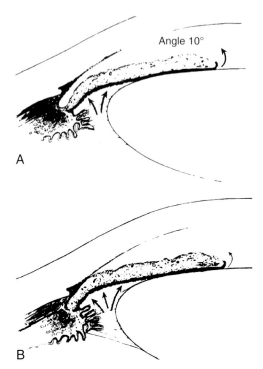

Fig. 16.4 Mechanism of relative pupillary block closure. **A,** Extremely narrow angle with resistance to aqueous flow between the iris and the lens, leading to increased posterior chamber pressure. **B,** Closed angle.

21. How would you treat the involved eye medically?

The "kitchen sink" approach is generally preferred, using some combination of the drugs listed later (Table 16.3). The use of miotics such as pilocarpine in narrow, potentially occludable, angles is a subject of some debate, even among glaucoma specialists. The rationale for miotic use is to pull the peripheral iris away from the TM, which opens the angle and prevents appositional closure. It may, however, make the angle narrower and potentially induce angle closure by causing the lens–iris diaphragm to move anteriorly with contraction of the ciliary muscle, which relaxes zonular tension and makes the pupillary block worse. If pilocarpine is used in such a patient, repeat gonioscopy should be performed 30 to 60 minutes after the initial drop. If the angle is not any wider, some would argue that a laser PI should be performed right away. If this is not feasible, consider adding a β-blocker to decrease aqueous secretion until the PI is performed.

- **Topical inhibitors of aqueous secretion:** β-Blockers, carbonic anhydrase inhibitors (CAIs), and α2-adrenergic agonists.
- **Uveoscleral outflow enhancers:** The prostaglandin analogs, as well as the α2-agonist brimonidine, increase uveoscleral outflow. Their use in angle closure has not been studied as extensively as some of the other agents, but they can also help lower the IOP. There is some theoretical concern that prostaglandin analogs could increase ocular inflammation. It should be remembered that miotics cause ciliary muscle contraction and decrease uveoscleral outflow.
- **CAIs:** In patients who are not nauseated, an oral CAI is administered. If intravenous (IV) medications are available and the patient is unable to tolerate oral medications, IV acetazolamide is preferred as an adjunct to topical therapy because of its faster onset of action.
- **Hyperosmotic agents:** Hyperosmotic therapy reduces vitreous volume and can be a very powerful weapon in lowering IOP and breaking an attack. Glycerin and isosorbide can be given orally. IV mannitol is the most potent agent for lowering IOP, but it also increases blood volume and should be used with caution, especially in patients with systemic medical issues such as congestive heart failure or kidney failure.
- **Topical steroids:** Topical steroids (e.g., prednisolone 1% qid) are a useful adjunct to control the usually concurrent intraocular inflammation that may or may not be clinically apparent.
- **Miotics:** Pilocarpine helps to break the attack by pulling the peripheral iris away from the TM and increasing trabecular outflow. However, the pupillary sphincter (but not the ciliary muscle) usually becomes ischemic at IOPs above 40 to 50 mm Hg and therefore unresponsive to miotics until the IOP is lowered with other

Table 16.3 Treatment of Angle-Closure Glaucoma

FIRST DAY OF PRESENTATION	IOP <40 mm Hg	IOP 40–60 mm Hg	IOP >60 OR >40 mm Hg WITH CUPPING
	• Topical pilocarpine 1%	• Topical pilocarpine 2%	• Topical α-agonist and β-blocker
	• Topical β-blocker and α-agonist (possible topical carbonic anhydrase inhibitor)	• Topical β-blocker and α-agonist	• Topical prednisolone 1%
		• Topical prednisolone 1%	• IV acetazolamide 500 mg
	• Recheck at 1 hour	• IV acetazolamide 500 mg	• Analgesics and antiemetics as needed
1 hour after presentation	• IOP < IOP of other eye	• IOP reduced 50% but > IOP of other eye	• IOP not reduced >50%
	• Topical β-blocker and α-agonist two times a day	• Topical pilocarpine 2%	• Topical pilocarpine 2%
	• Topical prednisolone 1% as needed	• Oral acetazolamide 500 mg	• Topical β-blocker and α-agonist
	• Recheck at 1 hour	• Recheck at 1 hour	• Oral glycerol 50% 1 mg/kg (or mannitol if vomiting)
2 hours after presentation	• IOP < IOP of other eye	• IOP reduced 50% but > IOP of the other eye	• IOP still not reduced 50%
	• Home on topical pilocarpine 1% two times a day and topical prednisolone 1% four times a day	• Topical pilocarpine 2% • Topical β-blocker and α-agonist • Oral glycerol 50% 1 mg/kg (or mannitol if vomiting) • Recheck at 1 hour	• Refer to specialist • Admit for IV mannitol • Maintain on oral acetazolamide 500 mg two times a day
	• Return the next day		• Topical agents, α-agonists, β-blockers two times a day
			• Keep NPO in preparation for surgery next day
			• If possible, have the specialist see the patient on same day
			• Do iridotomy or have specialist do iridoplasty (see "IOP elevated even after repeat mannitol"). In unlikely event that cornea is clear, do iridotomy

Continued on following page

Table 16.3 Treatment of Angle-Closure Glaucoma *(Continued)*

SECOND DAY	IOP < IOP OF OTHER EYE	IOP ELEVATED EVEN AFTER REPEAT MANNITOL
	• If eye uninflamed and cornea clear, do Nd:YAG peripheral iridotomy in the affected eye	• Clear the cornea with glycerin
	• If eye inflamed and cornea not clear, defer peripheral iridotomy in the affected eye and do peripheral iridotomy on the fellow eye	• Gonioscope again • Check disc
		• If peripheral iridotomy not already done, try to do if able to see adequately
		• If laser iridotomy already done and angle still closed, consider iridoplasty
		• If IOP falls >50% below presentation level, continue topical and oral medications and adjust therapy, depending on the amount of cupping and future course of glaucoma
		• If IOP does not fall >50% below level at presentation, patient probably needs guarded filtration procedure
		• If IOP falls >50% below the presentation level, continue topical and oral medications and adjust therapy, depending on the amount of cupping and future course of IOP
THIRD DAY		
	• Do Nd:YAG peripheral iridotomy on fellow eye if not already done	
	• Arrange follow-up	
	• Plan to do Nd:YAG laser iridotomy on the affected eye as soon as cornea is clear and eye quiet	

All topical medications apply to the affected eye. No therapy in the form of drops is to be used in the unaffected eye unless that eye also has glaucoma or other ocular problems. Specifically, pilocarpine is *not* to be used in the unaffected eye.
IOP, Intraocular pressure; *IV*, intravenous; *NPO*, nothing by mouth; *YAG*, yttrium, aluminum, and garnet.
From Glaucoma Service, Wills Eye Hospital/Jefferson Medical College.

medications. The duration of IOP elevation and sphincter ischemia ultimately determines whether the sphincter will respond to miotics even after the IOP is lowered. The usual concentration used is 1% or 2%. Pilocarpine should be used with caution to avoid cholinergic toxicity. Also keep in mind that it may make some cases of angle closure worse, as noted earlier. Some believe it should not be used in aphakic or pseudophakic pupillary block.
- **Topical glycerin:** Topical glycerin can be quite helpful to clear the cornea, which facilitates detailed examination of the eye and also laser treatment.
- **Others:** The α2-agonist brimonidine increases uveoscleral outflow, as do the prostaglandin analogs.

KEY POINTS: BASIC TREATMENT OF ACUTE PRIMARY ANGLE CLOSURE

1. "Kitchen sink" approach of maximal medical topical therapy plus oral acetazolamide if patient not nauseated.
2. Oral hyperosmotics if above not effective and the patient not nauseated, otherwise IV mannitol.
3. Laser PI.

22. **How would you treat the involved eye with laser?**
    Laser PI is the definitive procedure of choice to relieve pupillary block (Fig. 16.5). Angle closure from any etiology other than pupillary block will not respond to iridotomy. The argon or Q-switched yttrium, aluminum, and garnet (YAG) lasers

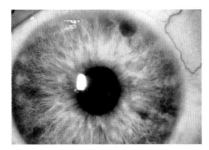

Fig. 16.5 Patent laser peripheral iridotomy.

are used. The Nd:YAG laser is preferred because it is faster and easier, requires fewer bursts with less energy (causing less inflammation), is not dependent on iris color, and is less likely to cause complications such as posterior synechiae. The argon laser's thermal effect can help prevent bleeding and facilitate penetration of thick irides.

There is also some difference of opinion regarding the timing of the laser PI in acute angle closure. If the IOP cannot be reasonably controlled medically, then the PI must be performed immediately. If the pressure can be reasonably controlled medically, it may be better to defer the iridotomy for a few days for the following reasons:
- Corneal edema from high pressure and Descemet's folds from the abrupt lowering of pressure can both make visualization and performing the iridotomy more difficult. In addition, because the AC is usually shallow, the corneal endothelium is closer to the point of laser energy focus and is more likely to be damaged from the concussion.
- The iris is usually somewhat congested, edematous, and inflamed during an attack. This can make the iridotomy more difficult to perform. More power may be required to successfully penetrate the iris, and this can be more uncomfortable for the patient than when the eye is not inflamed.

23. What are the most common complications of laser peripheral iridotomy?
    The most troublesome problem is a ghost image resulting from light that has entered through the PI.
    - **Argon:** Posterior synechiae and localized cataracts. Argon laser PIs are more likely to close than are Nd:YAG PIs.
    - **Nd:YAG:** A hemorrhage may occur in up to 50% of eyes. It is usually small and localized to the area of the PI, but sometimes can form a significant hyphema. The bleeding may be controlled by applying gentle pressure on the eye with the contact lens. Even relatively large hyphemas are almost always gone the next day.

      Transient IOP spikes of more than 6 mm Hg do occur in up to 40% of patients, most often within the first 1 to 2 hours. Perioperative treatment with apraclonidine decreases the incidence and severity of postlaser IOP spikes. β-Blockers and CAIs have been used, but with less success. The incidence and severity of postoperative IOP elevation are similar with argon and Nd:YAG lasers.

24. What if a peripheral iridotomy is unsuccessful? What other options are available for acute primary angle closure?
    I. Other laser treatments for APAC
        A. Laser iridoplasty: Using a goniolens, place spots of argon or diode laser at the peripheral iris to pull the iris away from the angle.
           One study showed that initial treatment with laser iridoplasty was more than one schedule or medicinal treatment in patients of Chinese extraction who developed acute primary angle-closure glaucoma. It is not known whether this conclusion holds in people of other ethnic extractions.
        B. Cyclophotocoagulation (CPC): Mild CPC using diode laser can abort cases of APAC refractory to medical and laser treatments (iridotomy and iridoplasty). It is not considered the first-line treatment for APAC but can be successful at aborting an episode of APAC when all options have failed before proceeding to surgery.
           In most cases of APAC, the IOP can be brought down successfully with medical treatment (usually requiring systemic medication) and laser treatment; surgery is rarely indicated in resolving IOP in the acute phase of APAC. It is not infrequent, however, that after a crisis of APAC, the IOP is elevated chronically (i.e., APAC progresses into PAC/PACG). Studies from recent years have demonstrated the benefit of removing the lens in the treatment of APAC, PAC, and PACG even when there is an absence of significant cataract.
    II. Surgical options for APAC
        A. Clear corneal peripheral iridectomy: This procedure was the treatment of choice for angle-closure glaucoma (acute or chronic) prior to the introduction of laser iridotomy. It is rarely performed today. However, if laser is not available or unable to be performed successfully, surgical iridectomy can be an option.
        B. Early cataract extraction for APAC: Recent studies demonstrated the benefit of lens extraction in patients with APAC, PAC, and PACG. Unlike in POAG, the IOP-lowering effect of cataract extraction alone is significant in all primary angle-closure cases (APAC, PAC, or PACG). A recent study compared the efficacy, safety,

and cost-effectiveness of laser PI to extraction of a clear lens as the initial treatment of primary angle-closure glaucoma and primary angle closure in association with an IOP above 29 mm Hg. A major conclusion was that control of IOP was minimally but statistically significantly better with lens extraction than laser iridotomy. Three years later, there was no difference detected in the visual field of the two groups. The importance of this study is that it indicates that lens extraction as well as laser iridotomy should be considered as initial treatment in patients with primary angle-closure glaucoma of mild or moderate severity, the choice depending on the particular aspects of each individual case.

C. Cataract extraction combined with goniosynechialysis: Mechanical pulling of PAS from the angle is performed at the end of cataract extraction surgery using a goniolens and a forceps of the surgeon's choice. The goal is to relieve the blockage of the TM from PAS and restore the outflow of aqueous humor. Some studies suggest that goniosynechialysis is more effective when the PAS are recent.

D. Cataract extraction combined with endocyclophotocoagulation (ECP): Laser treatment of the CB is performed at the time of cataract extraction using an endoscope equipped with a diode laser. Similar to CPC (which refers to external laser application on the CB), ECP coagulates the CB and reduces IOP. In addition, laser application shrinks the CB and opens the angle further, sometimes referred to as endocycloplasty. Currently, there is no evidence that cataract extraction combined with ECP or goniosynechialysis is superior to cataract extraction alone in the treatment of angle-closure diseases.

E. Trabeculectomy or tube shunts: Close to half the cases of APAC will progress into chronic PAC or PACG. In cases in which the IOP is consistently elevated despite laser iridotomy and medical treatment, lens extraction should be performed prior to filtering or tube shunt surgery, as the former carries fewer long-term complications and is often effective in reducing IOP. In advanced cases of PACG requiring very low IOP, combined lens extraction and filtering or tube surgery may be the best option.

When operating on these eyes, it is important to remember that they already have shallow chambers and are more likely to develop flat chambers and aqueous misdirection (malignant or ciliary block glaucoma). The use of miotics can also increase the chances of aqueous misdirection.

25. When can you consider an attack to be completely "broken"?

An attack can be considered "broken" when the IOP in the involved eye is lowered significantly and the patient's symptoms are resolved. However, many of these eyes will have chronically elevated IOP and require further medical and surgical treatment over the long term.

26. What are the chances of the same thing happening to the fellow eye?

There is a 40% to 80% chance of an acute attack in the fellow eye over the next 5 to 10 years.

27. What would you recommend for the fellow eye?

Prophylactic laser PI is recommended, if gonioscopic evaluation reveals a potentially occludable angle. It may be appropriate to treat the fellow eye first (if the angle is occludable) while waiting for the involved eye to quiet down and for the cornea to clear. The use of pilocarpine in the fellow eye to try to prevent angle closure by pulling the peripheral iris away from the TM until PI is performed is not without risk, as discussed in question 21.

28. Describe the short- and long-term sequelae to the various structures of the eye after an acute angle-closure attack.

- **Cornea:** Shortly after the IOP is lowered, the epithelial microcystic edema will resolve, and Descemet's folds may be seen from the acute reduction in IOP (Fig. 16.6). The stromal edema takes longer to resolve. In most cases, significant endothelial damage occurs. If the attack has caused enough endothelial injury, epithelial and stromal edema may persist. Endothelial pigment may result from the pigment released during iridotomy or from any ischemic atrophic regions of the iris.
- **AC:** Even after successful PI, the AC is usually still shallower than normal. Cataract extraction is the definitive treatment to deepen the AC.
- **Iris:** One may see a middilated, nonreactive, or sluggish pupil and sector atrophy and stromal necrosis from ischemia. Posterior synechiae may eventually develop long after a PI is performed owing to the alternate route available for aqueous humor flow. The pupil is often vertically oval.
- **Lens:** Glaukomflecken are small whitish anterior subcapsular opacities representing areas of necrotic lens epithelium with adjacent subcapsular cortical degeneration (see Fig. 16.6). Cataracts may develop or progress after an attack. Cataract extraction can be beneficial for IOP control in primary angle-closure glaucoma.
- **Zonules:** Zonular weakness may not manifest until much later, i.e., during cataract extraction or spontaneous subluxation or dislocation.
- **Gonioscopy:** PAS.
- **Optic nerve:** Disc congestion and swelling, if present, may take several days to resolve. Acute attacks typically produce more pallor than cupping. Chronic angle closure usually produces more cupping than pallor, similar to open-angle glaucoma. OCT may show a loss of ganglion cells and thinning of the retinal nerve fiber layer.
- **Retina:** "Decompression retinopathy" may be seen after rapid lowering of the IOP as scattered intraretinal hemorrhages concentrated more around the posterior pole and optic nerve. Peripapillary atrophy can also develop over time, along with focal nerve-fiber bundle defects, diffuse thinning of the retina, etc.

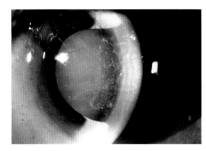

Fig. 16.6 Photograph of an eye after resolution of an acute angle-closure attack. Note the corneal Descemet's folds, the peripheral iridotomy at 12 o'clock at the upper edge of the photograph, and the lacy pattern of glaukomflecken under the anterior lens capsule.

29. What types of medications are contraindicated in narrow-angle glaucoma?

Topical and systemic sympathomimetic and anticholinergic medications should be avoided by people with eyes that have narrow and potentially occludable angles until a prophylactic laser iridotomy is performed. These are found in many over-the-counter antihistamine and cold remedies, antispasmodics for overactive bladder, and some antiparkinsonian agents. These medications are not contraindicated in patients with eyes that have narrow but not occludable angles, or eyes with a patent iridotomy, or in patients with open-angle glaucoma.

Use *miotics* with caution in patients with narrow angles, regardless of occludability, because of the risk of causing further narrowing by anterior displacement of the lens–iris diaphragm. These patients should at least have repeat gonioscopy after commencing miotic therapy to rule out this possibility. If the angles do become significantly narrower, one must consider discontinuation of miotic therapy or performing a prophylactic PI, in case there is a compelling reason for continuing miotic therapy.

KEY POINTS: LONG-TERM SEQUELAE OF AN ACUTE PRIMARY ANGLE-CLOSURE ATTACK

1. Corneal endothelial cell loss, endothelial pigment.
2. Permanently middilated and unreactive pupil.
3. Iris sector atrophy, posterior synechiae.
4. PAS in the angle.
5. Glaukomflecken, other cataractous changes.
6. Occasionally, lens zonular weakness (may be causative).
7. Optic nerve pallor out of proportion to cupping.

30. List some possible causes for persistent or recurrent intraocular pressure elevation after a successful PI.

- PAS formation and/or undetected injury to the TM during the period of angle closure
- Nonpupillary block angle closure (see question 10, classification, II.A.1 to 4.)
- Incomplete iridotomy will result in persistent IOP elevation. Occlusion of the iridotomy with debris or a membrane may cause a recurrent episode of pupillary block angle closure. Remember that transillumination does not equal patency.
- Underlying or residual TM dysfunction—chronic apposition of iris to the TM can induce trabecular dysfunction even in the absence of PAS.

PLATEAU IRIS

31. What is plateau iris configuration?

Anteriorly positioned (and sometimes larger than normal) ciliary processes push the peripheral iris more anteriorly than normal (Fig. 16.7). The central AC is usually slightly shallow or normal depth, but the angle recess is narrower than the depth of the AC would suggest. The iris has a relatively flat contour, with a sharp peripheral drop-off at the angle approach. This finding is designated "p" in our gonioscopic system. A component of pupillary block is frequently present. With dilation, the peripheral iris folds into the angle and occludes the TM.

32. How does plateau iris present clinically?

It may be noted on routine examination or present as an acute or chronic angle-closure glaucoma.

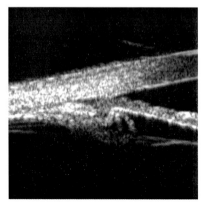

Fig. 16.7 Ultrasound biomicroscopy image of the anterior segment of an eye with plateau iris. Note the large ciliary processes causing anterior displacement of the peripheral iris and angle closure, whereas the central iris remains flat.

33. **Describe the epidemiology of plateau iris.**
   Traditional teachings describe patients with PIC as usually younger (typically fourth and fifth decades) and less hyperopic than patients with primary angle closure; they may even be myopic. With the advent of anterior segment imaging devices such as UBM, it has been found that PIC is quite common in both Asian patients and White patients—about 20% to 30% of the population has PIC. PIC refers to a narrow angle with steep iris on gonioscopy despite a patent iridotomy; however, the IOP is normal in the PIC. Eyes with PIC can develop elevated IOP acutely (APAC) or chronically (PAC). Traditionally, PIC eyes with elevated IOP, either acutely or chronically, are referred to as having plateau iris syndrome (PIS). It is unclear how many PIC eyes will progress to APAC or PAC. We suspect that only a small percentage of PIC patients will develop elevated IOP. However, we are still unable to identify which subset of PIC will progress to APAC or PAC.

34. **How can plateau iris be distinguished from relative pupillary block (primary) angle closure on slit lamp examination?**
   Primary angle closure normally presents with a shallow central AC and moderate to significant iris convexity, which is in contrast to the appearance of PIC noted earlier. With indentation gonioscopy, the angle is much harder to open and does not open as widely as a typical narrow angle. A "hills and valleys" profile may be seen when looking at the angle. In addition, indentation gonioscopy reveals the almost pathognomonic "double hump sign," characterized by posterior displacement of the midperipheral iris but a persistently anterior position of the peripheral iris. Persistence of the plateau iris appearance despite a patent iridotomy confirms the diagnosis clinically. High-resolution UBM can also confirm the diagnosis.

35. **What is plateau iris syndrome?**
   PIS is an acute or chronic angle closure that develops with dilation or, even spontaneously, in an eye with PIC and a patent PI.

36. **How is plateau iris syndrome treated?**
   PIC is a subset of PACS. PIS is APAC or PAC secondary to PIC. The treatment of PIC or PIS is similar to the treatment of PACS, PAC, or APAC.
   The primary procedure of choice in an eye with (or at risk for) angle closure is laser PI, to eliminate any component of pupillary block that may be present. In general, the older the patient, the more the pupillary block contributes, as a percentage, to the mechanism of angle closure. However, laser iridotomy is *not* adequate treatment in these cases; it is merely the necessary first step. Eyes with PIC often require other treatments to open the angle, especially if the patient has symptoms of intermittent angle closure or a positive prone darkroom test. It is essential to perform gonioscopy after the iridotomy to verify the angle status.
   Laser peripheral iridoplasty may be necessary in patients whose angle approach remains very narrow despite a patent PI. This technique uses the argon laser to apply burns circumferentially to the peripheral iris, which cause it to contract and pull away from the angle. Although the green wavelength is usually used, use of the yellow-green wavelength may improve absorption of laser energy in more lightly colored irides. One important potential complication that should always be discussed with the patient is the risk of a permanently larger pupil size postoperatively and its attendant potential to increase problems with glare. Avoiding vessels is also important to prevent anterior ischemia.
   Chronic miotic therapy can also be a useful alternative or adjunct to iridoplasty in eyes with a narrow approach despite a patent PI. With either method of therapy, the angle should be examined with gonioscopy after instillation of pilocarpine and at regular 6- to 12-month intervals afterward, to document the effect on angle configuration.

37. Are angles always open after a successful laser peripheral iridotomy?

No. About 20% to 40% of PACS eyes still have narrow angle even after a successful laser PI. To reiterate, PACS eyes do not have elevated IOP. Angles can remain narrow after a successful laser PI with normal IOP. The possible mechanisms of narrow angle after laser PI are PIC, thick peripheral iris (often found in Chinese PACS eyes), and lens-related mechanisms. Other secondary causes of angle narrowing should be sought as well. See question 10.

AQUEOUS MISDIRECTION SYNDROME (MALIGNANT/CILIARY BLOCK GLAUCOMA)

38. What is aqueous misdirection syndrome?

Posterior misdirection of aqueous into the vitreous cavity causes an anterior displacement of the lens–iris diaphragm. It most commonly occurs in eyes with narrow angles after ocular (typically glaucoma-filtering as well as cataract) surgery, but can occur after laser procedures or, rarely, spontaneously. Miotic use and previous angle-closure glaucoma increase the risk of occurrence. It typically presents within the first postoperative week with a shallow to flat AC and a high IOP, but the IOP may be normal in an eye with a functioning filter. Serous choroidal effusion/detachment, pupillary block, and SCH should be ruled out.

39. Why does aqueous misdirection occur? How does it present clinically?

It is still unclear why aqueous misdirection occurs. It is not an uncommon entity in glaucoma patients who undergo cataract or glaucoma surgery, especially in those with angle-closure glaucoma. It is hypothesized that a spontaneous or induced choroidal effusion in an eye with an impermeable vitreous can cause AC shallowing from a posterior pushing mechanism (the vitreous pushing the lens–iris diaphragm). This hypothesis makes clinical sense, as aqueous misdirection often occurs during the surgery when the AC volume is not maintained, leading to a transient hypotony.

Aqueous misdirection can occur during surgery or postoperatively. Patients will present with blurred vision with myopic shift (forward movement of lens). On slit lamp examination, the AC is diffusely shallow, both centrally and peripherally, in contrast to pupillary block, in which the AC is shallow more so peripherally than centrally. The IOP is usually high to normal.

40. How is aqueous misdirection treated medically?

- Cycloplegics relax the ciliary muscle, which increases zonular tension and pulls the lens–iris diaphragm posteriorly. Cycloplegics are also essential in the management of angle closure due to anterior rotation of the CB. They may be required indefinitely.
- Aqueous suppressants.
- Hyperosmotic agents.
- Miotics are contraindicated.

41. How can aqueous misdirection be treated with laser if it is unresponsive to medication?

The goal of therapy is to reestablish aqueous flow from the posterior chamber to the AC and to try to create a channel for aqueous flow from the posterior segment to the anterior segment.

- **Nd:YAG laser hyaloidotomy:** In pseudophakes and aphakes, using the Nd:YAG laser to disrupt the anterior vitreous face can be successful in resolving aqueous misdirection.
- **Argon laser treatment of ciliary processes:** Regardless of the lens status, this procedure can be done only if a surgical iridectomy or a relatively large laser iridotomy is present.

42. How can aqueous misdirection be treated surgically if it is refractory to medical therapy and/or laser?

The timing and mode of intervention depend on the following factors:

- Duration of misdirection without resolution.
- Degree and duration of shallowness or flatness of the AC. When there is contact between the corneal endothelium and the crystalline lens or an intraocular lens, surgical correction is urgent.
- IOP and optic nerve status.
    The treatment options are as follows:
- **AC reformation:** Occasionally, this can be performed at the slit lamp by injecting a small amount of air followed by viscoelastic through a peripheral corneal paracentesis wound. The initial air helps to confirm complete penetration of the needle through the cornea into the AC before injecting any viscoelastic. Because the IOP is almost always elevated with the aqueous misdirection syndrome, this is rarely an option.
- **Pars plana anterior or posterior vitrectomy (PPV):** Removing the vitreous is often the curative surgery for aqueous misdirection. Aqueous misdirection can occasionally persist or recur even after PPV, especially in phakic eyes.
- **Lens extraction:** This may be combined with vitrectomy. The posterior capsule and anterior hyaloid are usually incised to allow aqueous passage to the AC.
- **Iridozonulohyalovitrectomy:** This can be performed in phakic, pseudophakic, or aphakic eyes and consists of rendering the eye unicameral, by passing a vitrector either from the pars plana forward or from the AC posteriorly.

NEOVASCULAR GLAUCOMA

43. What typically causes neovascular glaucoma?

Posterior segment (retinal) ischemia results in the production of angiogenic factors that stimulate the formation of a neovascular membrane on the iris (NVI). Vascular endothelial growth factor (VEGF) has been shown to be the primary angiogenic factor. As the membrane first grows into the angle and across the scleral spur to the TM, the angle appears anatomically open. Later, the membrane contracts, pulling the peripheral iris up to the TM and peripheral cornea, creating PAS. This process can occur over significant areas of the angle very quickly (often in a few days), producing an acute angle-closure glaucoma (through an anterior pulling mechanism). Common causes of NVG are CRVO (one-third), proliferative diabetic retinopathy (one-third), and carotid occlusive disease (approximately 10%). Occasionally, CRAO, chronic uveitis, and intraocular tumor can cause NVG.

44. How is neovascular glaucoma treated?

- The underlying etiology of the neovascularization must be diagnosed and treated, usually with PRP or, if the lack of clear visualization of the retina precludes PRP, peripheral retinal cryotherapy for posterior segment ischemic processes. Anti-VEGF compounds injected into the vitreous or AC can produce a dramatic regression of NVI within 1 to 2 weeks. Patients should have repeat gonioscopy after an anti-VEGF injection, as the rapid contraction of the neovascular membrane may lead to further angle closure.
- **Medical treatment.** The percentage of angle that is closed with PAS as well as the outflow resistance of the TM still open will determine the potential for successfully treating the glaucoma medically. Even if the angle is completely closed, maximal tolerated aqueous suppressant and, if necessary, hyperosmotic therapy should be used in an attempt to temporize until surgery is performed. Miotics should not be used, because they decrease uveoscleral outflow and increase inflammation.
- **Surgical treatment.** One of the most important principles to remember when operating on these eyes, especially eyes with florid NVI, is to try to avoid rapid decompression of the eye. The fragile new vessels may rupture, creating a spontaneous hyphema that can significantly complicate subsequent management.
- **The guarded filtering procedure (trabeculectomy)** has been used to control the IOP in these eyes with poor results. The success rate is somewhat better if an adjunctive antimetabolite such as mitomycin C is used. The risk of filtration failure due to fibrosis is higher, presumably owing to the presence of angiogenic factors in the aqueous.
- **Aqueous tube shunts** have become the procedure of choice for many glaucoma surgeons, but still have success rates of only approximately 70%, owing to the often poor prognosis of the underlying pathologic process.
- **Laser CPC.** This may be a viable option in eyes with minimal visual potential, as an attempt to control IOP for long-term comfort and to prevent the need for enucleation for pain owing to high IOP. The diode laser is the preferred method of CPC. CPC by cryotherapy is seldom used nowadays because of postoperative pain, inflammation, and the risk of phthisis bulbi.

MISCELLANEOUS

45. What are the various mechanisms of producing angle closure secondary to ocular inflammation?

- PAS formation from any etiology
- Complete pupillary block (secluded pupil) from posterior synechiae, resulting in iris bombé
- Uveal effusion causing anterior rotation of the CB (uncommon)
- Exudative retinal detachment pushing the lens–iris diaphragm forward (rare)

N.B. Intraocular inflammation leads to elevated IOP mostly through open-angle mechanisms: blockage of the TM by debris or pigment and steroid-induced ocular hypertension.

46. Describe nanophthalmos.

Nanophthalmos is a bilateral condition in which the globes are significantly shorter than normal, with an axial length less than 20 mm (mean 18.8 mm), with a corresponding hyperopia. In addition, the corneal diameter is smaller (mean 10.5 mm vs. 12 mm for a normal adult) and the sclera is much thicker (often at least twice as thick) than normal. The unusually thick sclera creates an impediment to uveoscleral outflow that predisposes to choroidal effusions, either spontaneously or after surgery, and angle closure. Angle-closure glaucoma can also occur as a result of anterior-segment crowding without uveal effusions.

47. List one systemic medication that can cause angle closure by producing ciliochoroidal effusions and the principles for management of this type of angle closure.

Topiramate, a sulfa-derived antiepileptic medication whose indications have expanded to include the treatment of migraine headaches and obesity, has been reported to cause idiosyncratic ciliochoroidal effusions with acute-onset myopia and angle-closure glaucoma. Thus a careful and thorough history can be crucial in making the diagnosis. These changes do gradually resolve with discontinuation of the medication. Pupillary block is usually not present, and thus, laser PI is not helpful. Miotics will make the problem worse, as they cause anterior movement of the lens–iris diaphragm. The treatment includes topical and systemic aqueous suppressants, systemic hyperosmotics if necessary for IOP control, steroids, and cycloplegics to help pull the lens–iris diaphragm posteriorly.

WEBSITES

The Glaucoma Foundation:
1. www.glaucomafoundation.org
Glaucoma Research Foundation:
2. www.glaucoma.org
3. www.gonioscopy.org

BIBLIOGRAPHY

Albert D, Jakobiec F: Principles and practice of ophthalmology, ed 3, Philadelphia, 2008, W.B. Saunders.

American Academy of Ophthalmology: Basic and clinical science course: section 10, glaucoma, San Francisco, 2019, American Academy of Ophthalmology.

American Academy of Ophthalmology: Preferred practice pattern: primary angle closure glaucoma, San Francisco, 2020, American Academy of Ophthalmology.

Azuara-Blanco A, Burr J, Ramsey C, et al.: Effectiveness of early lens extraction for the treatment of primary angle closure glaucoma (EAGLE): a randomised controlled trial, Lancet 388;1389–1397, 2016.

Davidorf J, Baker N, Derick R: Treatment of the fellow eye in acute angle-closure glaucoma: a case report and survey of members of the American Glaucoma Society, J Glaucoma 5:228–232, 1996.

He M, Jiang Y, Huang S, et al.: Laser peripheral iridotomy for prevention of angle-closure; a single-centre, randomised, controlled trial, Lancet 393;1609–1618, 2019.

Husain R, Gazzard G, Aung T: Initial management of acute primary angle closure a randomized trial comparing phacoemulsification with laser peripheral iridotomy, Ophthalmology 119:2274–2281, 2012.

Lam DSC, Lai JSM, Tham CCY, et al.: Argon laser peripheral iridoplasty versus conventional systemic medical therapy in treatment of acute primary angle-closure glaucoma: a prospective, randomized, controlled trial, Ophthalmology, 109;1591–1596, 2002.

Lowe RF: Acute angle closure glaucoma the second eye: an analysis of 200 cases, Br J Ophthal 46:641–650, 1962.

Rhee DJ, Goldberg MJ, Parrish RK: Bilateral angle-closure glaucoma and ciliary body swelling from topiramate, Arch Ophthalmol 119:1721–1723, 2001.

Ritch R: The pilocarpine paradox [editorial], J Glaucoma 5:225–227, 1996.

Ritch R, Shields B, Krupin T: The glaucomas, ed 2, St. Louis, 1996, Mosby.

Spaeth GL, Idowu O, Seligsohn A, et al.: The effects of iridotomy size and position on symptoms following laser peripheral iridotomy, J Glaucoma 14:364–367, 2005.

CHAPTER 17

SECONDARY OPEN-ANGLE GLAUCOMA

Janice A. Gault

1. A 72-year-old man presents for a routine exam. He states that vision in the left eye is getting bad. On exam, he has vision of 20/30 in the right and counts fingers at 3 feet in the left. The intraocular pressure in the right eye is 25 mm Hg, and in the left eye, 42 mm Hg. The optic nerve appears somewhat cupped on the right, severely so on the left. Visual fields reveal a significant nasal step in the right eye and a temporal island on the left. He does not have pseudoexfoliation syndrome or a Krukenberg spindle in either eye. His angles are deep. What do you suspect?

   A history of trauma. The patient had been a boxer, and he was often hit in his eyes. Angle-recession glaucoma can be asymptomatic until many years later when visual loss occurs. On gonioscopy, the angle recession is determined by torn iris processes and posteriorly recessed iris, revealing a widened ciliary body band. Comparison with the other eye may help to identify this condition. Any patient with traumatic iritis or hyphema needs to be warned of this complication, which may occur many years later. Treatment is the same as with open-angle glaucoma except that miotic agents are ineffective and may even increase the intraocular pressure. Argon (ALT) or selective (SLT) laser trabeculoplasty is rarely effective.

2. What should you look for to make a diagnosis of pseudoexfoliation glaucoma?

   Fibrillar, "dandruff-like" material is deposited on the anterior lens capsule in a characteristic bull's-eye pattern, most easily seen after pupillary dilation. This material is also seen clinically in the angle and on the iris. Gonioscopy reveals a heavily pigmented trabecular meshwork and a Sampaolesi's line, which is pigment deposited anterior to the Schwalbe's line (Fig. 17.1).

   Pseudoexfoliation syndrome is thought to be part of generalized basement membrane disorder, because it can be found histologically in other parts of the body. It may be unilateral or bilateral with asymmetry. Although pseudoexfoliation is infrequent in the United States, it accounts for more than 50% of open-angle glaucoma in Scandinavia. The condition is often more resistant to medical therapy than primary open-angle glaucoma and may require ALT, SLT, or surgical therapy.

3. Is the condition cured after cataract extraction?

   No. The deposits continue, and cataract surgery has a higher risk in such patients. The zonules are weak, and synechiae are often present between the iris and the anterior lens capsule. There is an increased risk of posterior capsular rupture and zonular dialysis.

4. What is true exfoliative glaucoma?

   True exfoliative glaucoma is a capsular delamination caused typically by exposure to intense heat, as seen in glassblowers.

KEY POINTS: PSEUDOEXFOLIATION GLAUCOMA

1. Bull's-eye deposits on anterior lens capsule.
2. Sampaolesi's line on gonioscopy.
3. Less responsive to medical therapy.
4. Higher risk for complications in cataract surgery.

5. A 24-year-old man with sarcoidosis presents with an intraocular pressure of 35 mm Hg in the right eye and 32 mm Hg in the left eye. He notes mild pain and some decreased vision but is otherwise asymptomatic. On examination, you notice 2+ cell and flare in both eyes as well as significant posterior synechiae and mutton-fat keratic precipitates. Gonioscopy reveals an open angle with no peripheral anterior synechiae. A dilated exam reveals no significant cupping of either optic nerve. What do you do?

   Most likely, the inflammatory cells have clogged the trabecular meshwork. Intensive topical steroids and a cycloplegic should decrease the inflammatory load and break the synechiae to prevent angle closure from becoming an issue in the future. Antiglaucoma medications are also appropriate until the pressure decreases. However, miotics are contraindicated because they may cause further synechiae and precipitate angle closure. They also increase the permeability of blood vessels and may contribute to an increase in inflammation. Prostaglandin agonists or analogs may also increase inflammation and should be avoided. The aggressiveness with which the pressure is lowered depends a great deal on optic nerve cupping.

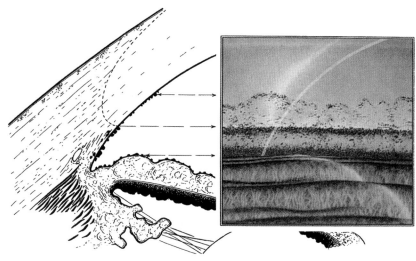

Fig. 17.1 The Sampaolesi's line is a scalloped band of pigmentation anterior to the Schwalbe's line. (From Alward WLM: *Color atlas of gonioscopy,* St. Louis, 1994, Mosby.)

6. **The same patient returns 14 days later with pressures of 40 and 45 mm Hg in the right and left eye, respectively. Exam reveals minimal cell and flare in each eye as well as a significant decrease in the keratic precipitates. He has been using prednisolone acetate 1% every hour and atropine 1% three times a day. What should you do?**
   A gonioscopy should be performed. The differential of increased intraocular pressure in this situation includes:
   - Steroid response. Decreasing steroids lowers the pressure if this is the cause.
   - Cellular blockage of the trabecular meshwork from the inflammatory cells. Increasing the steroids lowers the pressure if this is the cause.
   - Synechiae formation causing an element of secondary angle closure or blocking of the meshwork. Gonioscopy determines whether the angle is open. Increased steroids may melt the synechiae.

   Provided the angle is open and without neovascularization, the most likely cause is response to steroids. The increased intraocular pressure may occur anywhere from a few days to years after initiating therapy. Raised intraocular pressure has been seen with topical steroids in or around the eye, after oral and intravenous administration of steroids, and even with inhalers. Patients with Cushing's syndrome with excessive levels of endogenous steroids are also at risk. Optic nerve evaluation is crucial to determine the risks of damage. Decrease the steroid concentration or dosage and start antiglaucoma therapy. A topical nonsteroidal agent may help decrease inflammation without increasing intraocular pressure. Fluorometholone and loteprednol (Alrex, Lotemax) are also less likely to increase intraocular pressure than other formulations of steroids; however, they have less potency to decrease inflammation.

7. **What does Krukenberg's spindle look like? What does it mean?**
   Krukenberg's spindle is a vertical pigment band on the corneal endothelium (Fig. 17.2). It is typically found in patients with pigmentary dispersion syndrome. The iris is often bowed posteriorly and rubs against the lens

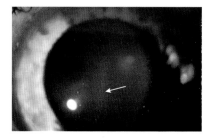

Fig. 17.2 A Krukenberg spindle *(arrow)* is made of pigment deposited on the endothelium in pigmentary dispersion syndrome. (From Alward WLM: Color atlas of gonioscopy, St. Louis, 1994, Mosby.)

zonules. This process causes midperipheral spokelike iris transillumination defects. Gonioscopy reveals a densely pigmented trabecular meshwork for 360 degrees. The patient is often asymptomatic but may notice blurred vision, eye pain, and halos around lights after exercise or pupillary dilation. Pigmentary dispersion syndrome is more common in young adults and white, myopic males. It is usually bilateral.

8. How is pigmentary dispersion treated?

If no optic disc damage is noted and the visual fields are normal, the patient may be observed. Treatment for intraocular pressure over 28 mm Hg is usually indicated, although this point is controversial. Once damage is noted, miotics may be the first line of therapy because they minimize contact between the zonules and the iris. However, miotics also cause myopic fluctuation and may not be practical in young patients, especially in myopes with lattice degeneration because of their increased risk of retinal detachment. Laser peripheral iridectomy has been recommended; it treats the posterior bowing of the iris and may theoretically cure the disorder. The pressures may still be elevated until the residual pigment in the trabecular meshwork is cleared. This treatment is controversial and seems to have fallen out of favor. Patients also respond well to ALT or SLT because of the increased pigment of the trabecular meshwork.

9. A 95-year-old woman presents with a markedly red, painful right eye of 2 days' duration. Her vision is hand motions at 1 foot and 20/400 in the right and left eye, respectively. Exam of the right eye reveals a steamy cornea with a pressure of 60 mm Hg and no view of the anterior chamber. The left eye has a brunescent cataract but appears to be deep and quiet with a pressure of 18 mm Hg. With topical glycerin, the cornea clears in the right eye to reveal iridescent particles floating in the anterior chamber with a morgagnian cataract. Gonioscopy reveals bilateral open angles. No view is obtained of either posterior chamber. What do you do now?

The patient denies a history of uveitis. A B-scan of both eyes reveals significant cataract without retinal detachment or intraocular tumor. The leakage of lens material through an intact lens capsule is obstructing the trabecular meshwork. If the diagnosis is in question, paracentesis may be done to examine the anterior chamber reaction microscopically. Macrophages are filled with lens cortical material (phacolytic glaucoma). Typically, the lens is hypermature, as in this patient. The intraocular pressure must be reduced and the inflammation controlled before surgical therapy is attempted. A steroid such as prednisolone acetate 1% every hour, a cycloplegic such as scopolamine 0.25% three times a day, and antiglaucoma medications are started immediately. Cataract extraction is performed in the next day or two once the eye is less inflamed.

10. A 64-year-old woman who had cataract surgery in the left eye 1 week ago presents to the emergency department complaining that the eye is red and painful with decreasing vision. What is your concern?

First, you must think of endophthalmitis. Any patient presenting after surgery with a red, painful eye with decreased vision must be presumed to have endophthalmitis until it is ruled out. The exam reveals vision of hand motions at 2 feet, a severely injected eye with corneal edema, 4+ cell and flare, and an intraocular pressure of 47 mm Hg. The anterior chamber is filled with lens cortical material, and a rupture in the posterior capsule is seen. A large chunk of nuclear material is in the vitreous. The optic nerve is mildly cupped.

Because the lens material is seen in the anterior chamber, treatment with steroids and antiglaucoma medications is appropriate, along with close observation. The diagnosis is most likely lens-particle glaucoma. The patient is started on prednisolone acetate 1% every 2 hours, scopolamine 0.25% three times a day, latanoprost once daily, a β-blocker twice daily, apraclonidine twice daily, and acetazolamide sequels twice daily. In addition, because her pressure is so high, mannitol is given. When the pressure improves to 25 mm Hg, she is sent home. The next day, she counts fingers at 5 feet, her intraocular inflammation is subsiding, and the pressure is 23 mm Hg. Once her eye is less inflamed and the pressure well controlled, she is scheduled for removal of the remaining lens material. If the retained lens material is minimal, patients sometimes can be maintained on medical therapy until the eye clears without surgery.

11. What other type of open-angle glaucoma can be caused by the lens?

Phacoanaphylactic glaucoma, which occurs after penetrating trauma or surgery. The patient is sensitized to the lens protein during a latent period and develops a granulomatous uveitis. This feature distinguishes it from lens-particle glaucoma. Patients are treated medically and may need surgery to remove the lens if they do not respond adequately.

12. What is Posner-Schlossman syndrome? Who gets it?

Patients are young to middle-aged. They notice unilateral attacks of mild pain, decreased vision, and halos around lights. Episodes tend to recur. Also known as glaucomatocyclitic crisis, this disorder is idiopathic. On exam, intraocular pressure is high, usually between 40 and 60 mm Hg. The angle is open on gonioscopy without synechiae, and the eye is minimally injected. Anterior chamber reaction is minimal. The corneal epithelium may be edematous because of the acute rise in pressure. A few fine keratic precipitates may be present on the corneal endothelium, often inferiorly. Treatment includes steroids and antiglaucoma medications to reduce aqueous production. A cycloplegic agent is necessary only if the patient is symptomatic. The attacks usually resolve in a few hours to a few weeks. No therapy is needed between attacks. However, the risk of chronic open-angle glaucoma is increased in both eyes.

13. **What is the classic triad of Fuchs' heterochromic iridocyclitis?**
This consists of heterochromia, cataract, and low-grade iritis. The iritis is mild and does not cause synechiae. Characteristic stellate, colorless keratic precipitates are seen over the inferior endothelium. Fine new vessels may be seen in the angle but do not cause closure. The glaucoma is difficult to control and often does not correspond to the degree of inflammation. Steroids are not often helpful.

14. **A patient reports for postoperative check-up 1 day after cataract surgery. The pressure in the operated eye is 40 mm Hg, and the patient complains of nausea. What is the most likely cause?**
Retained viscoelastic from surgery. The pressure usually increases 6 or 7 hours after surgery and normalizes within 24 to 48 hours, depending on the type of viscoelastic. Most eyes tolerate short-term pressures up to 30 mm Hg; of course, tolerance depends on preexisting optic nerve status. Medical treatment and paracentesis to remove the viscoelastic are indicated to decrease pressure quickly and relieve nausea. Paracentesis is somewhat controversial because of the small increased risk of endophthalmitis.

15. **What else can cause postoperative glaucoma?**
Hyphema, pigment dispersion, generalized inflammation, aphakic or pseudophakic pupillary block, malignant glaucoma (aqueous misdirection syndrome), and steroid-response glaucoma. In patients who have undergone an intracapsular cataract extraction, α-chymotrypsin is injected into the anterior chamber to dissolve the zonules. The zonular debris may block the trabecular meshwork postoperatively. Epithelial ingrowth may occur many months to years after surgery or trauma and block outflow.

16. **A patient had cataract surgery 1 year ago but continues to have episodes of anterior chamber cell and flare with increased intraocular pressure. Some of the cells are red blood cells. What is the diagnosis?**
The diagnosis is uveitis–glaucoma–hyphema syndrome. The cells may layer out to produce a hyphema, usually as a result of irritation from an anterior chamber intraocular lens, although a posterior chamber lens may be involved. Gonioscopy may reveal where the irritation is occurring, such as from a lens in the sulcus or a haptic causing iris chafing. Ultrasound biomicroscopy (UBM) can show intraocular lens position—one or both haptics may be in the sulcus, causing tilt and chafing of the iris and ciliary body. Treatment consists of atropine, topical steroids, and antiglaucoma medications until the pressure is reduced. Argon laser of the bleeding site, if it can be identified, may be curative. However, exchange or removal of the intraocular lens is often necessary especially if malpositioning is seen on UBM or gonioscopy.

17. **How can raised episcleral venous pressure cause glaucoma?**
Aqueous drains from the anterior chamber through the trabecular meshwork, Schlemm's canal, and intrascleral channels to the episcleral and conjunctival veins. Normal drainage depends on an episcleral venous pressure that is lower than the pressure of the eye. Usually, it ranges from 8 to 12 mm Hg. However, if it is higher than intraocular pressure, drainage does not occur. Blood will be seen in the Schlemm's canal on gonioscopy. Drugs that reduce aqueous humor formation are obviously the most effective medical treatment in these patients.

KEY POINTS: CAUSES OF RAISED EPISCLERAL VENOUS PRESSURE

1. Thyroid ophthalmopathy.
2. Carotid and dural fistulas.
3. Superior vena cava syndrome.
4. Retrobulbar tumors.
5. Orbital varices.
6. Sturge-Weber syndrome.

18. **A patient with long-standing diabetes has had recurrent vitreous hemorrhage. While you are observing him, waiting for the condition to clear, intraocular pressure increases to 35 mm Hg. What should you suspect?**
When intraocular hemorrhages clear, hemolytic or ghost-cell glaucoma may develop. Hemolytic glaucoma occurs because macrophages full of hemoglobin block the trabecular meshwork. Reddish cells can be seen in the anterior chamber. In ghost-cell glaucoma, degenerating red blood cells block the aqueous outflow. Khaki cells in the anterior chamber may layer out to form a pseudohypopyon. Both conditions can be treated medically until the hemorrhage clears. However, because the intraocular pressure may become markedly raised, washout of the anterior chamber and/or vitrectomy often becomes necessary. In addition, the patient may be developing neovascular glaucoma; thus, it is important to check the angles for new vessels and angle narrowing.

19. **What other conditions may cause open-angle glaucoma?**
   - Intraocular tumor may cause secondary open-angle glaucoma by invasion of the chamber angle or blockage of the trabecular meshwork by tumor debris.

- Siderosis (excess iron) or chalcosis (excess copper) from a retained metallic foreign body.
- Chemical injuries from acid or alkali can shrink the scleral collagen or cause direct damage to the trabecular meshwork.
- Posterior polymorphous dystrophy is a bilateral and autosomal dominant disease. Vesicles are seen at the Descemet's membrane. Corneal edema occurs in severe cases. Iridocorneal adhesions may occur. Glaucoma is associated in 15% of cases.
- Iridocorneal endothelial syndrome.

20. What is iridocorneal endothelial syndrome?

It is a spectrum of three entities that overlap considerably:
- **Essential iris atrophy:** Iris thinning leads to iris holes and pupillary distortion
- **Chandler's syndrome:** Mild iris thinning and distortion with hammered metal appearance of corneal endothelium
- **Cogan-Reese syndrome:** Pigmented nodules on the iris surface with variable iris atrophy

Such patients are generally asymptomatic, middle-aged adults. Usually, findings are unilateral with increased intraocular pressure and corneal edema. No treatment is necessary unless corneal edema and glaucoma are present.

21. What types of secondary open-angle glaucoma occur in children?

- Glaucoma associated with mesenchymal dysgenesis is a spectrum of disease, but two main categories are recognized:
  - Axenfeld's anomaly consists of a prominent Schwalbe's ring with attached iris strands. Axenfeld's syndrome is the anomaly with coincident glaucoma and occurs in 50% of cases. It is autosomal dominant or sporadic.
  - Rieger's anomaly is Axenfeld's anomaly plus iris thinning and distorted pupils. Sixty percent of patients develop glaucoma; it is also autosomal dominant or sporadic. Rieger's syndrome is the anomaly associated with dental, craniofacial, and skeletal abnormalities.
- Aniridia is a bilateral, near-total absence of the iris. The strands may be seen only by gonioscopy. Glaucoma, foveal hypoplasia, and nystagmus may occur. The disorder may be autosomal dominant or sporadic. Patients with sporadic inheritance need to be evaluated for Wilms' tumor, which is associated in 25% of cases.
- Oculocerebrorenal syndrome (Lowe) is an X-linked recessive disease. Patients have aminoaciduria, hypotonia, acidemia, cataracts, and glaucoma.
- Congenital rubella may be associated with cataracts and pigmented retinal lesions. Cardiac, auditory, and central nervous abnormalities are often coexistent.
- Sturge-Weber syndrome.
- Neurofibromatosis.
- Glaucoma is an ongoing risk in patients who have had cataract surgery as infants or small children.

BIBLIOGRAPHY

American Academy of Ophthalmology: Basic and clinical science course, section 10, San Francisco, 2020, American Academy of Ophthalmology.

Bagheri N, Wajda B, Calvo C, Durrani A: The wills eye manual: office and emergency room diagnosis and treatment of eye disease, ed 7, Philadelphia, 2016, Lippincott Williams & Wilkins.

Damji K, Freedman S, Moroi S, Rhee D, Shields MB: Shields textbook of glaucoma, ed 6, Baltimore, 2010, Lippincott Williams & Wilkins.

Danyluk AW, Paton D: Diagnosis and management of glaucoma, Clin Symp 43:2–32, 1991.

CHAPTER 18

MEDICAL TREATMENT OF GLAUCOMA

Joshua Paul, Upneet Bains, Warren Robinson, and Jeffrey D. Henderer

1. **What classes of medications are used to treat glaucoma?**
   See Table 18.1.

2. **How do these medications work?**
   - Adrenergic agonists work in a variety of pathways. Apraclonidine and brimonidine are the currently available adrenergic agonists, which predominantly work on alpha 2 adrenergic receptors and decrease aqueous production. Brimonidine may also increase uveoscleral outflow.
   - β-Blockers and carbonic anhydrase inhibitors (CAIs) decrease aqueous production. β-Blockers decrease aqueous humor secretion by inhibiting cyclic adenosine monophosphate production in the ciliary epithelium. CAIs decrease aqueous humor production by directly antagonizing carbonic anhydrase in the ciliary epithelium.
   - Hyperosmotic agents increase the osmolarity of the blood, which in turn draws fluid from the posterior chamber into the blood vessels of the ciliary body.
   - Miotics constrict the longitudinal muscle of the ciliary body, which is attached to the scleral spur anteriorly and to the choroid posteriorly. When the longitudinal muscle constricts, it pulls the scleral spur posteriorly, pulling open the spaces between the trabecular beams and mechanically increasing the capacity for aqueous outflow.
   - Prostaglandin analogs increase outflow through the uveoscleral outflow channels. Aqueous is absorbed into the face of the ciliary body and then flows posteriorly in several directions through the sclera, supraciliary and suprachoroidal spaces. The nitric oxide donating component of latanoprostene bunod increases outflow through the trabecular meshwork pathway.
   - Rho kinase inhibitors increase outflow through the trabecular meshwork by inhibiting smooth muscle contraction within the meshwork. They may also function to decrease aqueous production and episcleral venous pressure.

3. **For patients in good health with primary open-angle glaucoma, what is the first drug to try?**
   The short answer is that any of the topical medications can be used. The choice is based on the desired amount of intraocular pressure (IOP) reduction, the possible side effects, and the relative costs of the medicines. The advantage of having four commonly used classes of medications (β-blockers, prostaglandin analogs, topical CAIs, and adrenergic agonists) is that therapy can be customized for each patient. Prostaglandin analogs are the most commonly used first-line therapeutic agents because of their daily dosing, powerful hypotensive effect, and favorable side-effect profile. Prior to the development of prostaglandins, most ophthalmologists chose a β-blocker as first-line therapy.

   If a patient would not be a good candidate for a prostaglandin (see question 10), one of the other three classes of medicines can be used. Nonselective β-blockers are the most potent of the three. The cardioselective β-blocker (betaxolol), topical CAIs, and adrenergic agonists are all similar in hypotensive effect. When used alone, topical CAIs and α-adrenergic agonists should be used three times a day to prevent possible IOP fluctuation.

4. **What medicine should be used as second-line therapy? Third-line therapy?**
   As in the case of first-line therapy, any of the medicine classes can be used as second- or third-line therapy. With several options available, the physician can attempt to tailor the choice to the patient's particular situation. If a prostaglandin has been used as first-line therapy, a β-blocker is often chosen as second-line therapy, and vice versa. As these medicines are the most potent ones available and timolol can be used as a once-a-day medicine (most commonly a β-blocker once per day in the morning and prostaglandin once per day in the evening), this regimen typically results in a very good hypotensive effect for the number of drops used.

   The availability of the fixed combinations of timolol/dorzolamide and timolol/brimonidine makes it easy to add dorzolamide or brimonidine as a second-line agent after timolol. This reduces the drop count from three or four to two per day, and fewer drops per day are likely to result in greater compliance.

   Brimonidine or a topical CAI can be an excellent choice for additive therapy. In addition, the fixed combination of brimonidine/brinzolamide can play a role in simplifying the drop regimen, especially if the patient cannot tolerate a β-blocker.

   Miotics are uncommonly used today because of the drop frequency and side effects but can be quite effective, especially in aphakic (no crystalline lens in the eye) patients. In phakic patients with little remaining accommodation and little cataract, pilocarpine is often well tolerated. It provides a pinhole effect that gives an increased depth of field for most patients. Many patients can read without reading glasses when taking pilocarpine, and no one needs trifocals if the pupils are adequately miotic.

   Oral CAIs were once quite commonly used and are among the most potent of all hypotensive medications. Their side-effect profile and the availability of a variety of topical medicines limit their use today.

Table 18.1 Commonly Used Agents for Glaucoma Management

CHEMICAL NAME	COLOR TOP	STRENGTH	USUAL DOSAGE	SIZE (ML)
Adrenergic Agonists				
Apraclonidine hydrochloride	Purple	0.5%, 1%	Two to three times a day	5 (0.5%) 24 (1%)
Brimonidine tartrate	Purple	0.1%, 0.15%, 0.2%	Two to three times a day	5, 10, 15
β-Blockers				
Betaxolol hydrochloride suspension	Light blue	0.25%	Two times a day	10, 15
Betaxolol hydrochloride solution	Dark blue	0.50%	Two times a day	5, 10, 15
Carteolol hydrochloride	Yellow	1%	One to two times a day	5, 10, 15
Levobunolol hydrochloride	Yellow	0.5%	One to two times a day	5
Timolol maleate	Yellow	0.25%, 0.5%	One to two times a day	5, 10, 15
Timolol XE gel-forming solution	Yellow	0.25%, 0.5%	Daily	5
Carbonic Anhydrase Inhibitors				
Acetazolamide sodium (oral)	NA	125, 250 mg	Three to four times a day PO	NA
Acetazolamide sequels (oral)	NA	500 mg	Two times a day PO	NA
Methazolamide (oral)	NA	25, 50 mg	Two to four times a day PO	NA
Dorzolamide	Orange	2%	Two to three times a day	10
Brinzolamide	Orange	1%	Two to three times a day	10, 15
Hyperosmotic Agents				
Mannitol (IV)	NA	20% (IV)	0.5–1 g/kg over 30–60 minutes	NA
Miotics				
Pilocarpine hydrochloride	Green	1%, 2%, 4%	Two to four times a day	15
Prostaglandin Analogs				
Latanoprost	Teal	0.005%	Daily	2.5
Travoprost Z	Teal	0.004%	Daily	2.5, 5
Bimatoprost	Teal	0.01% 0.03%	Daily	2.5, 5, 7.5 2.5, 3, 5, 7.5
Tafluprost	Teal label, clear cap	0.0015%	Daily	One pack (30 each single use vials)
Latanoprostene bunod	Teal	0.024%	Daily	2.5, 5
Rho Kinase Inhibitors				
Netarsudil	White	0.02%	Daily	2.5
Fixed Combinations				
Timolol/dorzolamide	Dark blue	0.5%/2%	Two times a day	10
Brinzolamide/brimonidine tartrate	Pale green	1%/0.2%	Three times a day	8
Timolol/brimonidine tartrate	Dark blue	0.5%/0.2%	Two times a day	10, 15
Netarsudil/latanoprost	White	0.02%/0.005%	Daily	2.5

IV, Intravenous; *NA*, not applicable; *PO*, by mouth (orally).

5. What new medications are approved to treat glaucoma?

Netarsudil (Rhopressa), a rho kinase inhibitor, was approved in 2017. Latanoprostene bunod (Vyzultza), a nitric oxide donating prostaglandin analogue, was approved in 2017 after the APOLLO studies. Netarsudil/latanoprost (Rockalatan), a new combination drop, was approved in 2019 after the MERCURY 2 study.

6. How do the newer agents fit into the glaucoma treatment paradigm?

Early clinical trials have demonstrated significant IOP reduction and favorable side effect profiles (except for potential for red eye) in all three medications. In addition, the once-daily dosing afforded by all three medications will help patients reduce their drop burden and hopefully assist with compliance. At this time, the cost of these medications and the lack of insurance coverage limit their use. As the newer agents become more affordable and widespread, their role in glaucoma treatment will become more clearly defined.

7. What are some prescribing pearls and key side effects of adrenergic agonists (Table 18.2)?

Apraclonidine and brimonidine are α_2-selective agonists that are readily available.

The α-adrenergic compounds are characterized by a high allergic-reaction rate. Apraclonidine has an allergic rate of approximately 20% by 1 year. Because of its high rate of allergy and tachyphylaxis, apraclonidine is used almost exclusively for acute pressure control or to prevent acute pressure rise after laser procedures.

Brimonidine is less likely to cause an immediate allergic reaction, but many patients develop an intolerance or allergy months after starting the drug. Ocular adverse effects include contact blepharoconjunctivitis and follicular conjunctivitis. The generic form of brimonidine packaged with benzalkonium chloride (BAK) preservative is available in two concentrations—0.15% and 0.2%. The brand form of brimonidine (Alphagan-P 0.1%) is available in only one concentration. Though Alphagan-P has a lower concentration of brimonidine, it has a comparable IOP-lowering effect. Alphagan-P is packaged with a less allergy-provoking preservative (Purite) than generic brimonidine and has a reduced incidence of allergic side effects.

Brimonidine has a similar IOP-lowering effect as nonselective β-blocker activity at peak effect, although less at trough 6 to 12 hours later. Aside from allergy, it is well tolerated by the eye. Systemically, it can cause dry mouth and fatigue, which can be debilitating. Brimonidine is contraindicated in infants because it causes central nervous system (CNS) depression and apnea. Avoid coadministering brimonidine with a monoamine oxidase inhibitor or tricyclic antidepressant therapy, as potentiating or additive effects of CNS depression and/or adverse cardiovascular events can occur. There is some evidence from animal models of glaucoma that brimonidine may protect ganglion cells from death. There is no evidence of this property in humans, but this drug has sparked interest in treating glaucoma by mechanisms other than pressure reduction especially in low-tension glaucoma.

8. What are some prescribing pearls and key side effects of topical β-blockers (see Table 18.2)?

Timolol was the first β-blocker and is still considered the gold standard against which all other ocular hypotensive medications are judged. It has been formulated as both a nonviscous and a viscous drop. The viscous formulation remains in the tear film longer; consequently, intraocular absorption is greater, and systemic absorption is reduced. This drug provides the best diurnal curve for pressure control with once-daily dosing and can reduce the possibility of systemic side effects.

Nonselective β-blockers may be effective with the 0.25% dosage once daily for patients with light irides and the 0.5% dosage once daily for patients with dark irides. β-Blockers block intrinsic $\beta1$ and $\beta2$ receptor tone; thus, when patients are asleep, β-blockers are ineffective because there is little tone. However, because aqueous production also declines at night, this fact is usually considered inconsequential. Although β-blockers are labeled as twice a day and very frequently prescribed twice a day, many ophthalmologists will prescribe β-blockers once daily when patients awake in the morning to effectively minimize pressure rise as well as medication-induced nocturnal hypoperfusion to the optic nerve especially in patients with low-tension glaucoma. For patients with more advanced disease, a twice-daily regimen of 0.25% for lighter irides and 0.5% for darker irides is common. This regimen guards against going a full day without medication in patients who miss one prescribed drop.

Table 18.2 Common Side Effects of Topical Glaucoma Medications	
DRUG	SIDE EFFECT
Adrenergic agonists	Dry mouth, allergic conjunctivitis, fatigue, and headache.
β-Blockers	Bronchospasm, bradycardia, fatigue, poor exercise tolerance, depression, and decreased libido.
Carbonic anhydrase inhibitors	Stinging, metallic taste, rash, and nausea.
Prostaglandin analogs	Lash growth, iris and eyelid hyperpigmentation, allergic conjunctivitis, macular edema in pseudophakes, flu-like symptoms, and reactivation of herpetic keratitis.
Rho kinase inhibitors	Conjunctival hyperemia, corneal verticillata, conjunctival hemorrhage.

Betaxolol, a selective β1 antagonist, has far fewer systemic side effects than the nonselective β-blockers but is not as potent. Betaxolol 0.25% results in a 15%–20% drop in IOP, whereas nonselective β-blockers achieve about a 20%–30% reduction at peak.

In general, the side effects of this class of medications are identical to those of the oral β-blockers. Patients, and even physicians, often forget that eyedrops can have systemic effects. Physicians must remember to ask about eyedrops when taking a complete medical history.

β-Blockers can exacerbate asthma or chronic obstructive pulmonary disease and can cause arrhythmia, bradycardia, hypotension, increased heart block, lethargy, cardiac arrest, cardiac failure, alteration of serum lipids, exercise intolerance, impotence, altered mental status, and CNS depression. There is some evidence that there might not be as much impact on chronic obstructive pulmonary disease (COPD) patients as thought. The selective β-blocker betaxolol is much less likely to trigger bronchospasm but still must be used with caution. In diabetics, they may cause reduced glucose tolerance and mask the symptoms of hypoglycemia. In hyperthyroidism, symptoms can be exacerbated with abrupt withdrawal of ocular β-blocker use. β-Blockers have been linked with impaired neuromuscular transmission; thus, myasthenia gravis symptoms can be exacerbated. Ocular side effects include blurred vision, irritation, corneal anesthesia, punctate keratitis, and allergy. Long-term use of topical β-blockers may result in decreased effectiveness or tachyphylaxis.

Concomitant use of topical and systemic β-blockers should be done judiciously. Although it is not clear what the additive effects of systemic and topical use are, there have been reports of patients taking both systemic and topical β-blockers with reduced ocular hypotensive efficacy and greater systemic side effects compared with patients who were taking a systemic β-blocker and a different class of topical IOP-lowering agent. There is also some evidence that oral β-blockers can lower IOP. One of the concerning systemic side effects is the exacerbation of blood pressure fluctuation. Such fluctuations (especially in diastolic blood pressure) leading to hypoperfusion potentially reduce ocular perfusion and increase susceptibility of the optic nerve to relative ischemic injury.

9. What are some prescribing pearls and key side effects of carbonic anhydrase inhibitors (see Table 18.2)?

Topical CAIs took more than 40 years to develop and were particularly welcome, as oral CAIs cause a myriad of side effects. The most common complaints with oral CAIs are lack of energy and lethargy, lack of appetite and weight loss, nausea and/or an upset stomach, paresthesias of extremities, and a metallic taste to foods. CAIs are chemically derived from sulfa drugs and historically have been avoided in patients with known sulfa allergies because of the risk of skin rash or even Stevens-Johnson syndrome as well as anaphylaxis, although the evidence for this practice is not strong. The most dangerous side effect is hypokalemia, especially when a CAI is combined with a potassium-reducing diuretic. This combination is dangerous in patients taking digitalis. Severe mental depression, aplastic anemia, and kidney stones are other serious side effects. The same sort of side effects can be seen with the topical medications, but they are extremely rare. Because complaints are frequent with oral CAIs, most ophthalmologists rarely use them unless there is a need for acute pressure control, especially temporarily, or if topical CAIs are not effective. Systemic CAIs may provide additional reduction of aqueous humor formation by yielding a renal acidosis that further inhibits the ciliary epithelium. Of the two oral CAIs available, acetazolamide is excreted by the kidney while methazolamide is primarily metabolized by the liver. For this reason, more caution should be used with acetazolamide in the setting of renal issues. Acetazolamide is also more likely to cause kidney stones. Both oral CAIs should be avoided in patients with sickle cell trait or anemia as they can cause a metabolic acidosis and increase sickling.

Although topical CAIs have an IOP fluctuation when used twice daily, twice-daily usage gives an adequate response when combined with another aqueous suppressant, which diminishes the washout effect of aqueous production.

The two topical CAIs are equally effective, but brinzolamide is less irritating to the eye. Both topical CAIs are associated with worsening of corneal endothelial dysfunction; therefore, caution should be used with these agents in the setting of corneal edema, or corneal endothelial dystrophy. Dorzolamide has been reported to augment blood flow to the optic nerve. This may help reduce the impact of free radicals that have been postulated to be a cause of glaucoma.

10. What are some prescribing pearls and key side effects of prostaglandin analogs (see Table 18.2)?

The prostaglandin analogs available today are all extremely effective at lowering IOP and are generally used as first-line therapy. They can be additive with any medicine but tend not to work as well if added beyond second-line therapy.

Latanoprost was released first and remains the most commonly used of the five medicines. As a prostaglandin analog, latanoprost is a powerful ocular hypotensive agent. Travoprost is equally effective compared to latanoprost, with greater conjunctival erythema but less effect on increased iris pigmentation. Travoprost Z 0.004% (travatan) is made without BAK preservative and contains the less irritating preservative, SofZia. Tafluprost, a preservative-free alternative, which is packaged in single-use containers, is also available. Bimatoprost 0.01% and 0.03% appears to offer on average about 0.5 mm Hg greater IOP reduction than the other prostaglandins, and in selected individuals, it may be significantly more powerful. The increased concentration of bimatoprost is accompanied by greater local ocular side effects. In some patients, the side effects can be lessened with the use of bimatoprost 0.01%, without compromising IOP reduction. Latanoprostene bunod, a new prostaglandin analogue, includes a nitrous oxide component, and this combination provides additional IOP lowering than latanoprost alone. The donation of nitric oxide allows for additional enhanced outflow through the trabecular meshwork.

Although there have been rare reports of systemic side effects, such as flu-like symptoms, numerous ocular side effects can occur. The most common are conjunctival injection, increased pigmentation of the iris and eyelid skin, growth of eyelashes, and prostaglandin-associated periorbitopathy (PAP). PAP is a term used to describe the constellation of eyelid and periorbital changes that occur with chronic use of topical prostaglandins; such changes include upper lid ptosis, deepening of upper lid sulcus, periorbital fat atrophy, loss of lower eyelid fullness, and relative enophthalmos. These changes appear to be partially reversible with discontinuation of the medication. Increased iris pigmentation is the result of increased amount of melanin within iris melanocytes and is not reversible. This seems to occur much more frequently in patients with hazel irides or who have iris nevi. Ocular inflammation, including anterior uveitis and keratitis, has been rarely reported, so in patients with a history of uveitis, it may not be the drug of choice. Prostaglandin analogs have been associated with cystoid macular edema, especially in pseudophakic eyes. However, these eyes typically have other risk factors that may be responsible. Herpetic keratitis may be reactivated or exacerbated. It also has been reported to produce a herpes-like keratitis that clears when the drops are stopped. Rechallenging patients with the prostaglandin after a period of washout and recovery will help determine if the medication is causing this effect.

11. What are some prescribing pearls and key side effects of rho kinase inhibitors (see Table 18.2)?
    While much is still to be learned about this class of medications, clinical trials have demonstrated effective IOP reduction with minimal side effects. Rho kinase inhibitors have a unique mechanism of action. Inhibition of rho-associated protein kinase prevents contraction within the trabecular meshwork yielding enhanced outflow. They may also decrease aqueous production and episcleral venous pressure. IOP reduction is estimated to be 20%–25%, and the systemic side effect profile is minimal. Local side effects are reported at a higher rate compared to traditional therapies; however, most are not clinically significant. The most frequently reported side effect is intermittent conjunctival hyperemia, which was found in 50% of patients. Corneal verticillata were found in 25% of patients but did not affect vision and resolved with cessation of therapy. Lastly, 16% of patients developed small petechial conjunctival hemorrhages intermittently during treatment. The hemorrhages resolved while on therapy and did not interfere with visual acuity.

12. What are some prescribing pearls and key side effects of topical combination therapies?
    Many patients medically managed for glaucoma are treated with more than one drug class for IOP control. Combining two different topical drug classes in a single formulation provides the benefit of improved convenience and compliance, less exposure to preservatives, and reduced cost. However, combination therapies are not generally used as a first-line therapy to initially treat a patient with glaucoma.
    Combigan (brimonidine 0.2%/timolol 0.5%), Cosopt (dorzolamide 2%/timolol 0.5%), Simbrinza (brinzolamide 1%/brimonidine 0.2%), and Rockalatan (netarsudil 0.02%/latanoprost 0.005%) are fixed-combination therapies available in the United States. All have a greater IOP-lowering effect than their component medications dosed separately as a monotherapy. Combigan is clinically associated with 50% lower incidence in ocular allergy compared to monotherapy with brimonidine. Cosopt and Simbrinza have ocular side effects similar to both of their individual components. Other fixed-combination medications with prostaglandin analogs are available only outside of the United States: Xalacom (latanoprost 0.005%/timolol 0.5%), Ganfort (bimatoprost 0.03%/timolol 0.5%), and DuoTrav or Extravan (travoprost 0.004%/timolol 0.5%).

KEY POINTS: GLAUCOMA TOPICAL MEDICATIONS

1. Allow 5 minutes between drops to prevent one drug from washing the other out of the eye.
2. Punctal occlusion can dramatically reduce systemic side effects of glaucoma drugs.
3. A patient on glaucoma drugs with dry or irritated eyes may be developing a medication allergy. Check the conjunctiva of the lower lid for a follicular reaction.
4. Noncompliance is the most common cause of ineffective treatment response.

13. Are there alternative therapies or nontraditional medication options for treating glaucoma?
    At present, no non-pressure-lowering medication has been conclusively demonstrated to be helpful in treating glaucoma. Many drugs are under investigation for this purpose. Some data from neurologic studies indicate that antioxidants, such as ginkgo biloba and vitamin E, as well as free radical scavengers, may be helpful. Oral calcium-channel blockers have been demonstrated to have a limited effect on preserving visual function in some studies. Aminoguanidine, an inhibitor of nitric oxide synthase, was found to be helpful in a rat model of glaucoma. Agents that increase blood flow to the optic nerve and retina may also be useful.
    Other drugs that have been investigated for chronic neurologic disease are being evaluated for effectiveness in glaucoma. Retinal ganglion cell death in glaucoma occurs by apoptosis and in this way is similar to many chronic neurodegenerative diseases. Identifying the unique trigger in glaucoma and/or interfering with the mechanism of

apoptotic cell death might yield multiple ways to treat glaucoma beyond IOP reduction. The trick will be to selectively target the tissue of concern and devise a drug delivery system that can bypass the blood–ocular barrier. Memantine, an antiparkinsonian drug that blocks *N*-methyl-ᴅ-aspartate-receptor-induced glutamate toxicity, was viewed as a promising agent, but a recent paper describing the results of two clinical trials revealed there was no clear benefit in patients receiving memantine versus placebo. It is likely that some type of neuroprotective agent will become an important adjunctive therapy for glaucoma in the future.

The medical use of cannabinoids has been a topic widely discussed in the United States. Inhalation of cannabinoid has an IOP-lowering effect for a duration of 3 to 4 hours. The mechanism of action is not fully understood, and the short duration of action would mean the drug would need to be consumed frequently to have around-the-clock effectivity. The deleterious effects of this level of consumption (altered mental capacity, lung damage, etc.) limit its recommendation by most glaucoma specialists. Although a topical, oral, or sublingual preparation may avoid the pulmonary impact, they are limited by other systemic side effects. Canasol is a cannabinoid-based eyedrop, but there are no Food and Drug Administration (FDA) clinical trials ongoing or planned in the future.

Exercise has also garnered significant attention as another modifiable risk factor in the development and progression of glaucoma. Some have proposed that exercise may be associated with reduced IOP and visual field progression. Headstand positions in yoga have been shown to increase IOP and should be avoided in patients with severe visual field defects, especially those close to fixation. More evidence is needed to demonstrate the benefits.

Although antioxidants, vitamins, herbal supplements, exercise, etc., and their effects on IOP have been studied, currently, there is no significant research-based evidence to support the implementation of alternative therapies in the prevention or progression of glaucoma.

14. **How many eyedrops can be used?**
Most ophthalmologists believe that compliance becomes increasingly difficult the more medicines are used. Most consider a combination like a prostaglandin analog, timolol/dorzolamide, and brimonidine to represent maximum medical therapy (five drops per day). Laser and/or surgical options are generally considered at this point, if not earlier. In selected cases, additional medicines such as miotics or oral medication can be tried, especially to temporize prior to incisional surgery.

15. **What are the general rules for using eyedrops?**
- Allow at least 5 minutes between applying any two topical eye medications.
- Drops should be spaced at roughly stable intervals. Once-a-day medication should be used each evening or morning. Twice-a-day medicines should be used about 12 hours apart. It becomes harder to space three- and four-times-a-day medicines equally, but an effort should be made to try. An easy schedule to remember is breakfast, lunch, dinner and before bed.
- Topical medications all have systemic side effects. Punctal occlusion can reduce the systemic absorption to minimize these effects. The patient puts a finger adjacent to the nose where the two lids come together and pushes down on the bone. The drop is then instilled in the eye, and the lids are gently closed. This position is held for 3 minutes. This procedure dramatically reduces the amount of drug entering the system. Because a drug coming into contact with the nasal mucosa is absorbed rapidly and almost completely, it attains serum levels quite similar to those achieved by intravenous administration. Absorption through the nasal mucosa also prevents a first pass by hepatic enzymes, which gives the liver a chance to metabolize or detoxify the medication.
- A one-eyed therapeutic trial can help a physician decide on the utility of a medication and how well it is tolerated. Although there can be some crossover effect (about 1 to 2 mm Hg) in the fellow eye, the one-eyed therapeutic trial is the best way to determine the drug's effect. However, this is not used uniformly because, unfortunately, the response in the first eye does not always correlate with the response in the fellow eye once the drug is used bilaterally. Still, most glaucoma specialists believe that a therapeutic trial provides critical evidence to justify the use of a medication.

16. **Pilocarpine is often used in the treatment of angle-closure glaucoma. What is its effect on the anterior chamber?**
Pilocarpine contracts the longitudinal muscle of the ciliary body, pulling on the scleral spur and mechanically opening the trabecular meshwork. However, it also pulls the lens-iris diaphragm forward, shallowing the anterior chamber. The contraction of the circular muscle of the ciliary body relaxes the stress on the zonules, allowing the lens to become rounder, to float forward on a longer tether, and to act more like a natural cork in the pupil. This effect increases pupillary block and bows the peripheral iris closer to the trabecular meshwork. All of these effects tend to shallow the anterior chamber and narrow the anterior-chamber angle. Luckily, these effects are balanced by the miosis caused by the contraction of the sphincter muscle of the iris. Miosis pulls the peripheral iris away from the trabecular meshwork. In most patients, although the anterior-chamber depth is decreased by pilocarpine, the peripheral angle is slightly widened. In some patients, however, shallowing of the peripheral angle may be more of a problem than angle crowding. In such patients, pilocarpine may cause angle closure. Therefore, one should perform gonioscopy on all patients with a narrow angle for whom a miotic is prescribed, both initially and periodically thereafter.

It is important to keep in mind that pilocarpine is virtually ineffective in treating acute angle closure. During such acute cases of angle closure with markedly elevated IOP, the iris becomes ischemic and does not respond to the acute miotic effects of pilocarpine.

17. **If a patient does not show an expected response to a topical glaucoma medication, what should the ophthalmologist consider as the reason?**
    - Noncompliance: The most common cause for an ineffective medication is failure to take it. Kass et al. performed a study in which a microchip placed in the bottom of pilocarpine bottles recorded when the bottle was tipped upside down. The chip was camouflaged, and patients did not know that their drop use was being monitored. Overall, he found that 76% of the prescribed doses were taken. Six percent of patients took less than 25% of the drops, whereas 15% took only 50%. However, 97% of his patients reported that they were taking all of their medication. Not surprisingly, compliance was best on the day before the office visit. This behavior can explain why many patients have completely controlled IOPs in the ophthalmologist's office but evidence of progressive glaucoma damage.
    - Ineffective medication: You can attempt a one-eyed trial.
    - Inability to instill the drops properly: The patient may be compliant in taking the medications but may not be getting the drops into the eye. Watch the patient instill lubricating drops in the office to see if their technique is successful. Have the patient use a drop dispensing aid or have another individual administer the drops.
    - Inadequate interval between multiple drops: Make sure that patients wait at least 5 minutes between drops and that the drops are spread evenly over the course of the day. Some patients take all their drops at once and assume they are done for the day.
    - Concomitant use of IOP-elevating medications: Review the patient's list of active medication. Use of systemic or topical agents such as steroids can cause an elevated IOP.

18. **Many patients taking topical medications complain of dry or irritated eyes. What should the treating ophthalmologist include as a routine part of the examination of all patients taking topical medication?**
    The treating ophthalmologist should examine the lower lid and observe the conjunctiva. If only papillae are present, the patient does not have a chronic allergy. If there is a significant follicular reaction, especially if follicles are present on the bulbar conjunctiva, the patient is more than likely allergic to the topical drops. Ocular allergies can appear immediately upon using the drop or months later. Brimonidine is well known for this, but such a late reaction is commonly underappreciated and unrecognized. Pilocarpine is famous for causing symblepharon with chronic use. For patients with ocular surface disease, switching to preservative-free or at least avoiding medications preserved with BAK may be of benefit. Medications with non-BAK preservatives include Alphagan P 0.1% and Travatan Z. Preservative-free formulations are available for tafluprost, timolol, and timolol/dorzolamide.

19. **In a patient with an ocular allergy secondary to topical medication, which is the most likely offender?**
    Apraclonidine has the highest incidence of allergic reaction. As such, it went from being a regular in the topical glaucoma drop armory to limited use as a preoperative agent to prevent IOP spikes after laser procedures or for acute IOP control. Among the medications now in use, brimonidine (less with the 0.15% and 0.1% formulation) has the highest incidence of allergic reaction, followed by (in order) topical CAIs, prostaglandin analogs, β-blockers, and pilocarpine.

    Stopping the medicines in that order will usually help sort out which is the offender. Alternatively, have the patient instill one drop in one eye and a different one in the fellow eye.

    The availability of generic formulations has also had an impact on the prevalence of allergic reaction secondary to topical glaucoma medications. For example, brimonidine is available in 0.1%, 0.15%, and 0.2% formulations. The last two are more likely to induce an allergic reaction and are the two formulations available in generic form. As such, prescribers may see increased rates of allergic reaction from brimonidine due to prescribing patterns aimed at patients' cost savings.

20. **Are any of the glaucoma medications safe for use in pregnant women?**
    Few data exist regarding the safety of glaucoma medicines in pregnancy. Most specialists would strongly consider stopping all glaucoma medicines during pregnancy and either forgoing treatment for the duration or considering a laser or surgical option.

    Brimonidine is a class B medication; all others are class C. In the postpartum period, brimonidine is contraindicated as it is secreted in breast milk and can cause severe CNS depression in neonates. Topical CAIs and betaxolol may be useful, although both are secreted in breast milk and may affect the newborn. Topical CAIs in high doses have demonstrated harm to animal fetuses. Prostaglandin analogs, which are associated with a high incidence of miscarriage in animal studies, are probably not a good choice in pregnancy. Safety in pediatric and pregnant patients has not been established with rho kinase inhibitors.

21. **Are any of the glaucoma medications safe for use in children?**
    Glaucoma in children is principally a surgical disease. Medications are typically used to lower the IOP until an exam under anesthesia can be performed and surgery done if needed. Topical or oral CAIs are a good choice in this group. Because of systemic side effects, β-blockers are used with caution in children. Brimonidine is a dangerous medication in neonates and infants because of its association with profound CNS depression and apnea. It is contraindicated in children under the age of 3 years and probably should not be used in children under the age of 8. Pilocarpine is useful after goniotomy or trabeculotomy but is not frequently used on a chronic

basis. Prostaglandin analogs in theory would not be a good option because the uveoscleral outflow pathways may be compromised by the angle dysgenesis that is typical of infantile glaucoma. In juvenile glaucoma, however, their effect is highly variable, and they can be used after a successful therapeutic trial.

22. **Is there any evidence that lowering intraocular pressure helps treat glaucoma?**
Elevated IOP is not only the most important but also the sole modifiable risk factor in the development of glaucoma. Data from randomized, prospective controlled clinical trials such as the Collaborative Normal-Tension Glaucoma Study, the Advanced Glaucoma Intervention Study, the Ocular Hypertension Treatment Study, and the Early Manifest Glaucoma Study all indicate that IOP reduction reduces the number of eyes that have continued glaucoma deterioration. Limited data suggest that the manner in which the pressure is reduced may be important. The Glaucoma Laser Trial found that patients initially treated with laser had less worsening of visual fields than did patients who were initially treated with medication. This finding is probably due to the fact that the laser-first group had a 2-mm lower IOP on average, compared with the medicine-only group. On the other hand, the Collaborative Initial Glaucoma Treatment Study found no difference at 5 years of follow-up between medicine and trabeculectomy with regard to the rate of glaucoma worsening. These more recent data seem to support the current general approach that, in theory, it makes no difference how you lower pressure as long as you lower it adequately. There is no consensus as to how much pressure lowering is adequate. This depends on several factors such as the amount of disease, the rate of change of the glaucoma, the patient's wishes, and the life expectancy. Most glaucoma specialists would probably agree that, all things being equal, mild disease would require a 25% to 30% IOP reduction; moderate disease, a 30% to 40% reduction; and advanced disease, a 40% to 50% or more reduction.

BIBLIOGRAPHY

Chua B, Goldberg I: Neuroprotective agents in glaucoma therapy: recent developments and future directions, Expert Rev Ophthalmol 5(5):627–636, 2010.
Girkin CA, Bhorade AM, Crowston JG, et al.: Basic and clinical science course. 2019–2020—Glaucoma, China, 2019, American Academy of Ophthalmology.
Henderer JD, Rapuano CJ: Ocular pharmacology. In Brunton LL, Hilal-Dandan R, Knollman BC, editors: Goodman and Gilman's: the pharmacological basis of therapeutics, ed 13, New York, 2018, McGraw-Hill.
Kass MA, Meltzer DW, Gordon M, et al.: Compliance with topical pilocarpine treatment, Am J Ophthalmol 101:515–523, 1986.
Lee MJ, Wang J, Fridman DS, et al.: Greater physical activity is associated with slower visual field loss in glaucoma, Ophthalmology 126:958–964, 2019.
Novack GD: Cannabinoids for treatment of glaucoma, Curr Opin Ophthalmol 27(2):146–150, 2016.
Onishchenko AL, Kolbasko AV, Zakharova AV, Onishchenko EG, Zhilina NM: Ocular hypotensive effect of systemic beta-blockers in patients with primary glaucoma and arterial hypertension, Vestn Oftalmol 133(2):46–51, 2017.
Piltz J, Gross R, Shin DH, et al.: Contralateral effect of topical β-adrenergic antagonists in initial one-eyed trials in the ocular hypertension treatment study, Am J Ophthalmol 30:441–453, 2000.
Schmidl D, Schmetter, Garhofer G, et al.: Pharmacotherapy of glaucoma, J Ocul Pharmacol Ther 31(2):63–77, 2015.
Weinreb RN, Liebmann JM, Cioffi GA, et al.: Oral memantine for the treatment of glaucoma: design and results of 2 randomized, placebo-controlled, phase 3 studies, Ophthalmology 125(12):1874–1885, 2018.

TRABECULECTOMY SURGERY

Marlene R. Moster and Augusto Azuara-Blanco

CHAPTER 19

1. **What are the indications for trabeculectomy surgery?**
   Trabeculectomy is indicated when neither medical nor laser therapy sufficiently controls or is likely to control glaucoma progression, and that progression is likely to diminish a patient's quality of life. Because visual needs and vision-related quality-of-life characteristics differ, patients should be assessed individually before surgery is considered. Physicians should consider the likelihood of success and risk of complications from surgery prior to proceeding. Trabeculectomy surgery can also be considered as a primary treatment, especially in eyes with severe glaucoma at presentation. Quality of life and visual field outcomes from trials comparing primary trabeculectomy with medication were comparable, but intraocular pressure (IOP) was lower after surgery. Studies comparing trabeculectomy with glaucoma drainage devices reported lower IOP after trabeculectomy.[1,2]

2. **What is the goal of glaucoma surgery?**
   The goal of glaucoma surgery is to lower the IOP sufficiently to prevent or minimize further damage to the optic nerve and visual field while avoiding severe complications. The target reduction of IOP will depend on individual factors. In the Advanced Glaucoma Intervention Study (AGIS), patients with severe glaucoma with an average IOP of 12 mm Hg after surgery had stable visual function after long-term follow-up.[3] Because many patients with glaucoma do not have elevated IOP, the goal of glaucoma surgery is *not* to reduce IOP to less than 21 mm Hg but to tailor the target IOP to the patient's characteristics. Another goal of trabeculectomy surgery is to decrease topical medications, as a substantial number of patients become allergic to glaucoma medications over time. With successful trabeculectomy surgery and the decrease in topical medications, the lids and ocular surface can heal (Fig. 19.1).

3. **What are the risks of trabeculectomy surgery?**
   The risks and benefits of glaucoma surgery and alternative options must be carefully outlined to all patients in a language that is easily understood. It is imperative to explain clearly the remote possibility of blindness or loss of the eye due to hemorrhage or infection. In addition, the possibility of sudden or permanent visual loss, failure to control IOP (which may be too high or too low), need for repeated surgery, droopy lid, discomfort, and significant blurring (common for the first 2 weeks) should be elaborated. Failure to control the IOP and the need to restart medication is not uncommon. Late-onset risks include bleb-related infection and endophthalmitis (rare) or

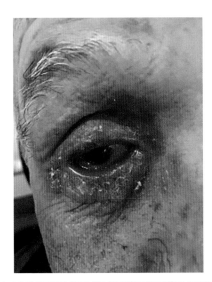

Fig. 19.1 Severe allergy to multiple classes of glaucoma drops. The lids and ocular surface reverted to normal following trabeculectomy and the decreased use of topical medications.

cataract (common). Patients should be aware that they will likely be needed to be seen frequently postoperatively in order to manage the healing process to allow for the best outcome in terms of IOP control and visual acuity.

4. Describe the factors associated with failure of glaucoma filtering surgery.
Unfavorable factors include pigmented skin (nonwhite), young age, intraocular inflammation, neovascular changes, previous trauma, dislocated lens, complicated cataract surgery, vitreous in the anterior chamber, inability to use corticosteroids, previous failed glaucoma surgery, previous retinal surgery, scarred or abnormal conjunctiva, and an inexperienced surgeon (Fig. 19.2).

5. Does a fornix versus a limbal–conjunctival approach affect outcome?
Fornix-based and limbal-based approaches produce similar results regarding IOP control. With a limbal-based approach, the risk of a wound leak is smaller (Fig. 19.3). However, this incision appears to increase the likelihood of having a thin avascular and localized filtering bleb (Fig. 19.4) and possible late-onset bleb-related infections. If a limbal-based flap is chosen, it should be made sufficiently posterior so that the closure is at least 10 mm or more from the limbus. If a fornix-based flap is chosen, it is imperative to ensure that the closure is watertight. There are many ways to close a fornix-based conjunctival flap and it depends on surgeon preference. Most commonly, individual 10-0 nylon mattress sutures are employed, or a running 8-0 vicryl suture can be used. After raising the filtering bleb at the end of the case, using a moistened fluorescein strip is helpful to check for aqueous leaks (Fig. 19.5).

6. What medications should be stopped before filtration surgery?
Patients should continue their systemic medications. Blood thinners do not necessarily need to be stopped. However, confirm that the anticoagulation levels are within therapeutic range for the patient's condition. If the surgeon desires to stop anticoagulants prior to surgery, it is imperative to discuss this with the patient's internist.

7. What are the choices of anesthesia?
General anesthesia is used in children and other patients unable to cooperate with a local anesthetic procedure. Intracameral, sub-Tenon's, and subconjunctival anesthesias are preferred choices. A detailed description of our current technique, "blitz" anesthesia, follows:
1. Place xylocaine 1% jelly or lidocaine hydrochloride 2% jelly in the fornix before surgery.
2. In the operating room, make a temporal paracentesis, release a small amount of aqueous from the anterior chamber, and inject 0.1 mL of 1% nonpreserved lidocaine on a cannula.

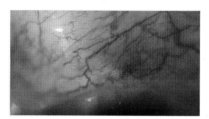

Fig. 19.2 Scarring of the sclera, Tenon's layer, and conjunctiva can cause bleb failure.

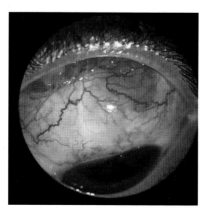

Fig. 19.3 Limbal-based conjunctival trabeculectomy closure 1 week following surgery.

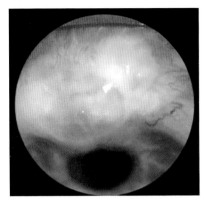

Fig. 19.4 A thin cystic bleb resulting from a limbal-based closure. These blebs are more prone to developing leaks over time.

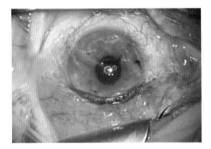

Fig. 19.5 Testing for a leak at the end of surgery is necessary to ensure a functioning, elevated bleb. This patient has a fornix-based flap seen as viewed through the operating microscope when sitting superiorly.

3. Inject a 1:1 mixture of 0.1 cc nonpreserved lidocaine 1% and 0.1 cc mitomycin C (MMC) (0.4 mg/cc) under the conjunctiva with a 30-gauge needle (Fig. 19.6). This injection proceeds the formation of either a limbal- or a fornix-based flap. If using this method, additional lidocaine is usually not necessary but can be used at the surgeon's discretion.
4. Inject 0.5 mL of lidocaine with a 30-gauge needle 10 mm posterior and parallel to the limbus, ballooning the Tenon's capsule and conjunctival space in both the nasal and temporal direction.
5. When closing the conjunctival incision, additional lidocaine 1% is irrigated with a cannula through the Tenon's capsule so that there is no sensation noted by the patient.

8. Does a triangular versus a rectangular flap affect outcome?
No. The shape of the scleral flap is surgeon dependent; there is no difference in clinical outcome with a triangular or rectangular flap. Although the shape of the flap is not important, its thickness may be. Very thin flaps should be avoided as it is necessary to be able to control the outflow and prevent overfiltration.

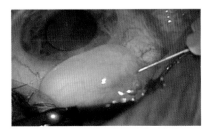

Fig. 19.6 0.2 cc subconjunctival lidocaine and mitomycin are injected prior to making either a fornix- or a limbal-based flap.

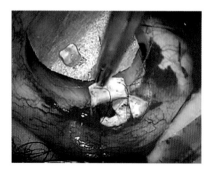

Fig. 19.7 Large internal block removed in a patient with normal tension glaucoma with high risk of scarring.

9. **Does the size of the internal block affect outcome?**
No. A small (e.g., 1-mm) excision is sufficient, although some surgeons choose to create larger fistulas. Increased filtration results when one edge of the fistula coincides with one edge of the scleral flap. The internal block can be removed with Vannas scissors or a punch (Fig. 19.7).

10. **Are an iridectomy and a paracentesis always necessary during filtration surgery?**
An iridectomy is always performed in angle-closure glaucoma to ensure that pupillary block does not occur. In addition, if the chamber shallows, the iris is less likely to occlude the ostium. However, iridectomy may not be always necessary in patients with open-angle glaucoma and particularly in pseudophakic eyes. A paracentesis is always done and can be made with either a sharp blade temporally or a 27-gauge needle on a syringe. A paracentesis is considered essential with each procedure because it allows reformation of the anterior chamber toward the end of surgery. By refilling the anterior chamber via the paracentesis, the surgeon has an appreciation of how much leakage is visible around the edges of the scleral flap. A paracentesis is useful in managing the patient in the office postoperatively, i.e., burping the anterior chamber if the IOP is high, and reforming the anterior chamber if it is flat.

11. **How tight should I make the scleral flap?**
The number of sutures and their tightness depend on the diagnosis, preoperative IOP, architecture of the scleral flap, location of the fistula, and how much leak is desired at the time of surgery. In general, those patients at high risk for complications associated with hypotony should have tighter scleral flaps. For example, patients with inordinately high IOP, shallow anterior chamber, angle-closure glaucoma, or increased episcleral venous pressure are more likely to develop complications if there is overdrainage.

With low-tension glaucoma, looser sutures with more flow may be indicated to ensure a low initial postoperative IOP. The sutures can be lysed with an argon laser anywhere from day 1 through the first 2 weeks or longer if antimetabolites are used.

12. **Are releasable sutures necessary?**
Although releasable sutures have some advantages, they are not necessary to achieve a good result. We tend to use additional releasable sutures (Fig. 19.8). The flap can be closed moderately loosely with permanent sutures, and the releasable sutures decrease the flow further, thus avoiding early hypotony. Selective suture removal between the first postoperative day and 1 month can easily be done at the slit lamp with the need for a laser.

13. **Does it matter how far I dissect the scleral flap anteriorly?**
We aim to open the fistula anterior to the trabecular meshwork. In large myopic eyes, a perpendicular incision just anterior to the corneoscleral sulcus carries the flap well anterior to the trabecular meshwork. In removing the internal block, a satisfactory anterior fistula results. In contrast, in small hyperopic eyes and those with angle-closure glaucoma or peripheral anterior synechiae, an incision at the same point terminates just in front of the iris root. In these patients, an anterior dissection well into the cornea is necessary both to ensure that the fistula will not be blocked by uveal tissue and to prevent bleeding (Fig. 19.9).

14. **Should atropine be used during the procedure?**
Atropine is needed only in patients with small eyes, shallow anterior chamber, or angle-closure glaucoma. Sterile 1% atropine drops are used during or at the end of the operation to dilate the pupil maximally and to move the lens iris diaphragm posteriorly. This technique decreases the likelihood of a flat anterior chamber in the early postoperative period. Care must be taken in those elderly patients with prostate or urinary problems so as not to precipitate kidney failure due to the anticholinergic properties of atropine.

15. **How often are steroids used in the postoperative period?**
It varies according to the surgeon's preference and the apparent inflammation, but at a minimum, they should be used four times a day for at least 1 month (e.g., prednisolone acetate 1%, difluprednate 0.05%, or betamethasone

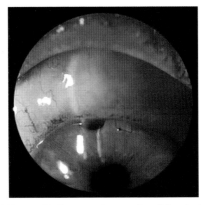

Fig. 19.8 Releasable sutures are helpful in controlling the egress of aqueous through the scleral flap in the postoperative period. They are usually removed within the first three postoperative weeks.

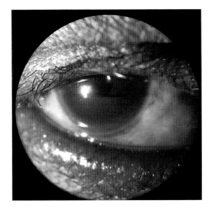

Fig. 19.9 Hyphema can be seen after trabeculectomy, especially in eyes with chronic angle closure and in patients on blood thinners.

0.1%). In phakic eyes, topical steroids are tapered quickly after 4–6 weeks to reduce the risk of cataract. In pseudophakic patients or eyes with signs of *increased* conjunctival or intraocular inflammation, the steroid treatment can be intensified and maintained for at least 2–3 months. Some surgeons prefer the addition of a nonsteroidal anti-inflammatory drug (NSAID) one time a day in conjunction with the steroids over a 1–2-month period. Longer and more intensive treatment is advisable in cases with high risk of failure, combined cataract extraction with trabeculectomy (phaco-trabeculectomy), and in those with a vascularized bleb.

16. How can you avoid a flat anterior chamber after trabeculectomy?
    The most useful strategy is to prevent overdrainage and hypotony. The amount of leakage underneath the scleral flap ultimately determines the postoperative pressure. To minimize the chance of a flat anterior chamber (Fig. 19.10), additional 10-0 nylon sutures, with or without releasable sutures, should be used to minimize the flow at the end of the procedure. Laser suture lysis may then be used to selectively increase the flow under the scleral flap and improve control. If the sutures are cut too aggressively, a flat anterior chamber may result.

17. What do you do when a wound leak occurs in the immediate postoperative period?
    Unless the leak is very brisk, it usually heals within the first few days. If the leak is near the limbus, a collagen shield or a bandage contact lens may help. If a leak is very brisk or associated with a flat filtering bleb or with a shallow anterior chamber, surgical closure is necessary. If the leak is located at the wound, restitching is indicated. If there is a buttonhole, close with a purse-string suture with 11-0 nylon on a round body needle to prevent further shredding of the tissue. Use a fluorescein strip to confirm that the wound and buttonhole are Seidel negative before ending the procedure.

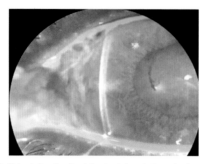

Fig. 19.10 Flat anterior chamber following trabeculectomy due to overfiltration.

KEY POINTS: HOW TO AVOID COMPLICATIONS OF TRABECULECTOMY

1. Identify high-risk conditions (e.g., angle-closure, elevated episcleral venous pressure, previous conjunctival surgery).
2. Minimize the risk of hypotony by avoiding a thin scleral flap and proper suturing of the scleral flap (with or without releasable sutures).
3. Excise the interior block to create the fistula anterior to trabecular meshwork.
4. Use the paracentesis to evaluate amount of filtration under the scleral flap and decide whether more or less sutures are required.
5. After closing the conjunctiva, inject balanced salt solution (BSS) into the anterior chamber to raise the bleb and confirm absence of leaks.

18. **What do you do if there is vitreous loss at the time of the trabeculectomy?**
A "dry" vitrectomy (without balanced salt solution [BSS] infusion) with viscoelastic can be very helpful. It can be done through the scleral flap and peripheral iridectomy. If an inordinate amount of vitreous is present, it is probably best to proceed with a full anterior vitrectomy. Vitreous loss is rare in phakic eyes that have no history of trauma, surgery, or other predilection toward lens dislocation. Vitreous loss is more frequent in eyes that are pseudophakic in the presence of zonular weakening (see next question). Nonpreserved triamcinolone injected into the anterior chamber can help visualize the vitreous strands if there is concern of blockage by vitreous within the trabeculectomy ostium. The vitreous strands are more easily removed when visualized in this way.

19. **Which ocular conditions may predispose to vitreous loss during trabeculectomy surgery?**
Previous ocular trauma, Marfan's syndrome, pseudoexfoliation, homocystinuria, complicated cataract surgery, and high myopia may predispose to vitreous loss during trabeculectomy surgery.

20. **Describe the indications of antimetabolites in trabeculectomy surgery**
Most surgeons routinely use MMC in trabeculectomy surgeries. Both 5-fluorouracil (5-FU) and MMC inhibit normal wound healing and facilitate the formation of highly functioning filtering blebs (Fig. 19.11). Although current antifibrotic agents improve surgical outcomes, they have associated complications.[4] The use of high dose of antimetabolites is advisable in eyes at high risk of failure, e.g., with scarring of the superior conjunctiva, previously failed filtering surgery, pseudophakia, ocular inflammation, or advanced optic nerve and visual field injury with desired postoperative pressure less than 14 mm Hg.

21. **How does 5-fluorouracil differ from mitomycin C?**
MMC (0.1–0.5 mg/mL) is 100 times more potent than 5-FU (25–50 mg/mL). Whereas 5-FU affects primarily the S-phase of the cell cycle, MMC inhibits fibroblastic proliferation regardless of the phase of the cell cycle. Most surgeons prefer intraoperative MMC. Intraoperative application is done with several Weck-cell sponges on the sclera under the conjunctiva and Tenon's capsule, treating a large area of the superior globe. The sponges are left in place for 1–5 minutes, depending on the perceived risk for failure. Alternatively, MMC can be injected subconjunctivally (0.1–0.3 mL of 0.2–0.4 mg/mL) at the beginning of the surgery, alone or combined with 0.1 mL of 1% nonpreserved xylocaine, and delivered in a 1-mL syringe with a 30-gauge needle, 10 mm from the limbus.

22. **Are antimetabolites indicated in primary filtering procedures?**
Yes, as they improve the outcome of the surgery. With modern surgical techniques, postoperative complications of hypotony (Fig. 19.12), suprachoroidal hemorrhage (Fig. 19.13), choroidal detachment, flat anterior chambers, and bleb leaks (Fig. 19.14) are uncommon and late endophthalmitis (Fig. 19.15) is rare.

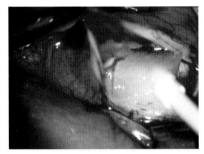

Fig. 19.11 Mitomycin C can be delivered directly via a sponge or injected under the conjunctiva and Tenon's capsule in order to provide a large surface area for adequate filtration.

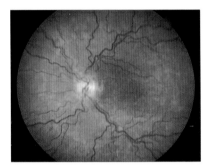

Fig. 19.12 Hypotony with chorioretinal folds at the macula. Intraocular pressure was 4 mm Hg.

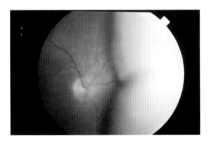

Fig. 19.13 Suprachoroidal hemorrhage 1 week after filtering surgery in a patient with known heart disease and previous heart valve replacement on blood thinners.

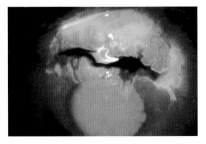

Fig. 19.14 Leaking bleb following a mitomycin C trabeculectomy 6 months after surgery.

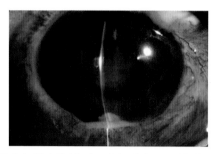

Fig. 19.15 Endophthalmitis following a trabeculectomy resulting in poor vision.

23. **What do you do when the iris blocks the trabeculectomy site in the immediate postoperative period?**
One option is to place Miochol or Miostat via the paracentesis into the anterior chamber in an attempt to constrict the pupil and dislodge it from the trabeculectomy site. A viscoelastic agent is then injected, and either a cannula or 30-gauge needle can be used to remove the iris carefully from the trabeculectomy site. On occasion, the iris does not occlude the ostium completely, and good filtration may occur around it.

24. **What if the ciliary processes roll anteriorly and block the trabeculectomy site during surgery?**
Ciliary processes may block the trabeculectomy site in small hyperopic eyes, and primary angle-closure glaucoma, and nanophthalmos, especially if the fistula is not done anteriorly to the trabecular meshwork. After the fistula is completed, the ciliary processes may roll into the filtering site. In most cases, closure of the scleral flap, reforming the anterior chamber, and reestablishing normal anatomy allow the ciliary processes to revert to their normal positions. If, after deepening the anterior chamber, the ciliary processes continue to block the trabeculectomy opening, they can be cauterized and cut away. Care must be taken not to disturb the vitreous face.

25. **When is it necessary to give postoperative 5-fluorouracil injections?**
Supplementary 5-FU injections, e.g., 0.1 mL (5 mg), may be given in the early postoperative period if the bleb is thickened, red, and vascularized. This option is left to the surgeon's discretion. This treatment is given to decrease the chances of bleb scarring and failure. When repeated injections are used, corneal epithelial toxicity may appear and should be monitored. If there are signs of keratopathy, 5-FU injections should be delayed (Fig. 19.16).

26. **What do you do if the bleb starts to fail?**
If the bleb is thick and injected, increase the topical steroid regimen and inject 5-FU. In addition, 2.5 mg bevacizumab (Avastin) can be injected into the bleb.[5] Digital massage in the early postoperative period increases the outflow, but it is not effective in the long-term to maintain the bleb function. Aggressive suture lysis should be considered. Sometimes, regardless of all efforts, the bleb fails and further glaucoma surgery may be required. Alternatively, bleb needling can be tried (see next question).

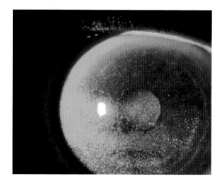

Fig. 19.16 Superficial punctuate keratopathy following repeated injections of 5-fluorouracil in a failing filter.

KEY POINTS: HOW TO IMPROVE YOUR SUCCESS RATE

1. Use intraoperative MMC.
2. Use postoperative 5-FU and increase topical steroids when the bleb has early signs of scarring and failure.
3. Cut or release sutures when function of filtering bleb is suboptimal.
4. Consider needling with 5-FU or MMC when the bleb has failed.

27. What is the technique of bleb needling?

It is important to detect where the resistance to filtration is occurring; thus, prior gonioscopy is essential. Although the needling procedure can be done at the slit lamp, we now prefer needling in the operating room as the situation is more controlled, bleeding can be handled more easily and everything is done under sterile conditions. If this is done in the office, a sterile technique is still required, including the use of topical diluted Betadine. Inject a 1:1 mixture of 0.1 cc nonpreserved lidocaine 1% and 0.1 cc MMC (0.4 mg/cc) under the conjunctiva or sub-Tenon's with a 30-gauge needle. The mixture is dispersed widely over the surgical area. After waiting a few minutes, proceed with needling. Most often, scarring at the scleral flap is responsible for bleb failure. In this case, a 27-gauge needle is introduced into the subconjunctival space 8–10 mm away from the scleral flap then directed toward the flap edge and, if possible, advanced under the scleral flap to ensure an outpouring of aqueous.[6] The surgeon can try to maximize the efficacy of the bleb revision with some careful movements of the needle. Postoperatively, use topical antibiotics and steroids and watch closely.

28. What is the differential diagnosis for a flat anterior chamber?

The most common cause of a flat chamber after glaucoma surgery is excessive filtration. Other possibilities include serous choroidal detachment, hemorrhagic choroidal detachment, pupillary block, and malignant glaucoma (Fig. 19.17 and Box 19.1). With excessive filtration and serous choroidal detachment, the IOP is low. With a hemorrhagic choroidal detachment, the IOP may be low, normal, or high and usually is associated with pain. With both pupillary block and malignant glaucoma, the IOP is typically elevated, and the cornea often edematous.

29. How urgent is the management of a flat anterior chamber?

Grade I (contact between the peripheral iris and the cornea) can be managed conservatively. If it is due to overfiltration, treatment includes use of cycloplegics, mydriatics, and careful observation. Improvement is usually spontaneous.

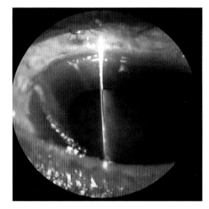

Fig. 19.17 Flat chamber seen in the presence of malignant glaucoma following trabeculectomy. The intraocular pressure was 48 mm Hg and required a vitrectomy to break the vitreous face and create a unicameral eye.

Box 19.1 Prevention of Malignant Glaucoma

1. Detect high-risk cases (angle-closure glaucoma, small, hyperopic eyes).
2. Minimize intraoperative shallowing of the anterior chamber.
3. Perform a large peripheral iridectomy.
4. Avoid overfiltration.
5. Cautious suture lysis.
6. Use cycloplegics, starting at the time of the surgery. Taper cycloplegics slowly.

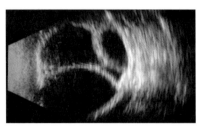

Fig. 19.18 Ultrasound of kissing choroidals following a filtering procedure in an eye with chronic angle closure.

Progression from grade I to grade II (contact between the peripheral and central iris and cornea) in spite of treatment may be a poor prognostic sign, especially if the pressure is falling and the bleb is flattening. Grade II may recover spontaneously or progress to grade III.

Grade III (contact between the corneal endothelium and lens) is an emergency and must be corrected promptly or the corneal endothelium will be damaged.

30. What are the indications to drain a choroidal detachment?
Whenever the pressure consistently falls, the bleb flattens, and the chamber shallows despite reformation with viscoelastic material, drainage of the associated choroidal detachment is indicated. Appositional "kissing" choroidal effusions that do not improve after a few days to weeks should also be drained (Fig. 19.18). A full-thickness scleral incision is made in one of the inferior quadrants to reach the suprachoroidal space. Reformation of the anterior chamber is done simultaneously with BSS through the paracentesis tract. If the choroidal detachment is hemorrhagic, it is recommended that at least 10 days should elapse so the blood can liquefy before drainage.

REFERENCES
1. Musch DC, Gillespie BW, Lichter PR, Niziol LM, Janz NK, CIGTS Study Investigators: Visual field progression in the Collaborative Initial Glaucoma Treatment Study the impact of treatment and other baseline factors, Ophthalmology 116:200–207, 2009.
2. Gedde SJ, Schiffman JC, Feuer WJ, Herndon LW, Brandt JD, Budenz DL; Tube versus Trabeculectomy Study Group: Treatment outcomes in the Tube Versus Trabeculectomy (TVT) study after five years of follow-up, Am J Ophthalmol 153:789–803, 2012.
3. The Advanced Glaucoma Intervention Study (AGIS): 7. The relationship between control of intraocular pressure and visual field deterioration, Am J Ophthalmol 130:429–440, 2000.
4. Wilkins M, Indar A, Wormald R: Intraoperative mitomycin C for glaucoma surgery, Cochrane Database Syst Rev (4):Art. No. CD002897, 2005.
5. Vandewalle E, Abegão Pinto L, Van Bergen T, et al.: Intracameral bevacizumab as an adjunct to trabeculectomy: a 1-year prospective, randomised study, Br J Ophthalmol 98:73–78, 2014.
6. Shetty RK, Warluft L, Moster MR: Slit-lamp needle revision of failed filtering blebs using high-dose mitomycin-C, J Glaucoma 14: 52–56, 2005.

CHAPTER 20

TRAUMATIC GLAUCOMA AND HYPHEMA

Douglas J. Rhee and Shipra Gupta

1. What is a hyphema?

   A hyphema is blood in the anterior chamber. The appearance of a hyphema may range from microscopic, seen only at the slit lamp as erythrocytes circulating in the aqueous, to a total hyphema that fills the entire anterior chamber.

2. List the causes of a hyphema.

   There are three major causes of hyphema: trauma to the globe, intraocular surgery, or spontaneous anterior segment hemorrhage in association with ocular or systemic conditions, such as neovascularization of the iris or anterior chamber angle, intraocular tumors, or clotting disorders (Table 20.1).

3. What is the most common cause of a traumatic hyphema?

   The most common cause of traumatic hyphema is blunt anterior segment trauma.

4. Describe the pathophysiology of a traumatic hyphema.

   Blunt ocular trauma results in ocular indentation, which causes a sudden expansion of ocular tissues and an immediate rise in the intraocular pressure (IOP). The sudden forceful displacement of the cornea and limbus posteriorly and peripherally may result in splitting or tearing of these tissues. As the tissues tear, blood vessels in the vicinity may rupture, resulting in a hyphema.

5. List the anterior segment structures that may split or tear in response to blunt ocular injury.
   - **Iris:** Sphincter tear ruptures a blood vessel within the iris
   - **Iris Root:** Iridodialysis, i.e., separation of the iris from ciliary body, causing rupturing blood vessels
   - **Anterior ciliary body:** Angle recession
   - **Separation of ciliary body from the scleral spur:** Cyclodialysis
   - **Trabecular meshwork:** Trabecular meshwork tear allows blood to reflux from the Schlemm's canal
   - **Zonules/lens:** Zonular tears with possible lens subluxation
   - **Separation of the retina from the ora serrata:** Retinal dialysis

6. When a patient presents with a hyphema due to blunt ocular trauma, which anterior segment structure is the most likely source of the hemorrhage?

   Hyphema as a result of blunt ocular trauma most commonly occurs as a result of angle recession, a tear in the anterior face of the ciliary body between the longitudinal and the circular ciliary body muscles. Rupture of the blood vessels in the vicinity of the tear results in a hyphema. The most frequently ruptured blood vessels include the major arterial circle of the iris, the arterial branches to the ciliary body, and the recurrent choroidal arteries and vein crossing between the ciliary body and the episcleral venous plexus.

7. What ocular injuries may be associated with a traumatic hyphema?
   - **Ocular wall:** Ruptured globe at the cornea, limbus, and/or sclera
   - **Cornea/conjunctiva:** Epithelial abrasion, laceration, subconjunctival hemorrhage
   - **Iris:** Sphincter tears, iridodialysis, mydriasis (long-term)
   - **Angle:** Angle recession, iris dialysis, cyclodialysis cleft
   - **Lens:** Traumatic cataract (acute, capsular rupture; chronic, direct injury), subluxation or total dislocation (damage of zonular attachments)
   - **Vitreous:** Vitreous detachment, vitreous prolapse
   - **Retina:** Retinal tear, detachment, and/or dialysis (vessel rupture, vascular occlusion)
   - **Retinal pigment epithelium and choroid:** Choroidal rupture
   - **Optic nerve:** Avulsion, optic nerve crush (chronic, glaucoma)
   - **Orbit:** Orbital wall/floor fractures with or without extraocular muscle entrapment
   - **Periorbital tissue:** edema, erythema, contusion, lid laceration

8. Describe an appropriate approach to the workup of a patient with a hyphema.

   The primary responsibility is to exclude a ruptured globe and search for an ocular foreign body in all patients who present with a traumatic hyphema. The color, character, and extent of the hyphema and associated ocular injuries, including potential corneal blood-staining, should be documented. Gonioscopy is usually best deferred, but, if necessary, it may be performed gently, taking care to avoid a rebleed. Before a possible rebleed obscures the view, a dilated lens and fundus examination should be performed without scleral depression. Computed tomography of

Table 20.1 Hyphema Classification by Etiology

I. Trauma
   A. Blunt—rupture of the iris or ciliary body blood vessels
   B. Penetrating—direct severing of blood vessels

II. Intraocular surgery
   A. Intraoperative bleeding
      1. Ciliary body or iris injury—most common when performing cyclodialysis, peripheral iridectomy, guarded filtration procedure, and cataract extraction
      2. Laser peripheral iridectomy—bleeding is more common with the YAG laser than with the argon laser
      3. Argon laser trabeculoplasty—rare
      4. Selective laser trabeculoplasty—extremely rare
      5. Cyclodestructive procedures—common, depending on the mechanism of elevated intraocular pressure (e.g., neovascular glaucoma)
   B. Early postoperative bleeding
      1. Dilation of a traumatized uveal vessel that was previously in spasm
      2. Conjunctival bleeding that enters the anterior chamber through a corneoscleral wound or a sclerostomy
   C. Late postoperative bleeding
      1. Disruption of new vessels growing across the corneoscleral wound
      2. Reopening of a uveal wound
      3. Chronic iris erosion from an intraocular lens causing fibrovascular tissue growth

III. Spontaneous
   A. Neovascularization of the iris secondary to (the conditions below cause the neovascularization):
      1. Retinal detachment
      2. Central retinal vein occlusion, central retinal artery occlusion, carotid occlusive disease
      3. Proliferative diabetic retinopathy
      4. Chronic uveitis
      5. Fuchs' heterochromic iridocyclitis
   B. Intraocular tumors
      1. Malignant melanoma
      2. Juvenile xanthogranuloma
      3. Retinoblastoma
      4. Metastatic tumors
   C. Iris microhemangiomas—may be associated with diabetes mellitus and myotonic dystrophy
   D. Clotting factor dysfunction
      1. Leukemia
      2. Hemophilia
      3. Anemias
      4. Aspirin
      5. Coumadin
      6. Ethanol
      7. Nonsteroidal anti-inflammatory drugs
      8. Vitamin C/gingko

IV. Indirect: spillover from vitreous hemorrhage

YAG, Yttrium, aluminum, and garnet.
Adapted from Gottsch JD: Hyphema: diagnosis and management, *Retina* 10:S65–S71, 1990.

the orbit can identify foreign bodies and associated bone injury and is highly suggestive of a ruptured globe if there is any alteration from the normal round shape of the eye.

Past medical and ocular history may identify risk factors for the bleeding episode and the chance of future complications. Persons with African or Latin ancestry as well as anyone with a positive family history should have a sickle cell test and Hgb electrophoresis. Establishing the exact nature of the trauma helps to estimate the likelihood of a possible ocular or orbital foreign body and/or ruptured globe. The exact timing of the injury is crucial in enabling one to predict when a patient will be at greatest risk for a rebleed and to help determine the expected time of clearing and the length of necessary treatment.

Four to six weeks after the injury, perform careful gonioscopy of the recovered eye to evaluate for angle recession. At this time, perform a dilated fundus examination with scleral depression to rule out peripheral retinal injury, such as described in Table 20.1.

KEY POINTS: TRAUMATIC HYPHEMA

1. All patients should be evaluated for systemic injuries (e.g., computed tomographic scans, x-rays).
2. All patients should be evaluated for intraocular foreign bodies and ruptured globes as well as other ocular injuries.
3. Recurrent hemorrhages occur in 0.4% to 35% of patients, usually 2 to 5 days after trauma.
4. Corneal blood staining occurs in 5%.

9. What are pertinent questions to ask a patient who presents with a traumatic hyphema? Why?
   - **When did your injury occur?** Establishing the exact time of the injury is important because there is an increased rate of rebleed in patients who present more than 24 hours after trauma, and it will help to determine how soon a patient will be at greatest risk for a rebleed.
   - **What type of injury did you sustain?** The type and severity of an injury is important to help assess the likelihood of associated systemic injuries, an ocular or intraorbital foreign body, and the possibility of a ruptured globe.
   - **Do you or any of your family members have a medical history of bleeding disorders or sickle cell disease?** The answer to this question may help to establish a possible etiology for the hyphema and to determine what type and how aggressive the treatment should be to control the IOP.
   - **What types of medications do you take (including alcohol intake)?** Antiplatelet or anticoagulant effects of aspirin, nonsteroidal anti-inflammatory drugs, warfarin (Coumadin) or other anticoagulants, and alcohol may predispose a patient to developing a hyphema or a rebleed after trauma and should be discontinued if possible.

10. How are hyphemas managed?
    There is no consensus regarding the appropriate treatment for hyphema. Traditionally, most patients with a hyphema were admitted to the hospital for bed rest and sedation and were given a monocular or binocular patch for approximately 5 days. Today, compliant patients with a microhyphema and a low risk for rebleed are usually followed as outpatients. It still appears prudent to hospitalize those patients who have a layered hyphema (Fig. 20.1), are at increased risk for rebleed, have a sickling hemoglobinopathy, or are noncompliant.
    Place a protective shield over the affected eye to decrease any inadvertent trauma and advise the patient to limit activity. The head is elevated (to allow the blood to layer inferiorly and thus assist with visual rehabilitation and prevent clot formation in the papillary aperture). Control systemic blood pressure to decrease the hydrostatic pressure in the traumatized blood vessels to minimize the risk of recurrent hemorrhage. Patients should be examined gently once or twice a day and check IOP.
    The medical management of hyphema includes the following:
    - Discontinuation of antiplatelet, anticoagulant, and nonsteroidal anti-inflammatory medications.
    - Treatment with cycloplegic drops, oral or topical steroids, antiemetics, and antifibrinolytics.
    - IOP control as necessary:
      - β-Blockers.
      - α-Agonists (avoid in young children because of the risk of bradycardia and hypotension).
      - Topical or systemic carbonic anhydrase inhibitors and hyperosmotics (except in patients with sickle hemo-globinopathies because of the risk of increased sickling with these medications).
      - Rho kinase inhibitors.
      - Prostaglandin analogues have the potential to increase intraocular inflammation but can be used with close monitoring.
      - Avoid miotics, as they might increase pupillary block and disrupt the blood–aqueous barrier.

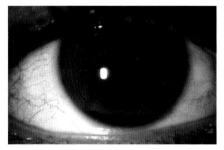

Fig. 20.1 Layered hyphema.

11. **Explain the rationale for the use of antifibrinolytic agents in the treatment of hyphema.**
Systemic antifibrinolytic agents are used in an effort to reduce the chance of recurrent hemorrhage. Their use is rare now, especially in populations with a low risk of rebleeding. Fibrinolysis of a clot that seals a recently ruptured blood vessel may result in a repeat hemorrhage from that site. Tranexamic acid and aminocaproic acid decrease the rate of clot hemolysis by inhibiting the conversion of plasminogen to plasmin, which results in stabilization of the clot that seals the ruptured blood vessel. The injured vessel now has more time to heal permanently prior to fibrinolysis of the clot, thus reducing the risk of recurrent hemorrhage. Topical aminocaproic acid shows promise but remains investigational at present.

12. **Name the most common adverse effects associated with aminocaproic acid treatment.**
Nausea, vomiting, and postural hypotension are frequent side effects of aminocaproic acid. Therefore, it is recommended that patients who receive aminocaproic acid be transported via wheelchair, particularly during the first 24 hours, to prevent possible complications from postural hypotension. Antiemetics may be used as necessary.

13. **Is aminocaproic acid contraindicated?**
Aminocaproic acid use is contraindicated in the presence of the following:
- Active intravascular clotting disorders, including cancer
- Hepatic disease
- Renal disease
- Pregnancy
     Cautious use is recommended in patients at risk for myocardial infarction, pulmonary embolus, and cerebrovascular disease.

14. **Why are patients with sickle cell disease or sickle cell trait at a higher risk for developing complications from a hyphema?**
Once pliable biconcave erythrocytes transform into elongated ridged sickle cells, they are unable to pass through the trabecular meshwork easily. The trabecular meshwork becomes obstructed with these inflexible cells, leading to a marked rise in IOP, even in the setting of a relatively small hyphema. Factors that encourage sickling include acidosis, hypoxia, and hemoconcentration. Vascular sludging of sickled cells may cause ischemia and microvascular infarction. Minimally elevated IOPs predispose patients with sickle cell to infarction of the optic nerve, retina, and anterior segment. Therefore, vigorous and aggressive therapy for IOP control is suggested for patients with sickle cell disease.

15. **How is IOP controlled in patients with sickle cell disease or sickle trait?**
β-Blockers, prostaglandin analogs and rho kinase inhibitors are the best choices as many glaucoma medications are generally avoided because they may increase sickling.
- Carbonic anhydrase inhibitors, particularly acetazolamide, increase the concentration of ascorbic acid in the aqueous. This decreases the pH, leading to increased sickling in the anterior chamber. Methazolamide may be a safer alternative because it causes less systemic acidosis than acetazolamide.
- Epinephrine compounds and α-agonists may cause vasoconstriction with subsequent deoxygenation, increasing intravascular and intracameral sickling.
- Hyperosmotics may cause hemoconcentration, leading to vascular sludging and sickling, increasing the risk of infarction in the eye and other organs.
- For these patients, there is a low threshold for surgical interventions; earlier and at lower IOPs than in people who do not have sickle cell trait or disease (see question 17).

KEY POINTS: TRAUMATIC HYPHEMA AND SICKLE CELL DISEASE

1. More aggressive management is required to prevent optic nerve damage and central retinal artery occlusion.
2. β-Blockers, prostaglandin analogs, and rho kinase inhibitors should be used as first line agents for IOP control.
3. Carbonic anhydrase inhibitors, epinephrine compounds, α-agonists, and hyperosmotics may increase sickling and are therefore contraindicated.

---

16. **What level of intraocular pressure is considered medically uncontrolled?**
An IOP that is considered uncontrolled depends upon the patient in question. (Some guidelines are included in subsequent discussions.) Surgery is generally not indicated in a patient with a healthy optic nerve unless the IOP is around 50 mm Hg for 5 days or greater than 35 mm Hg for a more prolonged period of time despite medical therapy. However, in the patient with previous glaucomatous optic nerve damage, the threshold for surgical intervention is lower and depends upon the level at which the IOP is likely to cause further optic nerve damage. In such patients, surgery may be appropriate within hours or days of the initial trauma. As previously discussed, aggressive therapy is required for patients with sickle cell disease, as these patients are predisposed to optic nerve damage and central retinal artery occlusion at minimally elevated IOPs. Surgery is generally indicated in a patient with sickle cell disease if the IOP exceeds 24 mm Hg for more than 24 hours despite medical therapy.

17. List the indications for surgical intervention in the management of a hyphema.
Approximately 5% of all traumatic hyphemas demand surgical management; however, as a rule, patients with true-eight ball hyphemas require prompt surgical intervention (see question 27).
   The Read Criteria for surgical intervention include the following:
- Microscopic corneal blood staining.
- Total hyphema with IOPs of 50 mm Hg or more for 5 days (to prevent optic nerve damage).
- Hyphema that is initially total and does not resolve below 50% at 6 days with IOPs of 25 mm Hg or more (to prevent corneal blood staining).
- Hyphema that remains unresolved for 9 days (to prevent peripheral anterior synechiae).

18. Name the major complications associated with a hyphema.
- Corneal blood staining.
- Recurrent hemorrhage.
- Secondary glaucoma.
- In addition to the preceding complications, patients with sickle cell anemia or sickle cell trait have a predisposition to central retinal artery occlusion and optic nerve damage at only minimally elevated IOP owing to vascular sludging of the sickled cells, which leads to ischemia and vasoocclusion.

19. What is corneal blood staining?
Endothelial cell decompensation results in the passage of erythrocyte-breakdown products (particularly iron from hemoglobin and lipid from cell membranes) into the stroma, creating a yellowish-brown discoloration of the posterior stroma. Corneal blood staining may resolve over months or years, first peripherally and then posteriorly.

20. What percentage of patients with a hyphema develop corneal blood staining?
Corneal blood staining will develop in 5% of hyphema patients.

21. In what settings is corneal blood staining most likely to occur?
- Recurrent hemorrhage
- Compromised endothelial cell function
- Larger hyphemas that are prolonged in duration
- Usually, but not always, in association with an elevated IOP

22. What is the differential diagnosis of the appearance of bright red blood in the anterior chamber within the first 5 days after a patient has suffered a traumatic hyphema?
- Recurrent hemorrhage
- Fibrinolysis and hemolysis of a clotted hyphema
   Recurrent hemorrhage must be differentiated from hemolysis that occurs as a clotted hyphema resorbs, particularly if the patient has been treated with aminocaproic acid. A rise in IOP associated with accelerated hemolysis can mimic a rebleed and may occur 24 to 96 hours after the use of aminocaproic acid has been discontinued.
   A patient who has been treated with aminocaproic acid should continue to have his or her IOP monitored several days after discontinuation of therapy in the event that there is a spike in IOP associated with accelerated hemolysis.

23. In the setting of a traumatic hyphema, when is a patient at greatest risk for developing a recurrent hemorrhage?
The greatest risk is between 2 and 5 days following blunt ocular trauma, perhaps owing to clot fibrinolysis and retraction.

24. How common is a recurrent hemorrhage?
A recurrent hemorrhage generally occurs in 0.4% to 35% of patients who suffer a traumatic hyphema.

25. What is the significance of a recurrent hemorrhage? Why is it important to try to prevent it?
A recurrent hemorrhage carries a poorer prognosis than the initial hyphema. Most rebleeds are larger than the initial hyphema and carry an increased risk of developing a secondary glaucoma and corneal blood staining; visual outcome is worse, and there is a more frequent need for surgical intervention.

26. List the risk factors that may be associated with an increased risk of developing a recurrent hemorrhage.
- Antiplatelet or anticoagulant ingestion
- Black or Hispanic race
- Hypotony
- Younger age
- Larger initial hyphema
- Systemic hypertension

27. What is an eight-ball hyphema?
An eight-ball or black-ball hyphema is a hyphema that has clotted and taken on a black or purple color (Fig. 20.2). The black or purple appearance of an eight-ball hyphema is due to impaired aqueous circulation, which leads to a

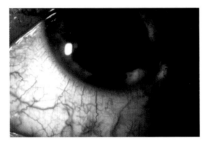

Fig. 20.2 Clotted hyphema.

subsequent decrease in the oxygenation of the intracameral blood and results in the characteristic black- or purple-colored clot. Impaired aqueous circulation occurs as a result of either pupillary block from the clot or a direct tamponade effect of the clot at the level of the trabecular meshwork. The impairment in aqueous circulation prevents the clotted black-ball hyphema from being reabsorbed. These hyphemas may have a higher chance of developing secondary glaucoma and corneal blood staining.

28. **How is an eight-ball hyphema different from a total or 100% hyphema?**
An eight-ball hyphema describes blood in the anterior chamber that has clotted and taken on a black or purple appearance. A total, or 100%, hyphema is one in which the blood filling the anterior chamber appears bright red. A hyphema that consists of bright red blood indicates that there is continuous aqueous circulation within the anterior chamber, which results in a significantly more favorable prognosis than an eight-ball hyphema.

29. **What is the prognosis for an eight-ball hyphema?**
Patients who develop an eight-ball hyphema carry a poor prognosis with respect to developing secondary glaucoma. Most, if not all, patients develop an elevated IOP that is usually severe and frequently difficult to control with medical therapy. Surgical intervention to evacuate the clot and/or decrease the IOP is generally required for most patients with an eight-ball hyphema.

30. **When is the optimal time to remove a clotted or eight-ball hyphema? Why?**
Optimal time for evacuation of a clotted hyphema is 4 to 7 days after the hemorrhage, because this time is when there is maximal consolidation and retraction of a clot from adjacent structures and thus a decreased risk of causing new bleeding. However, extremely high IOPs, with which vascular infarcts are a significant risk, are seen more commonly with eight-ball hyphema.

31. **What types of surgical techniques can be used to evacuate a hyphema?**
Surgical techniques in managing a hyphema include:
- Paracentesis and anterior-chamber washout alone or in association with a guarded filtration procedure (i.e., trabeculectomy).
- Clot expression with limbal delivery.
- Automated clot removal (hyphemectomy) with an automated vitrectomy instrument. (Take care to avoid lens and cornea; vasodilators can help maintain the chamber during removal of the clot. Keep the iris between the vitrectomy instrument and lens to minimize the risk of iatrogenic cataract).
- Peripheral iridectomy with or without a guarded filtration procedure to relieve pupillary block, which may be associated with an eight-ball hyphema.
  Fig. 20.3 provides an algorithm for the workup and management of a patient who presents with a hyphema.
- Trabecular gonioaspiration has been reported as a successful way of managing IOP elevation resulting from blood obstructing the trabecular meshwork in sickle cell patients.

32. **List the types of secondary glaucoma associated with a traumatic hyphema.**
An acute rise in IOP is generally due to obstruction of the trabecular meshwork by erythrocytes or their breakdown products. The IOP at which medical or surgical therapy is initiated should be individualized and depends upon the presence of previous glaucomatous optic nerve damage, corneal endothelial dysfunction, or sickle cell disease.

Late secondary glaucoma may develop weeks to years after a hyphema. Causes of late secondary glaucoma are listed in Table 20.2. In one retrospective case control study reviewing patients with open-globe injuries, 17% of patients developed ocular hypertension defined as IOP > 22 mm Hg at more than one visit or requiring treatment. A predictive risk factor includes the presence of hyphema, which reiterates the importance of monitoring IOP closely after trauma.

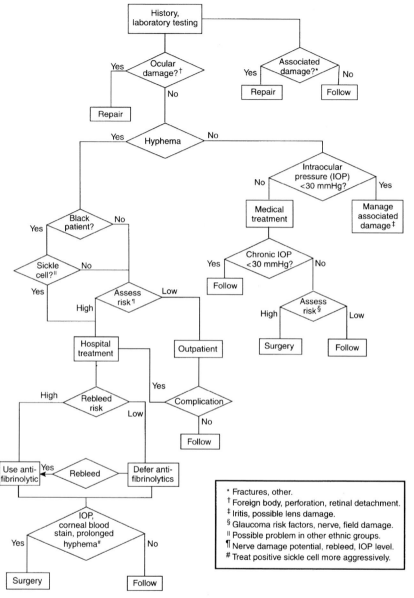

Fig. 20.3 Treatment algorithm for ocular trauma and glaucoma. (From Higginbottom EJ, Lee DA: Clinical guide to glaucoma management, Woburn, MA, 2004, Butterworth-Heinemann.)

33. **Is the chance of developing secondary glaucoma related to the size of the hyphema?**
    Although there are conflicting reports, the chance of developing a secondary glaucoma may be related to the size of the hyphema. Secondary glaucoma occurred in 13.5% of those eyes in which blood filled half of the anterior chamber, in 27% of those eyes in which blood filled greater than half of the anterior chamber, and in 52% of those eyes in which there was a total hyphema. However, the amount of blood may simply be an indirect marker of the degree of trauma.

    Recurrent hemorrhages are often larger than the initial hyphema and carry a greater risk for developing secondary glaucoma. Patients with eight-ball hyphemas develop glaucoma virtually 100% of the time.

Table 20.2 Secondary Glaucomas Associated With Traumatic Hyphema

A. Early
1. Trabecular meshwork obstruction with fresh red blood cells and fibrin, resulting in secondary open-angle glaucoma
2. Pupillary block by the blood clot, resulting in secondary angle-closure glaucoma
3. Hemolytic glaucoma
4. Steroid-induced glaucoma from treatment

B. Late
1. Angle-recession glaucoma
2. Ghost-cell glaucoma
3. Peripheral anterior synechiae formation, resulting in secondary angle-closure glaucoma
4. Posterior synechiae formation with iris bombé, resulting in secondary angle-closure glaucoma
5. Hemosiderotic or hemolytic glaucoma

---

34. **Why and when is it important to perform gonioscopy on patients who have suffered a hyphema?**

The gonioscopic appearance of angle recession may change with time. Immediately following blunt eye trauma, a hyphema may obscure adequate visualization of the angle. Thorough gonioscopic evaluation with indentation is recommended approximately 6 weeks after trauma, at which time the eye has recovered, the hyphema has resolved, and the risk of further injury has been minimized. Clues that may help the ophthalmologist diagnose an old angle recession include the presence of torn iris processes, depression or tears of the trabecular meshwork, and increased whitening of the scleral spur.

Up to 10% of patients with greater than 180 degrees of angle recession will eventually develop a chronic traumatic glaucoma. The term *angle-recession glaucoma* may also be used to describe the chronic traumatic glaucoma that occurs in association with an angle recession.

35. **Given a history of ocular trauma, how can one make the diagnosis of angle recession on gonioscopic examination?**

Angle recession can be diagnosed by careful gonioscopic examination of the injured eye and by comparing it with the fellow, nontraumatized eye. Gonioscopy may reveal an irregular widening of the ciliary body, indicating a tear between the longitudinal and the circular muscles of the ciliary body. A normal, nonrecessed ciliary body band is usually not as wide as the trabecular meshwork and should be roughly even in width throughout its entire circumference. Angle recession is found in 60% to 94% of patients with a traumatic hyphema (Fig. 20.4).

36. **Explain the difference between a cyclodialysis and an angle recession.**

Although not as common as angle recession, cyclodialysis can occur secondary to blunt compressive trauma. An angle recession is a tear within the ciliary body itself, whereas a cyclodialysis is a tear between the ciliary body and the scleral spur. Disinsertion of the uvea from the sclera allows free passage of the anterior chamber aqueous fluid to the suprachoroidal space, thus permitting direct access to the uveoscleral outflow pathway. Temporary or permanent hypotony is usual. A cyclodialysis cleft should be suspected and carefully searched for when the IOP remains low after ocular trauma. Other causes for a low IOP following trauma are retinal detachment and an inflammatory-mediated decrease in ciliary body production, i.e., ciliary body shutdown.

37. **Once a cyclodialysis cleft is suspected, how can it be diagnosed?**

A traumatic cyclodialysis cleft can be diagnosed by careful gonioscopic examination. Although the wall of the cyclodialysis cleft is white (i.e., sclera), it appears shaded, owing to the fact that one is looking down into a hole. This is opposed to the gonioscopic appearance of angle recession, which appears simply as an enlarged ciliary body band secondary to a tear in the ciliary body itself. Treatment for a cyclodialysis cleft includes atropine, laser, and surgical repair. Ultrasound biomicroscopy provides high-resolution (up to 50 μm) images of the anterior chamber angle, which can be particularly helpful if the cleft is small or as part of the preoperative evaluation to map the extent of a large cleft (see Fig. 20.4).

38. **How long after a traumatic hyphema is a patient at risk for developing angle-recession glaucoma?**

Angle-recession glaucoma may develop weeks to many years after blunt ocular trauma. Patients who develop traumatic or subsequent angle-recession glaucoma may have an underlying predisposition to primary open-angle glaucoma (POAG). It is believed that the trauma to a meshwork that is already predisposed to reduced aqueous outflow (POAG) may be just enough to push an already compromised trabecular meshwork over the edge, resulting in an angle-recession glaucoma. Evidence to support this underlying predisposition to reduced aqueous outflow includes an unusually high incidence of POAG in the nontraumatized fellow eye and an increased

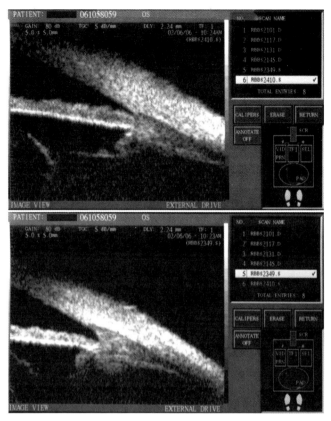

Fig. 20.4 Angle recession ultrasound biomicroscopy. **Top,** Normal angle. **Bottom,** Angle recession.

tendency for the IOP to be increased by topical corticosteroids. Therefore, management of patients with angle recession includes long-term follow-up of both the injured and the uninjured eye.

39. Explain the pathophysiology of angle-recession glaucoma. Is it a direct result of injury to the ciliary body?

No. Angle recession is merely a marker for anterior segment contusion injury, specifically injury to the trabecular meshwork. Angle-recession glaucoma is thought not to be due to the angle recession itself (i.e., a tear in the ciliary body) but rather due to (1) direct trabecular meshwork damage and subsequent inflammation from the blunt trauma or (2) an extension of a Descemet's-like membrane covering the trabecular meshwork. Both mechanisms may ultimately lead to chronic obstruction in the aqueous outflow pathway.

40. Describe the treatment for angle-recession glaucoma.

Eyes with secondary traumatic glaucoma have reduced conventional outflow owing to trabecular meshwork injury and may therefore shift over to primarily uveoscleral outflow. Miotics may actually paradoxically increase the IOP, possibly by decreasing uveoscleral outflow. Laser trabeculoplasty does not have a high rate of success in this setting. Prostaglandin analogs, β-blockers, carbonic anhydrase inhibitors, cycloplegics, and filtration surgery are the most effective treatments for angle-recession glaucoma.

BIBLIOGRAPHY

Berrios RR, Dreyer EB: Traumatic hyphema, Ophthalmol Clin 35:93–103, 1995.
Caprioli J, Sears ML: The histopathology of black-ball hyphema: a report of two cases, Ophthalmic Surg 15:491–495, 1984.
Chi TS, Netland PA: Angle recession of glaucoma, Int Ophthalmol Clin 35:117–126, 1995.
Coles WH: Traumatic hyphema: an analysis of 235 cases, South Med J 61:813, 1968.
Crouch ER, Frenkel M: Aminocaproic acid in the treatment of traumatic hyphema, Am J Ophthalmol 81:355–360, 1976.

Dietse MC, Hersh PS, Kylstra JA, et al.: Intraocular pressure increase associated with epsilon aminocaproic acid therapy or traumatic hyphema, Am J Ophthalmol 106:383–390, 1988.

Goldberg MF: Antifibrinolytic agents in the management of traumatic hyphema, Arch Ophthalmol 101:1029–1030, 1983.

Gottsch JD: Hyphema: diagnosis and management, Retina 10:S65–S71, 1990.

Herschler J: Trabecular damage due to blunt anterior segment injury and its relationship to traumatic glaucoma, Trans Am Ophthalmol Otolaryngol 83:239–248, 1977.

Kanski JJ, Bowling B: Clinical ophthalmology: a systematic approach, ed 9, Edinburgh, 2019, Elsevier Limited.

Kennedy RH, Brubaker RF: Traumatic hyphema in a defined population, Am J Ophthalmol 106:123–130, 1988.

Kutner B, Fourman S, Brein K, et al.: Aminocaproic acid reduces the risk of secondary hemorrhage in patients with traumatic hyphema, Arch Ophthalmol 105:206–208, 1987.

McGetrick JJ, Jampol LM, Goldberg MF, et al.: Aminocaproic acid decreases secondary hemorrhage after traumatic hyphema, Arch Ophthalmol 101:1031–1033, 1983.

Pandey P, Sung VS: Gonioaspiration for refractory glaucoma secondary to traumatic hyphema in patients with sickle cell trait, Ophthalmic Surg Lasers Imaging 41:386–389, 2010.

Parrish R, Bernardino V: Iridectomy in the surgical management of eight-ball hyphema, Arch Ophthalmol 100:435–437, 1982.

Read J, Goldberg MF: Blunt ocular trauma and hyphema, Int Ophthalmol Clin 14:57–97, 1974.

Ritch R, Shields MB, Krupin T: The glaucomas, ed 2, St. Louis, 1996, Mosby.

Sears ML: Surgical management of black-ball hyphema, Trans Am Acad Ophthalmol Otolaryngol 74:820–827, 1970.

Shields MB: Textbook of glaucoma, ed 7, Baltimore, 2020, Williams & Wilkins.

Shingleton BJ, Hersh PS, Kenyon KR: Eye trauma, St. Louis, 1991, Mosby.

Spaeth GL, Levy PM: Traumatic hyphema: its clinical characteristics and failure of estrogens to alter its course. A double-blind study, Am J Ophthalmol 62:1098–1106, 1966.

Tesluk GC, Spaeth GL: The occurrence of primary open-angle glaucoma in the fellow eye of patients with unilateral angle-cleavage glaucoma, Ophthalmology 92:904–912, 1985.

Turalba AV, Shah AS, Andreoli MT, Rhee DJ: Predictors and outcomes of ocular hypertension after open-globe injury, J Glaucoma 23: 5–10, 2014.

Volpe NJ, Larrison WI, Hersh PS, et al.: Secondary hemorrhage in traumatic hyphema, Am J Ophthalmol 112:507–513, 1991.

Wilson FM: Traumatic hyphema pathogenesis and management, Ophthalmology 87:910–919, 1980.

Wilson TW, Jeffers JB, Nelson LB: Aminocaproic acid prophylaxis in traumatic hyphema, Ophthalmic Surg 21:807–809, 1990.

Wolff SM, Zimmerman LE: Chronic secondary glaucoma, Am J Ophthalmol 54:547–562, 1962.

CHAPTER 21

CATARACTS

Richard Tipperman

CATARACTS

1. Explain the derivation of the word *cataract*.
   Cataract comes from the Greek word *cataractos*, which describes rapidly running water. Rapidly running water turns white, as do mature cataracts.

2. What is the leading cause of blindness worldwide?
   Believe it or not, cataracts, which are treatable, remain one of the leading causes of blindness worldwide.

3. What is a nuclear sclerotic cataract?
   A nuclear sclerotic cataract describes the sclerosis or darkening that is seen in the central portion of the lens nucleus. This type of cataract is typically seen in older patients. As the equatorial epithelial cells of the lens continue to divide, they produce compaction of the more central fibers and sclerosis.

4. What produces the brown color seen in cataracts?
   The brown color comes from urochrome pigment.

5. What is "second sight"? How is it associated with nuclear sclerotic cataracts?
   As patients develop nuclear sclerotic cataracts, the increased density of the lens causes the patient to become increasingly myopic. As a result of their nearsightedness, many patients who required spectacles to help them read find that they are able to read small print up close without glasses. In the past, this phenomenon was termed "second sight." Of interest, patients erroneously believe that their eyes are getting stronger or better, whereas the opposite is the case. Second sight indicates progression of the cataract.

6. What are the typical symptoms of nuclear sclerotic cataracts?
   In general, all types of cataracts cause decreased vision. Nuclear sclerotic cataracts tend to cause problems with distance vision but preserve reading vision because of the above-mentioned nearsightedness.

7. What are posterior subcapsular cataracts?
   Posterior subcapsular cataracts are granular opacities seen mainly in the central posterior cortex adjacent to the posterior capsule. They have a hyaline type of appearance.

8. What are the symptoms of posterior subcapsular cataracts?
   Unlike patients with nuclear sclerotic cataracts, patients with posterior subcapsular cataracts often have good distance vision but typically have blurred near vision. In addition, patients with posterior subcapsular cataracts often have extreme difficulty with glare so that in dim illumination they function well, whereas with bright illumination their vision decreases significantly. Patients complain of glare when driving at night.

9. What are the associated systemic findings in patients with cataracts?
   In general, **nuclear sclerotic cataracts** are seen in elderly patients, although they may occur in young patients as well. In younger patients, they are often associated with high myopia.
   Posterior subcapsular cataracts are common in patients with diabetes, patients who have taken steroids, and patients with a history of intraocular inflammation, such as uveitis.

10. What are the major potential causes of cataracts in infants?
    Common causes of congenital cataracts include familial inheritance, intrauterine infection (e.g., rubella), metabolic diseases (e.g., galactosemia), and chromosomal abnormalities. Complete evaluation by a pediatrician is mandatory for any infant with a congenital cataract.

11. What is a morgagnian cataract?
    A morgagnian cataract is a mature cataract in which the cortex liquefies and the mature central nucleus can be seen within the liquefied cortex.

12. What is phacolytic glaucoma?
    Phacolytic glaucoma may occur with morgagnian and mature cataracts. Liquefied cortex traverses the capsular membrane and enters the anterior chamber, producing an inflammatory response that clogs the trabecular meshwork and results in elevated intraocular pressure.

13. What is phacomorphic glaucoma?

   As the cataract matures, the lens becomes enlarged (intumescent). As the lens enlarges, it pushes the iris root and ciliary body forward, narrowing the angle between the iris and the peripheral cornea in the region of the trabecular meshwork. If the angle becomes narrow enough, the pressure may become elevated because of angle closure. Treatment involves removal of the cataract.

14. Can cataract surgery ever be an "emergency"?

   Both phacolytic glaucoma and phacomorphic glaucoma can be indications for "emergency" cataract surgery if the intraocular pressure is markedly elevated.

15. What is pseudoexfoliation? What is its relationship to cataracts?

   Pseudoexfoliation is a condition in which basement membrane material from the zonules and lens capsule is liberated onto the anterior lens capsule and anterior chamber. Patients with pseudoexfoliation have a predisposition for the development of glaucoma, presumably because of clogging of the trabecular meshwork by the exfoliated material. Patients with pseudoexfoliation often present a challenge for the cataract surgeon because their pupils tend to dilate poorly, and they often have weak or loose zonules that cause intraoperative complications with disinsertion of the zonules. Because of their propensity for developing glaucoma, patients often have postoperative pressure elevations.

16. A patient underwent successful and uncomplicated cataract surgery, and years after the surgery, the intraocular lens completely dislocated. What associated ophthalmic condition would the patient be likely to have?

   The patient would be likely to have pseudoexfoliation.

17. What is true exfoliation syndrome as opposed to pseudoexfoliation syndrome?

   True exfoliation is found in glassblowers who stand in front of hot furnaces throughout the day. Large sheets of material come off the anterior lens capsule. Such cataracts are termed **glassblower's cataracts**. With modern techniques of processing glass, they are no longer seen. Because the type of material produced in pseudoexfoliation seemed similar to the material produced in a glassblower's cataract, it was termed pseudoexfoliation to distinguish it from the exfoliative material produced by heat exposure.

18. What systemic syndromes should be considered in a patient with a spontaneously dislocated natural lens?

   In these patients, the zonular support system has been disrupted. Spontaneous dislocation of the lens is most common in Marfan's syndrome and homocystinuria. Typical patients with Marfan's syndrome are tall, thin, and lanky and exhibit arachnodactyly. The lenses in Marfan's syndrome tend to dislocate superiorly. In homocystinuria, the lenses tend to dislocate inferiorly. Trauma also should be considered in all patients with a dislocated lens. Rarely, pseudoexfoliation can be a cause.

KEY POINTS: DISLOCATED AND SUBLUXATED LENSES

1. Patients with a natural lens that is dislocated should be evaluated for trauma.
2. Marfan's syndrome most often causes lenses to dislocate superiorly. Patients need evaluation for possible cardiac and aortic abnormalities and retinal detachments.
3. Homocystinuria most often causes lenses to dislocate inferiorly. Patients have a high risk of thromboembolic events.

19. What other clinical findings are common in patients with a traumatic cataract?

   Blunt trauma may produce a cataract. Patients often have associated iris sphincter tears and may even have iridodialysis or angle recession. If the trauma has been severe, some or all of the zonules may be broken, causing the lens to be mobile within the eye. This phenomenon is called **phacodonesis**. Retinal detachment and optic neuropathy also may be present and cause decreased vision.

20. What are the indications for cataract surgery?

   The basic indication for cataract surgery is reduced visual function that interferes with activities of daily living. This indication obviously varies, depending on the patient's age and degree of activity. For instance, a 40-year-old accountant with an early posterior subcapsular cataract may be much more symptomatic than an 85-year-old who no longer reads or drives. Cases in which cataract surgery is medically necessary (e.g., phacomorphic and phacolytic glaucoma) are extremely uncommon. Patients with cataracts should be informed that cataract surgery is almost always an elective procedure and that leaving the cataract alone will not hurt or damage the eye. However, it is important to be aware of state standards of Snellen visual acuity and visual field for driving vision and to inform patients accordingly. They can be found in the Physicians' Desk Reference for ophthalmic medicines. In addition to noting Snellen acuity, it is important to formally document the patient's subjective visual difficulties such as "trouble driving at night" or "difficulty reading."

21. Does a cataract need to be "ripe"?

Many years ago, when cataract surgery was performed by removing the entire lens and leaving the patient aphakic, the cataract needed to be dense enough to remove in a single entire piece and to be causing sufficiently poor vision that the patient would benefit from cataract surgery.

Currently, "ripeness" of the cataract is no longer a consideration. The indications for cataract surgery in general are functional visual difficulties secondary to the cataract, interfering with the patient's day-to-day activities or overall quality of life. Typically, if the patient has a Snellen visual acuity (or glare disability) that reduces their vision to 20/50 or worse, they may be considered a candidate for cataract surgery.

22. What is aphakia? What are aphakic spectacles? What is pseudophakia?

Aphakia is the condition in which the patient's natural lens (*phakos*) has been removed surgically, leaving the patient without a lens. This is the result of intracapsular surgery. **Aphakic spectacles** are the heavy "Coke-bottle" glasses patients had to wear to achieve the needed focusing power of the eye with the natural lens missing. **Pseudophakia** or "artificial lens" is the term used to describe an eye with an intraocular lens (IOL).

23. How is the intraocular lens power determined? What is the most commonly used intraocular lens power?

The appropriate IOL power for a patient is determined by measuring the curvature of the patient's cornea (keratometry values) as well as the length of the eye (axial length measurement). These two measurements are then utilized by multivariable "IOL power equations" to help determine the most appropriate lens for the individual patient.

The most commonly used IOL power is 18 D.

24. What are multifocal intraocular lenses? How do multifocal intraocular lenses work?

With standard cataract surgery and conventional IOLs, there is only one fixed focal distance. Therefore, if a patient achieves good uncorrected distance vision after cataract surgery, he or she will not be able to see at near without correction because the artificial lens cannot accommodate to adjust its focal length the way a natural phakic lens can.

Multifocal IOLs now allow patients the ability to see both in the distance and up close by employing a number of optical strategies to achieve an increased optical range. Accommodating IOLs are designed to move or change shape much like the natural crystalline lens, although "real-world" technical difficulties make achieving this problematic. Extended depth of focus IOLs increase range of vision by elongating the focal range while diffractive IOLs increase the number of focal points by dividing light.

25. What is IFIS? What is a Flomax pupil?

IFIS is an acronym for intraoperative floppy iris syndrome. This condition occurs in patients who are taking tamsulosin (Flomax) for benign prostatic hypertrophy. Tamsulosin is a systemic sympathetic α1-A receptor blocker, which improves lower urinary tract flow by relaxing the neck of the bladder and prostatic smooth muscle.

Patients taking tamsulosin who undergo cataract surgery manifest pupillary abnormalities that include a flaccid iris, which undulates and billows in response to intraocular fluid currents. There is also a tendency for the iris to prolapse through both the phaco incision and the paracentesis. Last, there is typically a progressive intraoperative pupillary constriction despite apparent adequate pharmacologic dilation at the initiation of surgery. These iris abnormalities are believed to occur because the smooth muscle in the iris also has α1-adrenoreceptors that are affected by tamsulosin.

Because cataract surgery is more difficult in patients with poorly dilating pupils and the abnormalities noted above, cataract surgery in patients taking tamsulosin can be more difficult as well. Interestingly, even if the patient discontinues his tamsulosin for up to 4 weeks prior to cataract surgery, the pupil abnormalities persist. Surgical strategies for dealing with this situation include utilizing a highly cohesive viscoelastic agent and iris retractors. www.ascrs.org.

26. What is the difference between an anterior chamber lens and a posterior chamber lens? What is "the capsular bag"?

A posterior chamber lens is typically utilized in routine cataract surgery. During surgery, a circular opening termed a *capsulorrhexis* is made in the capsule that surrounds the cataractous lens. The cataract is removed and then the new lens is placed into the capsular bag, which is the membrane that is left behind once the cataract is removed. This region of the eye is termed the *posterior chamber*; hence, the IOL that resides there is termed a *posterior chamber lens*.

At times, it is not possible to place a posterior chamber lens because of either inherent weakness in the capsular bag or an intraoperative complication that disrupts its integrity. In these cases, one of the options is to place a lens in the front (or anterior) portion of the eye, hence the term *anterior chamber lens*. Anterior chamber lenses fixate in the eye by resting on the scleral spur. If not positioned correctly, these IOLs have the potential to chafe the sensitive uveal tissue in the iris and create complications.

27. What is posterior capsular opacification? What is a secondary membrane? Can a cataract grow back?

The new IOL replaces the cataractous lens by resting inside the capsular bag. Slowly, over time, residual epithelial cells in the capsular bag can grow across the posterior portion of the capsule and cause it to become hazy or cloudy. Over time, the capsule can become so cloudy it may seem as if the cataract has "come back." The cataract can never come back, but the secondary membrane can become cloudy, causing the vision to deteriorate as if the cataract were recurring.

28. What is a YAG capsulotomy?

When the reduced vision from the posterior capsular opacity becomes clinically significant, the patient may undergo an Nd:YAG capsulotomy. The initials are an acronym for neodymium, yttrium, aluminum, and garnet, which are the materials utilized to allow the laser to function properly and open the membrane.

29. What is the origin of the term laser?

Laser is actually an acronym for **l**ight **a**mplification by **s**timulated **e**mission of **r**adiation.

30. What is the difference between an "intracap" and an "extracap"?

An **intracap** describes intracapsular cataract extraction. This is the "old" type of cataract surgery back in the days when patients had a very large incision made at the corneoscleral limbus and the entire lens surrounded by the lens capsule was removed (usually with the aid of a freezing probe termed a *cryoprobe* as well as α-chymotrypsin to dissolve the zonules). In these cases, no lens was replaced and the patient was left aphakic.

In an **extracap** or extracapsular surgery, the capsule surrounding the lens is opened and the cataractous lens removed. The capsule, however, remains in the eye to support and hold the new posterior chamber IOL.

31. What is couching?

Couching describes an ancient technique for cataract surgery in which a needle was inserted into the eye and used to push the opaque cataract back into the vitreous cavity. Although the complication rate of this was extremely high and the visual result limited, in antiquity, it would allow patients with mature light perception cataracts to be able to regain a limited degree of vision.

BIBLIOGRAPHY

Datilles M: Clinical evaluation of cataracts. In Tasman W, Jaeger E, editors: Duane's clinical ophthalmology, vol. 1, Philadelphia, 2011, Lippincott-Raven, pp 1–15.

Datilles M, Kinoshita J: Pathogenesis of cataracts. In Tasman W, Jaeger E, editors: Duane's clinical ophthalmology, vol. 1, Philadelphia, 1996, Lippincott-Raven, pp 1–9.

Datilles M, Magno B: Cataract: clinical types. In Tasman W, Jaeger E, editors: Duane's clinical ophthalmology, vol. 1, Philadelphia, 1996, Lippincott-Raven, pp 1–25.

CHAPTER 22

TECHNIQUES OF CATARACT SURGERY

Sydney Tyson

1. **What are the indications for cataract surgery?**
   In general, the decision to have cataract surgery is elective. It is based on a patient's personal needs and the physician's judgment as to the probability of vision improvement. For some people, even a slight loss of vision is unacceptable. Others may choose to delay surgery because their cataracts do not seriously interfere with their lives. The key question is whether the patient perceives the cataract as interfering with his or her quality of life. Of course, the physician must be aware of state visual acuity requirements for driving.

2. **What are two nonsurgical methods of managing a cataract?**
   - **Refraction:** Patients with a cataract may experience a myopic (nearsighted) shift or so-called second sight. Occasionally, glasses can compensate for such shifts. However, if the shift is large and unilateral, binocular vision may be compromised by image size differences between the two eyes. This anisometropia may push patients to have surgery.
   - **Pupillary dilation:** An expanded pupil allows light rays to enter around a central cataract (such as a posterior subcapsular cataract) rather than be blocked by light rays that attempt to pass through a hazy cataract. This is not used clinically because chronic dilation causes patients issues with light sensitivity and glare.

3. **What preoperative tests are used to gauge visual impairment?**
   No single test adequately describes the effect of cataracts on a patient's visual functioning, but the most widely used tests are:
   - Snellen visual acuity (i.e., 20/20).
   - Potential acuity testing. This test estimates postoperative visual acuity by projecting a Snellen acuity chart through the patient's cataract. Most often, it is used to determine whether a patient's visual symptoms are due more to cataract or to retinal disease.
   - Glare/contrast sensitivity testing. This test simulates lighting conditions outdoors and determines a patient's vision when functioning under more normal conditions. The high-contrast situation in a Snellen test can overestimate a patient's abilities. A patient may have 20/40 acuity in a dark room but may have 20/100 with glare testing, which could significantly impair driving.

KEY POINTS: TESTS OF VISUAL IMPAIRMENT

1. Snellen visual acuity
2. Potential acuity testing
3. Glare testing
4. Contrast sensitivity testing

4. **What are the basic steps in removing a cataract?**
   1. The pupil is dilated with medications.
   2. The eye and eyelids are disinfected with an antiseptic, usually iodine based.
   3. The eye and eyelids are anesthetized, and a speculum is placed to keep the eyelids open.
   4. An incision is made into the anterior chamber (AC).
   5. A viscoelastic (viscous, protective gel) is injected into the AC.
   6. The anterior capsule is opened with a capsulotomy or capsulorrhexis to gain access to the lens mass.
   7. The nucleus is removed manually or by phacoemulsification.
   8. The residual cortex is removed.
   9. An intraocular lens (IOL) is inserted.
   10. The wound is closed.

5. **How is the eye anesthetized for surgery?**
   Most surgeons prefer local rather than general anesthesia for adult cataract surgery. Less commonly, facial akinesia with a short-acting agent such as lidocaine or hyaluronidase (a diffusion enhancer) may be given to prevent squeezing of the eyelids during surgery. There are three types of local anesthesia:
   - **Retrobulbar:** Anesthetic (usually a combination of a short- and a long-acting agent with hyaluronidase) is injected inside the muscle cone to achieve akinesia and anesthesia of the globe (Fig. 22.1).

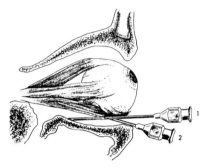

Fig. 22.1 Retrobulbar injection. If the tip of the needle strikes the floor of the orbit as it is inserted *(1)*, it is withdrawn slightly and directed more superiorly *(2)*. (From Jaffe NS, Jaffe MS, Jaffe GF: Cataract surgery and its complications, St. Louis, 1990, Mosby.)

- **Peribulbar:** Anesthetic is injected outside the muscle cone. Although this block takes longer to take effect (12 to 25 minutes), there are fewer potential complications because a shorter needle is used.
- **Topical:** Advances in technology have allowed skilled surgeons to perform the cataract procedure in 10 to 15 minutes. With such short operative times, prolonged anesthesia and akinesia become less critical. Topical drops or gels of short-acting agents such as lidocaine or tetracaine may be used to anesthetize the eye sufficiently to complete the procedure. The advantage to the patient is instantaneous binocular vision postoperatively without the risk of injection-related, potentially sight-threatening complications.
- **Intracameral:** As an adjunct to or substitute for topical anesthetics, intraocular administration of preservative-free lidocaine with or without dilating agents is being adopted by many surgeons.

6. What are the disadvantages of topical anesthesia for cataract surgery?
   - Because there is no akinesia, the eye can move during surgery.
   - Patient selection is crucial. Patients need to be able to follow the commands of the surgeon.

7. What is couching?
   Couching is one of the most ancient surgical procedures and it is the first known technique of cataract removal. Although the technique was first described by the Indian physician Susruta ca. 800 BC, copper surgical instruments that could have been used for couching have been found in the tomb of the Egyptian king Khasekhemwy ca. 2700 BC.[11] Popular in the United States until the 1850s, couching involves piercing the eye with a needle, then dislocating the entire lens backward and downward into the posterior chamber. Although it may seem crude by modern surgical standards and prone to myriad complications, it is still performed in the Third World, where advanced technology is not available, most commonly by traditional "healers."

8. What are the two most common ways to remove a cataract?
   - **Intracapsular surgery** was the procedure of choice from its discovery by Jacques Daviel in 1752 until the early 1970s. It is accomplished with a cryoprobe, an instrument that freezes the tissue. Intracapsular surgery is rarely performed in the United States today except in cases of dislocated lenses.
   - **Extracapsular cataract extraction (ECCE)** is the most popular technique. There are two types—manual extraction and phacoemulsification. Both methods require the use of an operating microscope that permits magnification. In extracapsular surgery, the anterior capsule of the lens is removed, the hard nucleus is expressed, and the remaining soft cortical fragments are removed with either an automated or a manual device (Fig. 22.2). The advantage of extracapsular surgery is preservation of the posterior capsule, which permits a pocket for an IOL. This method also minimizes the complications associated with vitreous loss.

9. What is phacoemulsification?
   Invented by the late Dr. Charles Kelman in 1967, phacoemulsification is a sophisticated form of extracapsular surgery that permits mechanical removal of a cataract through a 3.0-mm or smaller incision (Fig. 22.3). This reduction in incision size results in faster visual recovery and fewer complications, making phacoemulsification one of the most significant advances in cataract surgery. Conventional extracapsular surgery requires a wound size of 150 degrees (approximately 10 mm).

10. How does the phacoemulsification machine work?
    Although the machine is complex, its functions are simple: irrigation, aspiration, and ultrasonic vibration via a handpiece. The phacoemulsification handpiece consists of a hollow 1-mm titanium needle that fragments a cataract by vibrating at 40,000 times per second. The fragmented pieces are then aspirated through the tip of the needle into a drainage bag. An irrigation solution flows from a bottle suspended above the machine and into the eye through the needle. This fluid serves to cool the needle and to maintain proper AC depth.

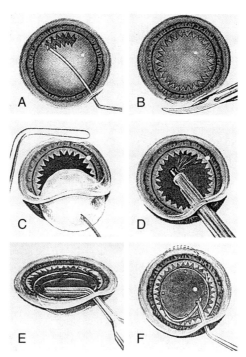

Fig. 22.2 Extracapsular extraction. **A,** Multiple small cuts are made in the anterior capsule. **B,** A full-thickness incision is completed with scissors. **C,** The nucleus is removed. **D,** The cortex is aspirated. **E,** The inferior haptic is inserted through the incision and passed under the iris. **F,** The tip of the superior haptic is grasped with a forceps and advanced into the anterior chamber; as the superior pole is clearing the edge of the pupil, the arm is pronated to ensure that when the haptic is released, it will spring open under the iris and not out of the incision. (From Kanski JJ: *Clinical ophthalmology: a systematic approach,* ed 2, Boston, 1989, Butterworth-Heinemann.)

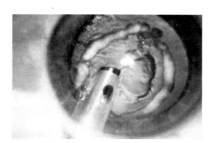

Fig. 22.3 Removal of nuclear material by phacoemulsification. (From Koch PS, Davidson JA: *Textbook of advanced phacoemulsification techniques,* Thorofare, NJ, 1991, Slack.)

11. What are the advantages and disadvantages of phacoemulsification?
    - **Advantages** are a small incision, fewer wound problems, less astigmatism, more rapid physical rehabilitation, and less risk of expulsive hemorrhage.
    - **Disadvantages** are machine dependency, a longer learning curve with complications while transitioning, and expensive equipment. Phacoemulsification is more difficult in patients with dense nuclei and/or poor pupillary dilation.

12. How is a capsulotomy performed?
    There are two types of capsulotomies: a can-opener capsulotomy and a continuous-curve capsulorrhexis (CCC). The can-opener capsulotomy is a series of jagged punctures performed with a bent needle. Although it is simple to perform, it is prone to peripheral extension of its jagged edges. The CCC is made by tearing the capsule so that the edges remain sharp, well demarcated, and strong. Forces are distributed more evenly and prevent an anterior

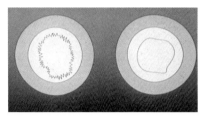

Fig. 22.4 Left, Can-opener capsulotomy. **Right,** Continuous-curve capsulorrhexis. (From Koch PS, Davidson JA: *Textbook of advanced phacoemulsification techniques,* Thorofare, NJ, 1991, Slack.)

capsule extension from becoming a posterior capsular tear. This approach permits safe utilization of phaco techniques that use shearing or rotational forces. Implants are held more securely and center better (Fig. 22.4).

13. Where is the nucleus phacoemulsified in the eye?

The nucleus can be disassembled in the AC or in the capsular bag. AC removal is less popular because of the higher risk of corneal endothelial damage. However, in cases with capsular rupture, this method of removal can prevent nuclear pieces from moving posteriorly into the vitreous.

14. Are there different ways to phacoemulsify the nucleus?

The nucleus can be disassembled as a whole (sculpting) or by first being split (nucleofractis) into pieces. Harder nuclei are more readily and safely removed with a splitting technique within the capsular bag. However, a capsulorrhexis is mandatory because the forces exerted during splitting may cause peripheral extension of a can-opener capsulotomy with possible posterior capsular rupture.

The type of capsulotomy and anticipated method of cataract extraction are closely interrelated. The planned location and technique of nucleus emulsification are affected by such variables as nucleus consistency (hard or soft lens), pupil size, zonular (lens ligament) integrity, and the presence of intraoperative complications.

15. Are lasers used to remove cataracts?

Patients love lasers, and this is a question they frequently ask. Femtosecond lasers can now assist or replace several aspects of manual cataract surgery. These include the creation of the initial incisions in the cornea, the creation of the capsulotomy, the reduction of preexisting astigmatism, and the initial disassembly of the lens. Phacoemulsification is still required to remove the partially disassembled, presoftened lens. The technology is purported to be safer and to deliver improved outcomes by many; however, further data will be required to prove these assertions. So far, data do not support this. The increased cost is a significant factor as well.

16. Once a cataract is removed (aphakia), what are the options to restore vision?

- **Thick aphakic glasses** are rarely used today because they create visually annoying magnification (approximately 25%) and distortion.
- **Contact lenses** are a better alternative to visual restoration (magnify only 7%), but many elderly patients do not possess the manual dexterity necessary to handle them. Long-term extended-wear lenses can help in this regard.
- **IOLs** are the best and most common alternative to restoration of normal vision after cataract surgery because they almost duplicate the aphakic eye. Magnification is minimal, and peripheral vision is normal. They are implanted in small children who need cataract surgery.

17. Who invented intraocular lenses?

In 1949, Sir Harold Ridley was the first person to insert an implant into the posterior chamber. Most authorities agree that this was one of the most significant advances in cataract surgery.

18. What are implants made of?

During World War I, it was noted that British Spitfire fighter pilots who had Plexiglas (polymethylmethacrylate [PMMA]) embedded in their eyes from shattered canopies tolerated the material well. PMMA lenses became the gold standard. Advances in technology led to the creation of soft or foldable materials made from silicone and acrylic materials. These materials have come into favor mainly because they can be inserted through much smaller incisions.

19. Describe the most common design and shape of IOLs.

Implants are composed of an optical portion called the "optic" and a nonoptical portion called the "haptic," which is used for fixating the IOL.

Most optic designs are unifocal (distance only). Multifocal and accommodating designs, which reduce or eliminate the need for computer and/or reading glasses, are now available. The multifocal lenses do have drawbacks, with some patients experiencing significant glare and haloes postoperatively. Toric IOLs, which can correct preexisting astigmatism, are also available. Optics can be round or oval, with or without positioning holes, and range in size from 5 to 7 mm. Lens haptics can be looped or plate style (mostly seen in foldable implants) and made of the same material as their optics or a different one. AC lenses are designed with special haptics that allow proper fixation in the delicate AC angle.

20. **What are the most common positions of IOLs?**
The most common positions are capsular bag, ciliary sulcus, and AC. Capsular bag fixation is preferred because it affords excellent lens stability far away from the corneal endothelium. In more complex cases with no means of capsular support, iris or scleral fixation of the IOL are reasonable options.

21. **Is an implant indicated in every aphakic patient?**
No. Implants are generally not used in babies or initially in eyes with severe anterior segment disease or inflammation. However, implants to treat older children who are aphakic are becoming more common.

22. **How is the power of an intraocular lens determined?**
The most common method of determining IOL power (P) uses a regression formula called SRK. The formula is $P = A - 2.5L - 0.9K$. The components of this formula include the axial length (length of the eye) measurement (L), which is determined by A-scan ultrasonography or more accurately by partial coherence interferometry; the average corneal curvature (K), which is determined by keratometry; and an A constant (A), which is specific for each lens type. The closer the implant is to the retina, the greater the A constant. Therefore, the A constant is larger for posterior chamber implants than for AC implants. Newer IOL calculation formulas have been gaining popularity. These third- and fourth-generation formulas, such as the SRK/T, Haigis, Olsen, and Holladay II formulas, have offered surgeons the ability to predict IOL powers with uncanny accuracy. Some formulas such as the Hill-RBF are dynamic and rely on radial basis function mathematics and continuously updated databases validated by artificial intelligence to achieve remarkable accuracy. These next-generation formulas are especially important in determining IOL power in extremely short or long eyes and in eyes that have had previous refractive surgery.

Intraoperative wavefront aberrometry with the ORA (Alcon, Inc.) device has added yet another dimension of precision and accuracy to these power determinations.

23. **How is the surgical wound closed?**
The need for wound closure is directly related to wound size and construction. Larger ECCE incisions can be reapproximated with 10-0 nylon sutures, in a radial, running, or combination technique. The major consideration with these closure techniques is postoperative astigmatism. The tighter sutures are tied, the greater the astigmatism and the more distorted the early postoperative vision. Phaco incisions are smaller and valvelike in construction. This makes them essentially self-sealing and astigmatism free, although some surgeons sleep better at night if at least one suture is placed. The Food and Drug Administration (FDA) recently approved the first synthetic gel sealant, ReSure (Ocular Therapeutix, Inc.), for surgical wound closure, obviating the need for sutures.

24. **How should patients be managed postoperatively?**
The postoperative patient is seen within the first 48 hours of surgery—preferably within 24 hours. Intraocular pressure, wound integrity, AC inflammation, and IOL positioning are assessed.

Typical postoperative medications include antibiotic solutions for infection control and steroids and/or nonsteroidal anti-inflammatory drugs for controlling the inflammation. A growing trend among some surgeons has been the elimination of postoperative drops altogether by infusing various combinations of steroids and/or antibiotics inside the eye at the end of the surgery. In this way, compliance, drop cost, and confusion issues for patients are eliminated. This is still under evaluation. Patients are then seen at 1 week, 1 month, and 3 to 6 months. In advanced small-incision surgeries, refractions are usually stable by 1 month. Eyeglasses may be given at this visit, if necessary.

25. **What are the most significant trends in cataract surgery?**
- Topical and intracameral versus needle anesthesia for cataract surgery.
- Diminished surgical incision size: microincisional cataract surgery allows an incision size reduction of 50% or more.
- Conversion to femtosecond from manual cataract surgery; again this is still under evaluation.
- Presbyopia- and astigmatism-correcting versus monofocal implants.
- Changing drug delivery methods with intracameral cocktails, pellets or implants. Recent FDA approval was granted for sustained-release dexamethasone intracanalicular plugs (Dextenza, Ocular Therapeutix, Inc.) and injections (DEXYCU, EyePoint Pharmaceuticals, Inc.) to treat pain and/or inflammation after cataract surgery.
- Sutureless wound closure with gel sealants.

26. **What does the future hold for cataract surgery?**
Improvements and advances in the way that cataracts are removed will continue. Important hardware and software advances in ultrasound technology will include new phaco needles, improved fluidics, and improved instrumentation, which will allow safer, more efficient removal of cataracts.

The role of the femtosecond laser in cataract surgery will continue to grow along with breakthroughs in IOL design and function. Different IOL materials, such as collamer and hydrogel, promise improved biocompatibility and reduced postoperative inflammatory response. These lenses are ideal for patients with iritis, glaucoma, or diabetes.

IOL designs are also available to correct for the eye's optical aberrations. The Tecnis Z9000 (Johnson & Johnson Vision, Inc.) is the first FDA-approved IOL designed to reduce these aberrations and improve the quality of vision by enhancing contrast sensitivity. IOL design will more closely mimic the natural lens. The Crystalens (Bausch & Lomb, Inc.) is the only FDA-approved accommodating IOL. This IOL theoretically restores accommodation by closely approximating the function of original lenses, thereby reducing or eliminating the need for reading glasses postoperatively. However, their clinical results are variable.

Other presbyopia-correcting lenses offer reduced dependence on glasses by utilizing extended depth of focus (Tecnis Symfony IOL, Johnson and Johnson Vision, Inc.) or bifocal and trifocal diffractive optic designs. The AcrySof IQ PanOptix IOL (Alcon, Inc.) is the first to offer the trifocal design in the United States. Finally, the light-adjustable IOL (RxSight, Alcon, Inc.) is a recently FDA-approved IOL design made of a light-absorbing polymer that allows precise and noninvasive postoperative modification of the lens power by applying ultraviolet (UV) light to the IOL.

One of the most interesting new refractive targeting options under development is the Perfect Lens (Perfect Lens, LLC). A femtosecond laser system is under development to modify the refractive power of any IOL that has already been implanted inside the eye. These novel approaches allow customization of vision after cataract surgery, including alterating spherical aberrations, asphericity, toricity, and multifocality in an in-office procedure.

IOL technology is evolving rapidly and there are now a multitude of choices we can offer our patients. The era of high-quality, spectacle-free postoperative vision is on the horizon.

BIBLIOGRAPHY

American Academy of Ophthalmology: Cataract in the otherwise healthy adult eye (preferred practice patterns), San Francisco, 2016, American Academy of Ophthalmology.

Ascaso FJ, Huerva V: The history of cataract surgery. In Zaidi F, editor: Cataract surgery, 2013. https://www.intechopen.com/chapters/42710. Accessed October 13, 2021. ISBN: 978-953-51-0975-4, InTech.

Boyd B: The art and science of cataract surgery, Highl Ophthalmol 2001.

Buratto L: Phacoemulsification: principles and techniques, Thorofare, NJ, 1997, Slack.

Gills J: Cataract surgery: the state of the art, Thorofare, NJ, 1997, Slack.

Jaffe N, Horowitz J: Lens and cataract. In Podos S, Yanoff M, editors: Textbook of ophthalmology, vol. 3, New York, 1992, Gower Medical Publishing.

Johnson S: Phacoemulsification. In: Focal points (clinical modules for ophthalmologists), vol. XII, San Francisco, 1994, American Academy of Ophthalmology.

Kratz R, Shammas H: Color atlas of ophthalmology: cataracts, Philadelphia, 1991, Lippincott Williams and Wilkins.

Maloney W, Grindle L: Textbook of phacoemulsification, Fallbrook, CA, 1988, Lasenda Publishers.

Stein H, Slatt B, Stein R: The ophthalmic assistant, ed 6, St. Louis, 1994, Mosby.

Steinert R: Cataract surgery: technique, complications, and management, Philadelphia, 2004, W.B. Saunders.

COMPLICATIONS OF CATARACT SURGERY

John D. Dugan Jr. and Robert S. Bailey Jr.

CHAPTER 23

1. **What complications may result from retrobulbar anesthesia for cataract surgery?**
   - **Retrobulbar hemorrhage** is the most common complication from retrobulbar injection. Blood collects in the retrobulbar space, often causing proptosis of the involved eye and a tense orbit. If not treated emergently, it may lead to severe, irreversible optic nerve ischemia.
   - **Ocular perforation** may occur if the needle perforates the globe. The risk of this complication is greatest in highly myopic eyes with long axial lengths.
   - **Optic nerve sheath hemorrhage** may occur if the needle penetrates the optic nerve. It may result in a secondary central retinal vein and/or central retinal artery occlusion.

   Most cataract surgeries are now performed using topical anesthesia. This has greatly reduced the frequency of the complications described earlier.

2. **How do you treat a retrobulbar hemorrhage?**
   Blood collecting in the retrobulbar space may cause a secondary increase in intraocular pressure from the pressure of the blood on the globe. It may also put pressure on the optic nerve, leading to optic nerve ischemia. When a retrobulbar hemorrhage occurs, apply intermittent pressure to the globe to tamponade the bleeding. Measure the intraocular pressure, check visual acuity, and assess optic nerve integrity. If a significant abnormality is identified, a lateral canthotomy should be performed. This technique is often successful in relieving the pressure on the globe and optic nerve. Surgery is usually canceled when a retrobulbar hemorrhage occurs.

KEY POINTS: MOST COMMON INTRAOPERATIVE COMPLICATIONS OF CATARACT SURGERY

1. Posterior capsule rupture
2. Dislocated lens fragment
3. Iris trauma
4. Thermal corneal injury
5. Descemet tear/detachment
6. Poor intraocular lens placement
7. Choroidal/expulsive hemorrhage

---

3. **What are the common complications related to the cataract wound?**
   - **Wound leak or dehiscence:** Occurs when apposition of the cataract wound is inadequate. Aqueous humor can be seen leaking from the involved area of the wound. If additional corneal hydration does not seal the wound, place one or more sutures until the wound no longer leaks.
   - **Wound burn:** Transfer of heat from the vibrating needle of the phacoemulsification instrument can induce an incision burn adversely affecting wound apposition. This is recognized as whitening and shrinkage of the corneal stroma. Stop phacoemulsification immediately to prevent further damage.
   - **Hypotony:** If a wound leak is present, the intraocular pressure is usually low.
   - **Flat anterior chamber:** If the wound leak is large enough, the anterior chamber shallows and may flatten with the iris contacting the cornea.

   Most wound leaks require repair in the operating room with additional sutures to achieve a watertight closure.

4. **What is iris prolapse? How is it treated?**
   Iris prolapse is when the iris presents outside the eye. Iris prolapse can occur both intraoperatively and postoperatively.

   Intraoperative iris prolapse is most commonly due to intraoperative floppy iris syndrome (IFIS) due to the urological drug Tamulosin or similar class medications. The use of an intraoperative iris ring is helpful in minimizing the likelihood of prolapse.

Iris prolapse is also more common with larger width incisions, especially with short transcorneal incisions that enter the eye too posteriorly. Iris prolapse at the conclusion of surgery is commonly related to over pressurizing the eye, especially with a poorly constructed incision. It is helpful to depressurize the eye prior to replacing the iris. Ensure a well-sealed incision with additional corneal hydration or suture placement. Intracameral miotics are also helpful in limiting iris prolapse.

Postoperative iris prolapse is always the result of a wound leak, either chronic from surgery or related to postoperative manipulation of the eye. When a wound leak is present, the iris can become incarcerated in the wound and may prolapse, leading to increased inflammation and an increased risk of infection. Prolapse requires repair in an operating room. If the iris is viable, it can be reposited in the eye; if not, it should be excised. Additional sutures are necessary in the area of the wound dehiscence.

5. What types of intraocular hemorrhage may occur during or after cataract surgery?
   - **Hyphema or blood in the anterior chamber** is seen as a layering or meniscus of blood in the anterior chamber. Blood vessels at the base of the cataract wound or possibly from the iris are usually the source of the blood. Most often, the blood clears spontaneously, and no treatment is required. The intraocular pressure needs to be monitored closely because secondary elevation may occur.
   - **Expulsive choroidal hemorrhage** is the most feared complication of cataract surgery and is caused by rupture of choroidal vessels, most often during surgery. The rupture causes a rapid rise in intraocular pressure with loss of the anterior chamber, iris prolapse, and possible prolapse of the entire intraocular contents if not recognized and treated promptly with aggressive suturing of the cataract incision. Fortunately, it is rare with an occurrence rate of 0.2%.

6. What are some of the risk factors for expulsive choroidal hemorrhage? How are they treated?
   Risk factors include advanced age, systemic hypertension, arteriosclerosis, glaucoma, and long axial-length. Time is of the essence in responding to this operating room emergency. The wound must be closed as quickly as possible; in fact, the surgeon may tamponade the wound with his or her thumb until a suture is ready. Sutures should be rapidly placed and the patient's eye closed. Some surgeons advocate performing posterior sclerotomies to release accumulated blood. The prognosis for visual outcome is usually quite poor.

7. What is the incidence of posterior capsule rupture for an experienced surgeon during cataract surgery?
   Most studies report between 1% and 3%.

8. What are the possible consequences of posterior capsule rupture?
   Posterior capsule rupture is often associated with vitreous loss. It may result in loss of lens material into the vitreous cavity (Fig. 23.1). It also increases the risk of endophthalmitis and retinal detachment.

KEY POINTS: POSTOPERATIVE CATARACT SURGERY COMPLICATIONS

1. Corneal edema
2. Cystoid macular edema
3. Inflammation/uveitis
4. Wrong intraocular lens power
5. Secondary membrane
6. Glaucoma/elevated intraocular pressure
7. Wound leak
8. Retinal detachment
9. Diplopia
10. Ischemic optic neuropathy
11. Ptosis

9. What are causes of postoperative inflammation?
   - **Operative trauma.** All eyes show some postoperative uveitis, characterized by cell and flare reaction in the anterior chamber. Despite individual variation, the degree of inflammation is usually proportionate to the degree of trauma induced by the surgical procedure. Procedures with longer surgical times and/or additional procedures (i.e., vitrectomy or iris manipulation) show greater amounts of inflammation.
   - **Retained lens material.** Fragments of lens material—either nuclear or cortical remnants—may cause inflammation. In almost all cases, cortical remnants resorb and require no additional treatment. Nuclear fragments may become a source of chronic inflammation that leads to macular edema. Most nuclear remnants require surgical removal.

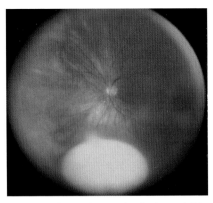

Fig. 23.1 Posterior capsule rupture may lead to loss of nuclear fragments into the vitreous. In this case nearly the entire lens "dropped" following a circumferential extension of a radial tear during capsulorrhexis.

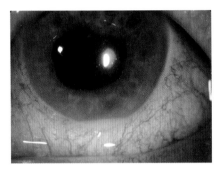

Fig. 23.2 A layered hypopyon is seen in this case of postoperative endophthalmitis.

- **Intraocular implant related.** This is more common when implants are poorly positioned, especially when they are in contact with uveal tissue. Some patients, particularly those with a history of uveitis, may react to the intraocular lens (IOL) material.

10. How does infectious endophthalmitis present? When does it usually occur?
   The classic presentation includes severe ocular pain, decreased vision, eyelid swelling, conjunctival chemosis, and hypopyon. Corneal edema and diminution or loss of the red reflex often occur. This condition must be suspected in any patient who presents with more inflammation than expected postoperatively. On average, patients developed signs and symptoms 6 days after surgery. More than three-fourths of patients developed signs and symptoms within 2 weeks (Fig. 23.2).

11. What are the common organisms cultured from the vitreous of endophthalmitis patients?
   In the Endophthalmitis Vitrectomy Study, the most common causative pathogens were gram-positive, coagulase-negative organisms (e.g., *Staphylococcus epidermidis*), followed by other gram-positive organisms, such as streptococci and *Staphylococcus aureus*.
   https://www.nei.nih.gov/news/clinicalalerts/alert-evs.

KEY POINTS: FINDINGS OF THE ENDOPHTHALMITIS VITRECTOMY STUDY

1. Systemic antibiotics provide *no* benefit in treating endophthalmitis.
2. Intravitreal antibiotics should be given to *all* endophthalmitis patients.
3. If vision is *better* than hand movements: intravitreal tap and biopsy.
4. If vision is *worse* than hand movements: full three-port pars plana vitrectomy.

12. What is toxic anterior segment syndrome?

It is sterile inflammation of the anterior segment after cataract surgery, but it has also been described after keratoplasty and posterior segment surgeries. The inflammation is usually mild but can be severe with significant corneal edema, anterior chamber cell and flare, and even hypopyon. The onset can be days or several months after surgery. A large case series revealed an incidence of 0.22%, but a significant number of cases occur in clusters.[1] It can be difficult to differentiate from bacterial endophthalmitis. Toxic anterior segment syndrome (TASS) does not respond to oral and fortified topical antibiotics but requires topical and/or systemic steroids. However, such patients must be treated initially as potentially infectious unless proven otherwise.

13. What causes toxic anterior segment syndrome?

In over half of cases, the cause may never be found. Thorough and prompt investigation of each case is critical to try to find a cause and prevent further outbreaks. Surgical instruments, viscoelastics, medications, drapes, and the sterilization systems must be investigated. Major reported causes include inadequate cleaning of surgical instruments, contamination of surgical instruments or IOLs, and adverse reactions to drugs. The American Society of Cataract and Refractive Surgery (ASCRS) TASS Task Force suggests that improper cleaning of surgical instruments is the most common cause.[1] Intracameral injections of medications with inadvertent dilution errors, preservatives, abnormal pH, and increased osmolality are also causes. Patients with diabetes mellitus, hypertension, hyperlipidemia, chronic ischemic heart disease, and chronic renal failure are also at increased risk.

14. What are the causes of corneal edema after cataract surgery?

Corneal edema frequently occurs adjacent to the cataract wound and usually resolves spontaneously. Surgical trauma, preexisting endothelial corneal dystrophy, and elevated intraocular pressure may cause central corneal edema. Treatment of elevated intraocular pressure and topical steroids, as necessary for inflammation, are important. Often, central edema resolves with time and topical steroids. Corneal or epithelial transplantation may be necessary for patients when corneal edema persists (Fig. 23.3). Evaluate for a Descemet's detachment if the edema does not clear or worsens.

15. What are the causes of vitreous loss during cataract surgery? Why is vitreous loss important?

Vitreous loss usually results from rupture of the posterior lens capsule during surgery or weakness or dehiscence of lens zonules. Zonular issues may be preexisting or occur during surgery. Vitreous loss increases the risk of retinal detachment, cystoid macular edema, and endophthalmitis. The additional surgical trauma may also lead to an increase in corneal trauma and secondary central corneal edema.

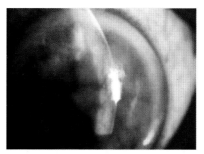

Fig. 23.3 Corneal edema such as this is characterized by thickening of the cornea with Descemet's folds and, frequently, microcystic epithelial changes. It is more commonly seen in patients with preexisting endothelial cell loss (Fuchs' dystrophy) or dysfunction.

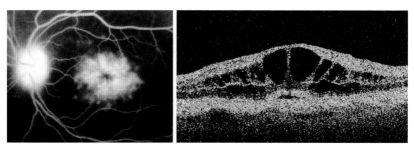

Fig. 23.4 Cystoid macular edema after cataract surgery (Irvine-Gass syndrome) has historically been documented with fluorescein angiography *(left)*, in which it has a classic petaloid appearance in late frames of the angiogram. Optical coherence tomography is increasingly being used to diagnose and follow macular edema *(right)*.

16. **How can vitreous loss be potentially minimized after capsular rupture?**
When capsular rupture is recognized, tamponade the vitreous and maintain intraocular pressure by filling the anterior chamber with viscoelastic prior to removing the phacoemulsification handpiece.

17. **What is the incidence of retinal detachment after cataract surgery? Which patients are at greater risk?**
Retinal detachment occurs in 1% to 2% of patients in most reported series. Patients predisposed to retinal detachment because of high myopia, lattice degeneration, and a history of retinal detachment in the fellow eye are at greatest risk. Vitreous loss at the time of surgery also raises the risk of retinal detachment. The risk of retinal detachment after cataract surgery has decreased with the advent of extracapsular cataract extraction, which has replaced intracapsular extraction.

18. **What is cystoid macular edema?**
Cystoid macular edema (CME) occurs when fluid accumulates extracellularly in and around the center of the macula, known as the fovea. The detection of CME can be diagnosed on clinical exam, with optical coherence tomography (OCT) imaging, or fluorescein angiography (FA) imaging. See Fig 23.4 OCT imaging is the most sensitive and least invasive tool for diagnosing CME and following treatment outcomes. A recent study found the incidence of OCT evidence of CME following cataract surgery with a reduction in vision to be up to 14%.[2]

19. **Which patients are likely to suffer from cystoid macular edema? How is it treated?**
Cystoid macular edema is more common after intracapsular than after extracapsular cataract extraction. It is also more common when vitreous loss occurs, especially if the vitreous or iris becomes incarcerated in the wound. However, it may occur even in uncomplicated cases.
    Treatment of CME is controversial because a significant percentage of cases resolve spontaneously. Initial treatment often includes topical steroids or topical nonsteroidal anti-inflammatory medications. Carbonic anhydrase inhibitors have also been shown to reduce edema in some cases and can be used both topically and orally (acetazolamide). More recently, periocular and intravitreal triamcinolone has been shown to help cystoid macular edema, although the improvement may be transient. Intravitreal anti–vascular endothelial growth factor (anti-VEGF) therapy has also been shown to be effective in refractory pseudophakic CME. When the vitreous or iris is adherent to the wound, lysis of vitreous strands with surgery, neodymium:yttrium–aluminum–garnet (Nd:YAG) laser, or wound revision may be beneficial. Pars plana vitrectomy has been used with success in some patients who suffer from chronic CME.

20. **What is a secondary membrane?**
A secondary or "after-cataract" membrane develops after extracapsular cataract surgery. The posterior capsule opacifies when persistent lens fibers adhere to the capsule or the remaining lens fibers undergo metaplasia. Patients typically present with progressive decrease in vision or problems with glare after surgery.

21. **When does a secondary membrane develop? How frequently does it occur?**
Usually, a secondary membrane begins to develop several months after surgery, although in many cases, the membrane may take 1 year or more to become visually significant. The opacification rate varies from 8% to 50% in various series. Recently, squared posterior optic edge designs have lowered this rate, particularly with acrylic material optics.

22. **How is a secondary membrane treated? What complications may occur?**
Surgical capsulotomy at the time of cataract surgery or post-operatively has been almost entirely replaced with Nd:YAG laser capsulotomy. Complications of laser capsulotomy include transient intraocular pressure rise, retinal detachment, and CME.

23. **What are the most common complications related to intraocular lens?**
    - Implantation of the wrong power IOL may result in an unacceptable refraction.
    - Decentration or dislocation of the IOL may produce unwanted optical images, including monocular double vision.
    - Mechanical chafing of the IOL against the iris or ciliary body may cause chronic inflammation. Chronic uveitis and secondary glaucoma, CME, or corneal decompensation may develop.
    - With astigmatism correcting toric IOLs, incorrect axis alignment or incorrect toric power may result in undercorrection or overcorrection of astigmatism.
    - With multifocal lenses, centration in the visual axis is critical. Even with a perfect surgical result, it is common for patients to note halos around lights in scotopic light conditions. This symptom is thought to lessen with time and neuroadaptation.
    Patients with these complications may require IOL repositioning or exchange.

24. **Why are patients with diabetes at greater risk when undergoing cataract surgery?**
Diabetic retinopathy may accelerate dramatically after cataract surgery. This risk is greatest if the posterior capsule ruptures.[3] Diabetics are more prone to the development of postoperative cystoid macular edema. Patients with preexisting macular edema are often treated shortly before and after surgery with steroid or anti-VEGF intravitreal injections.

25. **What are the major problems in managing patients with preexisting glaucoma and cataracts?**
    - In the past, many patients on glaucoma therapy were treated with miotics that constrict the pupil. Such therapy made cataract surgery more difficult and often required surgical maneuvers to enlarge the pupil. Thankfully, these miotics have been replaced by more effective medications without this unwanted side effect.
    - Postoperative pressure may rise because of retained viscoelastic material and inflammation. This elevation in pressure is often more severe and prolonged in patients with glaucoma. Elevation of pressure may cause additional optic nerve damage and visual field loss and result in loss of central vision in patients with advanced glaucoma. A glaucoma procedure may be combined with cataract surgery in patients with advanced or poorly controlled glaucoma to prevent a postoperative intraocular pressure spike as well as better intraocular pressure control in the long term.
    - Patients with glaucoma who have had previous filtration surgery and develop cataracts may require a different approach to cataract surgery. A shift in the location of the incision to avoid damage to the filtration site is often necessary. Inflammation from the surgical procedure may cause failure of a previously functioning filter postoperatively.

26. **What medication is associated with intraoperative floppy iris syndrome?**
    Tamsulosin (Flomax) is a systemic $\alpha 1$ antagonist medication used to treat prostatic hypertrophy. This drug relaxes the smooth muscle in the bladder neck and prostate. It is postulated that the same receptor is present in the iris dilator smooth muscle, resulting in loss of normal iris muscle tone.

27. **What can be done during cataract surgery in patients with intraoperative floppy iris syndrome?**
    The intraoperative placement of an iris stabilizing ring such as a Malyugen ring is often used to help with pupil dilation and to prevent iris prolapse. The use of a highly cohesive viscoelastic, such as Healon-5, may also assist with pupil dilation and tamponade of the iris to help minimize iris prolapse. Iris hooks are another option.

28. **What are the indications for capsular tension rings?**
    Capsular tension rings may be used in a variety of patients. Most frequently, they are used in patients with zonular laxity or instability such as in patients with pseudoexfoliation syndrome. It may also be a useful management tool in trauma cases or in patients who develop zonular dialysis as a result of the surgical procedure.

29. **What complications have been reported with femtosecond laser–assisted cataract surgery?**
    - Increased incidence of anterior capsule tears compared with traditional phacoemulsification cataract surgery. Laser anterior capsulotomy integrity seems to be compromised by postage-stamp-like perforations. This leads to an increased incidence of anterior capsule tears compared with manual continuous tear capsulorrhexis.
    - Incomplete anterior capsulotomy resulting in capsule tags or bridges.
    - Posterior capsule rupture possibly resulting in posterior dislocation of lens material.[4]
    - Incomplete procedure due to loss of interface suction/docking.

30. **What are the common reasons that patients may be unhappy with multifocal intraocular lenses?**
    - Uncorrected refractive error (either myopia, hyperopia, or astigmatism).
    - Ocular conditions that reduce contrast sensitivity or image quality that were undiagnosed prior to surgery, including but not limited to dry eye syndrome, anterior basement membrane dystrophy, macular degeneration, and/or epiretinal membrane.
    - Loss of contrast sensitivity related to IOL design with resulting image quality degradation.
    - Disabling glare or halos.
    - Intermediate vision complaints.
    - Decentered or tilted IOL.

31. **What is the difference between positive and negative dysphotopsia?**
    - Negative dysphotopsia represents an undesired optical phenomenon after cataract surgery. It is classically described as a dark temporal shadow. It is seen only with in-the-bag posterior chamber with overlap of the anterior capsulorrhexis onto the anterior surface of the IOL. If disabling to the patient, it has been successfully treated with two surgical strategies: reverse optic capture (the lens optic is moved anterior to the capsulotomy) and placement of a secondary piggyback IOL.
    - Positive dysphotopsia is characterized by light streaks, starbursts, or glare.

32. **What are the reasons for residual astigmatism following toric intraocular lens implantation?**
    - Implantation of a toric IOL on the wrong axis or rotation of the IOL off axis during the postoperative period.
    - An effect of posterior corneal astigmatism. A recent study showed that posterior corneal astigmatism, on average, will increase against-the-rule astigmatism and decrease with-the-rule astigmatism. Posterior corneal

astigmatism is difficult to measure with current preoperative tools, but intraoperative aberrometry can measure the total corneal power. The Cassini LED topographer does measure posterior corneal curvature preoperatively.

- Irregular astigmatism. Patients with irregular astigmatism from keratoconus, corneal scars, and other causes are not good toric IOL candidates. Attempted correction may result in undesirable postoperative results.[5]

REFERENCES

1. Park CY, Lee, JK, Chuck, RS: Toxic anterior segment syndrome—an updated review, BMC Ophthalmol 18:276–285, 2018.
2. Kim SJ, Belair ML, Bressler NM, et al.: A method of reporting macular edema after cataract surgery using optical coherence tomography, Retina 28:870–876, 2008.
3. Jaffe GJ, Burton TC, Kuhn E, et al.: Progression of nonproliferative diabetic retinopathy and visual outcome after extracapsular cataract extraction and intraocular lens implantation, Am J Ophthalmol 114:448–459, 1992.
4. Abell RG, Davies PE, Phelan D, Goemann K, McPherson ZE, Vote BJ: Anterior capsulotomy integrity after femtosecond laser-assisted cataract surgery, Ophthalmology 121(1):17–24, 2014.
5. Koch DD, Ali SF, Weikert MP, Shirayama M, Jenkins R, Wang LJ: Contribution of posterior corneal astigmatism to total corneal astigmatism, Cataract Refractive Surg 38(12): 2080–2087, 2012.

CHAPTER 24

AMBLYOPIA

Lauren B. Yeager and Steven E. Brooks

1. **What is amblyopia?**

   Amblyopia is a unilateral, or less commonly bilateral, loss of visual acuity and binocularity that results from inadequate or abnormal stimulation of the cortical visual system during the critical period of early visual development. The underlying causes can include optical blur, strabismus, or visual deprivation from pathologies such as ptosis, cataract, vitreous hemorrhage, or corneal opacity.

2. **Explain the concept of the "critical" or "sensitive" period.**

   This period is central to the concept of amblyopia. It refers to a developmental time frame early in life during which there is robust plasticity within the visual system, particularly the visual cortex. Although not precisely defined, this period extends from birth to approximately 8 to 10 years of age. During this period, the visual system is profoundly affected by the quality of visual stimulation it receives. Abnormal visual experience can lead to developmental abnormalities at both the structural and the functional level. If amblyopia occurs, it must be detected and treated during the critical period for vision to develop normally.[1]

3. **How is amblyopia classified?**

   Amblyopia is classified according to the underlying mechanism: strabismic, optical defocus or refractive, pattern or form deprivation, and organic.

   Strabismus can lead to amblyopia if one eye becomes strongly dominant. To avoid diplopia and visual confusion, the afferent input from the deviating, nondominant eye will be chronically suppressed at the level of the visual cortex, resulting in amblyopia. Optical defocus due to uncorrected refractive blur, including anisometropia as well as bilateral severe ametropia, represents another important and common cause of amblyopia. Pattern or form deprivation amblyopia, on the other hand, is caused by lesions that physically obstruct the visual axis, such as a congenital cataract, corneal opacity, vitreous hemorrhage, or ptosis. Organic amblyopia occurs secondary to a defined lesion of the visual pathways, such as a macular scar or coloboma. It is fundamentally different from the other types, because some or all of the vision loss is irreversible, and not simply a secondary effect on receptive fields in the lateral geniculate nuclei and visual cortex.

4. **How does strabismus cause amblyopia?**

   Manifest strabismus disrupts sensory fusion. As a result, the vision from one eye must be suppressed to avoid diplopia and visual confusion. If a child with strabismus develops a strong preference for the use of one eye over the other, or a dominant eye, the nondominant eye becomes amblyopic because of chronic suppression at the level of the visual cortex.

5. **What is anisometropia and how does it cause amblyopia?**

   Anisometropia is a difference in the state of refraction of at least one diopter between the two eyes. With significant anisometropia, the retinal image in one eye is always defocused and becomes incapable of processing high-resolution images. In addition, there is binocular rivalry between the blurred image in one eye and the clear image in the other eye. This leads to foveal suppression of the blurred image as a way to avoid visual confusion. The suppression affects the foveal region where high-grade visual acuity is processed and binocular rivalry is poorly tolerated. Patients with foveal suppression often display peripheral sensory fusion and gross stereopsis (monofixation syndrome) and maintain good ocular alignment.[2,3] Amblyopia caused purely by anisometropia has the best prognosis compared with other causes of amblyopia.

6. **What factors place children at increased risk for amblyopia?**
   - Developmental delay
   - Positive family history of amblyopia
   - Prematurity

     These factors lead to a twofold to sixfold increase in a child's chance of developing amblyopia.

7. **How prevalent is amblyopia?**

   The incidence of amblyopia is 2% to 4% in developed countries, and it is the most common cause of unilateral vision loss in children and young adults.

8. **What anatomic changes have been shown to occur in amblyopia?**

   Extensive animal studies have shown several neuroanatomic alterations in amblyopia. The primary abnormality appears to be the atrophy of cells in the layers of the lateral geniculate nucleus and visual cortex serving the amblyopic eye. These changes can be partially or wholly reversed if the amblyopia is successfully treated.[4–6]

9. How early should children be screened for amblyopia?

The American Association of Pediatric Ophthalmology and Strabismus recommends routine vision screening in children by a pediatrician or properly trained health care provider as follows:

- In newborns in the newborn nursery
- At each routine well visit from 1 month to 4 years of age
- A formal visual acuity should be documented by 5 years of age, or earlier if possible
- Repeat screening every 1 to 2 years after 5 years of age[7]

10. What are some clinical techniques to check for amblyopia in nonverbal children?

Fixation preference testing is especially useful. In strabismic patients, a lack of spontaneous alternation in visual fixation between the two eyes suggests amblyopia in the nonpreferred eye (Fig. 24.1). In patients with straight eyes or small-angle strabismus, the vertical prism, or induced tropia, test is used to determine fixation preference. A child who consistently objects to occlusion of one eye but not the other can be assumed to have decreased vision in the eye that they will allow to be covered. Visual evoked potentials and preferential looking (e.g., Teller acuity cards) tests can be used to measure visual acuity, or detect a disparity between the two eyes. The Bruckner test, comparing the quality and symmetry of the red reflex between the two eyes using a direct ophthalmoscope, can help detect small-angle strabismus or anisometropia.[8–10] Photoscreeners may also be used to assess for amblyopic risk factors in preverbal children, and utilize the red reflex in much the same way as the Bruckner test to detect media opacity, anisometropia, small angle strabismus, or significant ametropia of any form.

11. Describe photoscreening and its role in detecting amblyopia.

A photoscreener is a device used by pediatricians or other individuals to screen for amblyogenic risk factors in children. The photoscreener is a camera that takes multiple images of a child's undilated eyes to detect amblyogenic risk factors, including high refractive errors, anisometropia, anisocoria, and the presence of strabismus (Fig. 24.2). Children who are identified as having risk factors for amblyopia by the photoscreener should be referred to a pediatric

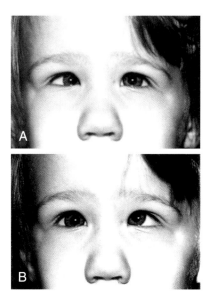

Fig. 24.1 Child with esotropia showing spontaneous alternation in fixation. **A,** The left eye is used for fixation. **B,** The right eye is used for fixation. Alternating fixation is good evidence against the presence of amblyopia in children with strabismus.

Fig. 24.2 Image taken from a commercially available photoscreening device. Similar to the Bruckner test, the red reflex is evaluated. Based on the shape, size, and location of the bright crescents in the pupillary light reflexes of the undilated pupils, a determination can be made as to whether the child has significant refractive error, anisometropia, or strabismus. Digital analysis software available in many of the commercially available devices can analyze the images and provide referral recommendations to the tester.

ophthalmologist for a complete examination. Photoscreeners may have significant advantages over traditional eye chart acuity screening, especially in younger children who are preverbal or may not be able or willing to participate in the eye chart acuity test.

12. **In addition to visual acuity, what other aspects of visual function may be affected in amblyopia?**
    - Binocular vision and stereoacuity
    - Contrast sensitivity
    - Motion perception and processing
    - Spatial localization

13. **What is more likely to cause amblyopia—hypermetropic or myopic anisometropia?**
    Hypermetropic anisometropia is more likely to cause amblyopia. In hypermetropic anisometropia, the more hypermetropic eye never receives clear and focused images. The fovea of the less hypermetropic eye is always dominant so there is no stimulus for added accommodative effort to adjust the focus of the more hypermetropic eye. In myopic anisometropia, the more myopic eye may receive clear and focused images at closer fixation distances, thereby avoiding chronic foveal suppression.

14. **Which is more likely to produce amblyopia—unilateral or bilateral ptosis? Why?**
    Unilateral ocular abnormalities are much more likely to lead to amblyopia than binocular ones. If one eye has a competitive advantage over the other, its afferent connections become stabilized and more numerous, while those of the other eye atrophy and retract. This competition also forms the basis for treating amblyopia. The amblyopic eye, by one means or another, must be given a temporary competitive advantage over the dominant eye.

KEY POINTS: AMBLYOPIA FUNDAMENTALS

1. Amblyopia is a potentially reversible loss of vision caused by abnormal visual stimulation during early visual development.
2. The critical period for amblyopia extends from birth to ages 8 to 10 years.
3. Etiologies of amblyopia include strabismus, optical defocus, pattern or form deprivation, as well as physical/organic pathologies within the retina or anterior visual pathways.
4. Amblyopia is characterized by functional and structural changes in the visual cortex and lateral geniculate nuclei.

---

15. **Describe the treatment of amblyopia.**
    The first step is to identify and treat any organic causes for vision loss. The second step is to ensure a clear visual axis. For example, this may require removal of a congenital cataract or vitreous hemorrhage. Significant refractive errors should also be corrected. The third step is to patch or penalize the dominant eye so that the nondominant eye receives the visual input. Of note, some cases of refractive amblyopia may be treated by wearing glasses alone, obviating or delaying the need for patching, or penalization therapy.[11] It is ideal to diagnose and treat amblyopia is as soon as it occurs, but it is critical to do so before the close of the critical period.

16. **How effective is part-time patching compared with full-time patching?**
    Part-time patching is equally effective as full-time patching in the treatment of amblyopia. Greater compliance is seen with part-time patching regimens. With full-time occlusion, there is a greater risk of amblyopia being induced in the sound eye. Children can safely receive full-time occlusion of the sound eye for up to 1 week per year of life before the next follow-up visit without significant risk of inducing occlusion amblyopia in the sound eye.

17. **What is penalization and how is it used to treat amblyopia?**
    Penalization refers to the intentional degradation of visual acuity in the sound eye by either optical or pharmacologic means. For example, the sound eye might be effectively blurred by intentional undercorrection of its refractive error, using atropine drops to prevent accommodation, or both. Translucent filters can be placed over the spectacle lens of the sound eye to degrade the vision. Penalization techniques are best suited for patients with a high degree of hyperopic refractive error in the sound eye and in whom the amblyopia is mild to moderate (20/100 or better).[12–15]

18. **At what point can amblyopia treatment be discontinued?**
    When the acuity in the treated eye is equal to that of the sound eye. The decision is less clear when there is some persistent deficit in visual acuity. If poor compliance can be ruled out, many practitioners continue to patch until no further improvement is noted after three consecutive treatment intervals (3 to 4 weeks per interval). The eye examination and refraction should also be repeated to detect uncorrected refractive error or structural lesions. Patching should be gradually decreased to decrease the chance of recurrence.

19. What are some of the factors affecting the success of amblyopia treatment?
    • Age of onset
    • Age at which treatment is initiated
    • Compliance with treatment regimen
    • Depth of amblyopia
    • Presence of associated ocular anomalies or injuries

20. Can the vision of an amblyopic eye improve after the critical period has ended?
    Treatment of amblyopia is most effective when children are under 7 years of age. However, studies have shown treatment response in older individuals, and children up to 13 years of age may show significant improvement with patching, particularly in cases of purely anisometropic amblyopia. However, these children may have a slower rate of response and require a higher dose of patching, and the extent of recovery may be less complete.[16]

21. Is color vision affected in amblyopia?
    Generally speaking, color vision is not affected by amblyopia.

22. Does amblyopia cause a relative afferent pupillary defect?
    Generally speaking, amblyopia does not cause an afferent pupillary defect (APD), because the pathologic changes in amblyopia are located in the posterior visual pathways, not in the retina or optic nerve. If an eye suspected of having amblyopia is found to have a relative APD, it is imperative that a retinal or optic nerve lesion is ruled out.[17]

23. In which of the following conditions is amblyopia most likely to occur: congenital esotropia, accommodative esotropia, or intermittent exotropia?
    Amblyopia is most likely to occur in accommodative esotropia. Patients with this condition, particularly if there is significant anisometropia, are less likely to alternate fixation than patients with congenital esotropia or exotropia. Patients with intermittent exotropia are unlikely to develop amblyopia because they spend a fair amount of time being bifoveal.

24. What is the effect of neutral density filters on the vision of an amblyopic eye compared with a normal eye?
    The visual acuity of a normal eye is progressively reduced by neutral density filters, whereas that of an amblyopic eye may remain unchanged or even improve slightly.

25. What is the crowding phenomenon? What is its significance in amblyopia?
    The crowding phenomenon refers to a loss of spatial acuity when optotypes are presented in close proximity, or surrounded by other visual details, rather than in isolation. The crowding phenomenon is seen in both normal and amblyopic eyes but tends to be much more pronounced in amblyopia. Because of this, measurement of acuity by isolated optotypes may overestimate acuity in amblyopia. In order to obtain the most accurate visual acuity, examiners should test patients with linear optotypes whenever possible.

26. What is eccentric fixation?
    Eccentric fixation is seen in severe amblyopia as well as other conditions in which foveal fixation is severely compromised. It refers to the use of nonfoveal areas of the retina for visual fixation. The fixation in such eyes is generally unsteady and poorly maintained. It appears as though the eye is looking elsewhere when, in fact, it is simply attempting to fixate using a nonfoveal area of the retina.

27. Can refractive surgery be used to treat anisometropic amblyopia in children?
    The role of refractive surgery to treat anisometropic amblyopia is quite controversial, and laser keratorefractive surgery for children remains an off-label use for these devices. Investigators have reported successfully performing photorefractive keratectomy in pediatric patients, and studies have shown that the procedure can be performed safely in children who are noncompliant with refractive correction. Best corrected visual acuity and stereopsis improved. While refractive procedures may have a future role in the management of amblyopia, they remain investigative at this time.[18]

KEY POINTS: AMBLYOPIA TREATMENT GUIDELINES

1. Part-time occlusion therapy can be as effective as full-time occlusion if compliance is good.
2. Atropine penalization is as effective as occlusion for treatment of amblyopia. In addition to daily atropine use, once-weekly atropine use is effective and may improve compliance.
3. Treatment of amblyopia is most successful in children under 7 years of age, but significant improvement can be seen in children up to 13 years of age.
4. Refractive errors in the amblyopic eye should be fully corrected during treatment.

28. When should strabismus surgery be performed in a patient with amblyopia?
    Traditional teaching dictates that amblyopia should be fully treated before strabismus surgery. Some, however, have suggested that surgery may be performed during the course of amblyopia treatment if the physician believes that recovery of binocular vision may be improved or treatment of the amblyopia facilitated. It is likely that the management of any given case will need to be determined individually and that both practice patterns can be effectively used.[19] It must be kept in mind that strabismus surgery is not used to treat amblyopia and that treatment must continue following surgery if amblyopia persists.

REFERENCES

1. von Noorden GK: Binocular vision and ocular motility, ed 6, St. Louis, 2001, Mosby.
2. Brooks SE, Johnson D, Fischer N: Anisometropia and binocularity, Ophthalmology 103:1139–1143, 1996.
3. Townsend AM, Holmes JM, Evans LS: Depth of anisometropic amblyopia and difference in refraction, Am J Ophthalmol 116: 431–436, 1993.
4. Harwerth RS, Smith EL III, Duncan GC, et al.: Multiple critical periods in the development of the primate visual system, Science 232:235–238, 1986.
5. Crawford ML, Harwerth RS: Ocular dominance column width and contrast sensitivity in monkeys reared with strabismus or anisometropia, Invest Ophthalmol Vis Sci 45:3036–3042, 2004.
6. Wiesel TN, Hubel DH: Single-cell responses in striate cortex of kittens deprived of vision in one eye, J Neurophysiol 26: 1003–1007, 1963.
7. American Academy of Ophthalmology, Board of Trustees: Joint policy statement: vision screening for infants and children, San Francisco, 2013, American Association for Pediatric Ophthalmology and Strabismus.
8. Fischer N, Brooks SE: Effect of fixation target on fixation preference testing, Am Orthoptic J 49:105–110, 1999.
9. Tongue AC, Cibis GW: Bruckner test, Ophthalmology 88:1041–1044, 1981.
10. Wright KW, Walonker F, Edelman P: 10-Diopter fixation test for amblyopia, Arch Ophthalmol 99:1242–1246, 1981.
11. Cotter SA, Edwards AR, Wallace DK, et al.: Pediatric Eye Disease Investigator Group: Treatment of anisometropic amblyopia in children with refractive correction, Ophthalmology 113(6):895–903, 2006.
12. Pediatric Eye Disease Investigator Group: A comparison of atropine and patching treatments for moderate amblyopia by patient age, cause of amblyopia, depth of amblyopia, and other factors, Ophthalmology 110:1632–1637, 2003.
13. Pediatric Eye Disease Investigator Group: The course of moderate amblyopia treated with atropine in children: experience of the amblyopia treatment study, Am J Ophthalmol 136:630–639, 2003.
14. Repka MX, Cotter SA, Beck RW, et al.: A randomized trial of atropine regimens for treatment of moderate amblyopia in children, Ophthalmology 111:2076–2085, 2004.
15. Repka MX, Kraker RT, Beck RW, et al.: Pediatric Eye Disease Investigator Group: A randomized trial of atropine vs patching for treatment of moderate amblyopia: follow-up at age 10 years, Arch Ophthalmol 126(8):1039–1044, 2008.
16. Holmes JM, Lazar EL, Melia BM, et al.: Pediatric Eye Investigator Group: Effect of age on response to amblyopia treatment in children, Arch Ophthalmol 129(11):1451–1457, 2011.
17. Greenwald MJ, Folk ER: Afferent pupillary defects in amblyopia, J Pediatr Ophthalmol Strabismus 20:63–67, 1983.
18. Paysee EA, Coats DK, Hussein MA, et al.: Long-term outcomes of photorefractive keratectomy for anisometropic amblyopia in children, Ophthalmology 113(2):169–176, 2006.
19. Lam GC, Repka MX, Guyton DL: Timing of amblyopia therapy relative to strabismus surgery, Ophthalmology 100:1751–1756, 1993.

CHAPTER 25

ESODEVIATIONS

Brooke D. Saffren, Scott E. Olitsky, and Leonard B. Nelson

1. What is an esodeviation?

   A convergent deviation, noted by crossing or in-turning of the eyes, is designated by the prefix *eso.*

2. What are the different types of esodeviations?

   - **Esophoria** is a latent tendency for the eyes to cross. This latent deviation is normally controlled by fusional mechanisms that provide binocular vision or avoid diplopia. The eye deviates only under certain conditions, such as fatigue, illness, stress, or tests that interfere with the maintenance of normal fusional abilities (e.g., covering one eye).
   - **Esotropia** is a manifest misalignment of the eyes. The condition may be alternating or unilateral, depending on the vision. In alternating strabismus, either eye may be used for fixation while the fellow eye deviates. In cases of unilateral esotropia, the deviating eye is noted in the description of the misalignment (left esotropia).

3. How common is esotropia in infants?

   Misalignment is common within the first 3 months of life; afterward, alignment should stabilize. Forty percent of newborn infants seem to have straight eyes, 33% may display exotropia, and approximately 3% may be esotropic.[1] Many infants have variable alignment and cannot easily be classified in any single category. The incidence of infantile esotropia is about 1%.[2] Few patients with an esotropia of 40 or more prism diopters that is constant at 10 weeks of age will demonstrate spontaneous resolution of their deviation.[3]

4. What is pseudoesotropia?

   Pseudoesotropia is the false appearance of esotropia when the visual axes are actually aligned. A flat, broad nasal bridge, prominent epicanthal folds, or a narrow interpupillary distance causes the observer to see less sclera nasally than expected. This creates the impression that the eye is turned in toward the nose.

5. What is congenital or infantile esotropia?

   Congenital or infantile esotropia is a convergent strabismus, with no identifiable cause, that develops in a child before the age of 6 months. Although the two terms are often used interchangeably, there is an important difference between them. A child with true congenital esotropia is born with strabismus, whereas a child with infantile esotropia will develop it during the first few months of life. The period of time during early infancy in which the eyes are straight may play an important role in the development of binocular vision after the eyes are aligned.

6. What are the characteristics of congenital esotropia?

   - **Large deviation:** The characteristic angle of congenital esotropia is considerably larger than angles of esotropia acquired later in life (Fig. 25.1). In most series reported in the literature, average deviations are between 40 and 60 prism diopters. The diagnosis of congenital esotropia should be reconsidered in a child with a relatively small deviation.
   - **Normal refractive error:** Children with congenital esotropia tend to have cycloplegic refractions similar to those of normal children of the same age.[4]

7. What is cross-fixation?

   - Children with equal vision and a large esotropia have no need to abduct either eye. They use the adducted, or crossed, eye to look to the opposite field of gaze. This is called cross-fixation.
   - In children with good vision in both eyes and who demonstrate cross-fixation, neither eye will appear to abduct. If amblyopia is present, only the eye that sees better will cross-fixate, making the amblyopic eye appear to have an abduction weakness.

8. How can a pseudoabduction deficit be distinguished from a true abduction deficit?

   - By rotating the infant's head, either with the infant sitting upright in a moveable chair or by using a doll's head maneuver
   - By patching one eye for a short period. The child will eventually demonstrate abduction

9. What is the differential diagnosis of an infant with esotropia?

   - Pseudoesotropia
   - Congenital sixth nerve palsy
   - Duane's retraction syndrome

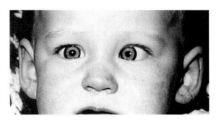

Fig. 25.1 A child with congenital esotropia. Note the characteristic large angle of crossing.

- Early-onset accommodative esotropia
- Möbius syndrome
- Sensory esotropia
- Nystagmus blockage syndrome
- Esotropia in the neurologically impaired

10. How is vision evaluated in a child with congenital esotropia?
    The following observations can be made to look for equal vision in a child with a large-angle esotropia:
    - Spontaneously alternates fixation
    - Holds fixation with either eye when one eye is covered and then uncovered
    - Cross-fixation present in both eyes

11. How common is amblyopia in congenital esotropia?
    Amblyopia may occur in as many as 19% to 72% of infants with congenital esotropia.

12. What are the goals in the treatment of congenital esotropia?
    - Development of normal sight in each eye
    - Reduction of distant and near deviation as close to orthotropia (straight eyes) as possible
    - Development of at least a rudimentary form of binocular vision

13. What level of binocular vision can develop in children with congenital esotropia?
    - Classically, it has been taught that patients with congenital esotropia do not develop bifoveal fixation (perfect binocular vision) regardless of their age at treatment.
    - Alignment within 10 prism diopters of orthotropia early in life is often associated with the attainment of some degree of binocular vision and stereopsis.
    - Some surgeons have suggested that surgery performed on a patient at a very early age can lead to the development of bifoveal fixation.

14. When is congenital esotropia treated?
    - The best results for treating surgically is to minimize the time between the onset of esotropia and when the procedure is done.
    - Operating on patients under 10 months of age improves sensory and motor outcome for certain patients.[5] Surgery at an even earlier age (3 to 4 months) is considered if the deviation is large and constant.[6]

15. Why is it important to treat amblyopia before surgical correction of congenital esotropia?
    - Treating amblyopia prior to surgery may increase the success.
    - Once the eyes are straight following surgery, amblyopia may be more difficult to detect in very young children.
    - Patients with congenital esotropia in general do not develop bifoveal fixation.

16. What other motility disorders are often associated with congenital esotropia?
    - **Inferior oblique overaction:** Elevation of the eye during adduction (Fig. 25.2); occurs in 78% of cases; most common in the second or third year of life; may require surgery
    - **Dissociated vertical deviation:** Slow upward deviation; occurs in 46% to 90% of cases; onset greatest in the second year of life; may require surgery
    - **Nystagmus:** Latent or rotary possible; occurs in 50% of cases; usually diminishes with time.[7]

17. What is accommodative esotropia?
    Accommodative esotropia is a convergent deviation of the eyes associated with activation of the accommodative reflex (Fig. 25.3).

18. At what age does accommodative esotropia develop?
    Accommodative esotropia usually occurs in a child between 2 and 3 years of age. Occasionally, children who are 1 year of age or younger present with all of the clinical features of accommodative esotropia.[8]

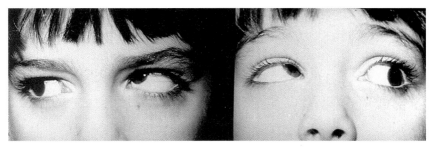

Fig. 25.2 Inferior oblique overaction. As the eye adducts (moves toward the nose), it elevates.

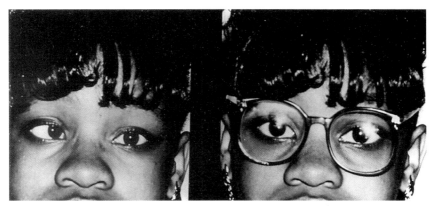

Fig. 25.3 Accommodative esotropia. As the child attempts to accommodate (focus), the eyes cross *(left)*. With glasses that eliminate the need to accommodate, the eyes are straight *(right)*.

19. What are the three types of accommodative esotropia?
    - Refractive
    - Nonrefractive
    - Partial or decompensated

20. What three factors influence the development of refractive accommodative esotropia?
    - Uncorrected hyperopia
    - Accommodative convergence
        - Sometimes, the esotropia is corrected at distance, but there is a residual esotropia at near. This can be treated with bifocals, but evidence for bifocals improving outcomes with stereopsis is lacking.[9]
        - Note: The accommodative convergence:accommodation (AC:A) ratio describes how many prism diopters a person's eyes converge for each diopter that he or she accommodates.
    - Insufficient fusional divergence[10]

21. How do the aforementioned three factors lead to accommodative esotropia?
    A hyperopic person must exert excessive accommodation to clear a blurred retinal image. This, in turn, stimulates excessive convergence. If the amplitude of fusional divergence is sufficient to correct the excessive convergence, no esotropia results. However, if the fusional divergence amplitudes are inadequate, or if motor fusion is altered by some sensory obstacle, esotropia results.

22. How is refractive accommodative esotropia treated?
    Spectacles correct the hyperopic refractive error. Generally, the full hyperopic correction as determined by cycloplegic refraction is given to the child.

23. What is the relationship between accommodative esotropia and congenital esotropia?
    Recurrent esotropia may occur in approximately 25% of patients who have been successfully treated for congenital esotropia. Most of these patients (80%) respond to correction of hyperopia, even if the level of hyperopia is small.

KEY POINTS: ESOTROPIA

1. Amblyopia is best treated before surgery for congenital esotropia.
2. The diagnosis of congenital esotropia should be reconsidered in the presence of a small-angle deviation.
3. A complete exam is required to rule out other disorders in all patients who present with early-onset esodeviation.
4. Refractive accommodative esotropia is treated with spectacles.
5. A neurologic workup should be considered for patients who present with an acute esotropia and normal levels of hyperopia.

24. **What is nonrefractive accommodative esotropia?**

Nonrefractive accommodative esotropia is associated with a high AC:A ratio. The effort to accommodate elicits an abnormally high accommodative convergence response. The amount of esotropia is greater at near deviation than at distance because of the additional accommodation required to maintain a clear image at near.

25. **How can nonrefractive accommodative esotropia be treated?**

- Bifocals eliminate the additional accommodative effort required at near and therefore reduce the near esotropia.
- Surgery may be performed to eliminate the esotropia at near and to correct the AC:A ratio permanently.
- Observation. Some ophthalmologists choose simply to observe patients as long as the patients' eyes remain straight at distance. The esotropia at near may resolve on its own as the AC:A ratio normalizes during childhood.

26. **What is partial or decompensated accommodative esotropia?**

Refractive or nonrefractive accommodative esotropias do not always occur in their "pure" forms. Glasses may reduce the esodeviation significantly. Sometimes, the esotropia may initially be eliminated with glasses, but a nonaccommodative portion slowly becomes evident despite the maximal amount of hyperopic correction consistent with good vision. The residual esodeviation that persists is called the deteriorated or nonaccommodative portion. This condition commonly occurs with a delay of months between onset of accommodative esotropia and antiaccommodative treatment.

27. **How is partial or decompensated accommodative esotropia treated?**

- Surgery may be indicated if the deviation is larger than an amount that allows the development of binocular vision.
- Surgery is generally performed for the nonaccommodative portion of the esotropia only, not for the full deviation that is present without glasses in place.

28. **What is cyclic esotropia?**

- A rare disorder that classically describes a large-angle esotropia alternating with orthophoria or a small-angle esodeviation on a 48-hour cycle
- It may result from an aberration in the biologic clock or a combination of defects in the clock, oculomotor nuclei, superior colliculi, or other nuclei
- Unpredictable response to various forms of therapy with the exception of surgery, which is usually curative

29. **What are the characteristics of acute acquired comitant esotropia?**

- A rare condition that occurs in older children and adults
- Dramatic onset of a large angle of esotropia with diplopia
- Normal levels of hyperopia
- Has been reported after periods of interruption of fusion, such as occlusion therapy for amblyopia

30. **How should patients with acute acquired comitant esotropia be managed?**

- A careful motility analysis to rule out a paretic deviation
- Consider further workup, including computed tomography or magnetic resonance imaging

REFERENCES

1. Nixon RB, Helveston EM, Miller K, Archer SM, Ellis FD: Incidence of strabismus in neonates, Am J Ophthalmol 100(6):798–801, 1985.
2. Magli A, Carelli R, Matarazzo F, Bruzzese D: Essential infantile esotropia: postoperative motor outcomes and inferential analysis of strabismus surgery, BMC Ophthalmol 14:35, 2014.
3. Pediatric Eye Disease Investigator G: Spontaneous resolution of early-onset esotropia: experience of the Congenital Esotropia Observational Study, Am J Ophthalmol 133(1):109–118, 2002.
4. Pediatric Eye Disease Investigator G: The clinical spectrum of early-onset esotropia: experience of the Congenital Esotropia Observational Study, Am J Ophthalmol 133(1):102–108, 2002.

5. Wong AM: Timing of surgery for infantile esotropia: sensory and motor outcomes, Can J Ophthalmol 43(6):643–651, 2008.
6. Hutcheson KA: Childhood esotropia, Curr Opin Ophthalmol 15(5):444–448, 2004.
7. Hiles DA, Watson BA, Biglan AW: Characteristics of infantile esotropia following early bimedial rectus recession, Arch Ophthalmol 98(4):697–703, 1980.
8. Coats DK, Avilla CW, Paysse EA, Sprunger DT, Steinkuller PG, Somaiya M: Early-onset refractive accommodative esotropia, J AAPOS 2(5):275–278, 1998.
9. Whitman MC, MacNeill K, Hunter DG: Bifocals fail to improve stereopsis outcomes in high AC/A accommodative esotropia, Ophthalmology 123(4):690–696, 2016.
10. Raab EL: Etiologic factors in accommodative esodeviation, Trans Am Ophthalmol Soc 80:657–694, 1982.

CHAPTER 26

MISCELLANEOUS OCULAR DEVIATIONS

Janice A. Gault

1. **What is the differential diagnosis of exotropia?**
   - Congenital exotropia
   - Sensory exotropia
   - Third-nerve palsy
   - Duane's syndrome
   - Craniofacial abnormalities with divergent orbit (e.g., Apert's syndrome or Crouzon's syndrome)
   - Myasthenia gravis
   - Thyroid disorder
   - Medial wall fracture
   - Slipped medial rectus muscle or excessively resected lateral rectus
   - Orbital inflammatory pseudotumor
   - Convergence insufficiency
   - Internuclear ophthalmoplegia

2. **A mother notices that her 4-month-old infant seems to be "wall-eyed." What is your concern as a physician?**
   First, check whether deviation or pseudostrabismus is present. A wide interpupillary distance or temporal dragging of the macula from retinopathy of prematurity or toxocariasis may cause pseudoexotropia. The light reflex test or cover testing elucidates this point. Make sure that the eyes move normally. Have the patient follow a light or a brightly colored toy to exclude paralysis or muscle restriction. If this test is normal and you notice true strabismus, quantify it with prisms at near and far. Check the cycloplegic refraction and do a complete dilated exam. Anisometropic amblyopia may cause an eye to deviate, but it usually presents as esotropia in the younger age group. A corneal lesion, cataract, glaucoma, or retinal lesion such as a toxoplasmosis scar or retinoblastoma may cause the deviation. These conditions must be ruled out.

   Once you have determined that the remainder of the exam is normal, you realize that the infant has an alternating exotropia of 40 prism diopters. Congenital exotropia is much rarer than congenital esotropia, but they have much in common. Both have a large angle of deviation and rarely develop amblyopia because of alternating fixation. The refractive error is normal. Early surgery is recommended to allow development of stereoacuity.

3. **A mother notices that her 2-year-old boy has a left eye that deviates outward when he is tired or has a fever. What is your concern as a physician?**
   Intermittent exotropia, which is the most common type of exotropia. The onset varies from infancy to 4 years of age. It may progress through the following three phases:
   - **Phase 1:** Exophoria at distance and orthophoria at near occur when the patient is fatigued or daydreaming. He has diplopia and often closes one eye. When aware of the deviation, he is easily able to straighten his eyes, often after a blink.
   - **Phase 2:** Exotropia at distance and exophoria at near. When the exotropia becomes more constant, suppression develops and the diplopia becomes less frequent. The exotropia remains after a blink.
   - **Phase 3:** The exotropia is constant at distance and near. There is no diplopia because of suppression.
   Vision must be equalized by correcting any significant refractive error and patching the nondeviating eye. Surgery should be done when the patient progresses beyond phase 1, but preferably before phase 3. There is controversy about timing of surgery—more studies are showing that fewer patients will need surgery than expected in the past. Patching and correcting refractive error are important, with surgery reserved for those who are losing binocularity and stereo acuity.

4. **An 18-year-old patient complains of blurred near vision and headaches while reading. Do you believe her, or is she just trying to get out of doing her homework?**
   Check her ocular deviations at near and far. She may be experiencing convergence insufficiency, which is common in teenagers and young adults. It is rare in children under 10 years of age. It is often idiopathic but may be exacerbated by fatigue, drugs, uveitis, or an Adie's tonic pupil. Exodeviation is greater at near than at distance and causes asthenopia. Exophoria at near may be all that is seen. The near point of convergence is more distant than normal (>3 to 6 cm for patients younger than age 20; >12 cm for patients older than age 40), and the amplitude of accommodation is reduced.

   Her fusional ability will be decreased. If you have her focus on a target at the reading distance that forces her to accommodate, you will see that she will have a low break point or a low recovery point when slowly increasing the amount of base-out prism in front of one eye. The break point is when she begins to see double vision with increasing prism; the recovery point is when she can fuse to single images working down from the higher amount of prism. Ten to 15 prism diopters is considered low.

Because she is symptomatic, treat her with base-in prisms for reading to help convergence. Near-point exercises or "pencil push-ups" can improve fusional amplitudes. These exercises are performed by having the patient slowly move a pencil from arm's length toward the face while focusing on the eraser. Have the patient concentrate on maintaining one image of the eraser. Repeat 10 times several times a day. Once this is mastered, pencil push-ups can be done while holding a 6-D base-out prism over one eye. Rarely, medial rectus resection may be necessary.

5. **What if the fusional capacities are normal and there is no exodeviation?**
The problem may be accommodative insufficiency, which has similar symptoms in the same age group. However, accommodation is reduced. First check the manifest and cycloplegic refraction. The patient may be underplussed and need a stronger hyperopic refraction. If refraction is normal, plus-lens reading glasses will help.

6. **How do you differentiate a patient with convergence insufficiency versus accommodative insufficiency clinically?**
In accommodative insufficiency, a 4-D base-in prism will cause blurring during reading, whereas patients with convergence insufficiency will note that print becomes clearer.

7. **Some patients have the opposite problem: esotropia that is worse at distance than at near. What is this condition called?**
This is divergence insufficiency. Fusional divergence is reduced. Treatment is with base-out prisms and, rarely, lateral rectus resections. However, divergence insufficiency is a diagnosis of exclusion, and divergence paralysis must be ruled out because it may be associated with pontine tumors, head trauma, and other neurologic abnormalities. Neuro-ophthalmic evaluation is necessary.

8. **What is Duane's syndrome? What are the different types of this disorder?**
Duane's syndrome is a congenital motility disorder characterized by limited abduction, limited adduction, or both. The globe retracts, and the palpebral fissure narrows on attempted adduction. A "leash effect" may cause upward deviation at the same time. There are three types of the syndrome:
- Type 1—limited abduction (most common) (Fig. 26.1)
- Type 2—limited adduction
- Type 3—both limited abduction and limited adduction (rarest type)

There are three females to every two males afflicted with Duane's syndrome. The left eye is involved in 60% of cases; in 18% of cases, both eyes are involved. Sixty percent of patients also have an associated esotropia, 15% have exotropia, and 25% are orthophoric. A and V patterns are common. Amblyopia, attributable to anisometropia, occurs in approximately one-third of cases. Surgery is done to correct a head turn, but resection should not be performed because it exacerbates the narrowing of the fissure and globe retraction.

9. **What is the cause of Duane's syndrome?**
The cause is unclear, but it appears that the lateral rectus muscle is innervated by the third nerve, causing cocontraction of the medial and lateral rectus muscles. This theory explains the globe retraction and fissure narrowing.

10. **What other features may be associated with Duane's syndrome?**
Goldenhar's syndrome, deafness, crocodile tears, and uveal colobomas.

11. **What is the differential diagnosis of hypertropia?**
- Myasthenia gravis
- Thyroid eye disease
- Orbital inflammatory pseudotumor
- Orbital trauma (may cause inferior rectus entrapment)
- Fourth cranial nerve palsy
- Pseudohypertropia
- Skew deviation—see Chapter 30

12. **What is the cause of Brown's syndrome?**
Brown's syndrome (Fig. 26.2) may be congenital or acquired. The cause may be related to mechanical restriction of the superior oblique tendon. Examples include trauma, surgery, or inflammation in the region near the trochlea.

13. **How is Brown's syndrome treated?**
Acquired cases may be observed because they may improve spontaneously. Some improve with steroid injections near the trochlea. If no improvement is seen by 6 months, the superior oblique muscle may be weakened with a tenotomy. Some surgeons recess the ipsilateral inferior oblique at the same time to prevent an inferior oblique overaction postoperatively. Patients need to be aware that they will never be able to elevate the affected eye normally in adduction.

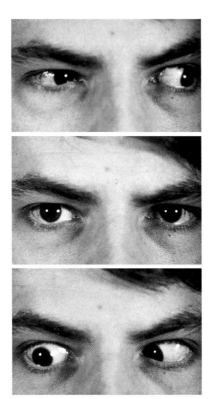

Fig. 26.1 Duane's syndrome affecting the right eye. In primary position *(middle)*, the eyes are aligned. There is a reduction in the right palpebral fissure height on left gaze *(top)* and right upper eyelid retraction as well as an abduction deficit on right gaze *(bottom)*. (From Burde RM, Savino PJ, Trobe JD: *Clinical decisions in neuro-ophthalmology,* ed 3, St. Louis, 2002, Mosby.)

KEY POINTS: BROWN'S SYNDROME

1. Inability to elevate the affected eye when adducted.
2. Hypertropia may be present in primary gaze.
3. The patient may turn their head away from the affected eye with a chin-up position.
4. Ten percent of cases are bilateral.
5. Forced adduction reveals superior oblique muscle restriction.

14. What is the differential diagnosis of Brown's syndrome?
    - **Inferior oblique palsy:** The three-step test reveals a superior oblique overaction that is not present in Brown's syndrome. In patients with diplopia, vertical deviations in primary gaze, or an abnormal head position, a superior oblique tenotomy or recession of the contralateral superior rectus is done. Forced ductions reveal no restriction.
    - **Double elevator palsy:** Patients cannot elevate the affected eye in any field of gaze (Fig. 26.3). Ptosis or pseudoptosis may be seen. A chin-up position helps to maintain fusion if a hypotropia is present in primary gaze. If no chin-up position is seen with hypotropia, amblyopia is present. Treatment for a large vertical deviation or an abnormal head position is inferior rectus recession, if the inferior rectus is restricted. If no restriction is present, transposition of the medial and lateral rectus toward the superior rectus (Knapp procedure) is indicated.
    - **Blow-out fracture with entrapment of the inferior rectus muscle:** History elucidates this injury and forced ductions show restriction. Confirm with an orbital computed tomographic (CT) scan.
    - **Thyroid disease:** Restriction is found on forced ductions, the strabismus is acquired and incomitant, lid retraction also may be noted. A CT scan reveals enlarged extraocular muscles.

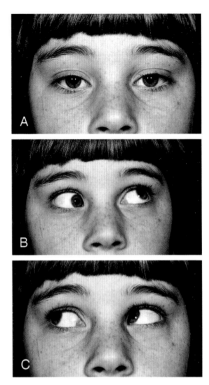

Fig. 26.2 Brown's syndrome affecting the right eye. **A,** Usually straight in the primary position. **B,** Limited right elevation in adduction and occasionally also in the midline. **C,** Usually normal right elevation in abduction. (From Kanski JJ: *Clinical ophthalmology: a systematic approach,* ed 5, Butterworth-Heinemann, 2003, New York.)

15. What is Möbius syndrome?

    This is a congenital syndrome with varying abnormalities of the fifth through twelfth cranial nerves. Patients may have a unilateral or bilateral esotropia with inability to abduct the eyes even on doll's head maneuvers. Patients also may exhibit limb, chest, and tongue defects and may have significant feeding difficulties.

16. A 48-year-old man undergoes medial rectus resection and lateral rectus recession for a sensory exotropia of 35 prism diopters in the left eye. He presents the next day with an exotropia of 60 prism diopters in primary position and an inability to abduct the eye. What is your diagnosis?

    The diagnosis is a slipped or lost medial rectus muscle. It is important to double-lock the suture through the tendon and muscle when reattaching the rectus muscle to the globe to prevent this complication. Reoperation is necessary to find the muscle and reattach it in the appropriate position. If you cannot locate the muscle, a transposition of the superior and inferior rectus muscles helps to correct the exotropia.

17. A patient complains that her right eye is hypertropic. The light-reflex test and covering test show her to be orthophoric. What may be going on?

    Pseudohypertropia. She may have a vertically displaced macula from retinopathy of prematurity or toxocariasis. Eyelid retraction of the right eye may cause the right eye to appear hypertropic. Vertical displacement of the globe superiorly by a mass, such as a mucocele, may cause a similar appearance.

18. A young boy has developed chin-up position and seems to move his head rather than his eyes to locate objects. On examination, he has poor ductions and versions in all fields of gaze as well as bilateral ptosis. Forced ductions reveal restrictions in all extraocular muscles. What is your diagnosis?

    The diagnosis is congenital fibrosis syndrome. The normal muscle tissue is replaced by fibrous tissue to varying degrees. It may be unilateral or bilateral. The eyes may exhibit little to no vertical or horizontal movements, depending on the number of muscles involved, as well as esotropia or exotropia. Amblyopia is common. Ptosis with chin elevation is a frequent manifestation. The cause is unknown. The goal of surgery is to restore orthophoria in primary gaze.

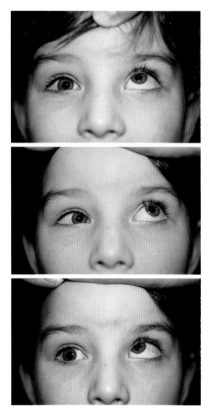

Fig. 26.3 Right monoelevation deficit showing defective elevation in all positions. (From Kanski JJ: *Clinical ophthalmology: a systematic approach,* ed 5, New York, 2003, Butterworth-Heinemann.)

19. A 20-year-old man with no history of strabismus complains that he cannot open his eyes well. You notice that ductions and versions are severely reduced and that he has bilateral ptosis. There is no restriction on forced ductions. What is your diagnosis?

    The diagnosis is chronic progressive external ophthalmoplegia (CPEO). This condition begins in childhood with ptosis and progresses slowly to total paresis of the eyelids and extraocular muscles (Fig. 26.4). It may be sporadic or familial. Patients usually do not have diplopia. A frontalis sling procedure may be necessary to elevate the eyelids.

20. What other evaluations are important?

    Check for retinal pigmentations, and order an electrocardiogram to check for heart block. The triad of CPEO, retinal pigmentary changes, and cardiomyopathy is known as Kearns-Sayre syndrome (Fig. 26.5). Patients may require pacemakers to prevent sudden death. Inheritance is by maternal mitochondrial DNA.

21. What other diseases may be associated with chronic progressive external ophthalmoplegia?

    • **Abetalipoproteinemia (Bassen-Kornzweig syndrome):** Patients have retinal pigmentary changes similar to retinitis pigmentosa (RP), diarrhea, ataxia, and other neurologic signs.
    • **Refsum's disease:** Patients have an RP-like syndrome with an increased phytanic acid level. They also may have neurologic signs.
    • **Ocular pharyngeal dystrophy:** Patients have difficulty with swallowing. The condition may be autosomal dominant.

22. What is congenital ocular motor apraxia?

    In this rare disorder, patients are unable to generate normal voluntary horizontal saccades. To change horizontal fixation, a head thrust that overshoots the target is made. The head is then rotated back in the opposite direction once fixation is established. Vertical saccades are normal, but vestibular and optokinetic nystagmus are impaired. Strabismus may be associated.

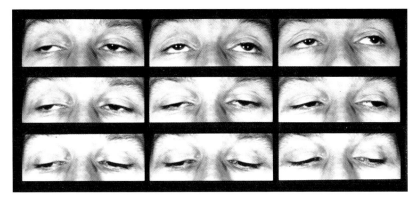

Fig. 26.4 Chronic progressive external ophthalmoplegia. (From Kanski JJ: *Clinical ophthalmology: a test yourself Atlas,* ed 2, New York, 2002, Butterworth-Heinemann.)

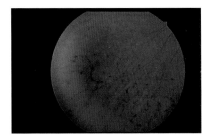

Fig. 26.5 Kearns-Sayre syndrome with retinal pigmentary changes. (From Kanski JJ: *Clinical ophthalmology: a test yourself Atlas,* ed 2, New York, 2002, Butterworth-Heinemann.)

23. A patient complains of diplopia. On examination, he has paresis of the third, fourth, and fifth cranial nerves on the right side. What can cause multiple ocular motor nerve palsies?

Anything that damages the cavernous sinus and/or superior orbital fissure, including the following:
- Arteriovenous fistula—carotid–cavernous sinus dural shunts
- Cavernous sinus thrombosis
- Tumors metastatic to cavernous sinus
- Skin malignancy with perineural spread to the cavernous sinus
- Pituitary apoplexy—patients often have extreme headaches with bilateral signs and decreased vision; need emergent intravenous steroids and neurosurgical consultation
- Intracavernous aneurysm
- Mucormycosis—more likely in diabetics, especially in ketoacidosis, and any debilitated or immunocompromised patient; look for an eschar in the nose and palate; emergent consultation with otolaryngology for débridement imperative
- Herpes zoster
- Tolosa-Hunt syndrome—acute idiopathic inflammation of the superior orbital fissure or anterior cavernous sinus (diagnosis of exclusion)
- Mucocele
- Meningioma
- Nasopharyngeal carcinoma

Multiple cranial nerve palsies also may occur with brain-stem lesions and carcinomatous meningitis. Other entities that can mimic multiple cranial nerve palsies include:
- Myasthenia gravis
- CPEO
- Orbital lesions such as thyroid disease, pseudotumor, or tumor
- Progressive supranuclear palsy
- Guillain-Barré's syndrome

24. **What is Parinaud's syndrome?**

Also known as dorsal midbrain syndrome, Parinaud's syndrome is characterized by a supranuclear gaze paresis with nuclear oculomotor paresis and pupillary abnormalities. Active upward gaze is diminished, but elevation is seen with a doll's head maneuver. Attempts at upward gaze cause retraction-convergence nystagmus and palpebral fissure widening (Collier's sign). Pupils are middilated and do not react to light but react normally to accommodation.

25. **What is the cause of Parinaud's syndrome?**

In children, pinealoma and aqueductal stenosis are the most common causes. In adults, demyelination, infarct, and tumor are most common.

26. **Describe the presentation of a patient with internuclear ophthalmoplegia.**

A young woman with a history of optic neuritis complains of double vision when looking to one side. She is unable to adduct on attempted contralateral gaze and exhibits horizontal nystagmus in the abducting eye. Adduction on convergence is normal. The condition may be unilateral or bilateral. Exotropia may be present if the condition is bilateral.

27. **Where is the causative lesion?**

The lesion is in the medial longitudinal fasciculus. Causes include multiple sclerosis, ischemic vascular disease, brainstem tumor, and trauma.

BIBLIOGRAPHY

American Academy of Ophthalmology: Basic and Clinical Science Course, Section 6: Pediatric ophthalmology and strabismus, San Francisco, 2019-2020, American Academy of Ophthalmology.

Gervasio K, Peck T: The Wills eye manual, ed 8, Philadelphia, 2021, Wolters Kluwer.

Nelson LB, Catalano RA: Atlas of ocular motility, Philadelphia, 1989, W.B. Saunders.

CHAPTER 27

STRABISMUS SURGERY

Bruce M. Schnall

1. **How are forced ductions performed?**

   Before beginning surgery, place an eyelid speculum in both eyes. Using one- or two-toothed forceps, grasp the conjunctiva at the limbus. Move the eye horizontally and vertically. The resistance encountered in moving the eye is compared with what normally would be expected, as well as with the resistance encountered in performing the same forced duction on the other eye.

2. **Why perform forced ductions?**

   Forced ductions are performed to detect "tight muscles" or restrictions in eye movement. If the forced ductions indicate that a muscle is restricted, the affected muscle should be recessed. For example, if a patient has a vertical deviation, the superior rectus on the hypertropic side or the inferior rectus on the fellow eye may be recessed. If forced ductions show resistance to elevating the fellow eye, the preferred surgery is recession of the inferior rectus.

3. **When correcting a horizontal or vertical strabismus, how do you decide how many muscles to recess or resect?**

   The angle of the deviation determines the number of muscles to recess or resect. Whereas a small-angle strabismus (<20 D) may be corrected by operating on one muscle only, a large deviation may require surgery on three or four rectus muscles. Most major texts contain tables that provide a guide as to how much surgery should be performed for the angle (measured in prism diopters) of strabismus. The tables indicate how many muscles should be operated on and the amount of recession or resection.

4. **When doing a recess–resect procedure, should you first perform the recession or the resection?**

   The recession is performed first. In a resection, the muscle is shortened and then brought forward to the insertion. This procedure creates tension on the resected muscle, making it difficult to bring the resected muscle to the insertion site. Initial recession of the antagonist muscle decreases the tension pulling the globe away from the resected muscle and makes it easier to bring the resected muscle to the insertion site and to tie the sutures tightly.

5. **When performing surgery on an oblique muscle and rectus muscle of the same eye, on which muscle do you operate first?**

   The oblique muscles are more difficult to identify and isolate on the muscle hook than the recti. Strabismus surgery creates swelling of the Tenon's capsule and bleeding, which can obscure the view and make identification of the oblique muscles difficult. Therefore, it is preferable to operate on the oblique muscles first when the Tenon's capsule and the tissues surrounding the oblique muscles are the least swollen and distorted. The recti are more easily hooked and identified. There should be no difficulty in isolating the correct rectus muscle, even in the presence of significant bleeding and swelling of the Tenon's capsule following oblique muscle surgery.

6. **What type of needle is used to suture the muscle to the sclera?**

   A spatulated needle has cutting surfaces only on the side and is flat on the bottom. This decreases the risk of perforating the globe. The sclera is thinnest just posterior to the insertion of the rectus muscles (0.3 mm).

7. **How long and how deep should the spatulated needle be passed though the sclera when suturing the muscle to the globe?**

   A scleral pass of 2 mm in length and 20% depth will adequately secure the muscle to the globe. The amount of force needed to rupture a scleral tunnel of 2 mm length and 20% depth would exceed that needed to break a 6-0 vicryl suture.

8. **What is an adjustable suture?**

   Various techniques of placing and tying scleral sutures allow the muscle to be moved forward or backward during the immediate postoperative period. If a patient has an immediate overcorrection or undercorrection, the muscle can be moved to improve the alignment. This suture adjustment is performed within 24 hours of the initial surgery, often in the office.

9. **When is an adjustable suture used?**

   The use of an adjustable suture is at the discretion of the surgeon. Some surgeons do not perform adjustable suture surgery, citing the fact that the correction seen immediately after strabismus surgery is variable and may not be indicative of the long-term result. Others use adjustable sutures in cases in which the results of strabismus surgery are difficult to predict, such as reoperations and restrictive or paralytic strabismus.

10. **What is a transposition procedure?**
In a transposition procedure, the direction the eye moves when the extraocular muscle contracts is changed. A transposition procedure usually involves placing the partial or entire tendon of the adjacent rectus muscles to the insertion of the palsied or underacting muscle. For instance, in double-elevator palsy, the tendon of the lateral and medial recti may be sutured to the nasal and temporal borders of the superior rectus insertion.

11. **When is a transposition procedure performed?**
A transposition procedure is the procedure of choice when the function of one or more rectus muscles is severely limited, as with third-nerve, sixth-nerve, or double-elevator palsy.

12. **When performing vertical rectus transposition to treat a sixth-nerve palsy, do you transpose both vertical recti or just one of the vertical recti?**
One or both vertical recti can be transposed. Historically, the superior and inferior recti are transposed temporally to treat a sixth-nerve palsy. More recently, superior rectus transposition with recession of the medial rectus has been shown to be effective in treatment of sixth-nerve palsy. Transposing only the superior rectus reduces the risk of anterior segment ischemia.

13. **How are A and V patterns of strabismus treated?**
In cases of oblique muscle overaction, the appropriate oblique muscle should be weakened. Weakening of the inferior oblique muscles corrects a V pattern, whereas weakening of the superior oblique muscles corrects an A pattern (Fig. 27.1). In patients with no oblique muscle dysfunction, the horizontal recti are supraplaced or infraplaced. The medial recti are displaced toward the point of the A or V pattern, whereas the lateral recti are moved in the opposite direction. A useful acronym is MALE, which stands for *m*edial recti to the *a*pex, *l*ateral recti to the *e*mpty space. For example, to treat a V-pattern esotropia without oblique muscle overaction, the medial recti are recessed and infraplaced (moved inferiorly) by half of the tendon width.

14. **What surgery can be done for Brown's syndrome?**
In Brown's syndrome, a congenitally short or tight superior oblique tendon creates a mechanical restriction of elevation when the eye is in adduction, as confirmed at surgery with forced duction testing. Brown's syndrome is treated surgically by superior oblique tenotomy, recession, or a tendon expander.

15. **What are the indications for surgery in Brown's syndrome?**
Hypotropia in primary gaze and abnormal head position (face-turn or chin-up position) are indications for surgery. A significant deviation in primary gaze or abnormal head posture is the indication for strabismus surgery in most incomitant strabismus (Brown's, Duane, superior oblique palsy, inferior oblique palsy, and monocular elevation deficit.)

16. **In strabismus surgery in patients with Duane's syndrome, is it better to recess or resect?**
Resection would increase the globe retraction; therefore, resections are avoided. Recessions or, less commonly, transposition procedures are performed.

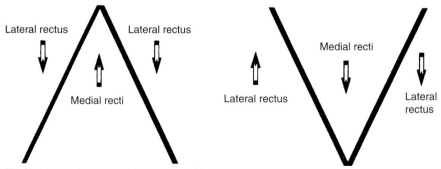

Fig. 27.1 Displacement of horizontal arch in the treatment of A- and V-pattern strabismus. *MALE, M*edial recti to the *a*pex, *l*ateral recti to *e*mpty space.

KEY POINTS: MOST COMMON COMPLICATIONS OF STRABISMUS SURGERY

1. Overcorrection or undercorrection
2. Anterior segment ischemia
3. Infection
4. Adherence syndrome
5. Diplopia
6. Scleral perforation
7. Slipped or lost muscle
8. Operating on the wrong muscle

17. **What are the signs of infection after strabismus surgery?**

    Signs of infection are cellulitis, subconjunctival abscess, or endophthalmitis. Cellulitis is most common, with an estimated incidence between 1 case in 1000 and 1 case in 1900 surgeries. It typically begins 1 to 7 days after surgery. The most common symptoms are marked swelling and pain. Suspected cellulitis requires prompt treatment with systemic antibiotics as well as careful examination to make certain that the patient does not develop endophthalmitis.

18. **What are the signs and symptoms of endophthalmitis after pediatric strabismus surgery?**

    The signs of endophthalmitis appear 1 to 7 days after surgery and include lethargy, asymmetric eye redness, eyelid swelling, and fever. Patients who develop endophthalmitis experience an increase in eyelid swelling and redness during the postoperative period rather than a decrease, as expected during a normal postoperative course. On examination, the patient has a decreased red reflex and signs of vitreal inflammation. Prompt evaluation and treatment are required if endophthalmitis is suspected.

19. **What should you do if you suspect that you perforated the globe when passing the scleral suture?**

    If a scleral perforation is suspected, indirect ophthalmoscopy should be performed in the operating room at completion of the strabismus surgery. If a retinal perforation is seen on ophthalmoscopy, retinal consultation or repeat examinations with the indirect ophthalmoscope are indicated. Treatment is controversial. Whereas some surgeons advocate treatment with cryotherapy or indirect laser, others simply observe the patient. The incidence of retinal detachment after scleral perforation is believed to be low. At the same time, cryotherapy may increase the incidence of retinal detachment by stimulating vitreous changes. In patients predisposed to retinal detachment (for example, high myopes), however, serious consideration should be given to treatment of a retinal perforation at the time of strabismus surgery. Some strabismus surgeons believe that scleral perforation increases the risk of endophthalmitis and therefore recommend a sub-Tenon's injection of prophylactic antibiotics if the globe is perforated.

20. **What is a slipped muscle?**

    The muscle is contained within a capsule. While operating on a rectus muscle, it is possible to mistakenly engage only the capsule on the suture. After the muscle is reattached to the eye, it may slip back within its capsule, which results in further weakening of the muscle and consecutive deviation. For instance, if a slipped muscle occurred in recessing a medial rectus muscle for esotropia, exotropia and limited adduction will develop in the involved eye over time.

21. **How is a slipped muscle prevented?**

    When placing the suture through the muscle, make locking bites on either end of the muscle. Locking bites are made by placing the suture through the muscle perpendicular to its insertion, engaging the tendon, rather than tangentially. Tangential placement may engage only the capsule.

22. **What is the adherence syndrome?**

    The orbital fat is separated from the globe by the Tenon's capsule. If an accidental opening is made in the portion of the Tenon's capsule that separates the orbital fat from the sclera, orbital fat may be pressed through the opening and adhere to the globe. This adherence often results in limited eye moments. It is best treated by prevention. Because the orbital fat comes forward around the equator of the globe to within 10 mm of the limbus, care should be taken not to cut the Tenon's capsule more than 10 mm from the limbus.

23. **How can strabismus surgery cause anterior segment ischemia?**

    The anterior ciliary arteries accompany the rectus muscles. They penetrate the sclera at the muscle's insertion site, contributing significantly to the blood supply of the anterior segment. In standard strabismus surgery, the anterior ciliary vessels are cut when the rectus muscle is disinserted.

24. How is anterior segment ischemia avoided?

Anterior segment ischemia is avoided by not operating on more than two rectus muscles in one eye at the same time. It is also possible to dissect the anterior ciliary vessels from the rectus muscle and preserve them. Surgery to preserve the anterior ciliary vessels is performed only when the risk of anterior segment ischemia is high, such as in older patients with cardiovascular disease or patients with a history of previous rectus muscle surgery.

BIBLIOGRAPHY

Awad AH, Mullaney PB, Al-Hazmi A, et al.: Recognized globe perforation during strabismus surgery: incidence, risk factors, and sequelae, J AAPOS 4:150–153, 2000.

Brooks SE: Securing extraocular muscles in strabismus surgery: how strong is the sclera? Ophthalmology 124(11):1712–1713, 2017.

Kivlin JD, Wilson ME, The Periocular Infection Study Group: Periocular infection after strabismus surgery, J Pediatr Ophthalmol Strabismus 32:42–49, 1995.

Mehendale RA, Dagi LE, Wu C, et al.: Superior rectus transposition and medial rectus recession for Duane syndrome and sixth nerve palsy, Arch Ophthalmol 130(2):195–201, 2012.

McKeown CA, Shore JW, Lambert HM: Preservation of the anterior ciliary vessels during extraocular muscle surgery, Ophthalmology 96:498–506, 1989.

Parks MM, Bloom JN: The "slipped muscle," Ophthalmology 86:1389–1396, 1979.

Recchia FM, Baumal CR, Sivalingam A, et al.: Endophthalmitis after pediatric strabismus surgery, Arch Ophthalmol 118:939–944, 2000.

Rubin SE, Nelson LB: Complications of strabismus surgery, Ophthalmol Clin North Am 5:157–164, 1992.

Schnall BM, Feingold A: Infection following strabismus surgery, Curr Opin Ophthalmol 29(5):407–401, 2018.

Sprunger DT, Klapper SR, Bonnis JM, Minturn JT: Management of experimental globe perforation during strabismus surgery, J Pediatr Ophthalmol Strabismus 33:140–143, 1996.

CHAPTER 28

NYSTAGMUS

Andrew P. Shyu and Jonathan H. Salvin

1. **What is nystagmus?**

   Nystagmus is an involuntary ocular movement of the eyes. Typically, it has a pathologic slow eye movement followed by a fast eye movement. The movements can be exclusively horizontal, vertical, torsional, or combinations of all three. Nystagmus may be congenital (present within the first 6–8 weeks of life), present in early childhood, or have acquired causes in adulthood.

2. **How is nystagmus generally classified?**

   Nystagmus can be classified based on movement, amplitude and frequency. Table 28.1 details some types of nystagmus based on their movement, amplitude, and waveform. It may be further broken down to early-onset nystagmus or acquired forms of nystagmus. If the amplitude of the oscillations differs, the nystagmus would be characterized as a disconjugate nystagmus. If the direction of the oscillations differs, the nystagmus is considered a disjunctive nystagmus. In this chapter, we will mainly focus on childhood nystagmus and a few key signs of acquired nystagmus.

3. **Can nystagmus be seen in patients without pathologic disease?**

   Yes—the most common forms are physiologic end-gaze nystagmus, caloric nystagmus, and optokinetic nystagmus (OKN). End-gaze nystagmus is an exhaustible horizontal nystagmus in extreme side gaze. The caloric nystagmus is stimulated when warm or cold water is placed in the ear canal to activate the horizontal semicircles. Cold water stimulates a jerk nystagmus to the opposite side of the ear, whereas warm water stimulates a jerk nystagmus to the same side. In OKN, a nystagmus can be seen when a patient follows large moving objects. If an OKN drum was turned to the right, one would see a slow movement to the right and a jerk nystagmus to the left.

4. **Do nystagmus patients see well?**

   It varies based on if there is an underlying sensory or motor cause of the nystagmus. Many of these patients have underlying eye pathology that affects sensory visual input such as cataracts, optic nerve hypoplasia,

Table 28.1 Nystagmus Classifications		
	AMPLITUDE	**WAVEFORM**
Jerk nystagmus	Slow wave followed by fast wave	Linear
Pendular nystagmus	Slow wave followed by slow wave	
Saccadic intrusions	Fast wave followed by fast wave	(Square wave jerk)

Table 28.2	Evolution of Different Nystagmus Movements
AGE	**ACTION**
6 weeks	Wide pendular movements with apparent poor visual behavior
6–8 months	Smaller pendular waveforms
18–24 months	Jerk type movements with possible formation of a null point

albinism, or other intraocular disease that cause decreased acuity and subsequent development of nystagmus. In those who do not have other eye disease (primary motor nystagmus), the nystagmus itself limits fixation time (foveation) and thus may decrease visual acuity.

5. Do affected patients see the world moving constantly?
Oscillopsia is the symptomatic perception of the visual world moving from variable eye movements. In early-onset nystagmus, most patients do not experience oscillopsia. It has been speculated that retinal information is only sampled during foveation and suppressive mechanisms are in place during eye motion—like a strobe light effect. In some forms of adult acquired nystagmus and other irregular eye movement disorders (such as opsoclonus), there may be symptomatic oscillopsia.

6. Are patients with well-adapted nystagmus (i.e., no oscillopsia or diplopia) able to see their own eyes move when they look in a mirror?
No, they cannot see their own eyes move in a mirror. The presumption is that the eye movements match the mirrored image, so they do not see it. A video of the eye movements may be shown to show a patient what he or she looks like to others.

7. Is photophobia common with nystagmus?
If photophobia is associated with nystagmus, primary sensory nystagmus should be considered. Patients with achromatopsia or albinism may have photophobia and present with nystagmus. However, congenital motor nystagmus generally does not present with photophobia.

8. What is the null point in nystagmus?
The null point is the direction of gaze in respect to orbital coordinates that minimize the amplitude and frequency of nystagmus. Because a position of gaze that minimizes the nystagmus allows better vision, it is common for patients to seek out the null zone with an anomalous head position if the null point is not in primary gaze.

9. What is nystagmus blockage syndrome?
Patients find that convergence dampens their nystagmus and manifest a large angle esotropia as their null point. They may manifest a face turn toward the fixating adducted eye and may alternate face turn with alternating fixation.

10. What is the infantile nystagmus syndrome?
Typically, this is a binocular conjugate horizontal nystagmus that tends to stay horizontal in all gazes. It can be categorized as a primary sensory nystagmus associated with visual impairments such as optic nerve hypoplasia, albinism, congenital cataracts, retinopathy of prematurity, or other intraocular pathology. When it is unrelated to any other eye pathology, it can be considered a primary motor nystagmus. Table 28.2 details the evolution of different nystagmus movements that may be seen in infantile nystagmus syndrome (INS) as patients get older.

11. What are the most common underlying sensory defects in infantile nystagmus syndrome?
Please refer to Table 28.3.

12. Does infantile nystagmus syndrome ever disappear spontaneously?
Generally no. However, entities such as spasmus nutans can resolve (see question 21 for further details.)

13. What would be observed in patients with congenital nystagmus and an optokinetic nystagmus drum rotating to the left?
In patients with INS, a reversal of the normal OKN would be observed. Therefore, one would see a left beating nystagmus if the OKN drum is rotating to the left. In addition, there is also an exponential increase in the slow phase of the eye movement in congenital nystagmus.

14. Should a magnetic resonance imaging be obtained in patients with infantile nystagmus syndrome?
A full ophthalmologic examination should be performed looking for an intraocular cause of the nystagmus. Neuroimaging of the brain and visual pathways should be obtained if no intraocular cause is found or if there are findings consistent with neurologic deficits with central nervous system (CNS) comorbities. For example, if optic nerve hypoplasia is found, imaging should be ordered to evaluate for other midline CNS defects. If there is optic atrophy or pallor found, then a magnetic resonance imaging (MRI) is indicated to look for midbrain lesion. If

Table 28.3 Sensory Defects in Infantile Nystagmus Syndrome	
ABNORMALITY	**DEFECT**
Bilateral anterior segment abnormalities	Congenital cataract Congenital glaucoma Iridocorneal dysgenesis
Primary retinal abnormalities	Leber congenital amaurosis Achromatopsia Blue-cone monochromatism Congenital stationary night blindness
Bilateral vitreoretinal abnormalities	Severe ROP Chorioretinal or optic nerve coloboma Retinoblastoma Familial exudative vitreoretinopathy Norrie disease Retinal dysplasia TORCH
Foveal hypoplasia	Albinism Aniridia Isolated foveal hypoplasia
Bilateral optic nerve disorders	Optic nerve hypoplasia Optic nerve coloboma

ROP, Retinopathy of prematurity; *TORCH*, TORCH is an acronym for (T)oxoplasmosis, (O)ther agents, (R)ubella, (C)ytomegalovirus, and (H)erpes Simplex.

spasmus nutans is considered, then an MRI of the brain should also be obtained to look for conditions that can present similarly and have a very different prognosis and treatment (see question 21).

15. Most patients with infantile nystagmus syndrome have vision that is better at near than at distance. Why?
    Most patients have an accommodative convergence:accommodation (AC:A) ratio that results in exophoria at near. The patient uses fusional convergence to overcome the exophoria. Fusional convergence dampens the nystagmus amplitude and frequency and in so doing improves the vision.

16. Because convergence improves vision, should minus lenses be used to stimulate accommodative convergence?
    No. Only fusional convergence (i.e., overcoming exophoria) dampens nystagmus. Accommodative convergence does not dampen nystagmus and even works against the patient by increasing accommodative demands and may cause the near point to recede with reduced visual acuity at near.

17. Do contact lenses help with nystagmus?
    There have been reports of decreased nystagmus with contact lens use. Many patients with nystagmus have significant astigmatism. Those that do may be helped with toric contact lenses, particularly if the null point is eccentric at points where spectacles distort the images. However, the nystagmus may make toric contact lens fitting difficult because of the constant eye movements causing shifting of the lens off axis.

18. Aside from using a full screen of letters, what should one do when checking the visual acuity of a nystagmus patient with unexpected poor vision?
    Be sure to measure binocular visual acuity first. If binocular vision is better, try blurring the nonfixing eye with a high plus (+6.00 or higher) lens and ask the patient to read with the opposite eye. Many patients will have worsening nystagmus with monocular occlusion (latent nystagmus), which makes measuring monocular acuity difficult.

19. What nonsurgical treatment options should be considered for these patients?
    Try glasses first to maximize the visual acuity. Many of these patients will have high astigmatic errors that should be corrected. Prisms (with the apices pointed towards the null point) can be used in the glasses to attempt to shift the eyes into the null position. Prisms can also be used to stimulate convergence, which can sometimes dampen nystagmus.

20. What surgical treatment options should be considered?
    If the patient has an anomalous head position, performing a Kestenbaum-Anderson recession-resection procedure will rotate the eyes toward the direction of the head turn (away from the null position). Recession of all

four horizontal recti muscles to positions behind the equator has been reported to be effective in improving visual function without significant face turns. Disinsertion and reattachment to the original insertion has been reported to have similar effects.

21. **What is spasmus nutans and what are the characteristics of the condition?**
    Spasmus nutans is an acquired form of nystagmus that arises in the first 2 years of life. It is a benign condition that generally resolves by 3–4 years of age. It consists of the triad of (1) high-frequency, small-amplitude shimmering nystagmus, (2) head nodding, and (3) torticollis. It can be monocular or asymmetric and multiplanar. CNS MRI should be obtained to look for lesions that can mimic it, such as pontine gliomas.

22. **What is a monocular vertical pendular nystagmus that can also mimic spasmas mutans?**
    Heimann-Bielschowsky is a monocular nystagmus that occurs in eyes with poor vision due to optic nerve gliomas, amblyopia, or other causes. Because of this, an MRI of the brain is always indicated in spasmas mutans to rule out optic nerve glioma or other midbrain pathology.

23. **What is latent nystagmus (also known as fusion maldevelopment nystagmus)?**
    This is a jerk nystagmus that is evident only with monocular occlusion. It is typically associated with other pathology that results in poor fusion development early in life, such as strabismus or significant amblyopia. Latent nystagmus can decompensate to manifest nystagmus present even when the patient is viewing things binocularly.

24. **Clinically, how do you distinguish manifest latent nystagmus from infantile nystagmus syndrome?**
    As you occlude each eye in manifest latent nystagmus (MLN), the direction of the jerk changes toward the fixing eye. With INS, the direction of the nystagmus remains constant on covering either eye, but the direction of the nystagmus fast phase changes when you cross to the other side of the null zone. In addition, there is an exponential decrease in the slow phase velocity in MLN, whereas congenital motor nystagmus in INS may have an exponential increase in the slow phase velocity.

25. **Are there distinctive patterns of nystagmus associated with specific ocular pathology?**
    Achromatopsia is somewhat distinctive as it evolves to an oblique direction from a horizontal pendular direction. Acquired downbeat nystagmus is generally medication induced (alcohol, anticonvulsants, lithium) or localized to a cervicomedullary lesion. Acquired upbeat nystagmus is generally localized to a cerebellar or medullary lesion. See-saw nystagmus is generally localized to a suprasellar lesion.

26. **What is alternating in periodic alternating nystagmus?**
    Periodic alternating nystagmus, or central vestibular instability nystagmus, is a horizontal nystagmus that alternates in the direction of the fast phase. Patients may develop alternating head turns toward the fast phase to compensate for the changing direction of the null position.

27. **What is the time cycle of period alternating nystagmus?**
    60–90 seconds with intervals of 10–20 seconds without nystagmus in between alternations.

28. **Is congenital periodic alternating nystagmus commonly associated with any other ocular problem?**
    Oculocutaneous albinism is the most common association—and most commonly overlooked.

29. **Does acquired periodic alternating nystagmus imply central nervous system pathology?**
    Midbrain and cervicomedullary pathologies are the most common etiologies in acquired alternating nystagmus. In addition, the nystagmus is often overlooked if the patient compensates well by changing head position.

KEY POINTS: REFRACTION FOR NYSTAGMUS

To get the best visual acuity in a patient with nystagmus:
1. Use careful dry and cycloplegic refraction.
2. Correct all astigmatism.
3. Use top line of full projector screen.
4. Watch for latent nystagmus—add +4.00 to +6.00 to the nonfixating eye to blur rather than occluding.

BIBLIOGRAPHY

Abadi RV, Whittle JP, Worfolk R: Oscillopsia and tolerance to retinal Image movement in congenital nystagmus, Invest Ophthalmol Vest Sci 40:339–345, 1999.
Barot N, McLean RJ, Gottlob I, Proudlock FA: Reading performance in infantile nystamgus, Ophthalmology 2013; 120:1232–1238.
Childhood nystagmus. In Basic and Clinical Science Course Section 6: Pediatric Ophthalmology, 2018, Academy of Ophthalmology, pp 147–158.

Felius J, Muhanna ZA: Visual deprivation and foveation characteristics both underlie visual acuity deficits in idiopathic infantile nystagmus, Invest Ophthalmol Vis Sci 54:3520–3525, 2013.

Gottlob I: Nystagmus, Curr Opin Ophthalmol 9:V32–V38, 1998.

Gottlob I: Eye movement abnormalities in carriers of the blue cone monochromatism, Invest Ophthalmol Vest Sci 35:3556–3560, 1994.

Gottlob I, Proudlock FA: Aetiology of infantile nystagmus, Curr Opin Neurol 27:83–91, 2014.

Gradstein L, Reinecke RD, Wizov SS, Goldstein HP: Congenital periodic alternating nystagmus, Ophthalmology 104:918–929, 1997.

Hertle RW, National Eye Institute Sponsored Classification of Eye Movement Abnormalities and Strabismus Working Group: A next step in naming and classification of eye movement disorders and strabismus, J AAPOS 6(4):201–202, 2002.

Jacob FD, Ramaswamy V, Goez HR: Acquired monocular nystagmus as the initial presenting sign of a chiasmal glioma, Can J Neurol Sci 37(1):96–97, 2010.

Jacobson L: Visual dysfunction and ocular signs associated with periventricular leukomalacia in children born preterm, Acta Ophthalmol Scand 77:365–366, 1999.

Healey N, McLoone E, Mahon G, Jackson AJ, Saunders KJ, McClelland JF.: Investigating the relationship between foveal morphology and refractive error in a population with infantile nystagmus syndrome, Invest Ophthalmol Vis Sci 54:2934–2939, 2013.

Kerrison J, Koenekoop RK, Arnould VJ, et al.: Clinical features of autosomal dominant congenital nystagmus linked to chromosome 6p12, Am J Ophthalmol 125:64–70, 1998.

Kerrison J, Vagefi MR, Barmada MM, Maumenee IH: Congenital motor nystagmus linked to Xq26-q27, Am J Human Genet 64:600–607, 1999.

Maybodi M: Infantile-onset nystagmus, Curr Opin in Ophthalmol 14:276–285, 2003.

Mellott ML, Brown J Jr., Fingert JH, et al.: Clinical characterization and linkage analysis of a family with congenital x-linked nystagmus and deuteranomaly, Arch Ophthalmol 117:1630–1633, 1999.

Reinecke RD: Idiopathic infantile nystagmus: diagnosis and treatment, AAPOS 1:67–82, 1997.

Smith JL, Flynn JT, Spiro HJ: Monocular vertical oscillations of amblyopia. The Heimann-Bielschowsky phenomenon, J Clin Neuroophthalmol 2(2):85–91, 1982.

Stahl J, Averbuch-Heller L, Leigh RJL: Acquired nystagmus, Arch Ophthalmol 118:544–549, 2000.

Strupp M, Kremmyda O, Brandt T: Pharmacotherapy of vestibular disorders and nystagmus, Semin Neurol 33:286–296, 2013.

Sprunger DT, Wasserman BN, Stidham DB: The relationship between nystagmus and survival outcome in congenital esotropia, J AAPOS 4:21–24, 2000.

The patient with nystagmus or spontaneous eye movement disorders. In: Basic and clinical science course (BCSC) Section 5: Neuro-Ophthalmology, 2018, Academy of Ophthalmology, pp 233–252.

CHAPTER 29

THE PUPIL

Archana Srinivasan and Mark L. Moster

1. **What muscles control the size of the pupil? Describe their innervation.**
   The iris sphincter muscle causes pupillary constriction and is innervated by the parasympathetic nervous system. The iris dilator muscle causes pupillary dilation and is innervated by the sympathetic nervous system. Thus, when sympathetic tone is increased, the pupil is larger, and when parasympathetic tone is increased, the pupil is smaller.

2. **Trace the pathway of the parasympathetic innervation of the pupil.**
   Parasympathetic fibers begin in the Edinger-Westphal nucleus in the oculomotor nuclear complex. With cranial nerve (CN) III, they exit the midbrain and travel in the subarachnoid space and cavernous sinus. They follow the inferior division of CN III into the orbit, where they synapse at the ciliary ganglion. Postganglionic fibers are then distributed to the iris sphincter and ciliary body via the short ciliary nerves.

3. **Trace the pathway of the sympathetic innervation of the pupil.**
   The first-order neuron begins in the posterior hypothalamus. The fibers travel caudally to terminate in the intermediolateral cell column of the spinal cord at levels C8–T1, otherwise known as the ciliospinal center of Budge. Pupillomotor fibers exit from the spinal cord and ascend with the sympathetic chain to synapse in the superior cervical ganglion, constituting the second-order (or preganglionic) neuron. The third-order neuron begins with postganglionic fibers of the superior cervical ganglion. These fibers travel with the internal carotid artery to enter the cranial vault. In the cavernous sinus the fibers leave the carotid artery to join the ophthalmic division of CN V and enter the orbit through the superior orbital fissure. The sympathetic fibers reach the ciliary body and dilator of the iris by passing through the nasociliary nerve and long posterior ciliary nerves.

4. **Trace the pathway of the pupillary light reflex.**
   The pupillary light response begins with the rods and cones of the retina. Afferent pupillomotor fibers travel through the optic nerves. Slightly greater than 50% decussate at the optic chiasm. They follow the optic tracts and exit before the lateral geniculate body to enter the brain stem via the brachium of the superior colliculus. Pupillomotor fibers synapse in the pretectal nuclei and then project equally to the ipsilateral and contralateral Edinger-Westphal nuclei. The pupillary fibers travel with CN III to innervate the iris sphincter and cause pupillary constriction, as described in question 2.

5. **What are intrinsically photosensitive retinal ganglion cells? What is their clinical significance?**
   Intrinsically photosensitive (ip) retinal ganglion cells (RGCs) are a small subset of RGCs that contain the photopigment melanopsin, believed to be the third photoreceptor in the human retina, in addition to rods and cones. These are mostly present in the inner plexiform and ganglion cell layers and constitute <1% of all RGCs. Ip RGCs play an important role in the non-image-forming visual functions of the eye, including pupillary light reflex and maintenance of circadian rhythm.
   Several studies in the last decade have shown a relative preservation of the melanopsin RGCs in patients with mitochondrial optic neuropathies, including Leber's hereditary optic neuropathy and dominant optic atrophy. This is responsible for sparing of the pupillary light response seen in some of these patients.

6. **What is an afferent pupillary defect? How should you examine for it?**
   The swinging flashlight test is used to elicit a relative afferent pupillary defect (RAPD). If you shine a light into one eye of a normal subject, both pupils constrict to the same degree. If you swing the light over to the other eye, the pupil stays the same size or constricts minimally. In patients with RAPD, the affected eye behaves as if it perceives a dimmer light than the normal eye; therefore, both pupils constrict to a lesser degree when the light is shone in the affected eye. Thus, if you shine the light in the right eye of a patient with left RAPD, both pupils constrict. If you swing the light to the left eye, it is perceived as dimmer and the pupils dilate. Note that this is a *relative* APD and signifies a difference in the pupillary response between the two eyes. However, if both eyes are equally abnormal, there may be no RAPD (Fig. 29.1).

7. **Damage in which anatomic areas may cause an afferent pupillary defect?**
   A lesion anywhere in the afferent pupillary pathway may cause an RAPD—that is, retina, optic nerve, optic chiasm, optic tract, or along the course of pupillary fibers from the optic tract to the pretectal nuclei. Pupillary fibers leave the optic tract prior to the lateral geniculate body. Therefore, any lesion from the lateral geniculate body posteriorly does not cause an RAPD. A retinal lesion causes an RAPD only if it is rather large. An optic nerve

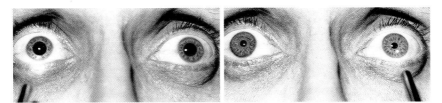

Fig. 29.1 Demonstration of a large afferent defect in the right eye. This is best demonstrated when the light is alternated from eye to eye at a steady rate. The light is kept just below the visual axis and 1 to 2 in (3 to 5 cm) from each eye. Each eye is illuminated for approximately 1 second, then the light is switched quickly to the other eye. This technique allows comparison of the initial direct pupil contraction with light in each eye. (From Kardon RH: The pupil. In Yanoff M, Duker JS, editors: Ophthalmology, ed 2, St. Louis, 2004, Mosby, pp 1360–1369.)

lesion causes an RAPD in the ipsilateral eye. A lesion in the optic chiasm may cause an RAPD if fibers from one optic nerve are affected more than those from the other. An optic tract lesion causes an RAPD in the eye with the most visual field loss. Typically, in patients with a mass lesion of the optic tract, an RAPD is produced in the ipsilateral eye because of ipsilateral optic nerve compression, but an ischemic lesion causes an RAPD in the contralateral eye because slightly more fibers cross than remain uncrossed. A lesion in the brain stem in the area of the pretectal nuclei may cause an RAPD without visual defects if the pupillomotor fibers are affected between the optic tract and the pretectal nuclei.

8. **What is anisocoria? How should one examine a patient with anisocoria?**
   Anisocoria is a difference in the size between the two pupils. In anyone who has anisocoria, the pupil size should be measured in both bright and dim light. If the anisocoria is greater in bright light, the larger pupil is abnormal and constricts poorly, which is usually caused by a defect in parasympathetic innervation. If the anisocoria is greater in dim light, the smaller pupil is abnormal because it dilates poorly, usually because of a defect in pupillary sympathetic innervation. If the relative difference in the size of the two pupils remains the same in bright and dim light, the anisocoria is probably physiologic and not pathologic.

9. **What is the differential diagnosis of a unilateral dilated, poorly reactive pupil?**
   - Third-nerve palsy
   - Pharmacologic paralysis (an anticholinergic medication such as atropine)
   - Adie's tonic pupil
   - Iris damage (e.g., sphincter tears secondary to trauma or posterior synechiae)

10. **What are the clinical findings in CN III palsy?**
    CN III innervates the superior, medial, and inferior recti and inferior oblique and levator palpebrae muscles. Therefore, in a complete CN III palsy, ptosis is complete, and the eye is in the down-and-out position; it does not move up, down, or medially. The parasympathetic nerves that innervate the pupillary sphincter travel with CN III; therefore, if those fibers are affected, the pupil will be dilated and nonreactive.

11. **What are some possible causes of third-nerve palsy?**
    In adults, the most common causes are microvascular ischemia in the nerve, aneurysm (usually of the posterior communicating artery [PCOM]), trauma, and neoplasm. In children, aneurysm is rare, and consideration must be given to ophthalmoplegic migraine although injury, infection, and tumor are more common.

12. **What is the significance of pupil involvement or pupil sparing in third-nerve palsy?**
    Pupil involvement in third-nerve palsy suggests a compressive lesion such as aneurysm or tumor. Pupil sparing is suggestive of microvascular ischemia. The parasympathetic fibers are on the outer portion of CN III and are more susceptible to external compression and less susceptible to ischemia, which is usually axial in the nerve.

13. **What is the appropriate workup for an isolated third-nerve palsy with or without pupillary sparing?**
    In elderly patients with vascular risk factors, the most likely cause is microvascular ischemia. The classic teaching has been that CN III palsy with complete pupillary sparing may simply be followed with the expectation that the ocular misalignment will improve. Although, that is occasionally still done, the recommendation has now evolved, such that all third-nerve palsy patients should have imaging with either magnetic resonance imaging (MRI)/magnetic resonance angiography (MRA) or computed tomography (CT)/computed tomography angiography (CTA) to exclude aneurysm. One must ensure that the radiology request form specifically notes the concern for a PCOM aneurysm rather than being vague about an intracranial pathology. When in doubt, talk to the radiologist directly to make sure the CTA/MRA has adequately excluded an aneurysm. A catheter arteriogram may be necessary if suspicion remains. A medical workup for hypertension or diabetes and giant cell arteritis is appropriate. If there is no improvement in 3 to 6 months, neuroimaging should be repeated. Patients too young

for the vasculopathic age group should all have an MRI and MRA scan. If the scan is negative, other hematologic investigations and lumbar puncture should be considered.

14. **What is an Adie's tonic pupil? What is its natural history?**
Adie's tonic pupil is a postganglionic defect in the parasympathetic innervation to the pupil. The clinical finding is a dilated pupil that is usually slightly irregular and shows segmental iris constriction at the slit lamp. There also is light/near dissociation, with characteristically slow and tonic constriction and redilation phases. This condition is benign and most commonly affects women in their second to fourth decades.

15. **How do you test for an Adie's pupil?**
An Adie's tonic pupil constricts to dilute pilocarpine 0.1% to 0.12%, whereas a normal pupil does not. This is a result of denervation hypersensitivity.

16. **What is Horner's syndrome?**
Horner's syndrome is a clinical syndrome characterized by ptosis, miosis, and occasionally anhidrosis (Fig. 29.2). Any lesion in the sympathetic innervation to the eye can cause this syndrome.

17. **What is the cause of ptosis in Horner's syndrome?**
Ptosis in Horner's syndrome is caused by decreased sympathetic tone in the Mueller's muscle. The Mueller's muscle is responsible for approximately 2 mm of elevation of the upper eyelid. Thus, the ptosis in Horner's syndrome is mild (approximately 2 mm).

18. **What are the possible causes of Horner's syndrome?**
The course of the sympathetic innervation to the eye was discussed in question 3. A lesion anywhere along this course may cause Horner's syndrome. Isolated third-order neuron lesions are concerning for a dissection of the internal carotid artery. Second-order neuron lesions may be caused by apical lung tumors. First-order neuron lesions are uncommon in isolation. They are found in demyelinating disease, cerebrovascular accidents, and neoplasms.

19. **How do you test for Horner's syndrome pharmacologically?**
A cocaine test has been the standard test for Horner's syndrome. Cocaine blocks the reuptake of norepinephrine. A normal pupil dilates in response to a drop of cocaine, whereas in Horner's syndrome, the pupil fails to dilate. Cocaine is often unavailable and has largely been replaced by the apraclonidine (iopidine) test. Apraclonidine, widely available as a glaucoma medication, has mild $\alpha 1$ agonist activity, usually too mild to cause pupillary dilation. However, with Horner's syndrome, there is sympathetic denervation of the pupil and it will dilate to topical stimulation with apraclonidine. Therefore, there will be a reversal of the anisocoria, with the miotic pupil now becoming larger. An additional finding is that the ptosis may resolve as well.

20. **What pharmacologic testing helps to localize the lesion in Horner's syndrome?**
Localization is important because the etiology and possibly the focus of the workup are quite different, depending on whether the lesion is a first-, second-, or third-order neuron. Hydroxyamphetamine 1% causes release of epinephrine from the third-order neuron junction with the iris. Thus, in third-order neuron lesions, there is no pupillary response to hydroxyamphetamine drops. In a first- or second-order neuron lesion, the pupil dilates in response to hydroxyamphetamine drops. Some concerns about hydroxyamphetamine drops include false positives, false negatives, and lack of availability.

21. **What is the appropriate evaluation for a patient with Horner's syndrome?**
Patients suspected of having Horner's syndrome should have apraclonidine or cocaine testing to confirm the diagnosis, unless the diagnosis is obvious. In first few days of an acute Horner's syndrome, pharmacologic testing may still be negative. If testing confirms the syndrome, imaging studies should be performed to evaluate the

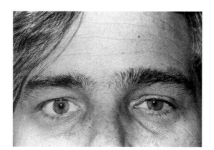

Fig. 29.2 Horner's syndrome with ptosis and miosis on the left. Note that the left lower eyelid is higher than the right lower eyelid. This inverse ptosis is a result of interruption of sympathetic innervation to the analog of the Mueller's muscle in the lower eyelid.

entire course of the sympathetic innervation of the eye, which would include head, neck, upper chest and the internal carotid artery. The protocol for this imaging varies by institution and should be coordinated with the neuroradiologist. Hydroxyamphetamine testing is helpful, but because there are false-positives and false-negatives, it should not be totally relied upon but may be used when it supports the rest of the clinical picture. Additionally, if the clinical symptoms point to a particular site of involvement, more selective imaging may be done.

22. What is light/near dissociation? What are its possible causes?
In light/near dissociation a pupil does not constrict well to light but will constrict better as part of the near response. Causes include Adie's syndrome, dorsal midbrain syndrome (Parinaud's syndrome), Argyll-Robertson pupils, diabetic neuropathy, prior CN III palsy with aberrant regeneration, and visual loss from any anterior afferent cause.

23. What is an Argyll-Robertson pupil?
Argyll-Robertson pupils are small, often irregular pupils that do not react to light but have a brisk near response. The cause of Argyll-Robertson pupils is almost always tertiary syphilis.

24. What is Parinaud's syndrome?
Found in dorsal midbrain disease, this syndrome is composed of light/near dissociation of the pupils, supranuclear paralysis of upward gaze, convergence–retraction nystagmus with attempted upward saccades, and eyelid retraction.

KEY POINTS: MANAGEMENT OF THIRD-NERVE PALSY

1. Pupil involvement in third-nerve palsy suggests a compressive lesion.
2. Pupil-involving third-nerve palsy requires immediate MRI and MRA or CT and CTA. If negative, conventional catheter angiography should be performed in cases in which the MRA or CTA does not fully rule out aneurysm.
3. Pupil-sparing third-nerve palsy in a patient in the vasculopathic age group should be worked up similarly to a pupil-involving CN III palsy with similar neuroimaging according to current thinking.

BIBLIOGRAPHY

Davagnanam I, Fraser L, Miszkiel K, et al.: Adult Horner's syndrome: a combined clinical, pharmacological, and imaging algorithm, Eye 27(3):291–298, 2013.
La Morgia C, Ross-Cisneros F, Hannibal J, et al.: Melanopsin-expressing retinal ganglion cells: implications for human diseases, Vision Res 51(2):296–302, 2011.
Lee A: Third cranial nerve (oculomotor nerve) palsy in adults, Basow DS, editor. Waltham, MA, 2009, UpToDate.
Liu GT, Volpe NJ, Galetta SL: Neuro-ophthalmology, diagnosis and management, ed 3, Philadelphia, PA, 2018, Elsevier.
Miller NR, Newman NJ, Biousse V, Kerrison JB: Walsh and Hoyt's clinical neuro-ophthalmology, 6th ed, Philadelphia, PA, 2005, Lippincott Williams & Wilkins.
Mughal M, Longmuir R: Current pharmacologic testing for Horner syndrome, Curr Neuro Neurosci Rep 9(5):384–389, 2009.
Yanoff M, Duker JS: Ophthalmology, ed 5, Philadelphia, PA, 2018, Elsevier.

CHAPTER 30

DIPLOPIA

Tal J. Rubinstein and Julian D. Perry

1. **What is diplopia?**
   Diplopia is a condition in which the patient perceives two images of a single object. Diplopia may be monocular or binocular, constant or intermittent. Check if the double vision resolves with each eye closed. If it does not, the patient has monocular diplopia. If it does, the patient has binocular diplopia.

2. **List the causes of monocular diplopia.**
   - Refractive error: astigmatism is the most common cause of monocular diplopia
   - Chalazion or other eyelid tumor producing irregular astigmatism
   - Keratopathy: dry eyes, keratoconus, irregular astigmatism (use a retinoscope to see scissoring reflex)
   - Iris atrophy, polycoria, large nonreactive pupil
   - Cataract, subluxated lens, intraocular lens decentration, capsular opacity
   - Retinal disease may produce metamorphopsia or aniseikonia; also consider a psychogenic etiology

3. **What are the causes of binocular diplopia?**
   Causes of binocular diplopia may be grouped into three general categories:
   1. Neuropathic: The pathology may be supranuclear, nuclear, or infranuclear. Specific neuropathic causes include traumatic, vaso-occlusive infarction, compression from a mass, inflammation, infection, demyelination, degeneration, decompensated phorias, spasm of the near reflex, and neuromyotonia.
   2. Myopathic: The pathology is within the extraocular muscles. Causes include inflammatory pseudotumor or myositis and thyroid-related eye disease (TED).
   3. Neuromuscular junction disorders. The major etiology in this category is myasthenia gravis (MG).

4. **What is the most important sign to check for in a third-nerve (oculomotor) palsy?**
   Check for the presence of a dilated, poorly reactive, or nonreactive pupil. A pupil-involving oculomotor palsy is an emergency. An aneurysm must be ruled out. One should be suspicious in a patient with mild anisocoria if the larger pupil is ipsilateral to the side of oculomotor nerve dysfunction. Note that diabetic patients without an aneurysm may nonetheless have pupil-involving third-nerve palsy.

KEY POINTS: CRANIAL NERVE PALSIES

1. A pupil-sparing palsy is probably vasculopathic in adults. In children, obtain a magnetic resonance image or angiography to rule out tumor and aneurysm.
2. To test for trochlear nerve palsy in a patient with an oculomotor palsy, have the patient look down and in to check for intorsion.
3. Primary oculomotor aberrant regeneration (oculomotor synkinesis) suggests a compressive lesion.
4. Sixth-nerve palsy may be a false-localizing sign of elevated intracranial pressure.
5. Always rule out trapdoor, "white-eyed" muscle entrapment in a pediatric facial trauma patient with otherwise seemingly normal-looking eyes.

5. **What is the workup of a pupil-involving third-nerve palsy?**
   In adults, perform magnetic resonance imaging/angiography (MRI/MRA) or spiral computed tomography (CT) angiography. If the results are consistent with an aneurysm or even if the results are negative, consider performing angiography after discussion with neuroradiology and neurosurgery. In children, perform MRI/MRA regardless of the state of the pupil. If the results are negative, children usually do not need an angiogram.

6. **Why do aneurysms involve the pupil in oculomotor nerve palsies, whereas infarctions generally do not?**
   Pupillary parasympathetic fibers travel superficially and dorsomedially in the third nerve as it traverses the subarachnoid space. These fibers are often affected first in a compressive lesion. Ischemic infarction often occurs in the center of the nerve, so the superficial fibers remain unaffected.

7. **What is the workup of an isolated pupil-sparing but otherwise complete oculomotor nerve palsy in the vasculopathic age group?**
   A lesion that compresses the central third-nerve fibers sufficiently to produce a complete paresis should affect the peripheral pupillary fibers sufficiently to produce at least some degree of pupil involvement. If not, the

likelihood of an aneurysm or other compressive etiology is extremely low. The patient may be treated for an assumed vaso-occlusive etiology. At a minimum, diagnostic workup includes measuring systemic blood pressure, a lipid panel, and fasting blood glucose and/or hemoglobin A_1c. If the patient has symptoms of giant cell arteritis, check for an elevated erythrocyte sedimentation rate, C-reactive protein, and platelet count; administer corticosteroids; and perform a temporal artery biopsy; otherwise, the patient may be seen again in 6 weeks. Some physicians reexamine the patient within 5 days to ensure the pupil remains uninvolved. If no resolution of symptoms occurs over 3 months, neuroimaging with an MRI is generally performed.

8. **What is primary oculomotor aberrant regeneration?**
   After injury to the oculomotor nerve, fibers can regrow to supply muscles other than the inferior oblique, medial rectus, superior rectus, levator palpebrae, and parasympathetically innervated iris sphincter. When the oculomotor nerve fires, the aberrant regeneration causes involuntary cocontraction of the lid, other extraocular muscles, or pupil. For example, the upper lid may elevate on downgaze or adduction, the globe may retract on attempted upgaze, or the pupil may constrict on eye movement. It is also known as oculomotor synkinesis. It occurs in about 15% of patients after acute oculomotor nerve injury. Patients should be evaluated with a brain MRI and angiography to rule out a compression lesion or aneurysm.

9. **What are the causes of isolated cranial neuropathies?**
   Many cranial neuropathies are idiopathic, but the causes of isolated cranial neuropathies are summarized in Table 30.1.

10. **How do you test for a trochlear nerve palsy in the presence of an oculomotor nerve palsy?**
    It is important to specifically test trochlear, abducens, and trigeminal nerve function in a patient with an oculomotor nerve palsy to localize the lesion. Because the third-nerve palsy may prevent adduction, it may be difficult to test fourth-nerve function. When the patient attempts to look down and in with the paretic eye, you will observe intorsion if the trochlear nerve is intact. This can be done by telling the patient to look at his or her nose.

11. **Describe the three-step test.**
    This is a test to determine if a hypertropia is due to superior oblique palsy or other causes (Fig. 30.1).
    Step 1: Which eye is hyperdeviated? A right hyperdeviation could be caused by palsy of any of the muscles circled in Fig. 30.1A. Determine which muscles might cause this.
    Step 2: Is the hyperdeviation worse in the right gaze or the left gaze? Isolate these muscles. A right superior oblique palsy reveals worsening of the right hyperdeviation in the left gaze (Fig. 30.1B).
    Step 3: Is the hyperdeviation worse on right head tilt or left head tilt (Fig. 30.1C)? The muscle isolated in all three steps is the palsied muscle. A right superior oblique palsy reveals increased hyperdeviation upon head tilt to the right. A double Maddox rod can then be used to determine if the trochlear nerve palsy is bilateral. If excyclotorsion is more than 10 degrees, bilateral superior oblique palsies exist.

12. **What is the best procedure to treat unresolved superior oblique palsy? Does one have to memorize Knapp's rules?**
    Knapp published his treatment scheme some years ago, and many surgeons use similar schemes. It is not necessary to memorize his particular scheme, but the principles should be understood. Generally, there are three possible surgical approaches:
    1. Strengthen (tuck) the palsied superior oblique muscle.
    2. Weaken (recess or myectomize) the antagonist ipsilateral inferior oblique muscle.
    3. Weaken the yoke contralateral inferior rectus muscle.
       Typically, the surgeon operates on the muscle or muscles that act in the field of gaze where the diplopia is worst. For example, if the left hyperdeviation in a left superior oblique (LSO) palsy is worse in downgaze, one would consider an LSO tuck or a right inferior rectus recession. The latter procedure may be favored because an adjustable suture technique can be used and there is no chance of producing an iatrogenic Brown's syndrome.

Table 30.1 Causes of Isolated Cranial Neuropathies

CRANIAL NEUROPATHY	CAUSE
III (pupil-sparing)	Adults: infarction, trauma, giant cell arteritis (GCA), tumor; rarely, an aneurysm. Children: congenital, trauma, tumor, aneurysm, migraine
III (pupil-involving)	Usually posterior communicating artery aneurysm (rarely, basilar artery)
IV	Adults: trauma, infarction, congenital, GCA Children: congenital, trauma
VI	Adults: infarction, tumor, trauma, multiple sclerosis, Wernicke's encephalopathy, sarcoidosis, GCA, herpes zoster, Lyme disease, increased intracranial pressure as in pseudotumor cerebri Children: trauma, tumor, post–viral infection

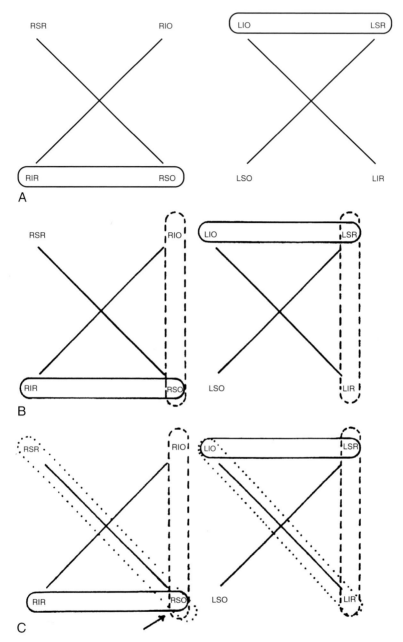

Fig. 30.1 The three-step test to determine if hypertropia is a result of superior oblique palsy or other causes. **A,** Step 1. **B,** Step 2. **C,** Step 3. (See question 10 for explanations.) (Reproduced, with permission, from Hered RW, Basic and Clinical Science Course: Section 6: Pediatric Ophthalmology and Strabismus, American Academy of Ophthalmology, 2019-2020.)

13. Explain the Harada-Ito procedure.
    The Harada-Ito procedure involves anterior and lateral displacement of the anterior portion of the palsied superior oblique muscle. This procedure is used primarily for correction of excyclotorsion but will correct a small degree of hyperdeviation. The amount of incyclotorsion created is variable, but the procedure is generally successful, especially in patients with <10 degrees of preoperative torsion.

14. What else should you know about trochlear nerve palsy?
    • It is the longest and most commonly injured cranial nerve in trauma.
    • It crosses to the contralateral side as it exits the dorsal midbrain.
    • About 60% are vascular in cause, 20% traumatic, with much fewer due to brain lesions or decompensation. Recovery rate, although dependent on etiology, is about 80%.
    • Patients of all ages with trochlear nerve palsy and increased vertical fusional amplitudes do not need further evaluation; they have decompensated "congenital" trochlear nerve palsies.
    • Always consider MG and TED in the evaluation of diplopia, even if the palsy "maps out" to a specific cranial nerve.

15. List the major causes of abduction deficit other than cranial neuropathy.
    • Restricted medial rectus muscle
    • Trauma (entrapment, damage)
    • Inflammatory pseudotumor or myositis
    • TED
    • Spasm of the near reflex
    • MG
    • Prior strabismus surgery (slipped lateral rectus, highly recessed lateral rectus)

16. How do you treat an unresolved abducens nerve palsy?
    • Weaken the ipsilateral medial rectus with strengthening of the ipsilateral lateral rectus muscle.
    • Vertical transposition procedure.
    • Botulinum toxin (Botox) injections may be used with the above procedures or alone.

17. What else should you know about abducens nerve palsy?
    • It may occur as a nonspecific sign of increased intracranial pressure. It may also occur after lumbar puncture.
    • In the case of bilateral abducens paresis, you must consider tumor, multiple sclerosis, subarachnoid hemorrhage, or infection.
    • In children with bilateral abducens paresis, reconsider strabismus and check for "doll's eyes." Doll's eyes should be incomplete in a paretic disorder.
    • Third-order sympathetic fibers briefly join the abducens nerve in the cavernous sinus. Horner's syndrome with an abducens nerve palsy localizes to this region.
    • Always consider MG and TED in the evaluation of diplopia, even if the palsy "maps out" to a specific cranial nerve. (Sound familiar?)

18. What are the localizing symptom complexes of nerve palsy?
    See Table 30.2.

19. What is internuclear ophthalmoplegia?
    The medial longitudinal fasciculus carries nerve fibers from the abducens nucleus on each side to the contralateral medial rectus subnucleus to coordinate horizontal gaze. This area of the brainstem may be damaged by demyelination,

Table 30.2 Localizing Symptom Complexes of Nerve Palsy		
SYMPTOMS/SIGNS	**SYNDROME**	**ANATOMIC LOCATION**
Ipsilateral III-nerve palsy with a contralateral hemiplegia	Weber's syndrome	Midbrain—third nerve and cerebral peduncle
Ipsilateral III-nerve palsy with contralateral choreiform movement	Benedikt's syndrome	Midbrain—third nerve fascicle and red nucleus
Ipsilateral VI-nerve palsy with hearing loss and facial pain	Gradenigo's syndrome	Petrous apex
Ipsilateral gaze palsy with facial palsy, Horner's syndrome, and deafness	Foville's syndrome	Dorsolateral pons
Ipsilateral VI- and VII-nerve palsies with contralateral hemiparesis	Millard-Gubler syndrome	Ventral pons
III-, IV-, VI-nerve (and V_1, V_2) palsies with Horner's syndrome	Cavernous sinus syndrome	Cavernous sinus
II-, III-, IV-, and VI-nerve (and V_1) palsies, often with proptosis	Orbital apex syndrome	Orbital apex
V-, VI-, VII-, and VIII-nerve palsies	Cerebellopontine angle syndrome	Cerebellopontine angle (often tumor)

ischemia, or tumor. Ipsilateral decreased adduction and contralateral abduction nystagmus are observed on attempted contralateral gaze. Saccadic velocity may be decreased in the adducting eye and may be the only sign of a subtle internuclear ophthalmoplegia (INO). Skew deviation (see later) may be observed. Bilateral INO often presents with esotropia and upward-beating nystagmus on attempted convergence in addition to the previous findings.

20. **What is ocular myasthenia gravis?**
    Intermittent diplopia and ptosis are common symptoms of this condition, and diurnal variability increases suspicion. On exam, ptosis will frequently worsen with prolonged upgaze, and obicularis strength is frequently affected. Myasthenia may mimic any isolated ocular motor nerve palsy or an INO. Both eyes may be affected differently at different times.

21. **What is the workup for myasthenia gravis?**
    Three types of acetylcholine receptor antibody tests are available for diagnosis: binding, blocking, and modulating. Binding antibodies are found in more than 80% of generalized MG, but in about 50% of the ocular type. Anti-MuSK antibodies may be found in generalized MG negative for acetylcholine receptor antibodies. Electrophysiologic tests such as repetitive nerve stimulation and single-fiber electromyography (EMG) assist in diagnosis. Workup additionally includes MRI of the chest and thyroid studies to rule out associated thymomas and hyperthyroidism. Myasthenia that is purely ocular after 2 years is likely to remain so.

22. **What is the Tensilon test?**
    Tensilon (edrophonium chloride) is a short-acting anticholinesterase that can cause improvement of symptoms and signs of MG by competing with acetylcholine for enzyme degradation. Intravenous Tensilon is administered. A positive test shows improved facial expression, lid position, or double vision within 3 minutes of injection. A positive test is quite specific for the diagnosis of MG; however, false-negative tests occur. An EMG may also show improvement after Tensilon administration. Atropine must be readily available in case adverse reactions occur (abdominal cramps and bradycardia are common).

23. **What is convergence insufficiency?**
    Typical convergence insufficiency presents with asthenopia and double vision at near. It is diagnosed by observing an exotropia near an abnormally remote near point of convergence and inadequate amplitudes of fusion. Patients can fully adduct during conjugate gaze movements, and the deviation is comitant for a given distance. The isolated condition is rarely associated with tumor or other serious pathology. Patients are treated with near-point exercises such as focusing on the end of a pencil while moving from arm's length toward the face.

24. **What is skew deviation?**
    Skew deviation is a vertical deviation that is caused by a prenuclear disturbance and cannot be isolated to a single extraocular muscle or muscles. It is distinguished from a superior oblique palsy in that it is associated with incyclotorsion, rather than excyclotorsion, as seen in a superior oblique palsy. It is associated with other manifestations of posterior fossa disease.

25. **What other supranuclear conditions commonly produce diplopia?**
    Progressive supranuclear palsy produces a variety of systemic and ocular motility disturbances, including bradykinesia, axial rigidity, and difficulty with vertical eye movements. If diplopia is present, it is typically caused by convergence difficulty. Similarly, patients with Parkinsonism, Huntington's disease, and Parinaud's dorsal midbrain syndrome may also have diplopia at near owing to convergence difficulty.

26. **Explain divergence paresis.**
    Patients with divergence paresis present with an esodeviation at distance causing diplopia. Patients are able to fuse at near. The esodeviation is comitant, and horizontal versions are normal. This condition tends to be benign and self-limited; however, it may be associated with infection, demyelinating disease, and tumor. A thorough neurologic evaluation should be performed, and consideration should be given to MRI, especially if any neurologic signs or symptoms are present.

27. **Do vaso-occlusive nerve palsies present with aberrant regeneration?**
    No. Aberrant regeneration of the third nerve does not occur after a vaso-occlusive (e.g., diabetic) third-nerve palsy. Primary oculomotor aberrant regeneration is highly suggestive of a lesion that is slowly compressing the third nerve, such as an intracavernous meningioma or aneurysm.

28. **To what anatomic region does Horner's syndrome with an abducens nerve palsy localize?**
    It localizes to the cavernous sinus. Third-order sympathetic fibers briefly join the abducens nerve in the cavernous sinus. Often, however, diseases of the cavernous sinus such as a carotid cavernous fistula or cavernous sinus thrombosis cause cranial nerve III, IV, and VI deficits in addition to proptosis, elevated intraocular pressure, conjunctival hyperemia, and reduced vision.

29. **What is the ice test?**
    The ice test is a noninvasive test for MG. The palpebral fissure is measured before and immediately after a 2-minute application of ice to the ptotic eyelid. Many patients with MG will show an improvement in the ptosis

after ice application. The sensitivity of the ice test in patients with complete ptosis decreases considerably. It may be more sensitive when performed following the sustained upgaze test.

KEY POINTS: MYASTHENIA GRAVIS

1. Always suspect MG in any patient with diplopia, especially if it is variable and associated with ptosis.
2. Have atropine available for adverse reactions if Tensilon tests are performed.
3. If a patient has classic MG symptoms and signs but negative acetylcholine receptor antibodies, consider checking for anti-MuSK or obtaining electrophysiological studies.
4. Thymomas and hyperthyroidism are common in patients with MG. Patients need a chest MRI and thyroid function tests.
5. Consider MG in patients with autoimmune hyperthyroidism who have ptosis rather than eyelid retraction.

30. Why is a trapdoor orbital fracture important to recognize?

A trapdoor fracture occurs when an orbital wall, most often the floor, breaks and then springs back together, entrapping a herniated extraocular muscle within it. This is more often seen in pediatric patients who may otherwise appear to have minimal ocular or adnexal trauma ("white-eyed" fracture). Examination of the extraocular muscles reveals restrictive deficits and diplopia at gaze opposite the fracture. CT scan of the orbits may reveal a fracture with entrapped muscle, but this may be easily missed. This type of fracture with muscle entrapment requires urgent surgical repair as ischemic damage and fibrosis of the muscle may occur if not treated promptly.

31. In facial trauma involving orbital fractures, what are indications for repair?

Emergent repair is indicated for globe luxation into the maxillary sinus or if an oculocardiac reflex is observed. Urgent repair is recommended for muscle entrapment due to trapdoor fractures. Repair within 1 to 2 weeks is often suggested in patients with sustained diplopia due to non-trapdoor entrapment, early enophthalmos of more than 3 mm, significant hypoglobus, large orbital wall fractures that will probably cause enophthalmos, or associated rim or other facial fractures. Indications for observation include no diplopia, diplopia that is improving, no enophthalmos, and small fractures with low risk of future enophthalmos. Despite these recommendations, there is a growing body of literature that good functional and aesthetic outcomes can be achieved in non-trapdoor fractures that are observed for several months and repaired late, or not repaired at all.

32. What is, and what causes, silent sinus syndrome?

Silent sinus syndrome is a slow, indolent process leading to enophthalmos of usually one eye, with hypoglobus and binocular diplopia. This may be a consequence of prior trauma and is caused by an impacted maxillary sinus with chronic sinusitis and atelectasis, creating a negative pressure pull of the orbital floor downward. Treatment requires simultaneous or stages functional endoscopic sinus surgery and orbital floor repair.

33. If a patient or the physician chooses against surgical therapy for binocular diplopia, what are some nonsurgical approaches?

- Occlusion or blurring of one eye
- Orthoptic or computer-based exercises good for <15 prism diopters diplopia, intermittent exotropia, or convergence insufficiency
- Prism treatment—Fresnel press-on prisms or ground in—to maximize binocular vision at primary gaze and downgaze, if possible

BIBLIOGRAPHY

Azarmina M, Azarmina H: The six syndromes of the sixth cranial nerve, J Ophthalmic Vis Res 8 (2)160–171, 2013.
Bagheri A, Babsharif B, Abrishami M, Salour H, Aletaha M: Outcomes of surgical and non-surgical treatment for sixth nerve palsy, J Ophthalmic Vis Res 5(1):32–37, 2010.
Bartiss MJ: Nonsurgical treatment of diplopia, Curr Opin Ophthalmol 29(5):381–384, 2018.
Bellusci C: Paralytic strabismus, Curr Opin Ophthalmol 12:368–372, 2001.
Bradfield YS, Struck MC, Kushner BJ, Neely DE, Plager DA, Gangnon RE: Outcomes of Harada-Ito surgery for acquired torsional diplopia, J AAPOS 16(5):453–457, 2012.
Burde RM, Savino PJ, Trobe JD: Clinical decisions in neuro-ophthalmology, ed 3, St. Louis, 2002, Mosby.
Brazis PW, Masdeu JC, Biller J: Localization in clinical neurology, ed 6, Lippincott Williams & Wilkins: Philadelphia.
Elrod RD, Weinberg DA: Ocular myasthenia gravis, Ophthalmol Clin North Am 17(3):275–309, 2004.
Fakiri MO, Tavy DL, Hama-Amin AD, Wirtz PW: Accuracy of the ice test in the diagnosis of myasthenia gravis in patients with ptosis, Muscle Nerve 48(6):902–904, 2013.
Golnik KC, Pena R, Lee AG, Eggenberger ER: An ice test for the diagnosis of myasthenia gravis, Ophthalmology 106(7):1282–1286, 1999.
Hamilton SR: Neuro-ophthalmology of eye-movement disorders, Curr Opin Ophthalmol 10(6):405–410, 1999.
Harada M, Ito Y: Surgical correction of cyclophoria, Jpn J Ophthalmol 8:88–92, 1964.

Holmes JM, Beck RW, Kip KE, et al.: Botulinum toxin treatment versus conservative management in acute traumatic sixth nerve palsy or paresis, J AAPOS 4(3):145–149, 2000.

Jordan DR, Mawn L: Blowout fractures of the orbit. In Black EH, Nesi FA, Calvano CJ, Gladstone GJ, Levine MR, editors: Smith and Nesi's ophthalmic plastic and reconstructive surgery, ed 3, New York, NY, 2012, Springer Science, pp 243–263.

Karmani TA, Schmidt J, Crowson CS, et al.: Utility of erythrocyte sedimentation rate and C-reactive protein for the diagnosis of giant cell arteritis, Semin Arthritis Rheum 41(6):866–871, 2012.

Kee HJ, Yang HK, Hwang JM, Park KS: Evaluation and validation of sustained upgaze combined with the ice-pack test for ocular myasthenia gravis in Asians, Neuromuscul Disord 29(4):296–301, 2019.

Kersten RC, Vagefi MR, Bartley GB: Orbital "blowout" fractures: time for a new paradigm, Ophthalmology 125(6):796–798, 2018.

Larner AJ: False localizing signs, J Neurol Neurosurg Psychiatry 74(4):415–418, 2003.

Larner AJ, Thomas JD: Can myasthenia gravis be diagnosed with the "ice pack test"? A cautionary note, Postgrad Med J 76:162–163, 2000.

Li Y, Arora Y, Levin K: Myasthenia gravis: newer therapies offer sustained improvement, Cleve Clin J Med 80(11):711–721, 2013.

Mein J, Trimble R: Diagnosis and management of ocular motility disorders, ed 2, London, 1991, Blackwell Scientific Publications.

Miller NR, Newman NJ: Walsh and Hoyts' clinical neuro-ophthalmology, ed 6, 2005, Baltimore, Williams & Wilkins.

North American Neuro-Ophthalmology Society: www.nanosweb.org.

Oh SY Oh SY: Clinical outcomes and aetiology of fourth cranial nerve palsy with acute vertical diplopia in adults, Eye (London) 34:1842–1847, 2020.

Wladis EJ, Kersten RC, Vagefi MR, Pinheiro-Neto C, Shinder R, Kim HJ: Clinical features and outcomes of post-traumatic silent sinus syndrome, Ophthalmic Plast Reconstr Surg 34(4):378–380, 2018.

CHAPTER 31

OPTIC NEURITIS

Archana Srinivasan and Mark L. Moster

1. What is optic neuritis?

   Optic neuritis is an inflammation of the optic nerve. It may be idiopathic or associated with systemic disease.

2. Which systemic diseases are associated with optic neuritis?

   The most common disease associated with "typical" optic neuritis is multiple sclerosis (MS). Recently, some of the immune mediated inflammatory disorders of the central nervous system such as neuromyelitis optica spectrum disorders (NMOSDs) and anti–myelin oligodendrocyte glycoprotein (anti-MOG) syndromes have been described as causes of "atypical" optic neuritis. Other less common associations include sarcoidosis, syphilis, Lyme disease, and collagen vascular diseases including granulomatosis with polyangiitis (GPA) and systemic lupus erythematosus (SLE).

3. What are the antibodies associated with neuromyelitis optica spectrum disorder?

   Majority of patients with NMOSD have antibodies targeted against aquaporin 4 (AQP4), a water channel present on the end-feet processes of astrocytes. Autoantibodies against MOG (MOG-IgG) have been identified in a subset of patients with AQP4-negative NMOSD. However, it is likely that the anti-MOG syndrome is a distinct entity with a wider clinical phenotype not limited to NMOSD.

4. Who most commonly gets optic neuritis?

   Women between the ages of 15 and 45 years are most commonly affected by typical optic neuritis.

5. What are the typical clinical findings in optic neuritis?

   Typical optic neuritis causes acute or subacute visual loss that is preceded or accompanied by pain on eye movement and that may progress over 10 to 14 days. Visual acuity may range from 20/20 to no light perception. However, even if visual acuity is 20/20, the patient usually has a defect in color vision, contrast sensitivity, and visual field. If the neuritis is unilateral, an afferent pupillary defect is present. The optic disc may be normal or swollen.

6. Which clinical test is most sensitive for patients with optic neuritis?

   The most sensitive test, that is, the test most likely to be abnormal in a patient with optic neuritis is contrast sensitivity.

7. How common is pain on eye movement in patients with optic neuritis?

   Pain around the eye or pain exacerbated with eye movement was present in 92% of patients in the Optic Neuritis Treatment Trial (ONTT).

8. What visual field defects are found in patients with optic neuritis?

   The classic visual field defect in optic neuritis is central scotoma. However, results of the ONTT showed that any optic nerve visual field defect is compatible with optic neuritis, including altitudinal defects and arcuate defects as well as diffuse visual field defects.

9. What is the natural history of optic neuritis?

   The visual loss of typical optic neuritis may progress over 10 to 14 days. At that point, it should stabilize and shortly thereafter begin to improve.

10. What is the expected visual outcome for patients with optic neuritis?

    The ONTT found that at 12 months, 93% of patients were 20/40 or better, 69% were 20/20 or better, and 3% were 20/200 or worse. At 10 years, 91% of patients had acuity of 20/40 or better and 74% were 20/20. At 15 years, 66% had visual acuity of 20/20 or better in both eyes. On average, visual acuity was worse in those who developed MS.

11. Are there any predictors of poor visual outcome?

    The ONTT found that the only predictor for poor visual outcome was poor visual acuity at presentation. Nevertheless, all patients with an initial visual acuity of 20/200 or less showed some improvement. However, 5% of the patients were still 20/200 or less at 6 months.

12. What were the objectives of the Optic Neuritis Treatment Trial?

    The ONTT was a multicenter, randomized, prospective clinical trial to determine whether corticosteroid treatment of optic neuritis was beneficial for visual outcome. A secondary objective was to determine the risk of developing

MS in patients with optic neuritis. The patients who participated in the ONTT were randomized to three treatment arms. One group of patients received oral placebo; another group received oral prednisone, 1 mg/kg for 14 days; and the third group received intravenous (IV) methylprednisolone (Solu-Medrol), 250 mg every 6 hours for 3 days, followed by oral prednisone, 1 mg/kg for 11 days.

13. What were the conclusions of the ONTT regarding treatment of optic neuritis?
No treatment group had statistically significantly better visual acuity at 6 months. However, patients treated with IV methylprednisolone began to recover vision more quickly. The surprising result was that patients treated with oral prednisone, 1 mg/kg for 14 days, had an increased incidence (2×) of recurrence of optic neuritis in the affected or contralateral eye. The researchers concluded that oral prednisone at a dose of 1 mg/kg is contraindicated in the treatment of optic neuritis.

14. What was the strongest predictor for the development of multiple sclerosis?
An abnormal brain magnetic resonance imaging (MRI) scan (Fig. 31.1) was the strongest predictor for the development of clinically definite MS at 2 years. Placebo-treated patients whose MRI scan at study entry showed two or more periventricular white matter lesions >3 mm had a 36% chance of developing MS within 2 years. Patients with one lesion had a 17% chance, and patients with no signal abnormalities had only a 3% chance.

15. What were the other predictors for developing multiple sclerosis?
Previous optic neuritis in the fellow eye, previous nonspecific neurologic symptoms, race (white), and family history of MS were associated with an increased risk of developing MS. Although young age and female gender have been reported to be risk factors for MS, they were not shown to increase the risk within 2 years in the ONTT.

16. What were the conclusions of the Optic Neuritis Treatment Trial about the effect of treatment on the risk of developing multiple sclerosis?
The results of the ONTT showed that IV methylprednisolone significantly decreased the risk of developing MS at 2 years. Most of the beneficial effect was seen in patients with abnormal MRI scans, because patients with normal MRI scans had a low incidence of MS, regardless of treatment. Among patients with two or more signal abnormalities on MRI, MS developed in 36% treated with placebo, 32% treated with prednisone, and 16% treated with IV methylprednisolone. Thus, the risk of developing MS at 2 years was cut in half by treatment with IV methylprednisolone. After 2 years, the beneficial effect wore off, and at 3 years and beyond, the three groups had a similar incidence of MS.

17. What is the 15-year risk of developing multiple sclerosis after optic neuritis?
A total of 50% of patients enrolled in the ONTT developed MS in a 15-year period. White matter lesions on MRI were the most potent predictor of MS. Patients with one or more lesions had an incidence of MS of 72%. Those with no lesions on MRI had a 25% incidence of MS.

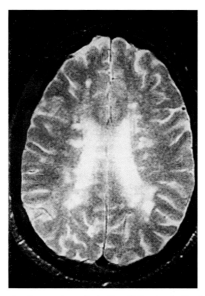

Fig. 31.1 Abnormal magnetic resonance imaging scan in a patient with multiple sclerosis. Classic periventricular white matter lesions appear bright on T2-weighted image.

18. **What is the 10-year risk of recurrence of optic neuritis?**

A total of 35% of patients in the ONTT who completed the examination at 10 years had a documented recurrence of optic neuritis in the previously affected eye or an attack in the fellow eye. Patients who had a diagnosis of MS had a higher recurrence rate (43%) than those who did not have MS (24%).

19. **Are there any other medications that may influence the risk of developing multiple sclerosis?**

Numerous medications approved for the treatment of MS have been shown to decrease the progression to MS in patients with optic neuritis or other clinically isolated syndromes (CIS). These include the agents taken orally, by injection and by infusion.

20. **What are the ocular adverse effects of multiple sclerosis medications?**

Macular edema is a well-reported adverse effect of fingolimod (Gilenya), a sphingosine 1 phosphate receptor modulator used for the treatment of relapsing MS. The incidence of macular edema is dose dependent; pooled data from major clinical trials and extension studies showed a higher incidence rate in the higher dose group when compared with patients who received the Food and Drug Administration (FDA) approved clinical dose of 0.5 mg (1.5% vs. 0.3% cumulative incidence). Diabetes and prior history of uveitis are known risk factors. All patients should undergo ophthalmic evaluation prior to or shortly after starting therapy and 3 to 4 months after starting therapy.

Alemtuzumab (Lemtrada) is associated with autoimmune thyroid dysfunction. The incidence varies from 17% to 41% according to different studies. Most cases develop after the last dose of alemtuzumab. Therefore, management is the same as non–alemtuzumab-associated thyroid eye disease.

21. **Describe the appropriate workup and treatment for patients with optic neuritis.**

All patients presenting with optic neuritis should have an MRI scan of the brain and orbits. Almost all patients will have enhancement of the optic nerve on the orbital MRI and many will have demyelinating brain lesions. The pattern of optic nerve enhancement in NMOSD and MOG-IgG diseases may be distinct from that seen in MS. Optic neuritis lesions in NMOSD and MOG-IgG are longitudinally extensive, often involving at least three optic nerve segments. Perineural enhancement is a distinguishing feature of MOG-IgG optic neuritis. Patients with typical optic neuritis and normal brain MRI may be monitored with sequential follow-up. However, high-dose steroids should be administered in all atypical cases. On the other hand, if the brain MRI shows white matter lesions consistent with demyelination, the patient should be offered high-dose IV methylprednisone and referred to the neurologist for further management.

With the recent discovery of NMOSD and anti-MOG optic neuritis, there is no clear consensus yet among experts if the initial evaluation in all patients with optic neuritis should include testing for AQP4 and MOG-IgG antibodies.

22. **When should I consider alternate diagnoses for optic neuritis?**

Atypical features such as severe vision loss, poor visual recovery, simultaneous bilateral optic neuritis, and sequential or early recurrence of optic neuritis are highly suggestive of AQP4+ NMO or MOG-IgG disease. In general, patients with MOG-IgG optic neuritis show excellent response to steroids and have better visual outcomes when compared to patients with AQP4+ NMO optic neuritis.

23. **What are the other central nervous system manifestations of neuromyelitis optica spectrum disorder and autoantibodies against myelin oligodendrocyte glycoprotein syndromes?**

NMOSD:
- Longitudinally extensive transverse myelitis (three or more vertebral segments) characterized by symmetric paraparesis or quadriparesis, bladder dysfunction, and sensory loss below the level of the spinal cord lesion.
- Area postrema syndrome characterized by intractable nausea with vomiting or hiccups.
- Hypothalamic dysfunction causing symptomatic narcolepsy, obesity, and various autonomic manifestations such as hypotension, bradycardia, and hypothermia.

MOG-IgG syndrome:
- Optic neuritis is the most common presenting phenotype in adults, followed by transverse myelitis.
- Acute disseminated encephalomyelitis (ADEM) is more common in children.

24. What are the management options for neuromyelitis optica spectrum disorder and autoantibodies against myelin oligodendrocyte glycoprotein optic neuritis?

NMOSD:

- For acute optic neuritis, high-dose IV steroids are used first. If recovery does not immediately occur, plasmapheresis is administered.
- Long-term immunosuppression is the mainstay of treatment for NMOSD. Eculizumab (Soliris) was recently approved by the FDA for AQP4+ NMO disease. Other options include rituximab, azathioprine, and mycophenolate.

MOG-IgG syndrome:

- High-dose IV methylprednisone followed by a slow taper of oral steroids over 1 to 3 months is the preferred treatment for acute cases of MOG-IgG optic neuritis. Plasma exchange or IV immunoglobulins are second-line options in resistant cases. Chronic immunotherapy may be required in relapsing cases.

25. What is chronic relapsing inflammatory optic neuropathy (CRION)?

The diagnostic criteria for CRION are as follows:

- Recurrent optic neuritis
- Objective evidence of loss of visual function
- Contrast enhancement of acutely inflamed optic nerves
- AQP4 and MOG seronegativity
- Response to steroids and relapse on withdrawal or dose reduction

BIBLIOGRAPHY

Beck R, Cleary P, Anderson M Jr., et al.: A randomized, controlled trial of corticosteroids in the treatment of acute optic neuritis, N Engl J Med 326(9):581–588, 1992.

Beck R, Clearly P, Trobe J, et al.: The effect of corticosteroids for acute optic neuritis on the subsequent development of multiple sclerosis, N Engl J Med 329(24):1764–1769, 1993.

Chen J, Pittock S, Flanagan E, et al.: Optic neuritis in the era of biomarkers, Surv Ophthalmol 65(1):12–17, 2020.

Glisson C: Neuromyelitis optica spectrum disorders. 2016. https://www.uptodate.com/contents/neuromyelitis-optica-spectrum-disorders.

Moss H: Visual consequences of medications for multiple sclerosis: the good, the bad, the ugly, and the unknown, Eye Brain 9:13, 2017.

Optic Neuritis Study Group: Multiple sclerosis risk after optic neuritis final Optic Neuritis Treatment Trial follow-up, Archiv Neurol 65(6):727–732, 2008.

Optic Neuritis Study Group: Visual function 15 years after optic neuritis: a final follow-up report from the Optic Neuritis Treatment Trial, Ophthalmology 115(6):1079–1082, 2008.

Pariani N, Willis M, Muller I, et al.: Alemtuzumab-induced thyroid dysfunction exhibits distinctive clinical and immunological features, J Clin Endocrinol Metab 103(8):3010–3018, 2018.

Petzold A, Plant G: Chronic relapsing inflammatory optic neuropathy: a systematic review of 122 cases reported, J Neurol 261(1):17–26, 2014.

Wynford-Thomas R, Jacob A, Tomassini V: Neurological update: MOG antibody disease, J Neurol 266(5):1280–1286, 2019.

Yanoff M, Duker JS: Ophthalmology: expert consult, ed 3, Philadelphia, PA, 2018, Elsevier.

Zarbin M, Jampol L, Jager R, et al.: Ophthalmic evaluations in clinical studies of fingolimod (FTY720) in multiple sclerosis, Ophthalmology 120(7):1432–1439, 2013.

MISCELLANEOUS OPTIC NEUROPATHIES AND NEUROLOGIC DISTURBANCES

Janice A. Gault

1. A young woman complains of headaches. Her vision is 20/20 in each eye with no evidence of afferent pupillary defect. She has a bitemporal visual-field cut. What do you suspect?
   A chiasmal lesion. Schedule a magnetic resonance imaging (MRI) scan to make an evaluation.

2. What may simulate a bitemporal field defect?
   A bitemporal field defect may be simulated by sector retinitis pigmentosa, coloboma, or a tilted disc.

3. A patient has 20/20 vision in her right eye and 20/400 in her left eye. Her left eye has an afferent pupillary defect and decreased color plates. What should you evaluate in her right eye?
   Check visual fields in *both* eyes. A central scotoma in one eye may be accompanied by a superior temporal field loss in the other. This condition, called a *junctional scotoma*, is also found in chiasmal lesions. See the chapter on visual fields (see Chapter 6).

KEY POINTS: DIFFERENTIAL DIAGNOSIS OF CHIASMAL VISUAL DEFECTS

1. Pituitary lesion—tumor or apoplexy
2. Craniopharyngioma
3. Meningioma
4. Glioma
5. Aneurysm
6. Trauma
7. Infection

4. Is there a difference in the treatment of secreting and nonsecreting symptomatic pituitary tumors?
   Yes. A prolactinoma secretes prolactin and may be treated successfully with bromocriptine. A nonsecreting tumor probably requires surgery. Of course, an endocrinologist should fully evaluate the patient for other hormonal imbalances.

5. What visual field is often seen in a toxic or metabolic optic neuropathy?
   Bilateral central or centrocecal scotomas. Optic nerves show temporal pallor (Fig. 32.1). Alcohol, tobacco, and vitamin B12 deficiency, as well as drugs such as chloramphenicol, ethambutol, digitalis, chloroquine, and isoniazid, have been implicated. Check for heavy metals and order a complete blood count as well as serum levels of vitamins B11, B12, and folate. Consider Leber's hereditary optic neuropathy (LHON) as a diagnosis.

6. A 60-year-old man presents with gradual vision loss to 20/400 in his right eye. On examination, the right optic nerve is pale and dot-and-blot retinal hemorrhages are seen. The left eye is normal. What history may be helpful?
   A history of radiation treatment. The patient reports radiation to his right frontal sinus 3 years earlier. There is no treatment for radiation optic neuropathy. Panretinal photocoagulation for neovascular disease and antivascular endothelial growth factor treatment is used for radiation retinopathy. This may prevent vitreous hemorrhage, macular edema, neovascular glaucoma, and ultimate loss of the eye.

7. What may cause a constricted visual field?
   - Retinitis pigmentosa
   - End-stage glaucoma
   - Thyroid ophthalmopathy
   - Optic nerve drusen
   - Vitamin A deficiency
   - Occipital strokes
   - Panretinal photocoagulation

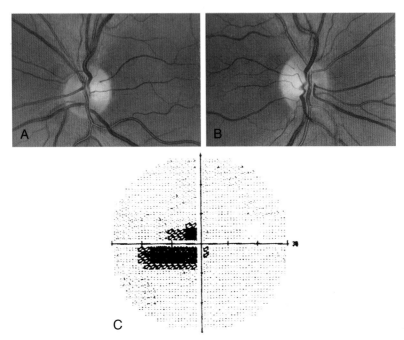

Fig. 32.1 Fundus views reveal mild temporal optic disc pallor in **(A)** right optic disc and **(B)** left optic disc. More interesting in **(B)** however, is the loss of the nerve fiber layer in the papillomacular bundle. This patient, who had tobacco–alcohol amblyopia (mixed toxic and nutritional deficiency optic neuropathy), also had a visual acuity of 20/400 in each eye, which recovered to only 20/100 after changes in habit and diet and vitamin therapy. In this class of optic neuropathies, relatively severely compromised visual acuity and dyschromatopsia often are found with minimal optic disc atrophy. **C,** Visual field exam reveals centrocecal scotoma. A lesion of the papillomacular bundle (nerve fiber layer or optic nerve) is the usual cause of this defect. (**A** and **B**, From Sadun AA, Gurkan S: Hereditary, nutritional, and toxic optic atrophies. In Yanoff M, Duker JS, editors: *Ophthalmology,* ed 2, St. Louis, 2004, Mosby, pp 1275–1278; **C** from Burde RM, Savino PJ, Trobe JD: Unexplained visual loss. In Burde RM, Savino PJ, Trobe JD, editors: *Clinical decisions in neuro-ophthalmology,* ed 3, St. Louis, 2002, Mosby, pp 1–26.)

- Hysteria
- Malingering

8. **How do you differentiate hysteria and malingering from real disease?**
   Have the patient do a tangent screen at two different distances. The closer the patient stands, the smaller the field should be. In a patient with nonphysiologic visual loss, the fields are often of equal size. Patients also may demonstrate spiraling with kinetic visual-field testing (see Chapter 6).

9. **A 55-year-old man notices that the vision in his left eye has worsened suddenly. He has 20/30 vision in his right eye and 20/100 in his left eye. The left eye also shows an afferent pupillary defect and decreased color plates. Visual-field examination reveals an inferior altitudinal defect on the left with a normal full field on the right. On fundus examination, the left optic nerve appears pale and swollen superiorly. He has a crowded disc in the right eye. What is your concern?**
   An altitudinal defect is a classic finding with ischemic optic neuropathy (ION). The two types are arteritic and nonarteritic (see Table 32.1). Because they are treated differently, you must differentiate the two. First, it is important to ask about symptoms of giant cell arteritis, such as weight loss, anorexia, fever, jaw claudication, headache, scalp tenderness, and proximal joint and muscle pain. Check for a palpable, tender, nonpulsatile temporal artery. Immediately order an erythrocyte sedimentation rate (ESR), a C-reactive protein (CRP), and a platelet count if you believe that giant cell arteritis is a consideration. The upper limits of normal for an ESR is age divided by 2 for men and age + 10 divided by 2 for women. The CRP is not affected by age and may be more sensitive than ESR. However, both are nonspecific tests; any inflammatory process can elevate them. Temporal arteritis patients have elevated platelet counts.
   The patient denied any of the symptoms, and his ESR was 20. He was diagnosed with nonarteritic ION. Because 50% of these patients have cardiovascular disease, diabetes, and/or hypertension, he was sent to his

Table 32.1 Nonarteritic and Arteritic Ischemic Optic Neuropathy

	NAION	AION
Age of onset	40–60 years	Usually older than 50 years
Gender	Either equally	More often female
Presenting visual acuity	May be better than 20/100	Often count fingers or worse
Visual-field defect	Altitudinal or involving central visual field	Altitudinal or involving central visual field
Ophthalmic exam	Hyperemic disc swelling, may be segmental with flame-shaped hemorrhages; later atrophy without cupping	Pale, swollen disc with few flame hemorrhages; later, optic atrophy and cupping
Symptoms	None	Jaw pain, scalp tenderness, night sweats, fever, weight loss
Systemic associations	Diabetes, hypertension, hyperlipidemia, sleep apnea; potential increase in use of erectile dysfunction drugs if a crowded disc initially	Polymyalgia rheumatica
Lab evaluation	Lab tests normal	Elevated ESR, C-reactive protein, and platelet counts. Disruption of internal elastic lamina on temporal artery biopsy

AION, Arteritic ischemic optic neuropathy; *ESR*, erythrocyte sedimentation rate; *NAION*, nonarteritic ischemic optic neuropathy.

internist. He was told that his prognosis for significantly improved vision was low. Forty percent of patients may have a mild improvement in vision over 6 months. However, some patients note an initial decrease in visual acuity and field, which is followed by a second decrease in visual acuity or field days to weeks later. Unfortunately, there is no proven treatment. Optic nerve sheath decompressions have not shown improvement. With time, the patient's optic nerve will atrophy in the area of damage. He has a 35% risk of involvement of the other eye. His blood pressure, blood sugars, and cholesterol should be optimized. Also, because of his crowded disc, he should be warned about the use of erectile dysfunction drugs and the risk of nonarteritic ION (NAION) in his other eye.

10. An 80-year-old man presents with the same history of sudden vision loss and the same visual field as the man in question 9. However, his vision consists of counting fingers at 10 ft, and his optic nerve is pale and swollen with flame-shaped hemorrhages. He admits to jaw pain when he chews, weight loss of 10 lb, and difficulty in getting up from a chair, suggesting polymyalgia rheumatica. He has a tender temporal artery without pulses. His erythrocyte sedimentation rate is 120. What do you do?

First, you make a diagnosis of giant cell arteritis and place him on 250 mg of methylprednisolone intravenously every 6 hours for 12 doses, followed by 80 to 100 mg/day of prednisone orally for 2 to 4 weeks after reversal of symptoms and normalization of ESR. Treatment may last for 1 year or more. (Evidence suggests that such high doses can prevent the same process in the other eye, of which there is a 30% risk.) The patient is then scheduled for temporal artery biopsy.

11. Should the biopsy be done before the steroids are started, to ensure that the diagnosis can be made?

Absolutely not. The steroids will not affect the biopsy results for at least 7 days, and it may be positive for up to a month after steroids. The therapeutic effect of the steroids is necessary immediately, because the second eye can become involved in as little as 24 hours. Patients are also at increased risk of stroke.

12. What biopsy finding makes the diagnosis?

Disruption of the internal elastic lamina. Giant cells are often present but are not necessary for the diagnosis.

13. What if the temporal artery biopsy is normal?

Giant cell arteritis is a diagnosis based mainly on symptoms. The ESR may be normal, and your suspicion should be extremely high because of the patient's history. Because skip areas also occur, make sure to get a significant length of artery for biopsy. Sometimes, it is necessary to also biopsy the other side. In a patient with less classic symptoms, a negative biopsy warrants discontinuing steroids. Ocular pneumoplethysmography may help with the diagnosis if it shows reduced ocular blood flow.

14. **What else may herald giant cell arteritis?**

Amaurosis fugax, cranial nerve palsies, or central retinal artery occlusion. Polymyalgia rheumatica and giant cell arteritis often occur together.

KEY POINTS: DIFFERENTIAL DIAGNOSIS OF OPTOCILIARY SHUNT VESSELS

1. Meningioma
2. Glaucoma
3. Old central retinal vein occlusion
4. Optic nerve glioma
5. Chronic papilledema
6. Idiopathic disease

15. **A 35-year-old woman says that she has binocular diplopia. On examination, you find weakness of adduction in her right eye and horizontal jerk nystagmus of the left eye with attempted abduction. What does she have? What should you do next?**

She has internuclear ophthalmoplegia. She also may have a skew deviation in which either eye can have a hypertropia that does not map to a specific muscle on the three-step test. She needs a scan of her brain and evaluation and further neurologic evaluation.

16. **Internuclear ophthalmoplegia can be bilateral or unilateral. What might you find in bilateral disease?**

You might find upbeat nystagmus in upgaze and exotropia.

17. **What causes internuclear ophthalmoplegia?**

Multiple sclerosis, ischemic vascular disease, or masses of the brain stem. The differential diagnoses that mimic weakness of inward eye movement include the following:

- **Myasthenia gravis:** Ptosis and orbicularis muscle weakness are common; symptoms worsen with fatigue. Results of a Tensilon test are often positive.
- **Orbital disease:** Nystagmus is usually not seen. Pain, ptosis, and/or globe displacement may coexist. Orbital computed tomography (CT) reveals the cause.

18. **An obese 30-year-old woman presents with severe headaches and occasional double vision. Her vision is 20/20 in both eyes. How do you evaluate her?**

Check pupillary responses, color plates, visual fields, and extraocular motility; do a full slit lamp and dilated examination. You notice that she has bilateral swollen optic nerves (Fig. 32.2).

19. **How do you differentiate between papilledema and pseudopapilledema?**

Pseudopapilledema is not true disc swelling. The vessels surrounding the disc are not obscured, the disc is not hyperemic, and the peripapillary nerve fiber layer is normal. Spontaneous venous pulsations, if present, strongly suggest pseudopapilledema. Nerve fiber layer hemorrhages are not present in pseudopapilledema. Causes of pseudopapilledema include optic nerve drusen and congenitally anomalous discs.

20. **What do you do after the evaluation?**

You must emergently evaluate the patient for increased intracranial pressure. First, she needs a CT or MRI of the head and orbit to rule out a mass or a cerebral venous sinus thrombosis. Provided the scan is normal, a lumbar puncture should follow. If the only abnormality is an increased opening pressure, the diagnosis is pseudotumor cerebri, also known as idiopathic intracranial hypertension.

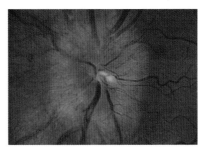

Fig. 32.2 Developed papilledema. This is the optic disc of a 30-year-old woman who suffered headaches and blurred vision for 2 months. Disc edema is fully developed. Note the engorged veins and peripapillary hemorrhages. (From Brodsky MC: Congenital optic disc anomalies. In Yanoff M, Duker JS, editors: *Ophthalmology*, ed 2, St. Louis, 2004, Mosby, pp 1255–1258.)

21. **How should the patient be treated?**
If she has no optic nerve damage on visual fields, encourage her to lose weight. If the headaches continue or she has evidence of decreased visual acuity or visual-field loss, treatment is indicated. Medications include a diuretic, such as acetazolamide, or systemic steroids. Optic nerve sheath decompression is used for worsening visual fields, and lumboperitoneal shunts have been used for headaches. The intraocular pressure should be treated if elevated.

KEY POINTS: CAUSES OF PSEUDOTUMOR CEREBRI

1. Obesity
2. Pregnancy
3. Drug use: Steroids (use or withdrawal), oral contraceptives, nalidixic acid, tetracycline, vitamin A
4. Idiopathic disease

22. **Why did the patient have double vision?**
Increased intracranial pressure may cause sixth-nerve palsies.

23. **A mother brings in her firstborn for his first exam. He is 6 months of age and appears not to see well. Dilated exam reveals optic nerve hypoplasia. What is the differential diagnosis?**
Optic nerve hypoplasia (Fig. 32.3) seems to occur in the firstborn of young mothers who may have diabetes or who may have used lysergic acid diethylamide (LSD), phenytoin, or alcohol during pregnancy. Patients also may have optic nerve hypoplasia in association with Goldenhar's syndrome or septo-optic dysplasia of de Morsier. The latter patients have seesaw nystagmus and chiasmal anomalies. Because of the risk of growth retardation, diabetes insipidus, and other pituitary abnormalities, patients with optic nerve hypoplasia should have a scan of the optic chiasm and an endocrine evaluation.

24. **A patient has a bilateral, right-sided superior field defect. Where do you suspect the lesion is located?**
A "pie-in-the-sky" defect is located in the temporal lobe. The inferior fibers loop around the temporal lobe (Meyer's loop).

25. **What other symptoms may the patient have?**
Formed hallucinations, déjà vu experiences, or uncinate fits (a form of temporal lobe epilepsy with hallucinations of taste and smell and inappropriate chewing movements).

26. **What if the patient has a bilateral, inferior right-sided visual-field loss?**
This "pie-on-the-floor" defect is typical for the parietal lobe. Patients have spasticity of conjugate gaze and optokinetic nystagmus abnormalities.

27. **A patient presents with the visual field illustrated in Fig. 32.4. Where is the lesion located?**
It is in the right occipital lobe. The more congruous the defect, the more posterior its location. Note the intact temporal crescent in the visual field in the contralateral eye because the nasal retina is larger. Macular sparing or splitting also may occur.

28. **What else may the patient experience?**
Patients with occipital lobe lesions often do not experience other neurologic abnormalities. If they do, they may have unformed hallucinations, dyschromatopsia (color vision deficiencies), prosopagnosia (inability to recognize familiar faces), and alexia without agraphia (patients can write but cannot read).

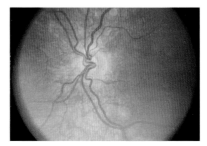

Fig. 32.3 Hypoplasia of the left optic nerve. Note the double ring sign. (From Sadun AA: Differentiation of optic nerve from retinal macular disease. In Yanoff M, Duker JS, editors: *Ophthalmology,* ed 2, St. Louis, 2004, Mosby, pp 1253–1254.)

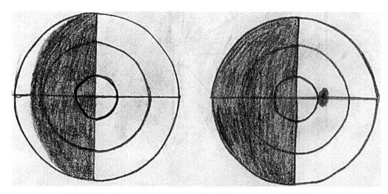

Fig. 32.4 Left homonymous hemianopia with temporal crescent in left eye.

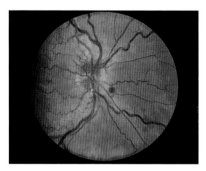

Fig. 32.5 Leber's optic neuropathy, acute. Note the hyperemic appearance of disc and opacification of the peripapillary nerve fiber layer. (From Burde RM, Savino PJ, Trobe JD: *Clinical decisions in neuro-ophthalmology,* ed 3, St. Louis, 2004, Mosby.)

29. **What causes pseudo–Foster Kennedy syndrome?**
    Pseudo–Foster Kennedy syndrome is optic atrophy with contralateral optic disc edema. A frontal lobe tumor causes true Foster Kennedy syndrome. The pseudosyndrome is usually the result of an acute ION in one eye with contralateral atrophy caused by a past episode of the same process. An olfactory groove meningioma also may cause the pseudosyndrome.

30. **An 18-year-old man presents with sudden vision loss in one eye, followed by the other eye within days. He denies pain. He has 20/20 vision in both eyes with decreased color plates and bilateral mild disc swelling with peripapillary telangiectatic microangiopathy (Fig. 32.5). Affected vessels do not leak on fluorescein angiography. What does he have?**
    LHON. The patient's history is typical. The disorder is transmitted by mitochondrial DNA; all female carriers transmit it to their offspring. Ten percent of daughters and 50% to 70% of sons manifest the disease. All daughters are carriers. None of the sons are carriers. Young men present with symptoms at 15 to 30 years of age. Some mutations are more likely to have spontaneous improvement than others; thus, genetic evaluation of the mitochondria is worthwhile. Because patients have a higher incidence of cardiac conduction defects, referral to a cardiologist is indicated.

    Recently elamipretide, a small mitochondrial-targeted tetrapetitide that reduces the production of toxic reactive oxygen species and stabilizes cardiolipin, has been given Fast Track designation for the treatment of LHON. Studies are ongoing.

BIBLIOGRAPHY

Gervasio K, Peck T, Fathy C, Sivalingham M: The Wills Eye Manual, ed 8, Philadelphia, 2022, Wolters Kluwer
Burde RM, Savino PJ, Trobe JD: Clinical decisions in neuro-ophthalmology, ed 3, St. Louis, 2002, Mosby.
Kline LB, Foroozan R: Neuro-ophthalmology review manual, ed 7, Thorofare, NJ, 2012, Slack.

CHAPTER 33

TEARING AND THE LACRIMAL SYSTEM

Nancy G. Swartz and Marc S. Cohen

OCULOPLASTICS

1. **What are the causes of tearing?**

   Tearing, also known as *epiphora,* occurs when there is an increase in the amount of tears produced or when there is a problem with the tear drainage system. We produce too many tears when the cornea is irritated. This tearing is adaptive, because if there is a foreign body present, it will wash it away. Acute corneal irritation typically results from mechanical irritants, such as an eyelash, or chemical irritants, such as the fumes from a freshly cut onion. Chronic tearing from irritation may also result from mechanical irritation as in entropion and trichiasis. However, it often occurs as a result of tear-film deficiencies (seen in dry eye syndrome and blepharitis), exposure keratopathy, or allergic conjunctivitis. When the production of tears is normal, tearing indicates an inadequate drainage of tears. A blockage at any point in the tear drainage system can cause tearing. Eyelid malpositions, such as lid and punctal ectropions, will also reduce the drainage of tears, as will lower eyelid laxity, which interferes with the eyelid's ability to pump the tears naturally through the lacrimal drainage system. For many patients, tearing is multifactorial.

KEY POINTS: COMMON CAUSES OF CHRONIC TEARING

1. Ocular irritation
   a. Dry eyes
   b. Allergies
   c. Computer vision syndrome
2. Tear-drainage dysfunction, such as from lower eyelid laxity
3. Blockage of the lacrimal drainage system, such as from a nasolacrimal duct obstruction

---

2. **Describe the normal path of tear drainage in the eyelids**

   The most important function of our tears is to lubricate the surface of the eye. Our tears travel across the cornea and conjunctiva, keeping them moist. Gravity then guides most tears to rest on the margin of the lower eyelid. Here, they are carried medially to the puncta, small openings in the eyelid located approximately 6 to 7 mm lateral to the medial canthal angle. Once inside the puncta, the tears enter the canaliculi, mucosa-lined ducts approximately 10 mm in length that carry the tears to the lacrimal sac. The first portion of each canaliculus is a 2-mm dilated, vertical segment called the ampulla. Distal to the ampulla, the canaliculus bends acutely and runs parallel to the eyelid margin toward the medial canthus. In 90% of the population, the upper and lower canaliculi join together, forming the common canaliculus before merging with the lacrimal sac. However, in 10% of the population, each canaliculus merges with the lacrimal sac independently.

3. **Where do tears go after leaving the eyelids?**

   The tears exit the canaliculi and enter the lacrimal sac, a mucosa-lined structure lying in a bony fossa in the medial orbit formed by the maxillary and lacrimal bones. The superior portion of the sac extends a few millimeters superior to the medial canthal tendon. It extends inferiorly approximately 10 mm and then continues as the nasolacrimal duct.

   Tears travel from the sac to the nasolacrimal duct. The first 12 mm of the duct lies in a bony canal in the maxillary bone. The duct then continues inferiorly for an additional 3 to 5 mm before opening into the inferior meatus of the nose. The tears exit the duct through its ostium into the nasal cavity. The ostium of the nasolacrimal duct can be found 30 mm posterior to the external nares in an adult. In young children, this distance is approximately 20 mm.

4. **What is the tear pump?**

   The tear pump is a muscular "pump" that drives the tears through the drainage system by peristalsis. Tears first enter the puncta by capillary action. During a blink, the orbicularis oculi muscle contracts, closing the puncta, shortening the canaliculi, and moving them medially, while dilating the lacrimal sac. As the sac dilates, it creates a vacuum, drawing in the tears from the canaliculi. When the orbicularis muscle relaxes, the lacrimal sac collapses, the canaliculi lengthen, and the puncta reopen. The valve of Rosenmüller sits between the canaliculi and the sac, preventing the tears from reentering the canaliculi. Thus, tears are forced to continue their course down the nasolacrimal duct into the nose.

5. How does lower eyelid laxity affect tear drainage?

Normal drainage of tears requires normal structure and function of the eyelids. The pretarsal orbicularis muscle surrounds the canaliculi and attaches to the wall of the lacrimal sac. Contraction and relaxation of this muscle help draw the tears into the canaliculus and the sac and eventually force the tears down the nasolacrimal duct. When lower eyelid laxity is present, contraction of the orbicularis muscle does not compresses the canaliculi or force open the lacrimal sac, and the lacrimal pump mechanism cannot function adequately.

6. How can you tell if a patient has lower eyelid laxity?

Stretching of the medial and/or lateral canthal tendon causes lower eyelid laxity. In the distraction test, if the lower eyelid can be pulled more than 6 mm from the globe, it is lax.

Poor orbicularis oculi tone, most obvious in patients with seventh cranial nerve palsy, also causes laxity of the lower eyelid. This is best demonstrated with the "snap-back" test, in which the lower eyelid is pulled down inferiorly and allowed to snap back into place. If the eyelid returns to its correct position immediately, the muscle tone is good. If the patient must blink to place the eyelid back in its normal position, eyelid tone is poor.

7. How do you correct lower eyelid laxity?

If there is laxity of the lateral canthal tendon, a horizontal lid shortening procedure is performed to tighten the eyelid. This is typically accomplished with a lateral tarsal strip procedure. In this operation, the inferior limb of the lateral canthal tendon is disinserted from the periosteum of the lateral orbital rim, a portion or the tendon is removed, and a new lateral canthal tendon is created from the lateral portion of the tarsus. The newly formed lateral canthal tendon is sutured back to the periosteum of the lateral orbital rim. This effectively shortens the lower eyelid, making the eyelid margin more stable and improving tear pump function.

8. Why do patients with dry eyes complain of tearing?

Patients tear when they have dry eyes for the same reason that they tear when cutting an onion. Onion fumes cause corneal irritation, which, in turn, causes reflex tearing.

Likewise, abnormalities in the tear film coating the cornea and conjunctiva cause irritation. Tear-film abnormalities can be caused by a decrease in the overall production of tears or by an imbalance in the composition of the tears. Inadequacies in any of the components of the tears cause a tear-film deficiency that can result in tearing.

9. What is computer vision syndrome?

Computer vision syndrome refers to a group of symptoms including tearing, eyestrain, and pain experienced by computer users. According to the National Institute of Occupational Safety and Health, computer vision syndrome affects some 90% of the people who spend 3 hours or more a day at a computer. Many of the symptoms relate to corneal exposure, poor or decreased blinking, and the resultant dryness that occurs when extended time is spent staring at a computer screen.

10. Of what are tears composed?

Tears are composed of three layers. *Mucin*, made by the conjunctival goblet cells found mainly in the conjunctival fornices, covers the epithelium, ensuring a smooth, uniform tear film. The middle *aqueous* layer, made by the main lacrimal gland and accessory glands of Krause and Wolfring, provides hydration, oxygen, and nutrients. On the surface is the *lipid* layer, made in the meibomian, Zeis, and Moll glands of the eyelids. It prevents rapid evaporation of the tears and provides a smooth surface for the eyelids to glide across the cornea with each blink.

11. How can you determine if a patient produces enough tears?

The volume of tears can be indirectly assessed by visualization of the tear meniscus, the tear layer resting on the lower eyelid adjacent to the globe, which should be approximately 1 mm in height. However, the tear meniscus is also affected by tear drainage. The Schirmer test directly tests production. In the Schirmer test, the palpebral conjunctiva is gently dried with a cotton swab. The small, folded end of a 5-mm-wide strip of Whatman No. 41 filter paper is placed into the inferior conjunctival fornix at the junction of the middle and lateral third of the lower eyelid. In 5 minutes, the amount of wetting of the filter paper is measured. When performed on an anesthetized cornea, it measures basal tear secretion. A normal result is 10 mm or greater. When performed on a nonanesthetized cornea, it measures both basal and reflex tearing. In this instance, normal wetting is 15 mm or greater.

Studies are ongoing to evaluate the clinical usefulness of ultrahigh-resolution special domain optical coherence tomography to measure tear meniscus height.

12. How do you know if the tear composition is inadequate?

A decrease in the tear break-up time or the presence of protein, mucus, or debris in the tears indicates a tear inadequacy. The tear break-up time is the time it takes after a blink to develop a dry spot on the cornea. It is measured by touching the palpebral conjunctiva with a moistened fluorescein strip and observing the tear film through the slit lamp with a cobalt-blue filter. It is important to avoid using other eyedrops mixed with fluorescein because this will change the composition of the tear film you observe. Once the patient blinks, the time is measured until the tear film begins to break up on the cornea, forming a dry spot. Less than 10 seconds is considered abnormal.

13. **What are ectropion and entropion? How do they cause tearing?**
They are both lid malpositions. Ectropion is an outward rotation of the eyelid margin. Entropion is an inward rotation of the eyelid margin. When either is present, patients tear. This occurs because both can cause corneal irritation with its associated reflex tearing, and both displace the punctum, so tears do not enter the tear-drainage system. The normal tear pumping mechanism is not functioning normally.

KEY POINTS: TESTING PATIENTS WITH CHRONIC TEARING

1. Tear quantity and quality evaluation
2. Evaluation of eyelid position
3. Evaluation of eyelid laxity
4. Probing and irrigation of lacrimal drainage system

14. **What causes obstructions of the punctum, canaliculus, or lacrimal sac?**
Complete and partial obstructions can occur anywhere in the lacrimal drainage system and may be caused by congenital agenesis, inflammation, infection, autoimmune disease, trauma, malignancy, radiation, and the toxic effects of medication. Here are the more common causes by location:
   - **Punctal obstructions** are most commonly seen in congenital agenesis, herpetic infections, iatrogenic closure in the treatment of dry eyes, and mechanical obstruction in the setting of conjunctivochalasis.
   - **Canalicular obstructions** can occur in one or both canaliculi or in the common canaliculus. These are often acquired from trauma, cicatrizing mucosal diseases such as Stevens-Johnson syndrome and ocular cicatricial pemphigoid, herpetic infections, canaliculitis associated with *Actinomyces israelii*, chemotherapeutic agents such as 5-fluorouracil and docetaxel, or long-term use of topical medications such as pilocarpine, epinephrine, phospholine iodide, and idoxuridine. Foreign bodies, such as silicone punctal and canalicular plugs, are used to iatrogenically occlude the canaliculi in patients with dry eye due to decreased tear production.
   - **Lacrimal sac obstructions** occur most frequently from scarring as a result of a prior infection. Dacryoliths may develop from infections or chronic use of topical medications. Lacrimal sac tumors are rare.

15. **What causes nasolacrimal duct obstructions?**
Congenital nasolacrimal duct obstructions are found in 6% of normal newborns, and approximately 90% resolve spontaneously in the first year of life. In adults, primary acquired nasolacrimal duct obstruction is the most common cause of these obstructions. The cause of these is not well understood. However, it is commonly believed that obstruction of the ostium of the duct most likely is caused by inflammation of the lining of the duct and nasal mucosa. Dacryocystitis commonly causes scarring, which leads to nasolacrimal duct obstructions. Abnormalities in adjacent structures are often associated with these obstructions, such as nasal polyps, sinus disease, trauma, and deviated septa.

16. **How do you evaluate the lacrimal system for obstructions?**
Obstructions can occur anywhere in the lacrimal system. Punctal obstructions can be visualized on examination. To determine the presence of an obstruction in the canaliculus, lacrimal sac, and nasolacrimal duct, a dye-disappearance test or a Jones dye test can be performed (see later).
   Obstruction in the canaliculus can also be determined directly by probing the canaliculus and feeling for partial and complete obstructions. Irrigation of the system will uncover obstructions in the lacrimal sac and nasolacrimal duct.
   Imaging techniques of the lacrimal system, including ultrasound, computed tomographic scans, contrast dacryocystography, and radionuclide dacryoscintigraphy, are rarely necessary.

17. **What is a dye-disappearance test?**
In the dye-disappearance test, a drop of fluorescein is placed in the inferior conjunctival fornix. After 5 minutes, the amount present in the tear lake is assessed using a cobalt-blue light. The presence of little or no fluorescein indicates a normal functioning system. If most of the fluorescein remains, the system is not functioning properly.

18. **What is a primary Jones dye test?**
A primary Jones dye test involves placing fluorescein in the inferior conjunctival fornix. A cotton swab is placed under the inferior turbinate at 2 and 5 minutes. If dye is recovered on the swab, the system is patent and functioning well. If no dye is recovered, this indicates a poorly functioning system.

19. **What is a secondary Jones dye test?**
A secondary Jones dye test is performed when no dye is recovered during the primary test. In a secondary Jones dye test, the inferior fornix is first irrigated to remove all residual fluorescein from the primary test. Clear saline is then irrigated through the canaliculus with a cannula. If fluorescein-stained fluid is recovered from the nose, the fluorescein must have passed freely through the punctum and canaliculus and to the lacrimal sac during the primary Jones test, indicating a partial blockage of the nasolacrimal duct. If clear fluid is recovered, a partial obstruction or functional disorder of the punctum or canaliculus is indicated. If no fluid is recovered from the nose

but instead regurgitates from the adjacent punctum, an obstruction at or distal to the common canaliculus is present.

20. **How do you treat obstructions of the eyelid portion of the lacrimal system?**
When the punctum is not patent, this can frequently be opened with a sharp probe or cut-down procedure to find the proximal canaliculus. In most patients, placement of a temporary silicone stent is helpful to prevent the punctum from reclosing. This office-based procedure is performed with local infiltrative anesthesia. If the canaliculus is stenotic but not completely occluded, dilation with silicone intubation is typically performed. If the canaliculus is completely occluded, a canaliculodacryocystorhinostomy (CDCR) is performed. In this surgery, a fistula is created between the caruncle and the nasal mucosa and a permanent glass tube (Jones tube) is placed in this tract to maintain its patency. A CDCR can be performed on an outpatient basis under general anesthesia or with monitored sedation.

21. **How do you treat obstructions of the nasolacrimal duct?**
The majority of lacrimal system obstructions occur in the nasolacrimal duct, which connects the lacrimal sac to the nose. When a nasolacrimal duct obstruction is present, a dacryocystorhinostomy (DCR) is performed. In this procedure, the lacrimal sac is marsupialized to the nasal passages, so the tears can bypass the blocked nasolacrimal duct and drain directly from the lacrimal sac into the nose.

22. **Describe acute dacryocystitis.**
An acute infection of the lacrimal sac is called *dacryocystitis*. Patients typically present with a painful, erythematous swelling in the medial canthus just inferior to the medial canthal tendon. A purulent discharge from the punctum can often be seen with gentle pressure on the lacrimal sac. Acute dacryocystitis is nearly always the result of a blocked nasolacrimal duct.

23. **What is the appropriate treatment for acute dacryocystitis?**
Dacryocystitis is a serious infection that must be treated as an emergency. If not adequately treated, an orbital cellulitis may develop. There is also the potential for the infection to spread intracranially. Appropriate systemic antibiotics should be given, and warm compresses should be applied to the medial canthus. Patients should be watched carefully to assure improvement. After resolution of the acute infection, unless the nasolacrimal duct is patent, a DCR should be performed to avoid recurrent infections.

24. **What are the signs of congenital nasolacrimal duct obstructions?**
Approximately 6% of newborns have a congenital obstruction of the nasolacrimal system. Infants may present with epiphora, conjunctivitis, amniocele formation, or dacryocystitis. The lacrimal drainage system begins embryologically as a cord in the medial canthus that expands laterally to the punctum and inferiorly to the nasal mucosa of the inferior meatus. The lumen first develops in the medial canthal portion of the system, and canalization progresses laterally and inferiorly. The distal end of the duct is the last portion to canalize. This may not yet be patent at birth and is the most common site of congenital obstructions.

KEY POINTS: TREATMENT OF CONGENITAL EPIPHORA

1. Treat initially with massage.
2. If it persists in patients younger than 13 months, probe the nasolacrimal duct under anesthesia, often with balloon dacryoplasty.
3. If this is unsuccessful, repeat step 2 and use silicone intubation.
4. If this also is unsuccessful, perform a DCR.

25. **How are congenital obstructions first managed?**
Most clinicians recommend massaging the infant's lacrimal sac (in the medial canthus) in an inferior direction to increase the hydrostatic pressure in the nasolacrimal duct and, it is hoped, force open any obstruction. If there is an associated conjunctivitis or discharge, topical antibiotics are also used. When dacryocystitis is present, systemic antibiotics are used, followed by a DCR.

26. **What if this does not work?**
If a child has a persistent tearing because of blockage of the nasolacrimal duct, a probing of the system should be performed in the first 13 months of life. Katowitz and Welsh have shown that the success rate of probing drops significantly if performed after 13 months of age. In this procedure, the child is placed under general anesthesia and a Bowman probe is passed into the punctum, through the lacrimal system, and out through the nasolacrimal duct. Some surgeons elect to perform a balloon dacryoplasty at the time of the initial probing. Here, a deflated balloon is passed into the duct and then inflated to dilate the duct and the ostium.

27. **What if the tearing is still present after a probing?**
Symptoms resolve in 90% to 95% of infants who undergo a nasolacrimal duct probing. When the problem persists after probing or balloon dacryoplasty, intubation with silicone tubes is indicated. Tubes are generally left

in place for approximately 6 months and serve to keep the passageway patent. Durso et al. reported an 84% success rate for patients intubated for nasolacrimal duct obstruction. When probing and intubation are unsuccessful, a DCR is performed.

BIBLIOGRAPHY

Blehm C, Vishnu S, Khattak A, Mitra S, Yee RW: Computer vision syndrome: a review, Surv Ophthalmol 50(3):253–262, 2005.
Durso F, Hand SI Jr, Ellis FD, Helveston EM: Silicone intubation in children with nasolacrimal obstruction, J Pediatr Ophthalmol Strabismus 17:389–393, 1980.
Kanski JJ: Clinical ophthalmology, ed 9, Oxford, England, 2019, Butterworth-Heinemann.
Katowitz JA, Welsh MG: Timing of initial probing and irrigation in congenital nasolacrimal duct obstruction, Ophthalmology 94:698–705, 1987.
Welham RAN, Hughes SM: Lacrimal surgery in children, Am J Ophthalmol 99:27–34, 1985.

CHAPTER 34

PROPTOSIS

David G. Buerger

1. What is proptosis?
   Proptosis is a forward protrusion of one or both eyeballs. Unilateral proptosis is frequently defined as asymmetric protrusion of one eye by at least 2 mm. Normal upper limits for proptosis are approximately 22 mm in White American and 24 mm in Black Americans.

2. How is proptosis diagnosed?
   Clinically, proptosis can be recognized best by observing the globes from above, over the patient's forehead, or from below with the head tilted back. It is measured with an exophthalmometer based at the lateral orbital rim. The amount of proptosis can also be quantified by measuring globe protrusion on a computed tomographic (CT) or magnetic resonance imaging (MRI) scan (Fig. 34.1).

3. List the common problems associated with proptosis.
   - **Exposure keratopathy** frequently develops secondary to a poor blink mechanism over the protruding globe. Patients can have mild symptoms of irritation and foreign body sensation, or they may experience more severe symptoms associated with corneal abrasions and ulcers (Fig. 34.2).
   - **Diplopia** (double vision) can result from unilateral or bilateral proptosis with displacement of the globes or poor extraocular muscle function.
   - **Optic nerve compression** can occur with space-occupying lesions of the orbit, which cause proptosis. Indications of nerve compression include decreased visual acuity, relative afferent pupillary defect, color vision deficit, and visual field defect of the affected eye. This is a medical emergency and requires prompt therapeutic intervention, surgically or medically.

4. What is the most common cause of unilateral proptosis?
   Thyroid eye disease.

5. What is the most common cause of bilateral proptosis?
   Thyroid eye disease.

6. What are other causes of proptosis?
   - Idiopathic orbital inflammatory disease (orbital pseudotumor)
   - Orbital infectious cellulitis
   - Orbital tumors (benign or malignant)
   - Lacrimal gland tumors
   - Trauma (retrobulbar hemorrhage)
   - Orbital vasculitis (i.e., polyarteritis nodosa, Wegener granulomatosis)
   - Mucormycosis
   - Carotid–cavernous fistula
   - Orbital varix

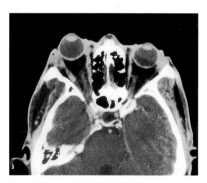

Fig. 34.1 Computed tomographic scan demonstrating proptosis of the right globe secondary to thyroid-related enlargement of the rectus muscles.

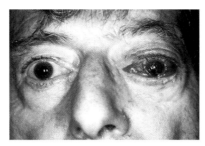

Fig. 34.2 Severe conjunctival chemosis with corneal erosion secondary to proptosis caused by an orbital lymphoma.

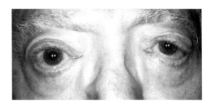

Fig. 34.3 Patient with enophthalmos of the left eye secondary to old trauma, which is causing apparent proptosis of the right eye.

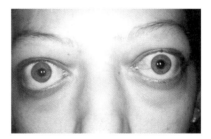

Fig. 34.4 Proptosis and eyelid retraction caused by thyroid ophthalmopathy.

7. List the causes of pseudoproptosis.
   • Unilateral high axial myopia can mimic proptosis, owing to the increased length of the myopic eye.
   • Actual enophthalmos of one eye may cause apparent proptosis of the contralateral eye (Fig. 34.3).
   • Upper eyelid retraction produces a more prominent-appearing eye. This often coexists in cases of thyroid ophthalmopathy.

8. Which neuroimaging test is best to evaluate the etiology of proptosis?
   CT scans are superior in most cases of proptosis because the relationship of the orbital process to the orbital bones is better visualized. MRI may be desirable in certain cases when optic nerve dysfunction is present. Plain films are not used for diagnostic accuracy in cases of proptosis.

9. What clinical entity is frequently associated with unilateral or bilateral painless proptosis, eyelid retraction, eyelid lag on downward gaze, and motility disturbances?
   Thyroid ophthalmopathy (Fig. 34.4) is a complex, multisystem, autoimmune disorder. Patients can be hyperthyroid, hypothyroid, or euthyroid when manifesting ophthalmic symptoms. Eye problems develop as a result of inflammation and enlargement of various extraocular muscles (most frequently the inferior rectus and medial rectus) and peribulbar tissues. CT scan or MRI results often show fusiform enlargement of the involved extraocular muscles with sparing of the tendon that attaches the muscle to the globe. Proptosis and eyelid retraction cause corneal problems. Muscle enlargement in the orbit causes diplopia and possibly optic nerve compression. Treatment is in stages, depending on the severity of the eye disease. Systemic and laboratory evaluation is mandatory. See Chapter 35.

KEY POINTS: CLINICAL SIGNS OF THYROID OPHTHALMOLOPATHY

1. Unilateral or bilateral proptosis
2. Eyelid retraction with lateral flare
3. Lagophthalmos
4. Diplopia
5. Pretibial myxedema

10. **What clinical entity is frequently associated with unilateral proptosis, pain, conjunctival injection, and motility disturbances in an adult?**
Orbital inflammatory disease (orbital pseudotumor) is a nonspecific idiopathic inflammatory disease of the orbit. Inflammation may be localized to a muscle, the lacrimal gland, or sclera or may be diffuse. Other possible signs include eyelid erythema or edema, palpable mass, decreased vision, uveitis, hyperopic shift, and optic nerve edema. Bilateral disease is more common in children. CT scan results may show thickening of one or more extraocular muscles (including the tendons), lacrimal gland enlargement, or thickening of the posterior sclera. Treatment is primarily with corticosteroids and possibly radiation therapy.

11. **What clinical entity is characterized by unilateral proptosis, pain, fever, decreased ocular motility, erythema, and edema of the eyelids?**
Infectious orbital cellulitis involves an infection (usually bacterial) that has extended posterior to the orbital septum. Once past the orbital septum barrier, infection can spread rapidly and cause serious complications such as meningitis or cavernous sinus thrombosis. The most common organisms include staphylococci, streptococci, anaerobes, and *Haemophilus influenzae* (in children younger than 5 years of age). The most common source of infectious spread to the orbit is an ethmoid sinusitis. Treatment is with intravenous antibiotics.

12. **What should be done for persistent proptosis or progression of infection despite adequate antibiotic treatment in a case of orbital cellulitis?**
The situation is highly suggestive of an orbital subperiosteal abscess. CT scanning should be performed to confirm this diagnosis and locate the abscess. Definitive treatment consists of surgical drainage and continued intravenous antibiotics.

13. **What clinical entity is characterized by a child younger than 6 years of age with gradual, painless, progressive, unilateral axial proptosis with visual loss?**
Optic nerve glioma (juvenile pilocytic astrocytoma) is a slow-growing tumor of the optic nerve that causes axial proptosis. Decreased visual acuity is usually associated with a relative afferent pupillary defect. CT scan or MRI results show fusiform enlargement of the optic nerve. Many cases are associated with neurofibromatosis and may be bilateral. Systemic evaluation and genetic counseling for neurofibromatosis are essential.

14. **What clinical entity is characterized by a child with rapidly progressive unilateral proptosis, displacement of the globe inferiorly, and edema of the upper eyelid?**
Rhabdomyosarcoma is the most common primary orbital malignancy of childhood. This malignant growth of striated muscle tissue typically produces a rapidly progressive mass in the superior orbit with proptosis, globe displacement, and eyelid swelling. The average age of presentation is 7 years. Prompt diagnosis with orbitotomy and biopsy is crucial, because *overall mortality is 60%* once the disease has extended to the orbital bones. Current treatment strategies with radiation and chemotherapy have lowered mortality rates to 5% to 10% for orbital rhabdomyosarcoma.

15. **What is the most common benign orbital tumor in adults that causes unilateral proptosis?**
The cavernous hemangioma (Fig. 34.5) is a slow-growing vascular tumor that is usually diagnosed in young adulthood to middle age. CT scanning usually shows a well-defined orbital mass within the ocular muscle cone. Visual acuity is often not affected. Treatment is observation or surgical excision.

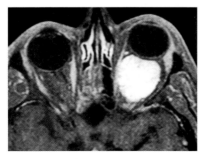

Fig. 34.5 Cavernous hemangioma of the left orbit, which is causing proptosis.

16. What is the most common malignant orbital tumor in adults that causes unilateral proptosis?

    Orbital lymphomas typically develop in the superior orbit with a slow onset and progression. These lesions may be associated with a subconjunctival "salmon-colored" mass in the fornix. CT scanning shows a poorly defined mass conforming to the shape of the orbital bones and globe without bony erosion. Diagnosis is made following orbital biopsy, and definitive treatment is radiation therapy. Orbital lymphoma can be associated with systemic lymphoma; therefore a medical consult and systemic evaluation are necessary for all patients.

17. Of the various orbital tumors causing proptosis, list those tumors that are encapsulated or appear well circumscribed on neuroimaging.
    - Cavernous hemangioma
    - Fibrohistiocytoma
    - Hemangiopericytoma
    - Schwannoma
    - Neurofibroma

BIBLIOGRAPHY

Dolman PJ, Glazer LC, Harris GJ, et al.: Mechanisms of visual loss in severe proptosis, Ophthal Plast Reconstr Surg 7:256–260, 1991.

Frueh BR, Garber F, Grill R, Musch DC: Positional effects on exophthalmometric readings in Graves' eye disease, Arch Ophthalmol 103:1355–1356, 1985.

Frueh BR, Musch DC, Garber FW: Exophthalmometer readings in patients with Graves' eye disease, Ophthalmic Surg 17:37–40, 1986.

Henderson JW: Orbital tumors, ed 4, New York, 2006, Raven Press.

Hornblass A: Oculoplastic, orbital and reconstructive surgery, Baltimore, 1990, Williams & Wilkins.

McCord CD, Tannenbaum M, Nunery WR: Oculoplastic surgery, ed 3, New York, 1995, Lippincott Williams & Wilkins.

Rootman J: Diseases of the orbit, ed 2, Philadelphia, 2002, Lippincott Williams & Wilkins.

Shields JA, Shields CL: Rhabdomyosarcoma: review for the ophthalmologist, Surv Ophthalmol 48:39–57, 2003.

Zimmerman RA, Bilaniuk LT, Yanoff M, et al.: Orbital magnetic resonance imaging, Am J Ophthalmol 100:312–317, 1985.

CHAPTER 35

THYROID EYE DISEASE

Robert B. Penne

1. **What is thyroid eye disease?**
   Thyroid eye disease (TED) is a chronic inflammatory disease of the orbits that occurs most often in patients with a systemic thyroid imbalance. Chronic inflammation results in scarring and dysfunction of the orbit. The course and severity are variable.

2. **Who is at risk for thyroid eye disease?**
   TED occurs in a wide range of ages. It has been reported from 8 to 88 years of age, with the average age of onset in the 40s. Females are affected three to six times more often than males. Children are rarely affected.

3. **Is everyone with thyroid eye disease hyperthyroid?**
   Ninety percent of patients who develop TED have Graves' hyperthyroidism, 3% have Hashimoto thyroiditis, 1% have primary hypothyroidism, and 6% are euthyroid. As many as one-third of patients do not develop clinical hyperthyroidism for more than 6 months after the onset of symptoms of TED. Thus, a significant number of patients who present with TED have not yet developed hyperthyroidism.

4. **What causes thyroid eye disease?**
   We do not know. TED is an immune-mediated process with the orbital fibroblast as the primary target. Many theories link the orbit and thyroid gland by a shared antigen, the thyroid-stimulating hormone receptor. Research continues to try to better understand TED.

5. **Do environmental factors affect thyroid eye disease?**
   Smoking is the one environmental factor that has been shown to affect TED. Multiple studies have shown a higher incidence of smoking in patients with TED than in patients with Graves' disease who do not have TED. Research suggests that smokers with TED have more severe disease and the disease lasts longer than in nonsmokers. The effects of secondhand smoke are unclear.

6. **Does thyroid eye disease improve when the systemic thyroid imbalance is treated?**
   Treatment of the systemic thyroid dysfunction has little predictable effect on the course of TED. Posttreatment hypothyroidism may worsen TED, especially if the hypothyroidism is profound. Also debated is whether radioactive iodine (RAI), surgery, and medical treatment have different effects on the course of TED. A large study suggested that treatment with RAI has a greater chance of causing progression of TED. The study also showed that giving systemic steroids during the treatment decreases and may eliminate this increased risk.

7. **Should all patients who receive radioactive iodine be treated with systemic steroids?**
   Unless the patient has specific contraindications or until further studies show otherwise, we recommend that patients undergoing RAI treatment receive a course of systemic steroids. The dosage and length of treatment are controversial. The patients at the highest risk of worsening TED with RAI are smokers and patients with active disease.

8. **What are the early signs of thyroid eye disease?**
   Many patients initially present with intermittent eyelid swelling along with nonspecific ocular irritation, redness, and swelling (Fig. 35.1). Because all of these symptoms are nonspecific, early-onset TED is infrequently diagnosed. The disease is not recognized until the appearance of more obvious clinical signs, such as eyelid retraction, eyelid lag, or early proptosis (Fig. 35.2). Suspecting TED in patients with the aforementioned nonspecific symptoms is important, especially if they have symptoms or a history of a thyroid imbalance.

9. **What studies need to be done in the workup for thyroid eye disease?**
   The most effective screening tool for systemic thyroid imbalance in patients with TED is the level of thyroid-stimulating hormone. Thyroid stimulating immunoglobulin levels may also be helpful in suggesting increased immune activity in a patient. An internist or endocrinologist can do further evaluation and workup. Patients require a complete ophthalmic exam. Special attention should be paid to visual function, including acuity, pupils, color vision, and, if indicated, visual fields. In particular, the ophthalmic exam should include noting eyelid position, evaluation of ocular motility with note of any diplopia, and checking for corneal exposure and proptosis.

10. **Which patients require orbital imaging?**
    Not all patients with TED require orbital imaging. Indications for imaging include suspicion of optic nerve compression, evaluation for orbital decompression surgery and/or orbital irradiation, unclear diagnosis, and a need to rule out other orbital processes. We prefer a computed tomographic scan without contrast in patients with thyroid-related ophthalmopathy who require imaging.

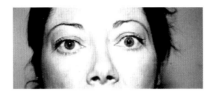

Fig. 35.1 Early thyroid eye disease with mild eyelid retraction of the left upper eyelid and the right lower eyelid.

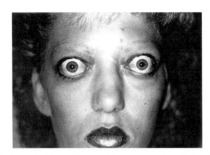

Fig. 35.2 Thyroid eye disease with proptosis and eyelid retraction.

11. **What findings are present on orbital imaging?**
    The classic finding is enlargement of the rectus muscle belly with sparing of the tendon (Fig. 35.3). The inferior rectus is the most commonly involved muscle, followed by the medial rectus and the superior rectus. The lateral rectus is least likely to be involved.

12. **Does everyone with proptosis have thyroid eye disease?**
    No. TED is the most common cause of both unilateral and bilateral proptosis in adults, but it is not the only cause. Patients with systemic thyroid disease may develop orbital tumors and nonthyroid orbital inflammation. TED is a bilateral disease, whereas most orbital tumors are unilateral. TED may present asymmetrically and appear unilateral, especially early in the disease. In rare cases, the disease may remain unilateral. If the entire clinical picture is not consistent with TED, orbital imaging is indicated.

13. **How do the tissues of the orbit change in thyroid eye disease?**
    The extraocular muscles, eyelid muscles, and orbital fat are the main tissues affected in TED. When stimulated, orbital fibroblasts secrete glycosaminoglycans, cytokines, and chemoattractants. Orbital and eyelid swelling are common early in the disease. Late in the disease, the inflammation resolves and the enlarged orbital tissues and muscles are left fibrotic and scarred.

14. **How long does the disease last?**
    Most patients go through a period of active inflammation, causing their eyes and orbital tissues to change. This period lasts from 6 months to more than 2 years. In some patients, the process may involve slow, mild changes over many months, whereas in others, the process is more acute with rapid changes over weeks. Once the disease activity has quieted and the eyes are stable, reactivation is possible but rare (5%–10%). Careful examinations that note changes in motility, eyelid position, proptosis, and general inflammation help to determine disease activity.

15. **Is everyone who develops thyroid eye disease affected in the same way?**
    No. There is a wide variation from mild irritation and eyelid retraction that totally resolve to severe orbital infiltration with visual loss. Visual loss may result from optic nerve compression or corneal scarring due to corneal exposure. More severe disease involves older patients (average age of 52 years vs. 36 years for milder disease) and has less of a gender difference (female-to-male ratio of 1.5:1 in severe disease vs. 8.6:1 in mild disease).

16. **What can be done to treat thyroid eye disease?**
    Many patients do not require any treatment, but monitoring during the active phase of the disease is important. Ocular lubrication often relieves symptoms. Systemic steroids decrease inflammation. Because of their side effects, systemic steroids are best used as a temporizing measure until more definitive treatment is given. Cessation of steroids generally results in return of orbital inflammation. Orbital irradiation may decrease inflammation in the orbit. Surgical treatment is also an option. At the time of writing, a new biologic drug has just been Food and Drug Administration (FDA) approved for the treatment of thyroid eye disease and offers great promise. See question 34.

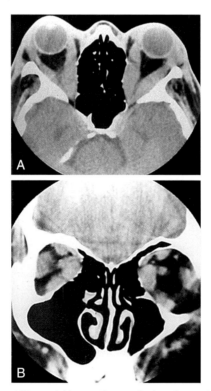

Fig. 35.3 Axial (**A**) and coronal (**B**) computed tomographic scans showing enlargement of all four rectus muscles.

17. **When are systemic steroids used?**
Systemic steroids are used to decrease orbital inflammation acutely, usually on a temporary basis until other treatment can be started. The most common indication is visual loss from optic nerve compression. Severe proptosis with resultant corneal exposure is a second indication. Both the short-term and long-term side effects of steroids limit their usefulness as long-term treatment. High-dose pulsed steroids have been studied, looking for any long-term improvement in TED. The results have been inconclusive.

18. **Is orbital irradiation standard treatment for thyroid eye disease?**
The use of orbital radiation is controversial. A study published in 2001 from the Mayo Clinic concluded that orbital irradiation does not improve TED. Subsequent smaller studies have shown stabilization of disease progression compared to controls. Many oculoplastic specialists believe that orbital irradiation has a role in the treatment of TED and that it stops progression of the disease but does not improve preexisting changes such as proptosis. Radiation may help stabilize ocular motility. How orbital radiation is used varies with the individual physician.

19. **How does orbital irradiation affect thyroid eye disease?**
The exact mechanism of action of irradiation in the orbit is unclear. Multiple theories of localized immunosuppression in the orbit have been postulated, but all remain unproven. Many patients have a definite decrease in orbital inflammation and edema after orbital irradiation. Irradiation seems to be most effective at stopping disease progression and less effective at reversing changes that have already occurred.

20. **Does orbital irradiation work immediately?**
No. It takes 2 to 4 weeks to see the initial effects of irradiation, and improvement may continue for 6 months. If steroids are stopped immediately after completion of irradiation, inflammation may recur rapidly.

21. **Which patients are candidates for orbital irradiation?**
Any patient with *active* TED is a candidate. The exception is patients with diabetes and vasculitic disease, as radiation may worsen their retinopathy. Early treatment, if effective, prevents the chronic orbital changes associated with TED. Later in the disease, irradiation can quiet the active disease and allows earlier and more

effective surgical rehabilitation. Orbital irradiation has resulted in fewer patients with severe TED when used in select patients.

22. **Which patients require surgery?**

Surgery may be indicated on an emergent basis because of optic nerve compression or corneal exposure. More often, patients require nonemergent surgery because of severe disfiguring proptosis, double vision from restrictive myopathy, or eyelid retraction.

23. **What kinds of surgery are done in patients with thyroid eye disease?**

Surgery falls into three basic categories: orbital decompression, eye muscle surgery, and eyelid surgery. Surgery needs to be done in this order because earlier surgeries affect the results of later surgeries. Decompression should be done before eye muscle surgery. Decompression affects ocular motility and may alter muscle surgery. Likewise, muscle surgery should be completed before eyelid surgery is done.

24. **What is orbital decompression?**

Orbital decompressive surgery involves removal of bone and/or fat to allow the eye to settle back in the orbit. Bone is removed from the inferior and medial walls of the orbit to let the expanded orbital tissue move partially into the sinus space. Lateral wall decompression can also be done. Removal of orbital fat has a decompressive effect to a much lesser degree. The amount of decompression is related to the amount of fat removed.

25. **Which patients require orbital decompression?**

Patients with optic nerve compression require decompressive surgery to relieve pressure on the optic nerve. Patients with severe proptosis resulting in corneal exposure or disfigurement are also candidates for orbital decompressive surgery.

26. **What is optic nerve compression?**

Optic nerve compression involves squeezing of the optic nerve at the apex of the orbit. When the extraocular muscles swell in TED, there is relatively little space at the apex of the orbit; therefore, enlargement of muscles exerts pressure on the nerve lying in the center of the muscles. Pressure decreases vision because the function of the optic nerve is affected. This loss of function can manifest as decreased vision, decreased color vision, or visual-field loss.

27. **What are the complications of orbital decompression?**

The most common complication is worsening of existing diplopia or new double vision. Patients with preexisting motility problems have a much higher risk of postoperative diplopia. Many patients have infraorbital hypesthesia postoperatively, but it usually improves with time. Risk of visual loss is small. Bleeding and infection, as with any surgery, must be considered.

28. **When do patients require muscle surgery?**

Patients with double vision in their functional field of vision require muscle surgery. Every effort must be made to ensure that the inflammation is quiet and the patient's motility pattern is stable. Repeated stable measurements over months help to ensure that motility is stable.

KEY POINTS: THYROID EYE DISEASE

1. Suspect the diagnosis of TED in nonspecific ocular irritation even without a systemic thyroid imbalance.
2. Eyelid retraction is often the earliest clinical sign of TED.
3. Monitor visual function closely in progressive TED.
4. Encourage patients who are smokers to stop smoking.
5. TED patients will take extra time during an office visit.

29. **What are the alternatives to muscle surgery?**

The use of prisms in glasses works for patients with double vision and relatively small deviations. Larger deviations or patterns of diplopia in which the deviation changes with small changes in the direction of gaze are poor candidates for prisms. It is also important that the motility is stable before prisms are prescribed. Temporary Fresnel prisms may be helpful during periods of instability.

30. **What type of muscle surgery is required?**

Recession of muscles, usually on an adjustable suture, is needed. Because the muscles are tight and scarred, resection is not done. The inferior and medial rectus muscles are the most common targets of surgery. Surgery can be done under local or general anesthesia with adjustment of the sutures later in the day or on the following day.

31. **Does eye muscle surgery affect the eyelids?**
    Recession of the tight inferior rectus muscle often improves upper eyelid retraction. The superior rectus muscle has to work against the tight inferior rectus; thus, the associated levator muscle is overactive, causing eyelid retraction. When the inferior muscle is recessed, the overactivity ends and often the upper eyelid retraction is less. Large recessions of the inferior rectus muscle may worsen inferior eyelid retraction.

32. **What kind of eyelid surgery is done?**
    Eyelid retraction is the main eyelid problem in patients with TED. In patients undergoing orbital decompression, the eye is lowered, often improving the lower eyelid retraction. For mild eyelid retraction, recession of the eyelid retractors (upper or lower) is adequate. For more severe retraction, spacers are needed, such as hard palate or acellular dermis in the lower eyelids. Patients also may require a blepharoplasty and/or brow lift to deal with the excessive skin that results from stretching caused by chronic swelling. This goal may be met at the time of eyelid repositioning or at a later date.

33. **How many surgeries do patients with thyroid eye disease require?**
    Most patients with TED do not require surgery. Patients who do need surgery may need from 1 to as many as 8 to 10 operations. Patients with severe disease may require many operations over 2 to 3 years of reconstruction.

34. **What is teprotumumab?**
    Teprotumumab is a human monoclonal antibody, insulin-like growth factor-1 receptor (IGF-1R) inhibitor that has completed phase 3 trials and was just FDA approved for the treatment of TED at the time of writing. Teprotumumab has the potential to dramatically improve treatment of moderate to severe TED. In phase 3 trials, it stopped the progression of TED, decreased proptosis, improved diplopia, and improved quality of life in a high percentage of patients when compared to placebo. It is given in eight IV infusions every 3 weeks for 24 weeks

35. **How will teprotumumab change the treatment of thyroid eye disease?**
    It is too early to say how well teprotumumab will work to treat TED, but there is potential to change the approach to TED. Instead of waiting for the disease to become inactive and then doing multiple surgeries to repair the damage, teprotumumab would stop the disease, avoid the progression, and the need for surgery. Time and experience with this newly approved medication will determine how well it works.

BIBLIOGRAPHY

Bartalena L, Marcocci C, Bogazzi F, et al.: Relation between therapy for hyperthyroidism and the course of Graves' ophthalmopathy, N Engl J Med 1338:73–78, 1998.

Bartley G, Fatourechi V, Kadrmas EF: The chronology of Graves' ophthalmopathy in an incidence cohort, Am J Ophthalmol 121:426–434, 1996.

Douglas RS, Kahaly JG, Patel A: Teprotumumab for the treatment of active thyroid eye disease, N Engl J Med 382:341–352, 2020.

Gorman CA, Garrity JA, Fatourechi V: A prospective, randomized, double-blind, placebo-controlled study of orbital radiotherapy for Graves' ophthalmopathy, Ophthalmology 108:1523–1534, 2001.

Holds JB, Buchanan AG: Graves' orbitopathy. Focal points: clinical modules for ophthalmologists, San Francisco, 2010, American Academy of Ophthalmology.

Mourits MP, van Kempen-Harteveld MI, Garcia MB, et al.: Radiotherapy for Graves' orbitopathy: randomized placebo-controlled study, Lancet 355(9412):1505–1509, 2000.

Rootman J, Stewart B, Goldberg RA: Orbital surgery: a conceptual approach, Philadelphia, 1995, Lippincott-Raven.

CHAPTER 36

ORBITAL INFLAMMATORY DISEASES

Nicole A. Langelier, Usiwoma Abugo, and Roberta E. Gausas

1. What is inflammation?

   The concept of inflammation is ancient and was used to describe a combination of rubor (redness), dolor (pain), tumor (swelling), calor (heat), and *functio laesa* (loss of function). We now recognize inflammation as a tissue response governed by multiple cellular processes.

2. How does inflammation affect the orbit?

   Inflammation is the most common problem that affects the adult orbit, leading to a spectrum of clinical presentations with variable onsets and variable orbital tissues affected, causing mass effect, inflammation, and/or infiltration resulting in variable deficits in function or vision.[1]

3. What are the best terms to describe orbital inflammation?

   For purposes of better understanding and better management, orbital inflammation should be classified based on pathology, anatomic location, and/or associated systemic disease as either specific or nonspecific in nature.

4. What is specific orbital inflammation?

   The diagnosis of specific orbital inflammation is based on the identification of a specific etiology causing the disorder, such as a specific pathogen (infection, as in orbital cellulitis), specific histopathology (granulomatous disease, as in sarcoidosis), or specific local and/or systemic constellation of findings that define a distinct entity (vasculitis, as in granulomatosis with polyangiitis [GPA]) (Box 36.1).[2]

5. How is nonspecific orbital inflammation different?

   Orbital inflammation that has no identifiable cause is considered nonspecific. It is a diagnosis of exclusion.

6. What is orbital pseudotumor?

   "Nonspecific orbital inflammation" (NSOI) and "idiopathic orbital inflammatory syndrome" are more accurate terms that replace orbital pseudotumor.

7. What, then, is the etiology of nonspecific orbital inflammation?

   The exact etiology is unknown, but it is generally believed to be an immune-mediated process, possibly related to previous bacterial or viral infection, previous trauma, or other autoimmune conditions, such as Crohn's disease, rheumatoid arthritis, and systemic lupus erythematosis.[3]

Box 36.1 Differential Diagnosis of Orbital Inflammation

Nonspecific Orbital Inflammation (NSOI)	Hypersensitivity angiitis
Diagnosis after exclusion of specific inflammations	Orbital vasculitis secondary to systemic lupus erythematosus
Specific Orbital Inflammation	Giant cell arteritis
Thyroid-associated orbitopathy	Granulomatous inflammation
Infection/infestation	Sarcoidosis/sarcoidal reactions
Bacterial	Xanthogranulomatous disorders of orbit
Contiguous spread from sinusitis	Foreign-body granuloma
Retained orbital foreign body	Erdheim-Chester disease
Fungal	Sjögren's syndrome
Rhino-orbital mucormycosis	**IgG4-related disease of the orbit**
Aspergillosis	**Sclerosing inflammation of the orbit**
Endogenous spread from septic emboli	**Idiopathic granulomatous inflammation**
Parasitic	**Nonspecific Orbital Inflammation (NSOI)**
Echinococcosis	**Noninflammatory Diseases of the Orbit that Mimic**
Cysticercosis	**Inflammation**
Tuberculosis and syphilis	**Vascular disorders**
Vasculitis	Dural–cavernous sinus arteriovenous fistula
Granulomatosis with polyangiitis	**Neoplasia**
Polyarteritis nodosa	Lymphoproliferative disorders

8. Describe a typical clinical presentation of nonspecific orbital inflammation.

Anterior orbital NSOI commonly presents as painful periorbital swelling and erythema, S-shaped eyelid deformity, and chemosis that may be unilateral or bilateral. Onset is typically acute (hours to days) or subacute (days to weeks) but can also be insidious or chronic (weeks to months). The symptoms and physical findings will vary based on the degree and anatomic location of the inflammation. Disease affecting the posterior orbit may present with proptosis and motility disturbances, and disease affecting the orbital apex may present with functional deficits and/or vision loss.

9. Is the symptom of pain necessary to make the diagnosis?

Although pain or discomfort is a typical symptom, absence of pain may occur less commonly.[4]

10. How is nonspecific orbital inflammation in children different?

In the pediatric population, bilateral manifestation is much more common, as well as concurrent uveitis, elevated erythrocyte sedimentation rate, and eosinophilia. When present, uveitis in particular appears to portend a poor outcome in children. Overall, NSOI in children is rare and cases should be monitored closely for future development of autoimmune disease.[5-7]

11. Name the five most common anatomic patterns of nonspecific orbital inflammation.

1. Extraocular muscle (myositis)
2. Lacrimal gland (dacryoadenitis)
3. Anterior orbit including scleritis
4. Orbital apex
5. Diffuse

12. How is the diagnosis of nonspecific orbital inflammation made?

Because NSOI is a diagnosis of exclusion, all known specific triggers of inflammation should be ruled out first. Ultimate diagnosis and treatment rely on complete history and detailed clinical examination, followed by judicious use of ancillary diagnostic testing, including neuroimaging, laboratory testing, and biopsy when appropriate.

13. What is the best imaging technique for nonspecific orbital inflammation?

Orbital computed tomography (CT), gadolinium-enhanced magnetic resonance imaging (MRI), or ultrasound can all provide useful information, but orbital MRI with fat saturation is the imaging study with the highest yield. Subtle edema of the retrobulbar fat is often one of the earliest changes seen in NSOI. The use of diffusion weighted imaging is helpful in differentiating NSOI from lymphoid lesions and orbital cellulitis.[8,9]

14. What blood tests can be ordered to evaluate nonspecific orbital inflammation?

Complete blood count, electrolytes, erythrocyte sedimentation rate, C-reactive protein, antinuclear antibody, anti-double-stranded DNA, anti-neutrophil cytoplasmic antibody (ANCA), angiotensin-converting enzyme level, rapid plasma reagin, and thyroid function tests.[10]

15. When should an orbital biopsy be performed?

Although the role of orbital biopsy has previously been an area of controversy, the only way to obtain an accurate and definitive diagnosis of an infiltrative lesion is through pathologic examination. Most orbital surgeons advocate biopsy, except for two clinical scenarios—that of orbital myositis, in which the clinical and radiographic findings are classic, and that of an orbital apex syndrome—in which the risk of biopsy must be weighed against the risk of a missed diagnosis. Empiric steroid treatment may be employed in such cases. However, recurrent or nonresponsive orbital myositis and orbital apex syndrome warrant orbital biopsy.[11]

16. What is the histopathology of nonspecific orbital inflammation?

In the acute phase, pathology reveals a diffuse polymorphous infiltrate composed of mature lymphocytes, plasma cells, macrophages, eosinophils, and polymorphonuclear leukocytes. In the subacute and chronic phases, an increasing amount of fibrovascular stroma is seen.

17. Name two histological subtypes of orbital inflammation.

A distinct sclerosing form of orbital inflammation exists, which is characterized by dense fibrous replacement. Clinically, the sclerosing subtype typically produces limited inflammatory signs and atypical pain.

Another distinct form displays granulomatous inflammation similar to sarcoidosis but is not associated with systemic sarcoidosis.

18. What is immunoglobulin G4–related disease?

Immunoglobulin G4 (IgG4)–related disease is a systemic fibroinflammatory condition that should be considered in patients with NSOI, particularly in cases with bilateral lacrimal gland involvement. Histology reveals IgG4-positive plasma cells and fibrosis, with or without obliterative phlebitis. Serum IgG4 is often elevated. Systemic manifestations of IgG4-related disease include sclerosing pancreatitis, retroperitoneal fibrosis, sclerosing cholangitis, Riedel's thyroiditis, and interstitial lung disease. IgG4-related orbital inflammation is typically exquisitely and rapidly responsive to steroid treatment.[12,13]

19. How is nonspecific orbital inflammation treated?

High-dose oral corticosteroids are the mainstay of treatment. The recommended starting dose for prednisone is 1.0 to 1.5 mg/kg/day, with a maximum adult dose of 60 to 80 mg/day for 1 to 2 weeks, then tapering off over the course of 6 to 12 weeks. For patients with vision loss or apical involvement, intravenous methylprednisone 1 mg/kg/day can be administered for 1 to 3 days. The response is usually quick, with resolution of pain and proptosis within 24 to 48 hours of onset of the treatment.[14]

20. What if a patient fails to respond to or is intolerant of steroids?

Alternative therapies include antimetabolites (azathioprine, methotrexate), T-cell inhibitors (cyclosporine), and alkylating agents (cyclophosphamide). Low-dose external beam radiation has also been shown to be effective.

Local injection of betamethasone can also be effective in treating acute idiopathic dacryoadenitis, myositis, and anterior diffuse orbital inflammation.[1,15]

KEY POINTS: NONSPECIFIC ORBITAL INFLAMMATION

1. NSOI is a diagnosis of exclusion.
2. Onset is usually acute and painful.
3. Inflammation may be unilateral or bilateral.
4. Children often have concurrent uveitis and eosinophilia.
5. Subtle edema of retrobulbar fat is an early finding on imaging.

21. What is the most common specific orbital inflammation?

Thyroid-associated orbitopathy.

22. Which extraocular muscle is most likely to be involved in thyroid eye disease?

The inferior rectus is the most likely. An easy-to-remember mnemonic is IMSLO, for the order of extraocular muscle involvement: inferior rectus, medial rectus, superior rectus, lateral rectus, and then the obliques.[16]

23. What infections can occur in the orbit?

The orbit may undergo bacterial (e.g., *Staphylococcus*, tuberculosis, syphilis), fungal (e.g., rhino-orbital mucormycosis, aspergillosis), parasitic (e.g., echinococcosis, cysticercosis, trichinosis), and viral (e.g., herpetic) infections.

24. Where do orbital infections originate?

- The most common source is contiguous spread of bacteria from the sinuses, often the ethmoid sinus.
- Direct inoculation following trauma or skin infection.
- Infection may spread endogenously from septic emboli.

25. In adults, what pathogens usually cause orbital cellulitis?

Staphylococcus aureus and streptococci are most common. It is important to note that adults need broad-spectrum antibiotics, because multiple organisms tend to be involved, versus children, in whom a single gram-positive organism is usually the culprit.[17]

26. In a 2-year-old patient, what pathogen might be a likely cause of orbital cellulitis?

Historically, it has been *Haemophilus influenza B* (Hib), but with the advent of the Hib vaccine, most pediatric cases are now the result of gram-positive cocci infection. Vaccination status is an important consideration.

27. How is orbital cellulitis treated?

Medical care consists of the proper use of the appropriate antibiotics. Preseptal cellulitis may be treated with oral antibiotics. Orbital cellulitis requires intravenous administration of antibiotics. Care must be taken to distinguish community-associated methicillin-resistant *S. aureus* (MRSA) from hospital-acquired MRSA, as the treatment differs and the potential for morbidity and long-term disability is significant.

28. When should surgery be undertaken?

If the response to appropriate antibiotic therapy is poor within 48 to 72 hours or if the CT scan shows the sinuses to be completely opacified, surgical drainage should be considered. Subperiosteal or intraorbital abscess formations are other indications for surgical drainage if there is a decrease in vision, development of an afferent pupillary defect, or failure of proptosis to resolve despite appropriate antibiotic therapy.

KEY POINTS: ORBITAL INFECTIONS

1. The most common source of an orbital infection is an adjacent sinus.
2. Bacterial infection is the most common cause of cellulitis.
3. The orbital septum defines preseptal versus orbital cellulitis.
4. Orbital cellulitis in adults is usually caused by multiple organisms vs. a single organism in children.
5. Intravenous antibiotics are required to treat orbital cellulitis.

29. What are the major categories of orbital vasculitis?
    GPA (formerly known as Wegener's granulomatosis), hypersensitivity vasculitis, polyarteritis nodosa, and Churg-Strauss syndrome.

30. What is Wegener's granulomatosis?
    Wegener's granulomatosis is an outdated term. The condition is now referred to as *granulomatosis with polyangiitis*, which provides a better description of the pathophysiology of the disease.

31. Is orbital and ocular involvement common in granulomatosis with polyangiitis?
    Yes, involvement is seen in approximately 50% of cases in both systemic and limited GPA.

32. Describe the features of orbital granulomatosis with polyangiitis.
    • **Clinical:** Bilaterality, respiratory tract/sinus/mastoid involvement, scleritis, limbal corneal infiltrates
    • **Imaging:** Three patterns; diffuse orbital involvement (may or may not be bilateral), lacrimal involvement, or midline involvement associated with bone erosion
    • **Laboratory:** Positive for ANCA (although initially not positive in limited form)
    • **Pathology:** Mixed inflammation, "cuffing" vessels, fat necrosis, lipid-laden macrophages, granulomatous microabscesses. Remember the commonly accepted triad of vasculitis, granulomatous inflammation (with or without giant cells), and tissue necrosis.[18,19]

ACKNOWLEDGMENTS

The authors recognize Madhura Tamhankar, MD, for her contributions to the previous edition of this chapter.

REFERENCES

1. Cockerham KP, Hong SH, Browne EE: Orbital inflammation, Curr Neurol Neurosci Rep 3:401–409, 2003.
2. Rootman J: Inflammatory diseases of the orbit. Highlights, J Fr Ophthalmol 24:155–161, 2001.
3. Espinoza GM: Orbital inflammatory pseudotumors: etiology, differential diagnosis, and management, Curr Rheumatol Rep 12: 437–443, 2010.
4. Mahr MA, Salomao DR, Garrity JA: Inflammatory orbital pseudotumor with extension beyond the orbit, Am J Ophthalmol 138: 396–400, 2004.
5. Bloom JN, Graviss ER, Byrne BJ: Orbital pseudotumor in the differential diagnosis of pediatric uveitis, J Pediatr Ophthalmol Strabismus 29:59–63, 1992.
6. Mottow-Lippa L, Jakobiec FA, Smith M: Idiopathic inflammatory orbital pseudotumor in childhood. II. Results of diagnostic tests and biopsies, Ophthalmology 88:565–574, 1981.
7. Yuen S, Rubin PD: Idiopathic orbital inflammation: distribution, clinical features, and treatment outcome, Arch Ophthalmol 121: 491–499, 2003.
8. Uehara F, Ohba N: Diagnostic imaging in patients with orbital cellulitis and inflammatory pseudotumor, Int Ophthalmol Clin 42: 133–142, 2002.
9. Kapur R, Sepahdari AR, Mafee MF, et al.: MR imaging of orbital inflammatory syndrome, orbital cellulitis, and orbital lymphoid lesions: the role of diffusion-weighted imaging, Am J Neuroradiol 30:64–70, 2009.
10. Gordon LK: Orbital inflammatory disease: a diagnostic and therapeutic challenge, Eye 20:1196–1206, 2006.
11. Papalkar D, Sharma S, Francis IC, et al.: A rapidly fatal case of T-cell lymphoma presenting as idiopathic orbital inflammation, Orbit 24:131–133, 2005.
12. Sato Y, Natohara K, Kojima M, et al.: IgG4 related disease: historical overview and pathology of hematological disorders, Pathol Int 60:247–258, 2010.
13. Linfield D, Attfield K, McElvanney A: Systemic immunoglobulin G4 (IgG4) disease and idiopathic orbital inflammation: removing 'idiopathic' from the nomenclature? Eye 26:623–629, 2012.
14. Harris GJ: Idiopathic orbital inflammation: a pathogenic construct and treatment strategy, Ophthal Plast Reconstr Surg 22:79–86, 2006.
15. Mohammed AA: Local steroid injection for management of different types of acute idiopathic orbital inflammation: an 8-year study, Ophthal Plast Reconstr Surg 29:286–289, 2013.
16. Bahn RS: Graves' ophthalmopathy, N Engl J Med 362:726–738, 2010.
17. Harris GJ: Subperiosteal abscess of the orbit. Age as a factor in the bacteriology and response to treatment, Ophthalmology 101:585–595, 1994.
18. Perry C, Shevland JJE: Limited Wegener's granulomatosis, Austral Radiol 28:106–113, 1984.
19. The Johns Hopkins Vasculitis Center: Wegener's granulomatosis, http://www.hopkinsvasculitis.org/types-vasculitis/wegeners-granulomatosis/.

CHAPTER 37

PTOSIS

Carolyn S. Repke

1. **How is ptosis defined and how is it different from dermatochalasis?**
   Ptosis is an abnormally low position of the upper eyelid margin, whereas dermatochalasis is excessive or redundant skin of the upper lid which can be present with or without ptosis (Fig. 37.1).

2. **What are the two muscles of eyelid elevation?**
   The two muscles that elevate the eyelid are the striated levator muscle, innervated by the superior division of the third nerve, and the smooth Muller's muscle, innervated by the sympathetic system.

3. **How is ptosis classified?**
   Ptosis is classified by either time of onset or etiology. By onset, ptosis is either congenital or acquired. By etiology, ptosis may be neurogenic, aponeurotic, mechanical, myogenic, or traumatic.

4. **What are the causes of acquired ptosis? What is the most common cause?**
   Acquired ptosis can be neurogenic (third nerve palsy, Horner's syndrome), mechanical (eyelid mass), myogenic (myasthenia gravis [MG], oculopharyngeal dystrophy, myotonic dystrophy, chronic progressive external ophthalmoplegia [CPEO]), or traumatic (injury to muscle or its innervation). However, of all causes, acquired ptosis is most often the result of disinsertion or attenuation of the levator aponeurosis, commonly related to aging but sometimes related to chronic ocular inflammation or eyelid edema (Fig. 37.2).

5. **What are the causes of congenital ptosis?**
   Congenital ptosis can be from maldevelopment of the levator muscle, blepharophimosis syndrome, congenital third nerve palsy, congenital Horner's syndrome, or Marcus Gunn jaw-winking syndrome.

6. **What clinical findings help to differentiate congenital ptosis from acquired aponeurotic ptosis?**
   Patients with aponeurotic ptosis have a ptotic eyelid in all positions of gaze. In downgaze, the ptotic eyelid remains ptotic. Patients with congenital ptosis, however, demonstrate eyelid lag in downgaze, causing the abnormal eyelid to ride higher in downgaze. This is caused by the maldevelopment of the levator muscle, with poor ability to contract in elevation as well as inability to relax in downgaze.

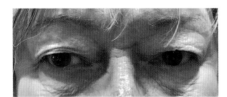

Fig. 37.1 Dermatochalasis causing the appearance of ptosis. (Courtesy Carolyn Repke, MD.)

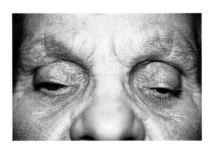

Fig. 37.2 Involutional (aponeurotic) ptosis is characteristically mild to moderate with high upper eyelid crease. Deep sulci are seen in severe cases. Levator function is essentially normal. (From Kanski JJ: *Clinical ophthalmology: a synopsis,* New York, 2004, Butterworth-Heinemann.)

KEY POINTS: FEATURES OF APONEUROTIC PTOSIS

1. High eyelid crease (>10 mm)
2. Moderate ptosis (3–4 mm)
3. Good levator function (>10 mm)
4. No eyelid lag on downgaze

7. **What are the features of congenital ptosis?**

Congenital ptosis is caused by a dystrophy or maldevelopment in the levator muscle/superior rectus complex (Fig. 37.3). Most patients demonstrate poor levator function on examination and, at surgery, have fatty infiltration of the levator muscle. This myogenic abnormality causes an inability of the levator to relax on downgaze, resulting in eyelid lag and, in some cases, lagophthalmos. Patients may or may not demonstrate motility defects because of superior rectus dysfunction (double elevator palsy with ptosis, vertical strabismus, and poor Bell's phenomenon). Approximately 75% of cases are unilateral.

With congenital ptosis, it is critical to evaluate visual function and refractive error as amblyopia will occur in up to 20% of cases.[1]

8. **What causes pseudoptosis?**

Causes of pseudoptosis (Fig. 37.4) include the following:
- Hypotropia on the ptotic side
- Eyelid retraction on the opposite side
- Enophthalmos/phthisis bulbi
- Anophthalmos/microphthalmos
- Severe dermatochalasis—with skin obscuring the position of the eyelid margin

9. **What is the primary cause of ptosis after intraocular surgery?**

Levator dehiscence likely causes the ptosis related to previous intraocular surgery. The exact etiology is uncertain; however, it has been linked to superior rectus bridal sutures (rarely used any longer), eyelid speculums, retrobulbar and peribulbar injections, and other draping maneuvers associated with manipulation of the eyelids. Affected patients probably had a tendency toward levator dehiscence preoperatively.

10. **What is the anatomic cause for the eyelid crease?**

The eyelid crease is formed by the levator aponeurotic attachments that travel through the orbicularis muscle to the skin. With aponeurotic ptosis, these attachments are disinserted, causing the eyelid crease to elevate.

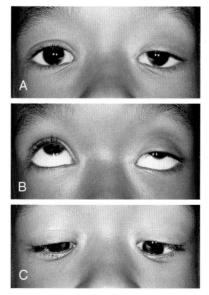

Fig. 37.3 Simple congenital ptosis. **A,** Decreased levator muscle function occurs along with an indistinct upper eyelid crease. **B,** The ptosis is exaggerated in upgaze because of the poor function of the levator muscle. **C,** In downgaze, the ptosis is reduced or absent because the fibrotic levator muscle cannot stretch. (From Custer PL: Blepharoptosis. In: Yanoff M, Duker JS, editors: *Ophthalmology*, ed 2, St. Louis, 2004, Mosby.)

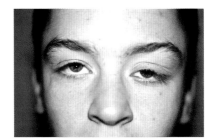

Fig. 37.4 Left pseudoptosis caused by ipsilateral hypotropia. (Kanski JJ: *Clinical ophthalmology: a systematic approach,* ed 5, New York, 2003, Butterworth-Heinemann.)

11. What neurologic conditions are associated with ptosis?
    Neurologic conditions that must be considered in a ptosis evaluation include third-nerve palsy, Horner's syndrome, Marcus Gunn's jaw-winking syndrome, ophthalmoplegic migraine, multiple sclerosis, and the Miller-Fisher syndrome, a variant of Guillain-Barre syndrome.

KEY POINTS: FEATURES OF THIRD-NERVE PALSY

1. Ptosis—mild to complete
2. Decreased elevation, adduction, and depression—may not all be present, depending on superior or inferior division involvement
3. Possible ipsilateral pupillary dilation—may be subtle to complete

12. What are the myogenic causes of ptosis?
    Muscular abnormalities associated with ptosis include MG, muscular dystrophies, CPEO, oculopharyngeal dystrophy, and congenital maldevelopment of the levator.

KEY POINTS: FEATURES OF CPEO

1. Slowly progressive ophthalmoplegia
2. Bilateral ptosis
3. Rarely have diplopia—owing to symmetry of disease
4. No variability (as in MG)

13. What are the features of blepharophimosis syndrome?
    Blepharophimosis syndrome (Fig. 37.5) is a congenital autosomal dominant disorder characterized by ptosis, epicanthus inversus, blepharophimosis (narrowing of the palpebral fissure in all dimensions), and telecanthus (widening of the distance between the medial canthi). Some patients also may demonstrate a flat nasal bridge, lower eyelid ectropions, and hypoplastic orbital rims.

14. What are the signs and symptoms of myasthenia gravis?
    The history of any patient with acquired ptosis should include questions searching for symptoms of MG. Patients may note variability in the degree of ptosis from day to day or morning to evening, with increased ptosis during

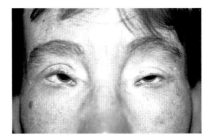

Fig. 37.5 Blepharophimosis with bilateral ptosis, eyelid phimosis, telecanthus, and epicanthus inversus. (From Kanski JJ: *Clinical ophthalmology: a test yourself atlas,* ed 2, New York, 2002, Butterworth-Heinemann.)

periods of fatigue. They may give a history of diplopia or difficulty with swallowing as well as dysphonia, dyspnea, and proximal muscle weakness.

On examination, patients may demonstrate eyelid fatigue on sustained upgaze, with curtaining of the eyelid on returning to the primary position. They also may demonstrate a Cogan's eyelid twitch after attempted upgaze. On return to primary position, the eyelid may show an upward twitch before it settles to its final resting place. Orbicularis strength may be weak, allowing the examiner to open the patient's eyelids even during attempted forceful closure.

KEY POINTS: FEATURES OF OCULAR MYASTHENIA GRAVIS

1. Ptosis—variable over time
2. Ocular misalignment
3. Fatigability of eyelids
4. Cogan's lid twitch
5. Orbicularis weakness

15. **What measurements should be taken during the preoperative examination of patients with ptosis?**
    - **Marginal reflex distance (MRD) 1:** The distance from the corneal light reflex in primary gaze to the upper eyelid margin; it demonstrates the distance of the upper eyelid from the visual axis; evaluated in primary position with the action of the frontalis muscle negated. The normal MRD is 4.0 to 4.5 mm.
    - **MRD2:** The distance between the corneal light reflex and the lower eyelid margin in primary gaze; evaluates for reverse ptosis (as seen in Horner's syndrome) or lower lid retraction
    - **Levator function:** Measures the entire excursion of the eyelid in millimeters from extreme downgaze to upgaze, with the action of the frontalis muscle manually negated; determines the surgical procedure to be performed; function is considered to be normal (>15 mm), good (>8 mm), fair (5 to 7 mm), or poor (>4 mm).
    - **Eyelid crease height:** The crease height is the distance from the eyelid margin to the skin crease. Normally, the crease height is 8 to 10 mm and is higher in women.
    - **Palpebral fissure width:** The distance between the upper and the lower lid margins (MRD1 + MRD2).

    Other critical parts of the preoperative evaluation include visual acuity, a careful pupillary examination for anisocoria, a cover test for strabismus, careful evaluation of ocular motility, and evaluation of corneal sensation and tear film (with further testing of tear osmolarity or Schirmer test if dry eye suspected). The lid position measurements are taken in primary position as well as in downgaze, looking for cyclid lag that suggests congenital ptosis or previous thyroid ophthalmopathy and in upgaze, looking for signs of muscle fatigue and curtaining, suggesting MG. The position of the eyebrows should be noted. The eyelids should be everted, especially in unilateral ptosis, looking for floppy eyelid structure, mass, or foreign body (i.e., lost contact lens). Proptosis or enophthalmos should be noted. Finally, it is important to document the presence of a good Bell's phenomenon (upshoot of the cornea with eyelid closure).[2] Surgical planning may include an automated visual field test to document loss of peripheral vision, an ice test (for MG), and a Neo-Synephrine test (to evaluate Muller's muscle response). A visual field test revealing field loss that resolves when repeated with the upper lids taped is documentation that the surgery is indicated for a medical issue rather than cosmetic.

16. **How does Hering's Law affect ptosis?**
    Hering's law of equivalent innervation of yoke muscles applies to the two levator muscles. It needs to be considered during the preoperative evaluation to determine accurately the degree of ptosis on each side. The eye with which the patient prefers to fixate affects the degree to which Hering's Law contributes to ptosis. If the ptotic eye is preferred for fixation, the opposite eyelid may develop a retracted position because of increased stimulation during attempts to open the ptotic eyelid. On occluding the ptotic fixating eye, the previously retracted eyelid may resume a more normal position.[3] Alternatively, the normal eyelid in a patient with unilateral ptosis may become ptotic when the ptotic eyelid is covered, breaking the bilateral stimulation.

17. **What are the surgical and nonsurgical approaches to the correction of ptosis?**
    The most common surgical approaches to ptosis correction include levator resection, from either an internal or an external approach; Muller's muscle resection; and frontalis suspension. A nonsurgical option is ptosis eyelid crutches, which may be secured to spectacle lenses. Although rarely used, spectacle adaptations are a reasonable option for patients with neurologic ptosis who have a poor Bell's phenomenon and are considered to be at high risk for exposure keratopathy after lid surgery.[4]

18. **What are the complications of ptosis surgery?**
    The most common complication is overcorrection or undercorrection of the ptosis and/or abnormalities in eyelid contour. Other complications include infection, scarring, wound dehiscence, eyelid crease asymmetry, loss of eyelashes, conjunctival prolapse, upper lid ectropion and/or tarsal eversion, eyelid lag on downgaze, and lagophthalmos on eyelid closure, leading to dry eyes or exposure keratopathy, corneal thinning, ulceration, and/or

scarring. In addition, the rare but vision-threatening complication of retrobulbar hemorrhage is a risk with all eyelid surgery, and precautions must be taken to discontinue all medications or supplements that may cause prolonged bleeding or clotting times.[5]

19. **What is Marcus Gunn's jaw-winking syndrome?**
Marcus Gunn's syndrome is a unilateral congenital ptosis with synkinetic innervation of the levator and ipsilateral pterygoid muscle. It is caused by aberrant connections between the motor division of cranial nerve V and the levator muscle. Patients demonstrate retraction of the ptotic eyelid on stimulation of the ipsilateral pterygoid muscles by either opening the mouth or moving the jaw to the opposite side.

20. **Describe the anatomy of Whitnall's ligament and its significance in ptosis.**
Whitnall's ligament, also known as the superior transverse ligament, is a condensation of collagen and elastic fibers on the anterior levator sheath as it changes from muscle to aponeurosis. It attaches medially near the trochlea and laterally traverses through the lacrimal gland, attaching to the lateral orbital wall approximately 10 mm above the lateral orbital tubercle. It serves as a suspensory ligament for the upper eyelid and is the point at which the vector forces of the levator muscle transfer from an anterior–posterior direction to a superior–inferior direction. It is an important landmark for performing large levator resections.[2]

21. **What is the concern when Horner's syndrome presents with pain?**
Patients with neck pain, facial pain, or headache and acute Horner's syndrome should be suspected of having a carotid artery dissection. Workup should be urgent and include magnetic resonance imaging (MRI)/magnetic resonance angiography (MRA) of the head and neck. Carotid Doppler sonography is not accurate in detecting carotid artery dissection. A carotid dissection usually requires urgent anticoagulation and neurovascular consultation.[6]

KEY POINTS: FEATURES OF HORNER'S SYNDROME (FIG. 37.6A)

1. Mild ptosis (1–2 mm)
2. Miosis
3. Anhidrosis
4. Reverse ptosis of the lower eyelid
5. Hypopigmentation of iris (congenital cases)

22. **What is the Neo-Synephrine test?**
The Neo-Synephrine test is an evaluation of the effect of Müller's muscle contraction on the degree of ptosis. One drop of 2.5% phenylephrine is placed in the eye. After 5 minutes, the degree of ptosis is reevaluated. The phenylephrine causes contraction of the sympathetic Horner's muscle, sometimes causing dramatic improvement in the degree of ptosis. If phenylephrine corrects the ptosis completely, many surgeons elect to perform a Müller's muscle resection as opposed to a levator resection (Fig. 37.6B).[7]

23. **Name some useful tests for diagnosing myasthenia gravis.**
   • Ice test (in office)
   • Blood tests:
   Acetylcholine receptor antibody test: Binding antibodies are detectable in up to 90% of patients with systemic MG and up to 70% of patients with ocular MG, with false-negative results in 50% of cases.
       MuSK antibodies: These are antibodies to muscle-specific kinase. In those patients with seronegative MG (no antibodies to acetylcholine receptors), testing for MuSK antibodies may be positive in 40% to 70%.
   • Edrophonium chloride (Tensilon) test
   • Single-fiber electromyography (orbicularis muscle)[8]

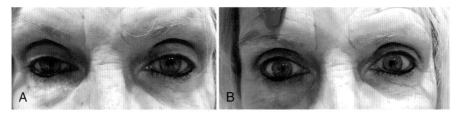

Fig. 37.6 A, Horner's syndrome demonstrating mild right ptosis and anisocoria. **B,** Positive Neo-Synephrine test with resolution of ptosis. (Courtesy Carolyn Repke, MD.)

24. Name some causes of acquired ptosis in young adults.

Levator aponeurosis dehiscence can certainly occur in a younger age group, but ptosis in younger adults should prompt thought of other causes as well. History and clinical exam should look for obvious neurologic, myogenic, and mechanical causes. Old photographs should be viewed to rule out a longstanding problem. In addition, consideration should be given to the following:

- Contact lens wear (ptosis from manipulation of eyelids or a lost lens under the eyelid, giant papillary conjunctivitis)
- Allergies, blepharochalasis, or other source of recurrent eyelid edema.
- Eyelid rubbing.
- Botox—ptosis is a possible side effect of treatment with all neuromodulators and is being seen more frequently owing to the rise in popularity of cosmetic treatments in younger patients. (Patients can be assured that the ptosis will resolve as the medication wears off.)
- Trauma—exposure of prominent preaponeurotic fat pads may suggest levator injury; may resolve spontaneously, so most wait 6 months before operating.[7]

25. Describe the ice test and its use in the diagnosis of ptosis

An ice pack is held over the ptotic eyelid for 2 to 5 minutes, and the patient is then reexamined. The cold temperature inhibits acetylcholinesterase at the neuromuscular junction, therefore enhancing neuromuscular transmission and raising the ptotic eyelid in myasthenics (poor man's Tensilon test). The test is 80% to 90% sensitive and 100% specific for MG. A positive result should prompt a further workup.[9]

26. How does prostaglandin-associated periorbitopathy affect eyelid position?

Prostaglandin eyedrop use (for glaucoma and possibly cosmetics for eyelash growth) can cause atrophy of fat cells in the periorbital area after as few as 3 weeks of use, causing the upper lids to become ptotic or giving the appearance of pseudoptosis owing to deepening of the superior sulcus. In addition, there may be lengthening of the lashes and darkening of the periorbital skin.[10]

27. What are the features of floppy eyelid syndrome?

Floppy eyelid syndrome is caused by decreased elastin in the tarsal plate with easy and sometimes spontaneous eversion of the upper lid. The upper eyelid can become ptotic, and the lashes themselves become ptotic with the direction of lash growth vertically downward, sometimes obstructing vision. In addition to lid and lash malposition, the patient may suffer chronic conjunctivitis with discharge and keratopathy. The syndrome is strongly associated with sleep apnea. All patients with floppy eyelid syndrome should be evaluated with sleep studies.

28. Compare and contrast the two most common types of ptosis surgical correction.

The two most common types of surgical correction are the external levator resection and the Müller's muscle resection (with or without skin resection).

The levator resection allows for the removal of skin and fat through the external incision. The contour and height of the eyelid are less predictable and are dependent on the placement of tarsal levator sutures. The reoperation rate is approximately 10% to 20%.

The Müller's muscle resection can be done from an internal or an external approach in those patients who respond positively to the Neo test. The external approach allows for removal of excess skin and fat, while the internal approach allows muscle resection without formation of an external scar. This can be desirable in younger patients in whom dermatochalasis does not coexist. The contour of the postoperative eyelid is generally excellent and the reoperation rate is low, approximately 3%.[11]

REFERENCES

1. Ahmadi AJ, Sires BS: Ptosis in infants and children, Int Ophthalmol Clin 42:15–29, 2002.
2. Kersten RA: Orbit, eyelids, and lacrimal system: basic and clinical science course, San Francisco, 2006, American Academy of Ophthalmology.
3. Gausas RE, Goldstein SM: Ptosis in the elderly patient, Int Ophthalmol Clin 42:61–74, 2002.
4. McCord CD Jr, Tannebaum M, Nunery WR: Oculoplastic surgery, ed 3, Philadelphia, 1995, Lippincott-Raven.
5. Schaefer AJ, Schaefer DP: Classification and correction of ptosis. In: Stewart WB, editor: Surgery of the eyelid, orbit, and lacrimal system, vol 2, San Francisco, 1994, American Academy of Ophthalmology, pp 128–131.
6. Chan C, Paine M, O'Day J: Carotid dissection: a common cause of Horner's syndrome, Clin Exper Ophthalmol 29:411–415, 2001.
7. Bassin RE, Putterman AM: Ptosis in young adults, Int Ophthalmol Clin 42:31–43, 2002.
8. Kerrison JB, Newman NJ: Five things oculoplastic surgeons should know about neuro-ophthalmology, Ophthal Plast Reconstr Surg 15:372–377, 2002.
9. Sethi KD, Rivner MH, Swift TR: Ice pack test for myasthenia gravis, Neurology 37:1383–1385, 1987.
10. Filippopoulos T, Paula JS, Torun N, et al. Periorbital changes associated with topical bimatoprost, Ophthal Plast Reconstr Surg 24:302–207, 2008.
11. Lewis K: Recognition and management of common eyelid malpositions, 2013, Audio Digest Foundation.

CHAPTER 38

EYELID TUMORS

Janice A. Gault

1. **What clues are helpful in determining whether an eyelid lesion is benign or malignant?**
   The size, location, age of onset, rate of growth, and presence of bleeding or ulceration; any color change; and a history of malignancy or prior radiation therapy are important. A thorough examination is necessary. Malignant or inflammatory lesions may cause loss of eyelashes and distortion of Meibomian gland orifices, but only malignant lesions destroy the orifices. If a lesion is near the lacrimal punctum, evaluate for invasion into the lacrimal system. Probing and irrigation may be necessary. Palpate lesions for fixation to deep tissues or bone. Examine regional lymph nodes for enlargement. Restriction of extraocular motility and proptosis are clues to localized invasion. If a sebaceous adenocarcinoma or melanoma is diagnosed, systemic evaluation should target lung, liver, bones, and neurologic systems. Photographic documentation is important for any lesion to be treated or observed.

2. **What is the difference between seborrheic keratosis and actinic keratosis?**
   Both are papillomas, an irregular frondlike projection of skin with a central vascular pedicle. These lesions are more common in elderly patients.
   - **Seborrheic keratosis** is pigmented, oily, and hyperkeratotic. It appears stuck onto the skin (Fig. 38.1). A shaved biopsy is all that is needed to diagnose and treat. It has no increased risk for malignant change.
   - **Actinic keratosis** is found in sun-exposed areas and appears as a flat, scaly, or papillary lesion (Fig. 38.2). This premalignant lesion may evolve into either a basal cell or a squamous cell carcinoma. Imiquimod is used to remove these before they become cancerous.

3. **What eyelid lesion is associated with a chronic follicular conjunctivitis?**
   Molluscum contagiosum. A virus causes the multiple waxy nodules with umbilicated centers. They may resolve spontaneously but frequently require surgical excision or cautery to prevent reinfection.

4. **What blood tests should you order in young patients with the lesions shown in Fig. 38.3?**
   The appropriate tests are cholesterol level, triglyceride level, and fasting blood sugar. Xanthelasma are yellowish plaques found at the medial canthal area of the upper and lower eyelids. They are collections of lipid. In older patients, xanthelasma are common and no cause for concern. In younger patients, they may be a sign of hypercholesterolemia, a congenital disorder of cholesterol metabolism, or diabetes mellitus. They may be removed for cosmetic purposes, but they can recur.

5. **What is a keratoacanthoma? What malignancy does it simulate?**
   A keratoacanthoma is a rapidly growing lesion that appears over several weeks. It is hyperkeratotic with a central crater that often resolves spontaneously (Fig. 38.4). Clinically, the lesion simulates a "rodent ulcer" basal cell carcinoma. Microscopically, the lesion appears similar to squamous cell carcinoma. It may occur near the edge of areas of chronic inflammation, such as a burn, or on the periphery of a true malignant neoplasm. If you are sure of the diagnosis, it is reasonable to observe. However, because it may cause destruction of the eyelid margin, lesions in this area are often removed surgically. In addition, steroids may be injected into the lesion to hasten resolution.

6. **What is the most common malignant eyelid tumor?**
   Basal cell carcinoma. It is most common in middle-aged or elderly patients.

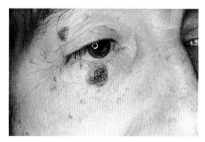

Fig. 38.1 Seborrheic keratosis is a greasy, brown, flat lesion with a verrucous surface and a "stuck-on" appearance. (From Kanski JJ: *Clinical ophthalmology: a synopsis,* New York, 2004, Butterworth-Heinemann.)

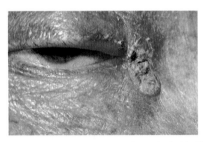

Fig. 38.2 Actinic keratosis is a dry, scaly lesion caused by sun exposure and occurring in fair-skinned people. (From Spalton DJ, Hitchings RA, Hunter PA: *Atlas of clinical ophthalmology,* ed 2, St. Louis, 1994, Mosby.)

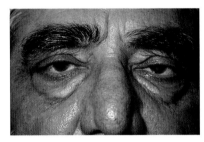

Fig. 38.3 Patient with xanthelasma. (From Kanski JJ: *Clinical ophthalmology: a systematic approach,* ed 5, New York, 2003, Butterworth-Heinemann.)

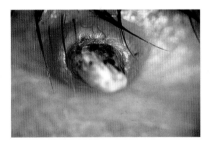

Fig. 38.4 Keratoacanthoma is a fast-growing nodule with a keratin-filled crater that spontaneously involutes after several months. (From Kanski JJ: *Clinical ophthalmology: a synopsis,* New York, 2004, Butterworth-Heinemann.)

7. **What are its two clinical presentations?**
   It presents as a nodular (Fig. 38.5) or morpheaform (Fig. 38.6) tumor. A nodular tumor is a firm, raised, pearly, discrete mass, often with telangiectasias over the tumor margins. If the center of the lesion is ulcerated, it is called a *rodent ulcer.* Morpheaform tumors are firm, flat lesions with indistinct borders. They tend to be more aggressive and have a worse prognosis than the nodular variety.

8. **In order of frequency, where do basal cell carcinomas present?**
   The most common location is the lower eyelid, followed by the medial canthus, lateral canthus, and upper eyelid.

9. **Do basal cell carcinomas metastasize?**
   Lesions grow only by local extension.

10. **If basal cell carcinomas do not metastasize, why be concerned with them?**
    Ocular adnexal basal cell carcinomas have a 3% mortality rate. The vast majority of these patients have canthal area disease, prior radiation therapy, or clinically neglected tumors. Tumors near the medial canthus may invade the orbit via the lacrimal drainage system. Rarely, extension can occur to the brain. Removal of the tumor can be quite disfiguring.

11. **How do you treat tumors with a suspicious lesion?**
    First, do an incisional biopsy of the lesion to confirm the diagnosis. Permanent sections must be done, not merely frozen sections. If a basal cell lesion is found, there are several possibilities for treatment.

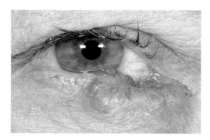

Fig. 38.5 Nodular basal cell carcinoma of the eyelid. A firm, pink-colored basal cell carcinoma of the left upper eyelid with raised border, superficial telangiectatic vessels, and characteristic central ulceration. These lesions are more commonly seen on the lower eyelid. (From Wojno TH: Eyelid abnormalities. In: Palay DA, Krachmer JH, editors: *Primary care ophthalmology,* ed 2, Philadelphia, 2005, Mosby, Fig. 4-13B.)

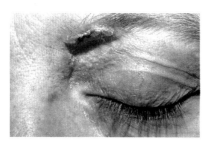

Fig. 38.6 Unlike nodular basal cell tumors, morpheaform basal cell carcinomas have less clearly defined surgical margins. (From Spalton DJ, Hitchings RA, Hunter PA: *Atlas of clinical ophthalmology,* ed 2, St. Louis, 1994, Mosby.)

- **Large surgical resection:** A large surgical resection with frozen sections is performed to confirm that the entire tumor has been removed. If the lacrimal system must be removed, do not perform a dacryocystorhinostomy at the same time as the primary surgery. Wait at least 1 year to prevent iatrogenic seeding of the nose.
- **Mohs' lamellar resection:** The complete tumor is removed, sparing as much healthy tissue as possible. The excised bits of tissue are sent to pathology during the procedure to confirm the presence or absence of tumor and therefore direct the subsequent course of the surgery. This procedure preserves a larger amount of normal tissue, allowing improved function and cosmesis. Sometimes, it even saves the globe, whereas conventional surgery may require exenteration. This time-consuming procedure is not available everywhere. After the tumor is completely removed and confirmed by pathology, the patient is sent to a plastic surgeon for reconstruction the same or the next day.
- **Radiation:** Basal cell carcinoma is radiosensitive, but treatment is not curative, only palliative (see question 10). Radiation should be reserved for elderly patients who are unable to undergo surgery.
- **Cryotherapy:** This treatment is not curative and should be used only palliatively.
- **Topical treatments:** Food and Drug Administration (FDA)–approved treatments for superficial basal cell include imiquimod (Aldara) and 5-fluorouracil (5-FU). Imiquimod activates the immune system via toll-like receptor 7 (TLR7) to activate the cell to secrete cytokines such as interferon-α (IFN-α), interleukin-6 (IL-6), and tumor necrosis factor-α (TNF-α) to attack the cancerous cells. 5-FU directly kills cancerous cells.
- **Oral medications:** Vismodegib (Erivedge) and Sonidegib (Odomzo) are FDA approved for rare cases of advanced basal cell carcinoma that are large, have penetrated deeply, metastasized or resistant multiple treatments and recurred. These block the "hedgehog" signaling pathway, which is relevant in more than 90% of basal-cell carcinomas.

12. How do you treat a recurrent tumor that has limited the extraocular motility from invasion of the orbit?

    It is treated with exenteration.

13. Describe basal cell nevus syndrome.

    This autosomal dominant disease is characterized by development of multiple basal cell carcinomas at an early age. Patients also have skeletal, endocrine, and neurologic abnormalities.

14. What are the complications of radiation to the area around the eye?

    Keratitis sicca (dry eye), cataracts, radiation retinopathy (if more than 3000 rads are used), optic neuropathy, entropion, lacrimal stenosis, and dermatitis. In young children, the bones of the orbit may not grow normally, causing a significant cosmetic deformity.

KEY POINTS: COMPLICATIONS OF RADIATION TREATMENT AROUND THE OCULAR AREA

1. Keratitis sicca (dry eye)
2. Cataracts
3. Radiation retinopathy
4. Optic neuropathy
5. Entropion
6. Lacrimal stenosis
7. Dermatitis
8. Cosmetic deformity in children (orbital bones may not develop normally)

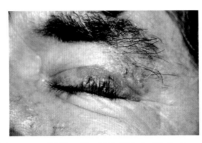

Fig. 38.7 Squamous cell carcinoma of the upper eyelid. (From Kanski JJ: *Clinical ophthalmology: a synopsis,* New York, 2004, Butterworth-Heinemann.)

15. **Where do squamous cell carcinomas usually present around the eye?**
    They usually present on the upper eyelid (Fig. 38.7). However, basal cell carcinomas are 40 times more common.

16. **How are patients with squamous cell carcinomas treated?**
    They are treated similar to patients with basal cell carcinomas. However, squamous cell carcinomas are more aggressive locally and metastasize via the blood or lymph system. Neuronal spread has been described and can be fatal. Exenteration is suggested for recurrences.

17. **A 60-year-old man has had a chalazion removed from his left upper eyelid three times. It has recurred yet again. How do you treat it?**
    A sebaceous gland carcinoma must be suspected. Such lesions arise from the Meibomian glands in the tarsal plate, Zeis' glands near the lashes, and sebaceous glands in the caruncle and brow. Any recurrent chalazia must be biopsied for pathologic evaluation. The lesion can mimic benign ocular diseases such as chronic blepharoconjunctivitis, corneal pannus, and superior limbic keratitis. Patients who do not respond to treatment should be biopsied, especially those with loss of lashes and destruction of Meibomian gland orifices.

18. **How is the biopsy performed? How is the specimen sent to the lab? What stains should be requested?**
    Sebaceous cell carcinoma is multicentric and undergoes pagetoid spread, that is, spreads from the bottom of the epidermis to the top. Multiple sites must be biopsied, including bulbar and palpebral conjunctiva, even if they appear uninvolved. A full-thickness biopsy may be necessary to make the diagnosis because the lesion originates deep in the tissues. The tissue should not be placed in alcohol, which will dissolve the fat from the specimen and make the diagnosis more difficult. Oil red O stain will stain the fat red.

19. **How are patients with sebaceous cell carcinoma treated?**
    Because sebaceous cell carcinoma is an aggressive and potentially fatal disease, wide surgical excision is mandatory. Some physicians prefer exenteration as a primary treatment. Mohs' microsurgery should be used with caution because the disease is multicentric with skip areas and some lesions may be missed. The tumor may spread hematogenously, lymphatically, or by direct extension.

20. **What is the most common type of malignant melanoma of the eyelid?**
    Superficial spreading melanoma accounts for 80% of cases; lentigo maligna and nodular melanoma each occur in 10% of cases. However, all are rare and represent less than 1% of eyelid tumors. Superficial spreading melanoma occurs both in sun-exposed and in nonexposed areas. Lentigo maligna, also known as melanotic freckle of Hutchinson, is sun induced. Both have a long horizontal growth phase before invading the deeper tissues. Nodular melanoma is more aggressive with earlier vertical invasion. Treatment is wide surgical excision and lymph node dissection if microscopic evidence of lymphatic or vascular involvement is noted.

21. How do you follow a patient who has had an eyelid malignancy?
Once the patient has healed from the initial treatment, reevaluate every 6 to 12 months. Patients are at risk for additional malignancies. A thorough examination by a dermatologist may reveal cutaneous malignancies elsewhere on the body, especially in sun-exposed areas. Patients with a history of cutaneous malignant melanoma and squamous cell carcinoma need periodic systemic evaluations for possible metastasis.

22. How can eyelid malignancies be prevented?
Use sunscreen to the face, limit sun exposure during 10 am and 4 pm and wear sunglasses and a hat. Yearly dermatologic evaluations should be scheduled for those at risk.

BIBLIOGRAPHY

Albert DM, Jakobiec FA: Principles and practice of ophthalmology, ed 3, vol 3, Philadelphia, 2008, W.B. Saunders.
American Academy of Ophthalmology: Basic and clinical science course on orbit, eyelids, and lacrimal system, San Francisco, 2008, American Academy of Ophthalmology.
Gervasio K, Peck T, Fathy C, Sivalingham M: The Wills Eye Manual, ed 8, Philadelphia, 2022, Wolters Kluwer.

CHAPTER 39

UVEITIS

Tamara R. Vrabec, Caroline R. Baumal, and Vincent F. Baldassano Jr.

UVEITIS IN THE IMMUNOCOMPETENT PATIENT

1. What is uveitis?
   Uveitis is inflammation of the uvea, or pigmented layer of the eye. It is classified as:
   - Anterior uveitis—inflammation predominantly affecting the iris with associated anterior chamber (AC) cells in the aqueous fluid
   - Intermediate uveitis (IU)—inflammation of the ciliary body and vitreous with vitreous cells but no retinal or choroidal involvement
   - Posterior uveitis—inflammation of the retina and/or choroid or sclera
   - Panuveitis—inflammation of both the anterior and the posterior segments
     The incidence of various uveitides may differ among populations. This chapter focuses on uveitis in the Western world.

ANTERIOR UVEITIS

2. Describe the presenting symptoms of acute and nonacute anterior uveitis.
   The typical symptoms of acute (sudden-onset) include pain, redness, and photophobia (sensitivity to light). Nonacute forms of anterior uveitis present with fewer symptoms or may be asymptomatic.

3. Name and describe the typical clinical signs of anterior uveitis.
   The hallmarks of anterior uveitis (a.k.a. iritis) are AC cell and flare, both of which are graded by amount.[1,2] Flare reflects protein leakage from inflamed, therefore more permeable, iris vessels. Keratic precipitates (KPs) are accumulations of white blood cells on the corneal endothelium. These may vary in size and distribution in different disease states (see later). Inflammatory material can create adhesions between the iris and the lens surface (posterior synechiae [PS]) and between the iris and the peripheral cornea (peripheral anterior synechiae [PAS]) in uveitis of longer duration and increased severity.

4. How is granulomatous uveitis distinguished from nongranulomatous uveitis?
   Granulomatous and nongranulomatous uveitis may be differentiated based on histopathologic and clinical features. The histopathologic features of granulomatous anterior uveitis (GAU) include nodular collections of epithelioid cells and giant cells surrounded by lymphocytes. In nongranulomatous uveitis, a diffuse infiltration of lymphocytes and plasma cells is present. Clinically, GAU usually has a subacute onset with a chronic course (greater than 4 months duration). On slit lamp exam, signs include large greasy "mutton-fat" KPs, nodules on the iris surface (Busacca nodules), and/or in the AC angle (Berlin nodules), PS, and PAS. AC cell and flare are also present (Table 39.1). Nongranulomatous anterior uveitis (NGAU) typically has an acute onset and self-limited course (less than 4 months' duration). At the slit lamp, clinical signs include fine KPs usually located on the inferior cornea and AC cells and flare. PS may or may not be present depending on the duration and severity of the inflammation. Certain forms of NGAU may present with hypopyon (Table 39.1).

5. Can iris nodules occur in nongranulomatous anterior uveitis?
   Koeppe nodules are grayish-white nodules at the pupillary margin. They may be present in either GAU or NGAU.

6. Can the shape and distribution of keratic precipitates be helpful in narrowing a differential diagnosis?
   Yes. Typically, KPs are located on the inferior cornea in an area referred to as the Arlt triangle (Fig. 39.1). In Fuchs' heterochromic iridocyclitis, the fine "stellate" KPs are found scattered diffusely on the entire posterior surface of the cornea. In herpes simplex keratouveitis, KPs are frequently localized to the area of corneal involvement.

7. Is a dilated fundus examination indicated in all patients with anterior uveitis?
   Yes. AC cells are present in panuveitis. Therefore, a dilated examination is imperative for all patients who appear to have anterior uveitis to identify potentially blinding posterior segment disease involving the choroid, retina, or vitreous. Posterior segment infection and severe forms of inflammatory posterior uveitis that require additional antibiotics/antivirals and/or local or systemic immunosuppression must be ruled out.

8. What is the most common cause of nongranulomatous anterior uveitis?
   Human leukocyte antigen (HLA)-B27-associated conditions account for approximately 45% of acute NGAU.[3] Although HLA-B27 can be seen in NGAU without systemic inflammatory disease, inflammatory

Table 39.1 Features of Granulomatous and Nongranulomatous Anterior Uveitis

FEATURES	GRANULOMATOUS	NONGRANULOMATOUS
Onset	Often insidious	Acute (usually)
Course	Chronic	Acute or chronic
Injection	+	+++ (usually)
Pain	+/−	+++ (usually)
Iris nodules	+++ (Busacca and Koeppe)	− (Koeppe on occasion)
Keratic precipitates	Large, mutton-fat	Small, fine
Other	Dense posterior synechiae	+/− posterior synechiae, hypopyon

+, Present; −, absent.

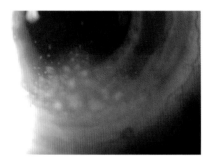

Fig. 39.1 Granulomatous keratic precipitates in the Arlt triangle.

Table 39.2 Differentiation of HLA-B27-Associated Conditions

HLA-B27-ASSOCIATED DISEASE	SYMPTOMS	SYSTEMIC CLINICAL FINDINGS
Ankylosing spondylitis	Stiffness and low back pain worsen with inactivity	Spinal fusion, sacroiliac joint disease; no skin findings; 25% develop NGAU
Reiter's disease	Same plus painless mouth ulcers, heel pain, painful urination	Keratoderma blennorrhagica, circinate balanitis, urethritis, polyarthritis; conjunctivitis is typically bilateral and papillary
Psoriatic arthritis	Skin rash, arthritis	Psoriasis
Inflammatory bowel disease	Gastrointestinal symptoms	Erythema nodosum

HLA, Human leukocyte antigen; NGAU, nongranulomatous anterior uveitis.

spondyloarthropathies including ankylosing spondylitis (AS), Reiter's disease, psoriatic arthritis, and inflammatory bowel disease are present in 50% to 80% of patients with HLA-B27-positive NGAU. A review of systems and appropriate imaging aids differentiation (Table 39.2).[4,5]

9. **Describe the typical findings and course of NGAU seen in HLA-B27 disease.**
   HLA-B27-related iritis is typically unilateral, acutely symptomatic, and self-limited. It may recur in the same or alternate eyes over time. A fibrinous response in the AC and, in some cases, hypopyon may occur.

10. **What is the incidence of HLA-B27 in the general population?**
    The incidence of HLA-B27 in the general population is 8%. However, it is present in 90% of patients with AS and 80% of those with Reiter's disease.

11. **What other conditions are in the differential diagnosis of acute NGAU?**
    More than 50% of cases are idiopathic. Other uveitides that may present with clinical findings consistent with NGAU are listed in Tables 39.3 and 39.4. Gout is the most common form of inflammatory arthritis in the United

Table 39.3 More Common Infectious Causes of Uveitis

DISEASE	GRANULOMATOUS VS. NONGRANULO-MATOUS	CLINICAL PRESENTATION	INFECTIOUS AGENT
Syphilis	Granulomatous[a]	Anterior, pan, or posterior	*Treponema pallidum*
Acute retinal necrosis	Granulomatous	Panuveitis	Herpes simplex or zoster virus
Chronic postoperative endophthalmitis	Granulomatous	Anterior or intermediate	*Propionibacterium acnes*
Lyme disease	Granulomatous[a]	Predominantly intermediate	*Borrelia burgdorferi* via *Ixodes* tick bite
Tuberculosis	Granulomatous	Panuveitis	*Mycobacterium tuberculosis*
Toxoplasmosis	Granulomatous[a]	Pan or posterior	*Toxoplasma gondii*
Cat-scratch disease	Granulomatous	Panuveitis	*Bartonella henselae*
Toxocariasis	Granulomatous	Panuveitis	*Toxocara canis*
Onchocerciasis	Nongranulomatous	Panuveitis	*Onchocerca volvulus*
Ocular histoplasmosis	No anterior chamber or vitreous cells	Posterior	*Histoplasma capsulatum*
Fungal choroiditis	Granulomatous	Predominantly posterior	*Cryptococcus, Aspergillus, Candida* species
Diffuse unilateral subacute neuroretinitis	Nongranulomatous	Posterior	*Baylisascaris procyonis*

[a]May also have nongranulomatous anterior uveitis.

States[6] and may cause recurrent inflammation of ocular tissues including iritis.[7,8] Note that certain forms of GAU (e.g., sarcoidosis, syphilis, Lyme disease, and toxoplasmosis) may at times present with nongranulomatous features, for example, fine KP instead of mutton-fat KP.

12. Discuss the most common cause of uveitis in children.

Juvenile idiopathic arthritis (JIA) is the most common identifiable cause of uveitis in children. Anterior uveitis occurs in up to 40% of JIA patients. Young girls (age 4 years) with pauciarticular JIA who are rheumatoid factor–negative and antinuclear antibody–positive are at highest risk. The uveitis is anterior and chronic and can lead to serious vision loss, although children often do not complain of symptoms and the parents are unaware because the eye is white and quiet. Consequently, diagnosis may be delayed. Children with JIA should be screened regularly for uveitis, more or less frequently depending on the number of previously mentioned risk factors for developing uveitis.[9] High-risk children are those who have rheumatoid factor negative, antinuclear antibody–positive pauciarticular arthritis, who are younger than 7 years of age at onset, or have JIA duration of 4 years or less. These patients should be screened at 3-month intervals. Low- or moderate-risk children with fewer risk factors should be screened at 6- to 12-month intervals. Boys may develop acute recurrent inflammation at a later age (9 years). A majority of these children with later-onset JIA are HLA-B27-positive and may develop AS later in life.

13. What condition may produce spontaneous hyphema in a child?

Juvenile xanthogranuloma (JXG) is a systemic condition that consists of one or more nonmalignant, inflammatory tumors consisting of histiocytes. Ocular lesions include iris nodules or masses, recurrent AC cellular reaction, and spontaneous hyphema (Fig. 39.2). Diagnosis is made with biopsy of the iris or similar lesions on the skin.[10,11]

14. What are the most common noninfectious and infectious causes of granulomatous anterior uveitis?

Sarcoidosis is the most common cause of GAU in adults over 60.[12] Differential diagnosis includes infectious causes of GAU, which includes syphilis, Lyme disease, tuberculosis, herpesvirus infection (varicella zoster virus [VZV], cytomegalovirus [CMV], and herpes simplex virus [HSV]), and *Propionibacterium acnes* (pseudophakic patients). Other more common causes are also listed in Tables 39.3 and 39.4. GAU may be present in multiple sclerosis (MS)–associated uveitis.[13]

Table 39.4 More Common Noninfectious Causes of Uveitis

DISEASE	GRANULOMATOUS VS. NONGRANULO-MATOUS	CLINICAL PRESENTATION	SECRETS
JIA	Nongranulomatous	Anterior	See text
HLA-B27-associated uveitis	Nongranulomatous	Anterior	See text
Fuchs' iridocyclitis	Nongranulomatous	Anterior	Iris heterochromia; no PAS/PS
Kawasaki syndrome	Nongranulomatous	Anterior	Rash, lymphadenopathy, fever, cardiac disease in children
TINU syndrome	Nongranulomatous	Anterior	Cellular casts in urine
Sarcoidosis	Chronic granulomatous; acute nongranulomatous	Anterior, posterior, or panuveitis	Clinical findings depend on age
Pars planitis	Nongranulomatous; if granulomatous, suspect MS	Intermediate	16% may develop MS
Juvenile xanthogranuloma	Nongranulomatous	Anterior or intermediate	See text
Phacoanaphylactic uveitis	Granulomatous	Intermediate uveitis	Autoimmunity to lens proteins after trauma or cataract surgery
Multifocal choroiditis	Nongranulomatous	Panuveitis	Myopia; 30% develop CNVM
Birdshot chorioretinitis	Nongranulomatous	Posterior or panuveitis	HLA-A29 in more than 90%
APMPPE	Nongranulomatous	Posterior or panuveitis	Young patients, viral prodrome, bilateral; recurrence and CNVM rare
MEWDS	Nongranulomatous	Posterior	IVFA wreath; hyperfluorescence
Serpiginous choroiditis	Nongranulomatous	Posterior	Older patients, lesions contiguous to disc, unilateral; recurrence common, CNVM 30%
Behçet's disease	Nongranulomatous	Anterior, posterior, or panuveitis	Hypopyon iritis
Vogt-Koyanagi-Harada syndrome	Granulomatous	Panuveitis	Starry sky
Sympathetic ophthalmia	Granulomatous	Panuveitis	See text

APMPPE, Acute posterior multifocal placoid pigment epitheliopathy; *CNVM,* choroidal neovascular membrane; *HLA,* human leukocyte antigen; *IVFA,* fluorescein angiography; *JIA,* juvenile idiopathic arthritis; *MEWDS,* multiple evanescent white dot syndrome; *MS,* multiple sclerosis; *PAS,* peripheral anterior synechiae; *PS,* posterior synechiae; *TINU,* tubulointerstitial nephritis–uveitis.

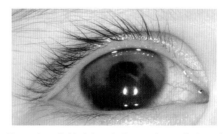

Fig. 39.2 Large, solitary juvenile xanthogranuloma that had given rise to a spontaneous hyphema in a 7-month-old patient. (Courtesy Carol Shields, MD.)

15. **When is a systemic workup indicated in anterior uveitis?**
A systemic evaluation should be performed in patients who have GAU, a second episode of NGAU, posterior uveitis, a positive review of systems for other systemic inflammatory symptoms, or severe disease that may require systemic immunosuppression.

16. **When should one consider checking human leukocyte antigen-B27 in cases of anterior uveitis?**
When a case of NGAU is acute in onset and especially if recurrent. It should also be checked in fibrinous anterior uveitis with or without hypopyon.

17. **What additional studies should be ordered?**
A chest x-ray for sarcoidosis and tuberculosis, fluorescent treponemal antibody absorption (FTA-ABS) or rapid plasmin reagin (RPR) test, urinalysis, erythrocyte sedimentation rate (ESR), and complete blood count should be considered in all patients. Additional diagnostic tests may be appropriate based on clinical history and ocular and physical examination and positive review of systems.

18. **When are ocular diagnostic imaging studies helpful?**
Ocular imaging including intravenous (IV) fluorescein angiography, indocyanine green angiography, B-scan ultrasound, ocular coherence tomography, and fundus autofluorescence may help to identify associated posterior segment findings including cystoid macular edema (CME) and to characterize forms of posterior uveitis.

19. **What is the role of ocular sampling techniques including paracentesis and vitrectomy?**
In cases of progressive sight-threatening uveitis in one or both eyes that is unresponsive to therapy or when unusual infections or masquerade syndrome are suspected and systemic antibody titers are not diagnostic, specimens from the iris, aqueous, vitreous, retina, or choroid may be obtained for evaluation, including antibody titers, polymerase chain reaction (PCR), histopathology, and flow cytometry. Because of its localized nature, an active intraocular infection is not always accompanied by a significant rise in systemic antibody titers. Furthermore, serology may be unreliable in immunocompromised patients or negative in masquerade syndrome. AC paracentesis with PCR testing is most often utilized in cases where viral etiology is suspected (e.g., HSV, CMV, or VZV) based on clinical findings. In cases of necrotizing retinitis, PCR for toxoplasmosis may be included. Goldman Witmer testing compares antibody levels from the aqueous to the serum for diagnosis.

INTERMEDIATE UVEITIS

20. **What is the most common intermediate uveitis?**
The most common cause of IU, pars planitis, is an inflammation of unknown etiology characterized by "snow bank" of inflammatory debris visible on the inferior pars plana. The clinical course is variable. IU may be also associated with systemic disease including sarcoidosis, post streptococcal infection, and renal diseases including tubulointerstitial nephritis and glomerulonephritis in children.[14] Although pars planitis is by definition idiopathic, approximately 16% of patients who have pars planitis may ultimately develop MS. HLA-DR15 may play a role in both diseases.[15]

21. **What are the infectious causes of intermediate uveitis?**
Approximately 10% of syphilitic uveitis may present as IU. Other infectious causes include Lyme disease and tuberculosis. These must be excluded before initiating treatment for presumed pars planitis. Human T-cell lymphotropic virus type 1 (HTLV-1), an exceptionally oncogenic human retrovirus, can cause adult T-cell leukemia (ATL) as well as systemic inflammatory syndromes, notably HAM/TSP (HTLV 1-associated myelopathy/spastic paresis, a progressive neurodegeneration that may be confused with MS). It is an emerging pathogen that may cause IU characterized by moderate or heavy lacework-like vitreous membranous opacities and vitreous cells.[16] Most prevalent in Japan, HTLV-1 has a worldwide distribution including Florida, West Africa, Western Europe, the Caribbean, and Brazil.[17]

22. **What are the causes of vision loss in pars planitis?**
CME is the most common cause of vision loss. Other causes include cataract, glaucoma, vitreous hemorrhage, epiretinal membrane, and tractional retinal detachment.

23. **What are the indications for treatment in pars planitis?**
CME with associated vision loss. Relative indications include vitreous floaters affecting vision.

POSTERIOR UVEITIS

INFECTIOUS POSTERIOR UVEITIS

24. **Describe the most common cause of posterior uveitis.**
Ocular toxoplasmosis is the most common cause of posterior uveitis. Most patients have asymptomatic inactive chorioretinal scarring. Active disease presents in most cases as a recurrent area of necrotizing retinochoroiditis, (a white infiltrate) adjacent to a pigmented retinal scar (previously healed retinitis). A diffuse dense vitritis may

limit visualization of the retinitis, which appears as a "headlight in the fog." In immunocompromised patients, including the elderly, diabetics, and those who have had intravitreal steroid injections, the retinitis may be multifocal and bilateral and may not be associated with a scar.[18,19]

25. **What are the risk factors for toxoplasmosis in the United States?**
Consumption of raw or rare pork, chicken, lamb or venison, raw beef, locally cured or dried meats, unpasteurized goat milk, raw shellfish, butchering or working with meats, and having three or more kittens.[20] Water or food contaminated with oocytes from cats may be causative, especially in outbreaks.

26. **Can toxoplasmosis be transmitted transplacentally?**
Yes. This is referred to as congentital toxoplasmosis.[21] Children may present with strabismus due to inactive macular chorioretinal scar.[22] Cases of retinochoroiditis, which tend to reactivate later in life, tend to occur when infection is acquired later in pregnancy. If infection occurs in earlier trimesters, more severe disease including blindness and neurologic and visceral involvement may occur.

27. **How is the diagnosis of ocular toxoplasmosis made?**
Diagnosis usually is based on clinical history and fundus examination. Positive immunoglobulin G (IgG) or IgM titers, even in very low concentrations (undiluted serum), are supportive of the diagnosis. IgG indicates congenital or previous infection, whereas IgM indicates recently acquired infection. Interpretation may be confounded by a high prevalence of positive titers in the population. A negative titer excludes the diagnosis except in severely immunosuppressed patients.[23]

28. **How is ocular toxoplasmosis managed?**
Treatment is recommended for active lesions that threaten the macula or optic nerve and for peripheral lesions with severe vitritis. Although systemic sulfonamides, pyrimethamine, folinic acid, azithromycin, clindamycin, and corticosteroids, as well as intravitreal clindamycin, have been used in various combinations, there is no universally accepted treatment regimen.[24] Duration of treatment is typically 4 to 6 weeks and treatment does not prevent recurrences. Steroids should never be used without concurrent antibiotic agents. Observation is recommended for small peripheral lesions.[25,26]

29. **What serious side effects may occur with oral antibiotic therapy for toxoplasmosis?**
   - Pseudomembranous colitis (systemic clindamycin)
   - Hematologic toxicity (pyrimethamine)
   - Erythema multiforme and Stevens-Johnson's reaction (sulfonamides)

30. **Name several other forms of infectious uveitis.**
Syphilis, histoplasmosis, Lyme disease, tuberculosis, acute retinal necrosis (ARN), and toxocariasis (in children).

31. **What are the features of ocular syphilis?**
Salt-and-pepper chorioretinitis, vitritis, iritis, and interstitial keratitis with AC cells typify congenital syphilis. Lens dislocation may occur. The clinical findings of acquired syphilis are protean. Anterior uveitis, vitritis, choroiditis, retinitis, retinal vasculitis, optic neuropathy, and Argyll Robertson pupils are most common. Others have been reported.[27] Syphilis is known as "The Great Pretender" as it mimics many other diseases.

32. **Which diagnostic tests are used to assess syphilitic uveitis?**
Nontreponemal tests, including serial venereal disease research laboratory (VDRL) titers, are useful in monitoring response to therapy but may be negative in late-stage syphilis. For this reason, syphilitic uveitis must be evaluated with specific treponemal tests, that is, FTA-ABS test or the microhemagglutination test. Examination of cerebrospinal fluid (CSF) for elevated protein, lymphocytic pleocytosis, or VDRL may reveal neurosyphilis, and hence, LP should be performed in all cases with ocular involvement. Human immunodeficiency virus (HIV) testing should be performed in all patients with ocular syphilis because these infections may be concurrent.[28]

33. **How is syphilitic uveitis treated?**
Ocular syphilis is treated as neurosyphilis with IV penicillin G, 12 to 24 million units/day for 14 days followed by intramuscular benzathine penicillin G, 2.4 million units/week for 3 weeks. Doxycycline, tetracycline, and erythromycin are used in penicillin-allergic patients.

34. **What are the most common features of ocular histoplasmosis?**
The most common features are peripapillary atrophy or pigmentation, peripheral punched out chorioretinal lesions, and macular choroidal neovascular membrane (ocular histoplasmosis triad). History often reveals exposure to fowl or bat waste. In the United States, prevalence is highest in the Ohio and Mississippi River valleys.

35. **Describe the ocular features of Lyme disease.**
Ocular Lyme disease is usually bilateral. In early or stage 1 disease, conjunctivitis may occur along with a migratory rash (erythema migrans) or arthritis. In later stages, an atypical IU with granulomatous KPs and PS may be present. Inflammation may affect almost any ocular tissue. Findings may include keratitis, multifocal choroiditis, exudative retinal detachment, neuroretinitis, optic neuritis, or edema.[29]

36. **How is an ocular Lyme disease diagnosis made?**
Diagnosis requires a history of outdoor activity in an endemic area in the late spring or summer and positive indirect immunofluorescent antibody and/or enzyme-linked immunosorbent assay. Western blot, which is very specific, may be confirmatory. False-negative results occur in the early stages or following incomplete antibiotic treatment. The spirochete may be identified in skin rash biopsy or CSF.[30,31]

37. **Describe the most common features of ocular tuberculosis.**
The most common feature of ocular tuberculosis is choroiditis, which may appear as a solitary granuloma or multifocal choroiditis or resemble serpiginous choroidopathy.[32] Inflammation is typically unilateral. Associated anterior uveitis is chronic and granulomatous. Ocular involvement may occur without signs of active pulmonary involvement.[33,34]

38. **Describe acute retinal necrosis syndrome.**
ARN is a clinical syndrome caused by herpesvirus infections (VZV and HSV type 1 in older and HSV type 2 in younger patients). The ARN triad includes peripheral retinitis, arteritis, and vitritis. Acute disease is also often associated with GAU. Optic neuropathy may occur. Long-term complications include retinal detachment resulting from multiple necrotic holes, glaucoma, cataract, and optic atrophy. IV acyclovir for 14 days, followed by 3 months of oral therapy, is recommended to limit retinal necrosis, as well as the occurrence of ARN in the fellow eye. Prophylactic laser photocoagulation to demarcate all areas of active and inactive disease from nonaffected retina may decrease the risk of secondary retinal detachment. ARN may occur in the fellow eye in approximately 30% of patients at an average interval of 4 weeks.[35] Extended treatment with antivirals for 6 weeks to 3 months after resolution may reduce the incidence of ARN in the fellow eye.

39. **What other types of necrotizing retinitis may have a similar clinical presentation?**
Toxoplasmosis (particularly in the elderly or otherwise immunocompromised), syphilis, Behçet's disease, *Aspergillus*, and lymphoma (masquerade syndrome) may have similar presentation.[36]

40. **What form of uveitis may present with enlarged lymph glands?**
Primary inoculation with *Bartonella henselae* produces regional lymphadenopathy and conjunctivitis (Parinaud's oculoglandular syndrome). Additional findings may include Leber's neuroretinitis and a retinal white-dot syndrome. Patients with sarcoidosis may also present with lymphadenopathy.[37]

NONINFECTIOUS POSTERIOR UVEITIS

41. **What are the major diagnostic characteristics of Behçet's disease?**
The major characteristics are uveitis, skin lesions (erythema nodosum, thrombophlebitis), genital ulcers, and painful oral ulcers. Vasculitis affecting all size arteries and veins is an underlying etiologic factor.

42. **How frequent is ocular involvement in Behçet's disease?**
Up to 70% may develop ocular disease, which may be the presenting manifestation in 10% of cases.

43. **What is the typical uveitis seen in Behçet's disease?**
NGAU (which may manifest as a mobile or shifting hypopyon in a white eye), vitritis, panuveitis, retinitis, and occlusive posterior vasculitis, which may involve both arteries and veins. Isolated anterior uveitis is uncommon.[38]

44. **What is unusual about the clinical course of Behçet's disease?**
Behçet's disease is characterized by periodic relapses with spontaneous remissions that occur even without treatment. Consequently, remissions may be misinterpreted as a therapeutic response to intermittent steroid therapy. Unlike most other causes of retinal vasculitis, Behçet's disease requires chronic systemic immunosuppression to prevent relapses that ultimately lead to blindness.

45. **What is Vogt-Koyanagi-Harada syndrome?**
Vogt-Koyanagi-Harada (VKH) syndrome is an idiopathic multisystem disorder that primarily affects more heavily pigmented individuals including Hispanic, Japanese, and American Indian. It is associated genetically with HLA-DR4. Symptoms in the early or prodromal phase include dysacusis, tinnitus, headache, and stiff neck. Evaluation of CSF at this stage may show a lymphocytosis. This is followed by the onset of acute granulomatous pan-uveitis involving choroidal infiltration with associated exudative retinal detachment. Fluorescein angiography is notable for a characteristic "starry sky" pattern of early hyperfluorescence. The convalescent phase includes skin and eyelash depigmentation (vitiligo, poliosis), alopecia, and depigmented fundus ("sunset glow" fundus). The chronic recurrent phase usually manifests as persistent anterior uveitis. Treatment usually requires systemic immune suppression.

46. **What is a Dalen Fuch's nodule?**
Small cream-colored lesions in the midperiphery and posterior fundus corresponding to sub–retinal pigment epithelium (RPE) infiltrates. They can be seen in VKH and sympathetic ophthalmia (see later).

47. **Name five other conditions that have uveitis and central nervous system manifestations.**
Sarcoidosis, syphilis, Behçet's disease, acute posterior multifocal placoid pigment epitheliopathy, and MS all have uveitis and central nervous system (CNS) manifestations. Although not associated with uveitis, Susac syndrome,

or retino-cochlear-cerebral vasculitis, is an autoimmune occlusive arteritis that affects the brain (with distinctive lesions in the corpus callosum), ear, and eye. Prompt diagnosis and immunosuppression may prevent serious CNS sequelae.[39,40]

48. **What is sympathetic ophthalmia?**
This is a bilateral, diffuse granulomatous T-cell–mediated uveitis that has been reported to occur between 5 days and many years after perforating ocular injury (0.2%) or ocular surgery (0.01%). Eighty percent of cases occur within 2 weeks to 3 months after the inciting event, but may occur years later. Clinical findings include panuveitis, papillitis, and in some cases exudative retinal detachment and Dalen-Fuchs nodules (see earlier). Treatment usually requires systemic immune suppression. Enucleation of the traumatized eye after the onset of the uveitis is not generally recommended.[41]

49. **What are the most common mechanisms of uveitic glaucoma?**
The most common mechanism of acute glaucoma is direct inflammation of the trabecular meshwork (TM) or trabeculitis, which occurs most often in herpetic viral uveitides. Chronic glaucoma may result from closure of the TM by PAS. Secondary angle closure glaucoma develops when 360 degrees of PS, which are adhesions between the iris pupillary margin and the lens, block fluid secreted behind the iris by the ciliary body, from exiting the eye by percolating around the lens and iris into the TM. The fluid buildup behind the iris causes iris bombé, a ballooning of the peripheral iris that elevates, narrows, and obstructs the angle, causing secondary angle closure glaucoma. In addition, topical, intraocular, and periocular corticosteroids can cause glaucoma in steroid responders.[42] However, increased cells in the AC can block the TM, increasing intraocular pressure (IOP). In these patients, increasing steroid dosage will decrease IOP.

50. **Name the uveitis entities that are associated with an acute elevation in intraocular pressure.**
Herpes simplex and herpes zoster, CMV, toxoplasmosis, and syphilis

51. **What are the clinical features of ocular sarcoidosis?**
The eye is involved in approximately 20% of cases of systemic sarcoidosis. Uveitis is the most common ocular manifestation. Anterior segment inflammation is classically bilateral, chronic, and granulomatous, although acute and asymmetric anterior uveitis may occur. Posterior segment inflammation including choroidal or optic nerve granuloma, vitritis, multifocal chorioretinitis, retinal vasculitis or vascular occlusions, exudative retinal detachment, and neovascularization are less common. Conjunctival and eyelid nodules and enlarged lacrimal glands may be found and are useful for confirmatory biopsy.

52. **How does the presentation of sarcoidosis differ with age?**
In children younger than 5 years, uveitis, arthritis, and skin rash are typical and the presentation may resemble JIA. In patients 20 to 40 years of age, bilateral chronic granulomatous iritis or panuveitis and hilar adenopathy are most common, whereas in elderly patients, lesions resembling multifocal choroiditis or birdshot chorioretinitis and interstitial lung disease may be seen.[43,44]

53. **What testing may be helpful in making the diagnosis of sarcoidosis?**
Chest x-ray is positive in 90% of patients with sarcoidosis.
Angiotensin-converting enzyme and lysozyme are moderately sensitive but not specific indicators of sarcoidosis. In cases with high suspicion and a negative chest x-ray, gallium scan (in children) and computed tomographic (CT) scan of the chest (adults) may be considered. Biopsy of normal-appearing conjunctiva in patients with presumed sarcoidosis is positive in 12% of cases. Lacrimal biopsy in presumed sarcoidosis is positive in 22% of cases.[45]

54. **According to the International Workshop on Ocular Sarcoidosis, what ocular findings are suggestive of sarcoidosis?**
Mutton fat KPs and/or iris nodules, tent-shape PAS, snowballs or "strings of pearls" in the vitreous, multiple peripheral chorioretinal lesions, periphlebitis, posterior pole granuloma, and bilateral disease are highly suggestive of ocular sarcoidosis.[46]

55. **How is a definitive diagnosis of ocular sarcoidosis made?**
A definitive diagnosis of ocular sarcoidosis requires a positive biopsy of skin, conjunctiva, or lacrimal gland in combination with suggestive uveitis. Without a positive biopsy, bilateral hilar adenopathy with suggestive ocular findings are diagnosed as presumed ocular sarcoidosis. Probable ocular sarcoidosis requires three intraocular signs suggestive for ocular sarcoidosis (see question 54) and two investigational tests supportive of ocular sarcoidosis (see question 53).

56. **What are three goals for the approach to treatment for uveitis?**
- Identify and treat the underlying causes. Exclude infections. This is especially important in immunocompromised individuals, in whom most uveitis cases are infectious.
- Prevent vision-threatening complications. Anti-inflammatory agents are the mainstay of treatment of noninfectious uveitis, or in some cases as an adjunct to antimicrobial therapy in infection cases to prevent or

reverse vision-threatening complications, including retinal ischemia, retinal scarring, cataract, and macular edema, among others.

- Relieve ocular discomfort and improve vision. Cycloplegic agents relax the ciliary body and reduce pain. In addition, they stabilize the blood–aqueous barrier and help to break or prevent PS that may lead to secondary glaucoma.

57. **What should be the general approach to the use of steroids to treat uveitis?**

High-dose corticosteroids should be used initially until inflammation is suppressed and then tapered. A common mistake is initial infrequent or low dosing, which results in a smoldering, extended course. Topical corticosteroids are best suited to anterior uveitis, as they do not reach the posterior segment in therapeutic levels. More potent topical preparations, that is, difluprednate, may penetrate more deeply. Prednisolone acetate achieves the highest AC concentrations. Posterior segment disease often requires treatment with periocular (posterior sub-Tenon or preseptal), intravitreal injection, intravitreal implant, and/or systemic corticosteroids. Systemic steroids are typically reserved for severe or bilateral disease. In patients incompletely responsive or made worse by steroids, one must suspect an infectious or neoplastic masquerade syndrome.

58. **Name the major categories of alternate (not steroids) immunosuppressives.**

- Antimetabolites (methotrexate, azathioprine, mycophenolate mofetil) are often used for their steroid-sparing effects.
- Calcineurin/T-cell inhibitors (cyclosporine, tacrolimus).
- Alkylating agents (cyclophosphamide, chorambucil) are typically reserved for severe, sight-threatening uveitis not adequately responsive to the aforementioned agents.
- Biologic agents. Tumor necrosis factor (TNF) inhibitors (adalimumab, infliximab, etanercept) and daclizumab, interferon a2α, and rituximab are examples of this expanding arsenal of immunosuppressant and anti-inflammatory agents.[47,48]

59. **Which biologic agent has been approved for the treatment of noninfectious intermediate, posterior, and pan uveitis?**

Adalimumab (Humira) has Food and Drug Administration (FDA) approval for these indications. It can be utilized alone or in conjunction with steroids and/or methotrexate in the proper clinical setting.

60. **Name three situations when a steroid sparing agent is indicated.**

- Systemic steroids required to suppress ocular inflammation are higher than can be safely administered over extended periods. This level varies but generally doses greater than or equal to 10 mg prednisone per day.
- Systemic or local steroids are causing intolerable side effects.
- Steroids do not significantly alter thc nature of the uveitis or underlying condition.

61. **In which diseases with uveitis or scleritis are immunosuppressive agents used alone or in addition to steroids?**

Immunosuppressive agents are indicated for the most severe types of uveitis, including Behçet's disease, granulomatosis with polyangiitis (formerly Wegener's granulomatosis), and rheumatoid arthritis–associated vasculitis. They are often required in cases of sympathetic ophthalmia, VKH syndrome, serpiginous choroiditis, birdshot retinochoroidopathy, and multifocal choroiditis. IU not amenable to steroid may require alternate immunosuppressives.

KEY POINTS: MOST COMMON FORMS OF UVEITIS

1. Children—JIA (chronic iridocyclitis)
2. NGAU—HLA-B27
3. GAU—sarcoidosis
4. IU—pars planitis
5. Posterior uveitis—toxoplasmosis

KEY POINTS: TREATMENT OF UVEITIS

1. Dilate all patients to rule out posterior segment disease.
2. Exclude infection before beginning anti-inflammatory treatment.
3. Recognize sight-threatening conditions that require immunosuppressive therapy.

MASQUERADE SYNDROMES

62. **Define "masquerade syndrome."**

The term *masquerade syndrome* refers to ophthalmic disorders that resemble uveitis clinically but are not primarily inflammatory in nature. Thus, they may be mistaken for, or masquerade as, either anterior or posterior uveitis (Table 39.5). Extensive evaluation is often initiated because patients manifest with atypical features, recurrent episodes of uveitis, or uveitis that is unresponsive to standard therapy.

63. In what age groups should one have the highest suspicion for masquerade syndromes?
One should suspect in the very young and in the elderly. They may occur at any age.

64. Describe the clinical features of retinoblastoma.
Retinoblastoma is the most common primary intraocular malignancy in children. It usually presents before age 2. The most common signs are leukocoria (white pupillary reflex) and strabismus. Occasionally, tumor necrosis may produce significant inflammation or discohesive tumor cells may layer in the AC, producing a pseudohypopyon (Fig. 39.3). Retinoblastoma cells in the vitreous (vitreous seeds) may simulate vitritis. Calcification on ultrasonography and magnetic resonance imaging (MRI) may help to differentiate retinoblastoma from various forms of childhood uveitis, including toxoplasmosis, toxocariasis, and pars planitis.[49]

Table 39.5 Most Common Masquerade Syndromes That May Mimic Uveitis

DISEASE	LOCATION	AGE (YEARS)	SIGNS OF INFLAMMATION	DIAGNOSTIC TESTS
Retinoblastoma	Anterior	<15	Flare, cells, pseudohypopyon	Aqueous tap for LDH levels and cytology
Leukemia	Anterior	<15	Flare, cells, heterochromia	Bone marrow, peripheral blood smear, aqueous cytology
Intraocular foreign body	Anterior	Any age	Flare, cells	X-ray, ultrasound, CT scan
Malignant melanoma	Anterior	Any age	Flare, cells	Angiography (fluorescein, ICG), ultrasound, MRI
Ocular ischemic syndrome	Anterior	50+	Cell, flare, redness	IVFA, carotid Doppler
Peripheral retinal detachment	Anterior	Any age	Flare, cells	Ophthalmoscopy, ultrasound
Retinitis pigmentosa	Posterior	Any age	Cells in vitreous	ERG, EOG, visual fields
Primary intraocular lymphoma	Posterior	15+	Vitreous cells, retinal hemorrhage or exudates, RPE infiltrates	Cytology of aqueous/vitreous fluid
Lymphoma	Posterior	15+	Retinal hemorrhage, exudates, vitreous cells	Biopsy of lymph node/ bone marrow, physical examination
Retinoblastoma	Posterior	<15	Vitreous cells, retinal exudate	Ultrasound, aqueous tap
Malignant melanoma	Posterior	15+	Vitreous cells	Fluorescein ultrasound

CT, Computed tomography; *ERG*, electroretinogram; *EOG*, electro-oculogram; *ICG*, indocyanine green; *IVFA*, intravenous fluorescein angiography; *LDH*, lactate dehydrogenase; *MRI*, magnetic resonance imaging; *RPE*, retinal pigment epithelium.
Adapted from American Academy of Ophthalmology: *Ophthalmology basic and clinical science course*, Section 6, San Francisco, 1997, American Academy of Ophthalmology.

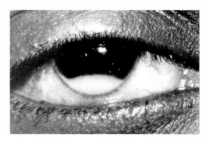

Fig. 39.3 Pseudohypopyon caused by seeding of retinoblastoma cells in the anterior chamber. (From Shields JA, Shields CL: *Intraocular tumors: a text and atlas*, Philadelphia, 1992, W.B. Saunders.)

65. What may present with chronic steroid-resistant panuveitis in a patient older than age 50?
    Primary intraocular lymphoma (Fig. 39.4) presents in persons over 60 with bilateral vitreous cells, AC reaction, and irregular patchy retinal or choroidal infiltrates.[50] When associated with hemorrhage and exudate, the retinal infiltrates may resemble infectious retinitis. Dense vitritis may be the only presenting sign. Most patients eventually develop some form of CNS involvement. CT or MRI may demonstrate CNS tumors. Vitreous aspirate or lumbar puncture may establish the diagnosis. Therapy may include ocular and CNS irradiation combined with intrathecal or intravitreal chemotherapy.[51–53]
    Interleukin 10 (IL-10) levels may be useful in aiding diagnosis and treatment response.[54]

66. Describe the ocular findings associated with leukemia.
    Leukemic cells may infiltrate any ocular tissue. Retinal findings (Fig. 39.5) include vascular dilation and tortuosity, retinal infiltrates composed of hemorrhages and cotton-wool spots (CWSs), and peripheral neovascularization. Roth spots are blot hemorrhages with white centers composed of leukemic cells or platelet–fibrin aggregates. Exudative retinal detachment may occur. Anterior segment findings include conjunctival mass, iris heterochromia, AC cell and flare, pseudohypopyon, spontaneous hyphema, and elevated IOP. Optic nerve infiltration and orbital involvement are also common.[55] Histopathologically, the choroid is the most commonly involved by leukemia infiltrate which leads to exudative retinal detachment. IV fluorescein angiogram (IVFA) demonstrates multiple pinpoint areas of hyperfluorescence similar to that found in VKH syndrome. Extended-depth optical coherence tomography (OCT) may be useful in detecting associated choroidal leukemic infiltrate and macular subretinal fluid.[56]

67. How does a malignant melanoma produce inflammatory signs?
    Necrotic tumors may elicit an intense inflammatory response or simulate uveitis with seeding of tumor cells into the vitreous cavity and anterior segment. Macrophages or tumor cells that contain melanin may produce a brown pseudohypopyon or block the TM, resulting in elevated IOP (melanocytic glaucoma). A necrotic tumor or one that invaded the retina may result in spontaneous vitreous hemorrhage. Other clinical findings include iris heterochromia and exudative retinal detachment with shifting subretinal fluid. Dilated examination, ultrasound, and IVFA help to establish the diagnosis.[57]

68. Describe two entities that can cause secondary anterior and/or posterior uveitis.
    • Long-standing peripheral rhegmatogenous retinal detachment may produce a cellular reaction in the anterior or posterior chamber as well as PS.

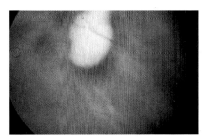

Fig. 39.4 Yellow-white chorioretinal infiltrates in intraocular lymphoma. (From Shields JA, Shields CL: *Intraocular tumors: a text and atlas,* Philadelphia, 1992, W.B. Saunders.)

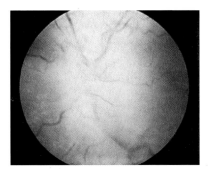

Fig. 39.5 Leukemic infiltration of the optic nerve head, retina, and choroid in an 8-year-old child. (From Shields JA, Shields CL: *Intraocular tumors: a text and atlas,* Philadelphia, 1992, W.B. Saunders.)

- Retained intraocular foreign bod**y** associated with trauma may cause persistent anterior and/or posterior segment inflammation. CT or ultrasonography results should demonstrate the abnormality. MRI is contraindicated if a metallic foreign body is suspected. Retained iron foreign bodies may lead to siderosis, retinal degeneration with an abnormal electroretinogram.

69. Describe another entity that could simulate uveitis.

Retinitis pigmentosa may present with anterior vitreous cells and posterior subcapsular cataract. The "bone spicule" pigment deposition in the retina, attenuated retinal vessels, mottling and atrophy of the RPE, and waxy pallor of the optic nerve help to distinguish this disease from other disorders. The diagnosis can be confirmed with an extinguished electroretinogram and ring scotoma on visual field testing.

KEY POINTS: COMMON MASQUERADE SYNDROMES

1. Retinoblastoma in children
2. Leukemia in children
3. Primary intraocular lymphoma in older adults
4. Ocular ischemic syndrome in the older adults
5. Peripheral retinal detachment in any age group

OCULAR MANIFESTATION OF ACQUIRED IMMUNE DEFICIENCY SYNDROME

70. Who is at greatest risk for developing AIDS-related eye disease?

Patients with severely reduced $CD4^+$ T-lymphocyte counts are most likely to develop acquired immune deficiency syndrome (AIDS)–related eye disease. For this reason, screening for opportunistic infections with dilated fundus examination is recommended every 3 months in patients with $CD4^+$ counts less than 100 cells/μL.[58]

71. What is the most common ocular manifestation of AIDS?

Retinal microvasculopathy, particularly CWSs, is the most common ocular manifestation (Fig. 39.6). Retinal microaneurysms and hemorrhages may be present. Most patients are asymptomatic. CWSs become more common as the $CD4^+$ T-lymphocyte count declines, reaching a prevalence of 45% in patients with counts less than 50 cells/μL.[59]

72. What is the most common ocular opportunistic infection in patients with AIDS?

CMV is the most common cause of opportunistic ocular infection and most frequently manifests as necrotizing retinitis (Fig. 39.7). "Frosted branch" angiitis and papillitis may occur. Varicella zoster, toxoplasmosis, and *Mycobacterium avium* are less frequent causes of posterior segment infection.

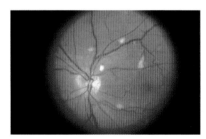

Fig. 39.6 Cotton-wool spots are infarcts of the nerve fiber layer. Unlike early infiltrates of cytomegalovirus retinitis, they do not enlarge, do not have associated hemorrhage, and may resolve in several weeks.

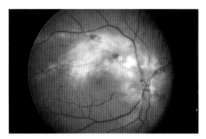

Fig. 39.7 Cytomegalovirus retinitis is characterized by areas of retinal infiltrate with associated hemorrhage. Note the optic nerve involvement.

73. **What is the incidence of cytomegalovirus retinitis?**
Among patients whose CD4+ count is less than 50 cells/μL, 20% per year develop CMV retinitis.

74. **Describe the early symptoms of cytomegalovirus retinitis.**
Floaters, described as numerous tiny black specks are often present early in the course of CMV retinitis. Pain and redness are not associated. Scotomas (blind spots) or visual loss may develop with more advanced stages of the disease.

75. **How does cytomegalovirus retinitis present clinically?**
Classic ophthalmologic findings of fulminant CMV retinitis include white areas of posterior retinal necrosis with associated hemorrhage and minimal vitreous inflammation (see Fig. 39.7). The indolent or granular form, which is often less symptomatic, is characterized by peripheral retinal whitening with minimal associated hemorrhage.[60]

76. **What are the more common entities in the differential diagnosis of cytomegalovirus retinitis?**
The more common entities are progressive outer retinal necrosis, toxoplasmosis, syphilis, HIV retinitis, and cotton wool spots.

77. **How is the diagnosis of cytomegalovirus retinitis made?**
The diagnosis of CMV retinitis is made clinically when characteristic findings of fulminant or indolent retinitis are found in an immunosuppressed patient with CD4+ count less than 100 cells/μL. In the unusual case in which the diagnosis is in question, a vitreous biopsy with or without retinal biopsy for PCR analysis may be performed.

78. **What is the initial treatment strategy for cytomegalovirus retinitis?**
Treatment of CMV retinitis is given in two stages. The first stage is 2 to 6 weeks of induction therapy with ganciclovir (Fig. 39.8), valganciclovir, foscarnet, or cidofovir. These are antiviral agents that inhibit the viral DNA polymerase. Induction is discontinued after a healing response (consolidation or stabilization of the margins) begins. The second stage, maintenance therapy, consists of a lower dose of the medication that is continued until relapse occurs.

79. **What is the strategy in the event of a relapse?**
Despite maintenance therapy, CMV retinitis will likely relapse in persons who remain immunosuppressed. The mean interval to relapse varies from 2 to 8 months and depends on the medication used and the route of administration. If relapse occurs in patients taking oral or IV medication, reinduction with the same medication (2 to 6 weeks of high-dose IV or multiple intraocular injections) is indicated.

80. **Does resistance to antiviral medication develop?**
Drug resistance is an emerging problem of great concern because of the limited number of available agents that are effective against CMV. Ganciclovir-resistant CMV has been reported in 27.5% of urine samples at 9 months. CMV UL97 mutation (a CMV DNA polymerase mutation that confers ganciclovir resistance) was detected in 30.8% of patients treated with ganciclovir over 3 months and in none treated less than 3 months. Resistance to foscarnet and cidofovir has also been reported. Owing to similarities in the mechanism of action, cross-resistance may develop with cidofovir and ganciclovir. Clinical resistance is defined as a lack of response to 6 weeks of induction therapy. A change in medication or combination therapy is indicated.[61,62]

81. **How long should treatment be continued in patients with cytomegalovirus retinitis?**
Length of therapy depends on the immune status of the patient. For patients who remain severely immunosuppressed (CD4+ count <100 cells/μL), treatment must be continued indefinitely. In patients whose immune status is improved by highly active antiretroviral therapy (HAART) (see question 83), maintenance therapy may be discontinued if certain criteria are met (see later).

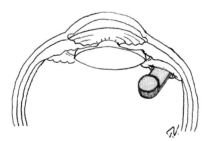

Fig. 39.8 The intraocular ganciclovir implant is sutured to the sclera and extends into the vitreous cavity. The drug delivery system slowly releases ganciclovir over 8 months. It may be replaced when the drug supply is exhausted. Although it is not associated with the systemic toxicity seen with oral or intravenous therapy, the implant provides no prophylaxis against systemic cytomegalovirus (CMV) or CMV retinitis in the fellow eye.

82. Name the main toxicities of the antiviral therapies.
    • Ganciclovir: bone marrow toxicity with neutropenia and/or thrombocytopenia.
    • Foscarnet: nephrotoxicity.
    • Cidofovir: nephrotoxicity, which may be ameliorated by concurrent probenecid and hypotony after either IV or intravitreal administration.

83. How has highly active antiretroviral therapy affected the natural history and treatment of cytomegalovirus retinitis?
    HAART causes significant and sustained increases in CD4[+] counts and remission of CMV retinitis. Discontinuation of maintenance therapy has been recommended for patients with completely quiescent retinitis and CD4[+] count greater than 100 cells/μL. Other criteria include CD4[+] elevation for at least 3 months, prolonged relapse-free intervals, HAART longer than 18 months, and reduced HIV and CMV viremia.[63,64]

84. What is immune recovery uveitis?
    Immune recovery uveitis (IRU) is intraocular inflammation that develops as systemic immunity recovers. It is hypothesized that immunologic improvement leads to an inflammatory response directed at the CMV antigen. IRU typically develops in 10% to 20% of eyes with CMV within 1 month after HAART is initiated but may occur up to 3 years later. Treatment of CMV retinitis with IV cidofovir and large CMV lesion size increase the risk. Vision-threatening complications include macular edema, epiretinal membrane, cataract, optic disc edema, retinal neovascularization, and neovascular glaucoma. Treatment depends on the location and severity of inflammation and the presence of complications and usually requires local and or systemic corticosteroids. On occasion, observation or antiviral therapy may be indicated.[65]

85. Can cytomegalovirus retinitis develop in other forms of immunosuppression other than AIDS?
    Yes. CMV is the most common retinitis among renal transplant patients. Unlike CMV in AIDS, the vitreous develops a pronounced inflammatory reaction (cells causing significant haze not unlike that seen in toxoplasmosis).

86. What is progressive outer retinal necrosis?
    Progressive outer retinal necrosis is an extremely aggressive form of retinitis in the AIDS population (Fig. 39.9). It primarily affects persons with CD4 counts less than 50 cell/μL. Caused by herpes zoster virus, it is temporally associated with herpes zoster skin lesions, which may or may not be in the periocular region. Prompt diagnosis and treatment are imperative to prevent blindness, which develops in greater than 80% of patients because of either relentless progression of infection or secondary retinal detachment.[66]

87. Why do retinal detachments develop in cases of infectious necrotizing retinitis? Who is at risk?
    Retinal infections may cause multiple necrotic retinal holes that over time lead to retinal detachment. Most AIDS-related retinal detachments develop as a complication of CMV retinitis and occur in 34% of patients with CMV. However, patients with progressive outer retinal necrosis are at highest risk; retinal detachments occur in 60% to 70% of these cases.

88. How are most AIDS-related retinal detachments repaired?
    Lasers may be used to demarcate or wall off macula-sparing retinal detachments, especially in patients who are not well enough to tolerate surgery. Vitrectomy with silicone oil injection is often required in cases in which the macula is detached or retinitis is active. The silicone oil replaces the vitreous and tamponades the multiple necrotic holes to prevent redetachment.[67,68]

89. Describe the unique characteristics of ocular syphilis in patients with AIDS.
    Syphilis is not considered an opportunistic infection by definition, because most patients have CD4[+] T-cell counts greater than 250 cell/μL. Ocular findings range from iritis to necrotizing retinitis. CNS syphilis is present in 85%

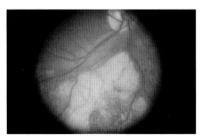

Fig. 39.9 Progressive outer retinal necrosis typically affects the outer retina with sparing of the retinal vessels. Note the areas of perivascular clearing and absence of associated hemorrhage.

of HIV-positive patients with ocular syphilis. Hence, evaluation of CSF is mandated for all HIV-positive patients with ocular syphilis. Syphilis may be seronegative (negative RPR despite active infection) in the AIDS population. Regardless of clinical findings, syphilis in patients with AIDS should be treated as a tertiary disease with a 10-day course of IV antibiotics. Although recurrent infection may occur, maintenance therapy is not currently recommended.[69]

KEY POINTS: OCULAR MANIFESTATIONS OF AIDS

1. Microvasculopathy (particularly CWSs) is the most common ocular manifestation.
2. CMV is the most common ocular opportunistic infection.
3. Progressive outer retinal necrosis is the most rapidly progressive and therefore potentially blinding ocular complication. Both CMV and progressive outer retinal necrosis typically occur when CD4 is <100.
4. Varicella zoster (ARN) is most likely to be complicated by retinal detachment and vision loss (>80%).
5. *Cryptococcus* is the most common cause of neuro-ophthalmologic abnormalities in ambulatory patients.

90. **What is the most common cause of neuro-ophthalmologic abnormalities in the ambulatory AIDS population, and what are the clinical findings?**
    Cryptococcal meningitis causes papilledema and cranial nerve palsies (Fig. 39.10). Papilledema is defined as disc swelling that is secondary to increased intracranial pressure. The central disc tissue remains pink. Early optic nerve dysfunction is minimal, and vision is usually preserved, in contrast to papillitis (see question 92). Other more common causes of papilledema include CNS infection by toxoplasmosis or malignancy (lymphoma).

91. **How should retrobulbar optic neuritis be diagnosed and managed in AIDS patients?**
    The etiology of retrobulbar optic neuritis in an AIDS patient is almost always infectious. Idiopathic optic neuritis is a diagnosis of exclusion. Prompt evaluation must include serology for *Cryptococcus*, syphilis, and varicella zoster virus. A lumbar puncture is also indicated. Patients should be questioned about the history of syphilis or previous varicella zoster infection, and a review of medications should be done. Ethambutol and didanosine may cause toxic optic neuropathy. Treatment with corticosteroids is contraindicated.

92. **What is papillitis?**
    Papillitis is an inflammation of the visible intraocular portion of the optic nerve. The optic nerve appears white and necrotic (Fig. 39.11), and vision is severely compromised. CMV may cause papillitis, often in association with adjacent retinitis. Vision may improve after treatment with antiviral medications.

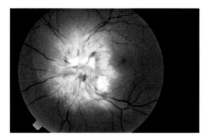

Fig. 39.10 Papilledema caused by cryptococcal meningitis is characterized by optic disc swelling and blurring of the disc margins.

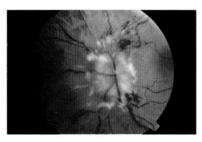

Fig. 39.11 Note white, necrotic appearance and associated hemorrhage of entire optic disc in this example of papillitis secondary to cytomegalovirus.

93. Which medications may be associated with ocular toxicity?

Rifabutin, when used in combination with clarithromycin and fluconazole, has been reported to cause severe hypopyon iritis and, in rare instances, sterile endophthalmitis. Ethambutol may cause optic neuropathy. Side effects of cidofovir include uveitis, hypotony, and nephrotoxicity.[70]

REFERENCES

1. Kopplin LJ, Mount G, Suhler EB: Review for disease of the year: epidemiology of HLA-B27 associated ocular disorders, Ocul Immunol Inflamm 24:470–475, 2016.
2. Angeles-Han ST, Ringold S, Beukelman T, et al.: 2019 American College of Rheumatology/Arthritis Foundation guideline for the screening, monitoring, and treatment of juvenile idiopathic arthritis–associated uveitis, Arthritis Care Res 71:703–716, 2019.
3. Kopplin LJ, Mount G, Suhler EB: Review for disease of the year: epidemiology of HLA-B27 associated ocular disorders, Ocul Immunol Inflamm 24:470–475, 2016.
4. Brewerton DA, Hart FD, Nicholls A, et al.: Ankylosing spondylitis and HLA B27, Lancet 1:904–907, 1973.
5. Tay-Kearney ML, Schwam BL, Lowder C, et al.: Clinical features and associated systemic diseases of HLA-B27 uveitis, Am J Ophthalmol 121:47–56, 1996.
6. Zhu Y, Pandya BJ, Choi HK: Prevalence of gout and hyperuricemia in the US general population: the National Health and Nutrition Examination Survey 2007–2008, Arthritis Rheum 63:3136–3141, 2011.
7. Hutchinson J: The Bowman lecture on the relation of certain diseases of the eye to gout, Br Med J 2:995–1000, 1884.
8. Ao J, Foldblatt F, Casson RJ: Review of the ophthalmic manifestations of gout and uric acid crystal deposition, Clin Exp Ophthalmol 45:73–80, 2017.
9. Angeles-Han ST, Ringold S, Beukelman T, et al.: 2019 American College of Rheumatology/Arthritis Foundation guideline for the screening, monitoring, and treatment of juvenile idiopathic arthritis–associated uveitis, Arthritis Care Res 71:703–716, 2019.
10. Clements DB: Juvenile xanthogranuloma treated with local steroids, Br J Ophthalmol 50:663–665, 1966.
11. Zimmerman LE: Ocular lesions of juvenile xanthogranuloma. Neoxanthoendothelioma, Trans Am Acad Ophthalmol Otolaryngol 69:412–439, 1965.
12. Grégoire MA, Kodjikian L, Varron L, Grange JD, Broussolle C, Seve P: Characteristics of uveitis presenting for the first time in the elderly: analysis of 91 patients in a tertiary center, Ocul Immunol Inflamm 19:219–226, 2011.
13. Zein G, Berta A, Foster CS: Multiple sclerosis–associated uveitis, Ocul Immunol Inflamm 12:137–142, 2004.
14. Babu M, Rathinam SR: Intermediate uveitis, Indian J Ophthalmol 58:21–27, 2010.
15. Raja SC, Jabs DA, Dunn JP, et al.: Pars planitis: clinical features and class II HLA associations, Ophthalmology 106:594–599, 1999.
16. Kamoi K, Mochizuki M: HTLV-1 uveitis, Front Microbiol 3:270, 2012.
17. Tagaya Y, Matsuoka M, Gallo R: 40 years of the human T-cell leukemia virus: past, present, and future. Version 1, F1000Res 8:F1000 Faculty Rev-228, 2019. Published online February 28, 2019. doi:10.12688/f1000research.17479.1
18. Smith JR, Cunningham ET Jr: Atypical presentations of ocular toxoplasmosis, Curr Opin Ophthalmol 13:387–392, 2002.
19. Rush R, Sheth S: Fulminant toxoplasmic retino-choroiditis following intravitreal triamcinolone administration, Indian J Ophthalmol 60:141–143, 2012.
20. Jones JL, Dargelas V, Roberts J, et al.: Risk factors for *Toxoplasma gondii* infection in the United States, Clin Infect Dis 49:878–884, 2009.
21. Melamed J, Eckert GU, Spadoni VS, Lago EG, Uberti F: Ocular manifestations of congenital toxoplasmosis, Eye 24:528–234, 2009.
22. Garza-Leon M, Garcia LA: Ocular toxoplasmosis: clinical characteristics in pediatric patients, Ocul Immunol Inflamm 20:130–138, 2012.
23. Weiss MJ, Velazquez N, Hofeldt AJ: Serologic tests in the diagnosis of presumed toxoplasmic retinochoroiditis, Am J Ophthalmol 109:407–411, 1990.
24. Harrell M, Carvounis PE: Current treatment of toxoplasma retinochoroiditis: an evidence-based review, J Ophthalmol 2014:273506, 2014. doi:10.1155/2014/273506
25. Kim SJ, Scott IU, Brown GC, et al.: Interventions for toxoplasma retinochoroiditis: a report by the American Academy of Ophthalmology, Ophthalmol 120:371–378, 2013.
26. Stanford MR, See SE, Jones LV, Gilbert RE: Antibiotics for toxoplasmic retinochoroiditis: an evidence-based systematic review, Ophthalmology 110:926–931, 2003.
27. Margo CE, Hamed LH: Ocular syphilis, Surv Ophthalmol 37:203–220, 1992.
28. Tramont EC, Syphilis in HIV-infected persons, AIDS Clin Rev 61–72, 1993–1994.
29. Raja H, Starr MR, Sophie J Bakri SJ: Ocular manifestations of tick-borne diseases, Surv Ophthalmol 61:726–744, 2016.
30. Aaberg TM: The expanding ophthalmologic spectrum of Lyme disease, Am J Ophthalmol 107:77–80, 1989.
31. Zaidman GW: The ocular manifestations of Lyme disease, Int Ophthalmol Clin 33:9–22, 1993.
32. Khanamiri HN, Rao NA: Serpiginous choroiditis and infectious multifocal serpiginoid choroiditis, Surv Ophthalmol 58:203–232, 2013.
33. Zhang M, Zhang J, Liu Y: Clinical presentations and therapeutic effect of presumed choroidal tuberculosis, Retina 32:805–813, 2012.
34. Yeh S, Sen HN, Colyer M, Zapor M, Wroblewski K: Update on ocular tuberculosis, Curr Opin Ophthalmol 23:551–556, 2012.
35. Duker JS, Blumenkranz MS: Diagnosis and management of the acute retinal necrosis (ARN) syndrome, Surv Ophthalmol 35:327–343, 1991.
36. Balansard B, Bodaghi B, Cassoux N, et al.: Necrotising retinopathies simulating acute retinal necrosis syndrome, Br J Ophthalmol 89:96–101, 2005.
37. Ormerod LD, Dailey JP: Ocular manifestations of cat-scratch disease, Curr Opin Ophthalmol 10:209–216, 1999.
38. Tugal-Tutkun I, Onal S, Altan-Yaycioglu R, Altunbas HH, Urgancioglu M: Uveitis in Behçet disease: an analysis of 880 patients, Am J Ophthalmol 138:373–380, 2004.
39. Susac JO: Susac's syndrome: the triad of microangiopathy of the brain and retina with hearing loss in young women, Neurology 44:591–593, 1994.
40. Papasavvas I, Teuchner B, Herbort CP: Susac syndrome (Retino-cochleo-cerebral vasculitis), the ophthalmologist in the role of the whistleblower, J Ophthal Inflamm Infect 10:Article 27, 2020. doi:10.1186/s12348-020-00217-z.

41. Chu DS, Foster CS: Sympathetic ophthalmia, Int Ophthalmol Clin 42:179–185, 2002.
42. Moorthy RS, Mermoud A, Baerveldt G, et al.: Glaucoma associated with uveitis, Surv Ophthalmol 41:361–394, 1997.
43. Iannuzzi MC, Fontana JR: Sarcoidosis: clinical presentation, immunopathogenesis, and therapeutics, JAMA 305:391–399, 2011.
44. Vrabec TR, Augsburger JJ, Fischer DH, et al.: Taches de bougie, Ophthalmology 102:1712–1721, 1995.
45. Weineb RN: Diagnosing sarcoidosis by transconjunctival biopsy of the lacrimal gland, Am J Ophthlamol 97:573–576, 1984.
46. Mochizuki M, Smith JR, Takase H, et al: International workshop on ocular sarcoidosis study group revised criteria of International Workshop on Ocular Sarcoidosis (IWOS) for the diagnosis of ocular sarcoidosis, Br J Ophthalmol 103:1418–1422, 2019.
47. Jabs DA, Rosenbaum JT, Foster CS, et al.: Guidelines for the use of immunosuppressive drugs in patients with ocular inflammatory disorders: recommendations of an expert panel, Am J Ophthalmol 130:492–513, 2000.
48. Jabs DA: Immunosuppression for the uveitides, Ophthalmology 125:193–202, 2018.
49. Shields JA, Augsburger JJ: Current approaches to the diagnosis and management of retinoblastoma, Surv Ophthalmol 25:347–372, 1981.
50. Char DH, Ljung BM, Miller T, Phillips T: Primary intraocular lymphoma (ocular reticulum cell sarcoma): diagnosis and management, Ophthalmology 95:625–630, 1988.
51. Frenkel S, Hendler K, Siegal T, Shalom E, Pe'er J, Intravitreal methotrexate for treating vitreoretinal lymphoma: 10 years of experience, Br J Ophthalmol 92:383–388, 2008.
52. Larkin KL, Saboo US, Comer GM, et al.: Use of intravitreal rituximab for treatment of vitreoretinal lymphoma, Br J Ophthalmol 98: 99–103, 2014.
53. Yeh S, Wilson D: Combination intravitreal rituximab and methotrexate for massive subretinal lymphoma, Eye 24:1625–1627, 2010.
54. Raja H, Snyder MR, Johnston PB, et al.: Effect of intravitreal methotrexate and rituximab on interleukin-10 levels in aqueous humor of treated eyes with vitreoretinal lymphoma, PLoS One 8(6):e65627, 2013. doi:10.1371/journal.pone.0065627
55. Kincaid MC, Green WR: Ocular and orbital involvement in leukemia, Surv Ophthalmol 27:211–232, 1983.
56. Adam MK, Pitcher JD, Shields CL, Maguire JI: Enhanced depth imaging optical coherence tomography of precursor cell leukemic choroidopathy before and after chemotherapy, Middle East Afr J Ophthalmol 22:249–52, 2015.
57. Fraser DJ Jr, Font RL: Ocular inflammation and hemorrhage as initial manifestations of uveal malignant melanoma: incidence and prognosis, Arch Ophthalmol 97:1311–1314, 1979.
58. Baldassano V, Dunn JP, Feinberg J, Dabs BA: Cytomegalovirus retinitis and low CD4$^+$ T-lymphocyte counts, N Engl J Med 333:670, 1995.
59. Freeman WR, Chen A, Henderly DE, et al.: Prevalence and significance of acquired immunodeficiency-related retinal microvasculopathy, Am J Ophthalmol 107:229–235, 1989.
60. Jabs DA, Enger C, Bartlett JG: Cytomegalovirus retinitis and acquired immunodeficiency syndrome, Arch Ophthalmol 107:75–80, 1989.
61. Gilbert C, Handfield J, Toma E, et al.: Emergence and prevalence of cytomegalovirus UL97 mutations associated with ganciclovir resistance in AIDS patients, AIDS 12:125–129, 1998.
62. Jabs DA, Enger C, Dunn JP, Forman M: Cytomegalovirus retinitis and viral resistance: ganciclovir resistance. CMV Retinitis and Viral Resistance Study Group, J Infect Dis 177:770–773, 1998.
63. Vrabec TR, Baldassano VF, Whitcup SM: Discontinuation of maintenance therapy in patients with quiescent CMV retinitis and elevated CD4$^+$ counts, Ophthalmology 105:1259–1264, 1998.
64. Holbrook JT, Colvin R, van Natta ML, et al.: Studies of Ocular Complications of AIDS (SOCA) Research Group. Evaluation of the United States public health service guidelines for discontinuation of anticytomegalovirus therapy after immune recovery in patients with cytomegalovirus retinitis, Am J Ophthalmol 152:628–637, 2011.
65. Figueiredo L, Rothwell R, Bilhoto M, et al.: Immune recovery uveitis masked as an endogenous endophthalmitis in a patient with active CMV retinitis, Case Rep Ophthalmol Med 462968, 2013.
66. Engstrom RE Jr, Holland GN, Margolis TP, et al.: Progressive outer retinal necrosis syndrome, Ophthalmology 101:1488–1502, 1994.
67. Baumal CR, Reichel E: Management of cytomegalovirus-related retinal detachments, Ophthalmic Surg Lasers 29:916–925, 1998.
68. Vrabec TR: Laser demarcation of macula-sparing cytomegalovirus-related retinal detachment, Ophthalmology 104:2062–2067, 1997.
69. Passo MS, Rosenbaum JT: Ocular syphilis in patients with human immunodeficiency virus infection, Am J Ophthalmol 106:1–6, 1988.
70. Saran BR, Maguire AM, Nichols C, et al.: Hypopyon uveitis in patients with AIDS treated for systemic *Mycobacterium avium* complex infection with rifabutin, Arch Ophthalmol 112:1159–1165, 1994.

TOXIC RETINOPATHIES

Priya Sharma Vakharia

1. Describe the clinical features of chloroquine/hydroxychloroquine retinopathy.
   Hydroxychloroquine (HCQ)/chloroquine (CQ) retinopathy can be insidious in onset, but early detection is imperative. Patients are usually asymptomatic initially. The visual acuity is typically normal in the early stages because the initial retinal changes are parafoveal and spare the central foveal area. Mild mottling of the perifoveal retinal pigment epithelium (RPE) is seen in conjunction with a reduced foveal reflex. Peripheral pigmentary changes often occur at this stage but may be overlooked. In late stages, as retinal atrophy progresses, patients may experience difficulties with reading due to paracentral scotomas or metamorphopsia. Nyctalopia, color vision defects, and blurred vision occur when the retinal epithelial atrophy extends to involve the fovea. These macular pigmentary changes progress to a classic bull's eye maculopathy (Fig. 40.1). In the later stages, generalized retinal pigmentary changes occur with vascular attenuation and optic disc pallor.

2. What doses of chloroquine and hydroxychloroquine cause retinopathy?
   Retinopathy is unlikely with a daily dose of <2.3 mg/kg real weight/day CQ or <5.0 mg/kg real weight/day HCQ. Patients taking <5.0 mg/kg real weight/day of HCQ have less than 1% risk of developing toxicity in the first 5 years of therapy, and less than 2% up to 10 years. After 20 years, the risk increases to approximately 20%. CQ toxicity has a similar dose-related effect.

3. What are the risk factors for chloroquine and hydroxychloroquine retinopathy?
   The cumulative dose is believed to be the most important risk factor. A cumulative dose of >1000 g of HCQ or >460 g of CQ is one of the largest risk factors for retinopathy. With daily doses of >5.0 mg/kg for HCQ and >2.3 mg/kg for CQ, accumulation of the drug may enhance the rate or degree of toxic retinopathy. CQ and HCQ are excreted by the kidney and liver. Therefore, hepatic and renal failure and disease are risk factors because they may contribute to increased blood levels of the drug. Other risk factors are age, tamoxifen use, genetic factors such as cytochrome P450 metabolism defects, and preexisting macular disease.

4. How should patients taking chloroquine and hydroxychloroquine be monitored?
   All patients starting CQ or HCQ therapy should have a baseline examination within the first year of the treatment. The baseline examination should include careful biomicroscopy with fundus examination to check for any preexisting macular pathology that may deter further use of HCQ or CQ. Baseline Humphrey visual field (HVF) and spectral-domain optical coherence tomography (SD-OCT) can be helpful but are not critical to obtain at baseline.
   In the absence of further risk factors and with correct dosing, annual screening can then be deferred until there has been 5 years of cumulative exposure. Screening can be done sooner per physician/patient preference or in a patient who is high risk. Screening at this time includes a full ocular examination with careful macular examination. Subjective testing should take place, which typically includes automated HVF testing with a white 10-2 protocol for the detection of paracentral scotomas, although wider test patterns (24-2 or 30-2) are needed for Asian patients who often manifest changes peripherally first. There should also be one or more objective tests for screening: SD-OCT, multifocal electroretinogram (mfERG), or fundus autofluorescence (FAF).

5. What does testing show in hydroxychloroquine/chloroquine retinopathy?
   In patients with early toxicity, automated HVF testing specifically looking at the pattern deviation often shows decreased sensitivity in the paracentral region, often with the inferotemporal region affected first. Asian patients can manifest changes peripherally first. The key is to retest any suspicious findings and compare to objective testing.
   SD-OCT shows attenuation or loss of ellipsoid layer in the parafoveal region of the macula. Similarly, the mfERG can show localized paracentral functional loss. FAF imaging may reveal paracentral foci of hyperfluorescence due to accumulation of outer segment debris within the RPE and hypofluorescent areas in the later stages due to RPE loss. Baseline color fundus photography may be useful for documentation.

6. What management is advised for chloroquine retinopathy?
   If retinal toxicity is present, HCQ or CQ should be stopped immediately. There is a stage of very early functional loss when the cessation of the drug will reverse the toxicity, but progression typically continues, although it is not clear if it is related to low excretion of the drug or to gradual decompensation of cells that were damaged during the period of drug exposure. If suggestive findings/visual symptoms occur, subjective tests should be repeated (automated fields, mfERG, SD-OCT, FAF). If toxicity is suspected, cessation of the CQ and HCQ followed by 3- to 6-monthly review is advised. Patients with probable toxicity (bilateral bull's eye scotoma, bilateral paracentral mfERG, SD-OCT/FAF abnormalities) should be closely monitored every 3 months.

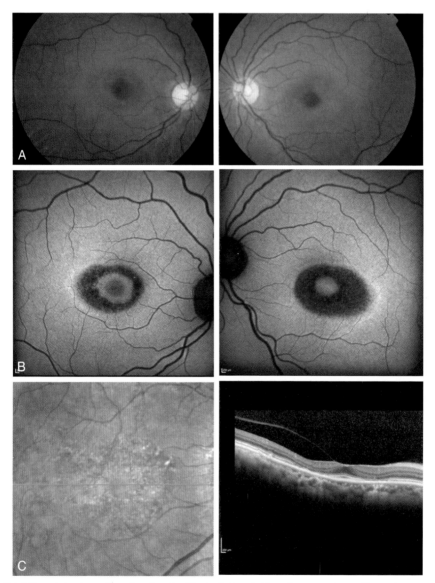

Fig. 40.1 Bull's eye lesion due to chloroquine retinopathy: **(A)** color photograph, **(B)** autofluorescence image, **(C)** magnified photograph of macula with associated spectral domain optical coherence tomography.

7. Is the pathogenesis of chloroquine and hydroxychloroquine retinopathy understood?

The pathogenesis is not completely understood. The earliest histopathologic changes of CQ retinopathy include membranous cytoplasmic bodies in ganglion cells and degenerative changes in the outer segments of the photoreceptors. However, CQ has a selective affinity for melanin, and it has been suggested that this affinity reduces the ability of melanin to combine with free radicals and protect visual cells from light and radiation toxicity. Other authors believe that the drug may directly damage photoreceptors.

8. How may thioridazine affect the retina?

Thioridazine (Mellaril) is a phenothiazine medication that is used as an antipsychotic. The exact mechanism of toxicity is unknown. It may cause nyctalopia, dyschromatopsia, blurred vision, and visual field defects. The earliest retinal changes are a fine mottling or granularity to the RPE posterior to the equator, which may progress to marked pigmentary atrophy and hypertrophic pigment plaques (Fig. 40.2). Vascular attenuation and optic atrophy may follow. Toxicity is said to be uncommon with daily doses <800 mg/day but may develop rapidly with doses over 1200 mg/day. Toxicity is more dependent on total daily dose than on cumulative dose. In perimetry, a nonspecific but most characteristic finding is a paracentral or ring scotoma. Fluorescein angiography reveals the loss of RPE and choriocapillaris within the areas of depigmentation.

9. **What other phenothiazines cause retinopathy?**
Retinal toxicity has been reported with other phenothiazines, including chlorpromazine. However, these compounds are less likely to cause retinopathy, probably because they lack the piperidinylethyl side group of thioridazine. It is thought that 1200 to 2400 g/day chlorpromazine for at least 12 months is required before toxicity occurs.

10. **How may quinine sulfate cause retinopathy?**
Quinine sulfate is used for nocturnal cramps and as a malarial prophylaxis. It may cause retinal toxicity after a single large ingestion (4 g). The therapeutic window is narrow, with some patients taking a daily dose of 2 g. Patients develop blurred vision, nyctalopia, nausea, tinnitus, dysacusis, and even coma within 2 to 4 hours of ingestion. The acute findings include dilated pupils, loss of retinal transparency caused by ganglion cell toxicity (Fig. 40.3), and dilated retinal vessels. As the acute phase resolves, vessel attenuation and optic disc pallor result. Visual acuity may improve after the acute phase.

11. **What are the retinal toxic effects of sildenafil (Viagra)?**
Sildenafil is an effective drug for erectile dysfunction, acting to inhibit phosphodiesterase type 5 (PDE-5) isoenzyme. It can also inhibit PDE-6 isoenzyme, an important enzyme in the retinal phototransduction cascade, and can cause reversible reduced amplitude of the a and b waves in an electroretinogram (ERG). Overall, 3% to 11% of patients may experience transient visual changes, such as tinting of vision or photosensitivity lasting minutes to hours after the ingestion of the drug. Serious and permanent side effects have been described, including retinal hemorrhages, branch retinal vein and artery occlusion, anterior ischemic optic neuropathy, and acceleration of proliferative diabetic retinopathy.

12. **How does cocaine abuse affect the retina?**
Cocaine has both dopaminergic and adrenomimetic effects. Dopamine is found in high concentrations in the retina and plays an important role in color vision. Cocaine-withdrawn patients have significantly reduced blue cone b-wave amplitude responses on the ERG and blue–yellow color vision defects. The adrenomimetic response and sudden increase in blood pressure associated with the intranasal use of cocaine may also cause retinal arterial occlusions.

13. **What is vigabatrin retinotoxicity?**
Vigabatrin (VGB) is an irreversible inhibitor of γ-aminobutyric acid transaminase and is a highly effective antiepileptic drug for treating partial-onset seizures and infantile spasms. It causes a characteristic form of peripheral retinal atrophy and nasal or "inverse" optic disc atrophy in approximately 10% of children being

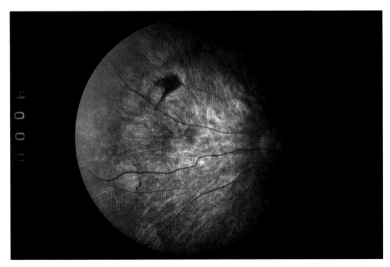

Fig. 40.2 Thioridazine retinopathy.

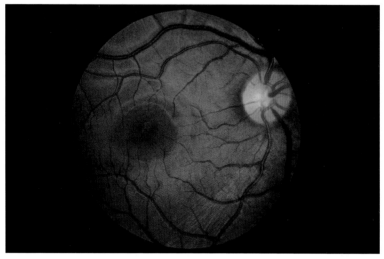

Fig. 40.3 Mild loss of retinal transparency caused by quinine sulfate toxicity.

treated with VGB, resulting in severely constricted visual fields. Strongly consider discontinuing VGB in these children.

14. **How does fetal alcohol syndrome affect the retina?**
   Alcohol-induced malformations include hypoplastic optic discs and tortuous retinal vessels.

15. **What is unusual about cystoid macular edema caused by nicotinic acid?**
   Nicotinic acid is used to reduce serum lipid and cholesterol levels in hyperlipidemia. In doses of >1.5 g/day, patients report blurred vision sometimes associated with paracentral scotoma or metamorphopsia. Although typical cystoid macular edema is seen clinically, fluorescein angiography shows no leakage, suggesting that the edema is caused by a toxic effect on Müller cells resulting in intracellular edema. The incidence is low (0.67%) and dose related. The cystoid macular edema is reversible.

16. **Name the substances that may cause crystalline retinopathy.**
   - Tamoxifen
   - Canthaxanthin
   - Nitrofurantoin
   - Anastrazole
   - Talc (often used with intravenous drug abuse) (Fig. 40.4)
   - Drugs that cause secondary oxalosis
     - Methoxyflurane anesthesia
     - Ethylene glycol
     - Salicylate ingestion in the presence of renal failure

17. **What is the mechanism of the retinopathy caused by talc?**
   Talc is used as filler in methylphenidate hydrochloride (Ritalin) and other pills that drug addicts may crush and inject intravenously. Initially, the talc particles embolize to the lungs, but after prolonged abuse, pulmonary arteriovenous shunts allow talc directly into the systemic circulation. Initially, talc particles in the retina appear as a crystalline retinopathy. Emboli to the retinal arterioles may lead to marked peripheral and posterior closure, resulting in retinal neovascularization, vitreous hemorrhage, and ischemic maculopathy.

18. **How should talc retinopathy be managed?**
   Immediate cessation of Ritalin abuse/intravenous drug abuse is essential. If retinal neovascularization and vitreous hemorrhage are present, peripheral panretinal photocoagulation should be considered. There is no effective treatment for ischemic maculopathy.

19. **What is xanthopsia? Which drug may cause it?**
   Xanthopsia is the unusual symptom of yellow vision. Along with hemeralopia (reduced visual acuity in the presence of increased background illumination), blurred vision, poor color vision, and paracentral scotomas, it is caused by digitalis toxicity.

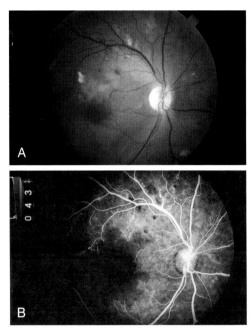

Fig. 40.4 Talc retinopathy showing fine perifoveal talc particles **(A)** and extensive resultant posterior pole retinal vascular closure on fluorescein angiography **(B)**.

20. What are the clinical features of tamoxifen retinopathy? How much drug is necessary to cause symptoms?

Tamoxifen is an antiestrogen drug commonly used to treat breast carcinoma. Patients are typically asymptomatic with inner retinal crystal deposits, although significantly reduced visual acuity has been reported in a subset of cases. Irreversible dot-like or refractile crystals are seen deposited in the inner retina and located predominantly in the paramacular region and often associated with macular edema. The cumulative dose of tamoxifen seems to be important, with retinal deposits occurring more frequently with higher doses (60–100 mg/day). The overall prevalence is 1% to 6%. No consistent ERG changes are seen. The risk of macular hole may be increased in patients taking tamoxifen and this can be evaluated with SD-OCT. Patients with documented visual loss or macular edema should discontinue the drug. Although vision may recover and macular edema resolve after cessation of tamoxifen, the retinal deposits will persist.

21. Can intraocular injection of antibiotics cause retinopathy?

Inadvertent intraocular injection of gentamicin may result in rapid onset of retinal whitening in the macular area, superficial and intraretinal hemorrhages, retinal edema cotton-wool spots, arteriolar narrowing, and venous beading. Optic atrophy and retinal pigment epithelial changes develop later. The visual prognosis is poor and neovascular glaucoma may develop. Fluorescein angiography reveals severe vascular nonperfusion in the acute stages. Macular infarction has been reported after intravitreal injections of 400 µg. Similar problems may occur with tobramycin and amikacin.

Intraocular vancomycin has also been reported to cause hemorrhagic-occlusive retinal vasculitis, especially after use as an intracameral agent following cataract surgery. It is thought to be due to a rare type of hypersensitivity response. Clinical examination shows a severe occlusive retinal vasculitis with vascular occlusion and retinal ischemia. Prognosis is often poor.

22. What is interferon retinopathy?

Interferon-associated retinopathy causes microvascular and ischemic changes to the retina. Ischemic retinopathy includes cotton-wool spots, retinal hemorrhages, cystoid macular edema, vascular occlusions, epiretinal membrane development, and optic disc edema. The mechanism may include immune complex deposition in the retinal vasculature and activated complement C5a followed by leukocyte infiltration and vascular closure, although the mechanism is still unclear. Fluorescein angiography demonstrates poorly perfused areas of retina. Changes typically appear a few weeks after taking the medication and can resolve upon cessation. Patients with underlying microvascular changes, such as diabetes and hypertension, are at higher risk for interferon retinopathy.

23. What is tacrolimus-associated retinopathy?

Tacrolimus is an effective immunosuppressive agent that inhibits cytokine synthesis and blocks T-cell development. Bilateral optic neuropathy and ischemic maculopathy were reported in patients after the use of tacrolimus. Rarely, tacrolimus toxicity may manifest as cotton-wool spots and superficial hemorrhages (Fig. 40.5). A direct neurotoxic effect on the RPE, cones, or rods has been hypothesized. The presentation is a gradual onset of bilateral blurred vision associated with nonspecific findings on OCT and fluorescein angiography but with a central scotoma on 10-2 threshold visual-field testing. Multifocal ERG has demonstrated foveal suppression in both eyes.

24. What effects may iron overload have on the retina?

A retained intraocular iron foreign body may lead to darkening of the iris, orange deposits in the anterior subcapsular region of the lens, anterior and posterior vitritis, pigmentary retinopathy, and progressive loss of visual field. The intraocular foreign body should be removed as soon as possible.

25. What drugs can cause retinal thromboembolic events?

Oral contraceptives have been associated with central, branch, and cilioretinal artery occlusions and central retinal vein occlusion. Considerable controversy surrounds the role of oral contraceptives in causing these events, but stopping the oral contraceptive seems advisable. Talc retinal emboli are discussed in questions 17 and 18. Periorbital steroid injection with inadvertent arterial penetration may result in extensive embolization of the retinal circulation.

26. What chelating agents may cause maculopathy?

The chelating agents deferoxamine and deferasirox are used routinely for iron overload, particularly in thalassemia major. Deferoxamine is a siderophore that has been commercially available for over 30 years and may cause blurred vision, nyctalopia, and ring scotoma. The fundus may show bilateral widespread retinal pigment derangement. Deferasirox is a highly protein-bound synthetic chelator that became available in 2005. Preclinical and clinical trials of deferasirox reported that it is well tolerated and does not cause toxic retinopathy, although one possible deferasirox-related retinopathy has been reported.

27. What is poppers maculopathy?

Poppers are a recreational inhaled substance of abuse belonging to the alkyl nitrite family of compounds. In the United Kingdom, the most commonly used compound is isopropyl nitrite, which can be purchased legally, but is illegal to sell for human consumption. These compounds are often inhaled to produce temporary euphoria. The exact mechanism of central photoreceptor damage is unknown. The patient presents with the symptoms of a central scotoma and distortion of central vision. Clinical signs range from a normal foveal appearance to yellow, dome-shaped lesions at the fovea. Disruption or loss of the presumed ellipsoid layer on SD-OCT is the characteristic feature (Fig. 40.6). Findings often resolve upon cessation of poppers use.

28. Which cancer therapy drugs can cause toxic retinopathies?

The retina is among the most metabolically active tissues in the body, making it vulnerable to unwanted side effects of chemotherapeutic agents.

The most common retinal side effect of chemotherapeutic drugs is caused by MEK inhibitors. These are agents that inhibit the MEK enzyme. The most common retinal side effect noted from MEK inhibitors is subfoveal serous detachments (Fig. 40.7) of bilateral multifocal serous retinal detachments. Onset occurs within days to weeks or initiation of therapy, and cessation of medication often leads to complete resolution. Visual symptoms are typically minimal.

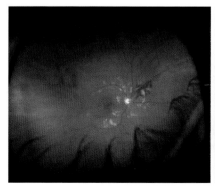
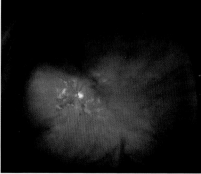

Fig. 40.5 Tacrolimus-associated retinopathy.

Biologic agents, small-molecule inhibitors, and chemotherapies can all cause toxic retinopathies. Clinical findings noted with monoclonal antibodies include choroidal neovascularization (ipilimumab) and macular edema, hemorrhages, and hard exudates (trastuzumab). Chemotherapies such as cisplatin may cause retinal/macular pigment changes or, rarely, retinal ischemia, neovascularization, intraretinal hemorrhages, and exudates. Retinoid acid derivatives such as isotretinoin may cause nyctalopia. Several agents also cause uveitis, including checkpoint inhibitors and BRAF inhibitors.

29. **What is pentosan polysulfate maculopathy?**
Pentosan polysulfate is a medication used for the treatment of interstitial cystitis that has recently been reported to cause a bilateral pigmentary maculopathy. Toxicity is reported after chronic use of the drug for over 15 years. Risk of toxicity increases in patients exposed to greater than 1500 g of cumulative use. Common symptoms include decreased visual acuity, metamorphosia, and scotomas. Imaging test reveals retinal pigment atrophy with outer retinal thinning, with classic speckled hyperautofluorescence on fundus autofluorescence (Fig. 40.8). Cessation of the medication is imperative but may not resolve visual issues.

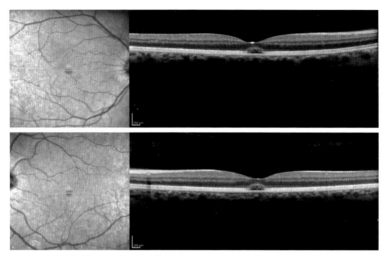

Fig. 40.6 Spectral-domain optical coherence tomography of poppers maculopathy.

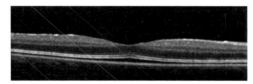

Fig. 40.7 Spectral-domain optical coherence tomography of MEK-inhibitor-associated serous retinal detachment.

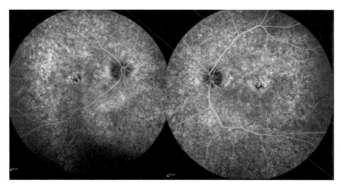

Fig. 40.8 Fundus autofluorescence of pentosan polysulfate maculopathy.

BIBLIOGRAPHY

Campochiaro PA, Lim JI: Aminoglycoside toxicity in the treatment of endophthalmitis. The Aminoglycoside Toxicity Study G, Arch Ophthalmol 112:48–53, 1994.

Dalvin LA, Shields CL, Orloff M, Sato T, Shields JA: Checkpoint inhibitor immune therapy: systemic indications and ophthalmic side effects, Retina 8(6):1063–1078, 2018.

Davies AJ, Kelly SP, Naylor SG, et al.: Adverse ophthalmic reactions in poppers users: case series of 'poppers maculopathy', Eye (Lond) 26(11):1479–1486, 2012.

Francis JH, Habib LA, Abramson DH, et al.: Clinical and morphologic characteristics of MEK inhibitor–associated retinopathy: differences from central serous chorioretinopathy, *Ophthalmology* 124(12):1788–1798, 2017.

Gass JDM: Toxic diseases affecting the pigment epithelium and retina. In Gass JDM, editor: Stereoscopic atlas of macular diseases, ed 4, St. Louis, 1997, Mosby, pp 775–808.

Gruener AM, Jeffriers MA, El Housseini Z, Whitefield L: Poppers maculopathy, Lancet 384(9954):1606, 2014.

Haimovici R, D'Amico DJ, Gragoudas ES, Sokol S, Deferoxamine Retinopathy Study Group: The expanded clinical spectrum of deferoxamine retinopathy, Ophthalmology 109:164–171, 2002.

Hanif AM, Armenti ST, Taylor SC, et al.: Phenotypic spectrum of pentosan polysulfate sodium-associated maculopathy: a multicenter study, JAMA Ophthalmol 137(11):1275–1282, 2019.

Kim HA, Lee S, Eah KS, Yoon YH: Prevalence and risk factors of tamoxifen retinopathy, Ophthalmology 127(4):555–557, 2019.

Laties A, Zrenner E: Viagra (sildenafil citrate) and ophthalmology, Prog Retin Eye Res 21:485–506, 2002.

Liu CY, Francis JH, Brodie SE, et al.: Retinal toxicities of cancer therapy drugs: biologics: small molecule inhibitors, and chemotherapies, Retina 34(7):1261–1280, 2014.

Marmor MF, Kellner U, Lai TYY, Melles RB, Mieler WF, for the American Academy of Ophthalmology: Recommendations on screening for chloroquine and hydroxychloroquine retinopathy, Ophthalmology 123:1386–1394, 2016.

Roy M, Roy A, Williams J, et al.: Reduced blue cone electroretinogram in cocaine-withdrawn patients, Arch Gen Psych 54:153–156, 1997.

Swartz M: Other diseases: drug toxicity, metabolic and nutritional conditions. In Ryan SJ, editor: Retina, ed 2, St. Louis, 1994, Mosby.

Urey JC: Some ocular manifestations of systemic drug abuse, J Am Optom Assoc 62:834–842, 1991.

van der Torren K, Graniewski-Wijnands HS, Polak BC: Visual field and electrophysiological abnormalities due to vigabatrin, Doc Ophthalmol 104:181–188, 2002.

Walia HS, Yan J. Reversible retinopathy associated with oral deferasirox therapy, BMJ Case Rep 2013:pii: bcr2013009205, 2013.

Wang D, Au A, Gunnemann F, et al.: Pentosan-associated maculopathy: prevalence, screening guidelines, and spectrum of findings based on prospective multimodal analysis, Can J Ophthalmol 55(2):116–125, 2020.

Weiner A, Sandberg MA, Gaudio AR, et al.: Hydroxychloroquine retinopathy, Am J Ophthalmol 112:528–534, 1991.

Witkin AJ, Shah AR, Engstrom RE, et al.: Postoperative hemorrhagic occlusive retinal vasculitis: expanding the clinical spectrum and possible associate with vancomycin, Ophthalmology 122(7):1438–1451, 2013.

CHAPTER 41

COATS' DISEASE

James Vander and William S. Tasman

1. What is Coats' disease?

   Exudation, retinal telangiectasia, and retinal aneurysms are hallmarks of the disorder. The British ophthalmologist George Coats first described this condition in 1908. It comes on painlessly and may be slow and insidious in its development. In many instances, Coats' disease is not discovered until the patient is beyond childhood.

2. List the clinical characteristics of Coats' disease.
   - It is a lifetime disease.
   - It occurs 80% to 90% of the time in young boys.
   - It is usually unilateral.
   - It is not familial.
   - Characteristic retinal vascular lesions are telangiectatic-like "light bulb" aneurysms that are associated with capillary dropout in the fundus periphery (Fig. 41.1B and D).
   - Intraretinal and subretinal exudation, a prominent feature, has a predilection to accumulate in the macular area (Fig. 41.1A and C); the exudate contains cholesterol crystals.
   - Coats' disease may lead to exudative retinal detachment, cataract, neovascular glaucoma, and phthisis bulbi.

3. What percentage of patients are girls?

   Between 8% and 10% of patients are girls.

4. What is the most common age at which Coats' disease becomes apparent?

   Coats' disease usually becomes apparent between 8 and 10 years of age. However, it can present in infancy and later in life. It is often much more severe when noted in infancy.

5. What percentage of cases are unilateral versus bilateral?

   Approximately 80% to 90% of the cases are unilateral. When bilateral cases do develop, there is usually asymmetry, with one eye being much more involved than the other.

6. Are the retinal vascular changes easy to detect?

   If the patient is cooperative, it is not hard to diagnose the peripheral retinal vascular changes. However, examination under general anesthesia may be necessary in younger patients.

7. How does this condition differ from Leber's miliary aneurysms?

   In 1912, Leber described retinal miliary aneurysms. He suggested that the conditions were one and the same as that reported by Coats, and that is the generally accepted thinking at the present time.

8. Do we know the etiology of Coats' disease?

   The precise etiology for Coats' disease has not been determined.

9. Are there any conditions with which Coats' disease can be confused?

   When there is exudation in the macula and peripheral telangiectasia, and no retinal detachment, Coats' disease can be diagnosed with confidence. There are a number of conditions to rule out, most notably retinoblastoma, the malignant intraocular tumor that occurs in infancy and childhood. It has been estimated that approximately 3.9% of eyes originally diagnosed as harboring retinoblastoma were subsequently discovered to have Coats' disease. See Table 41.1.

10. Can conditions other than retinoblastoma simulate Coats' disease?

    Angiomatosis retinae (von Hippel-Lindau syndrome), one of the phakomatoses, can cause exudation in the macula. This condition is inherited in an autosomal dominant fashion and has visceral and central nervous system hemangioblastomas as part of the syndrome. In addition, visceral cysts and tumors, including renal cell carcinoma, may occur. Early in its onset, the fundus picture is different from that of Coats' disease in that angiomatosis retinae demonstrates a dilated and tortuous afferent arteriole and an efferent draining venule that enters and leaves a reddish balloon-like mass, usually in the fundus periphery. If the capillary angioma is on the disc, it may be associated with macular exudation, making the differential diagnosis from Coats' disease more difficult. Other conditions to be considered in the diagnosis are familial exudative vitreoretinopathy (FEVR), persistent fetal vasculature (PVF), and retinopathy of prematurity (ROP). FEVR is a dominantly inherited condition that may have a Coats'-like response. PVF was previously known as persistent hyperplastic primary vitreous. It is usually unilateral and occurs in a microphthalmic eye. ROP may present with retinal detachment but usually occurs in patients with a history of significant prematurity.

11. Other than fluorescein angiography, what may be helpful in confirming the diagnosis?
    Ultrasonography and computed tomographic (CT) scans may help to differentiate between Coats' disease and retinoblastoma by detecting the presence or absence of subretinal calcifications. Calcification is found in retinoblastoma, but it is extremely rare in Coats' disease.

12. Can aspiration of subretinal exudates aid in diagnosis?
    The key diagnostic findings in the analysis of subretinal aspirates are the presence of cholesterol crystals and pigment-laden macrophages and the absence of tumor cells. This technique should be reserved for patients in whom retinoblastoma has been ruled out by all other noninvasive means, because tumor seeding may occur.

13. How is Coats' disease managed?
    If possible, it is desirable to treat the condition before exudate accumulates in the macular area. Treatment is directed at the peripheral vascular abnormalities. Photocoagulation can be used to eliminate these abnormal vessels. In patients with exudation under the peripheral vascular telangiectasia, cryotherapy may be preferable (Fig. 41.1D). Elimination of the defective vessels prevents further leakage and is followed by resorption of the exudate over ensuing months. Because patients have been found to have elevated levels of vascular endothelial growth factor (VEGF), bevacizumab, triamcinolone, and dexamethasone have been injected intravitreally. Most of

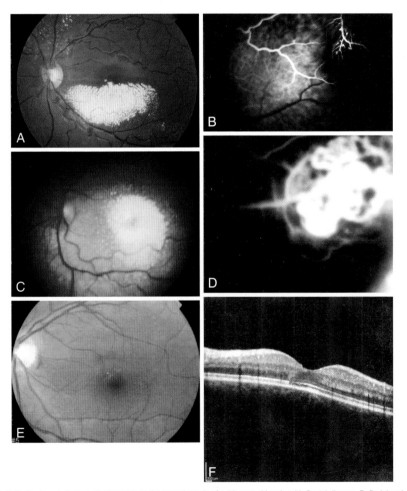

Fig. 41.1 A, Pretreatment photograph of exudate in the posterior pole of a 10-year-old male with Coats' disease. **B,** Peripheral vascular retinal changes of patient shown in A. **C,** Although Coats' disease predominantly affects males, females may also develop the disease, as seen in this 9-month-old girl. **D,** Peripheral retinal vascular changes are present in the temporal periphery of the patient shown in C. **E,** The 9-month-old baby girl is now 22 years of age and has not had a recurrence. **F,** After resorption of the exudate in the patient shown in E, the optical coherence tomography shows a normal macular contour, but there is irregularity of the ellipsoid layer and best corrected vision is only 20/200 despite patching in childhood.

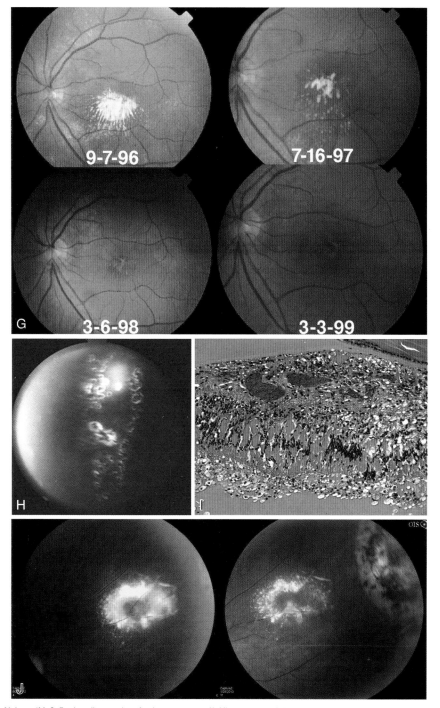

Fig. 41.1, cont'd G, Exudate disappearing after laser treatment. **H,** Microaneurysmal changes in a patient with Coats' disease. **I,** Histopathologic section of the retina in a patient with Coats' disease with bullous retinal detachment almost touching the posterior lens capsule secondary. Aneurysmal changes can be seen in the nerve fiber layer. **J,** Recurrent Coats in a 26-year-old male diagnosed at 5 years of age. Exudate is beginning to diminish 3 months after retreatment.

Continued

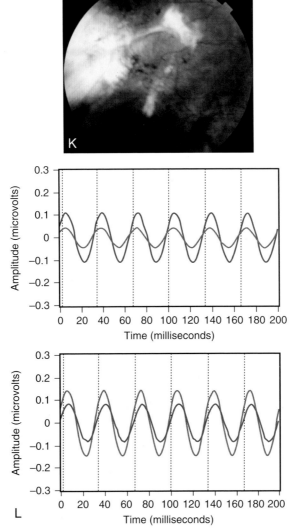

Fig. 41.1, cont'd K, 27-year-old male with retinitis pigmentosa and Coats' disease. **L,** The patient in J has reduced and delayed hertz (Hz) cone electroretinogram both eyes compatible with retinitis pigmentosa. (**I,** Courtesy Dr. Ralph Eagle.)

the time, these drugs are used as adjuvants to laser or cryotherapy. However, dramatic improvement has occasionally been reported when bevacizumab has been used as the primary mode of therapy. With the use of steroids, cataract has to be considered as a potential complication.

14. How long does it take for the exudate to disappear?
   Resorption of the exudate may take up to a year or more before it is completely gone. Its disappearance becomes apparent in the first few months after treatment. Solid masses of exudate take on a more speckled appearance as the exudate goes away.

15. Is more than one treatment necessary?
   If more than two quadrants have retinal telangiectasia, two or three treatments may be required.

16. Once the abnormal vessels are gone, is the patient considered cured?
   Recurrence, which is usually heralded by the reappearance of exudate and is almost always associated with new vascular abnormalities, can occur even many years later. It is recommended that patients be scheduled for follow-up appointments at 6- to 12-month intervals throughout their lifetime. See Table 41.2.

Table 41.1 Differential Diagnosis of Coats' Disease

1. Retinoblastoma
2. Familial exudative vitreoretinopathy
3. Von Hippel-Lindau disease
4. Retinopathy of prematurity
5. Persistent fetal vasculature

Table 41.2 Recurrence of Coats' Disease

Number of patients: 13
- Males: 11 (85%)
- Females: 2 (15%)

Average follow-up: 12.4 years
- Range: 4 to 58 years

Average number of recurrences: 3.3
Oldest patient at time of recurrence: 58 years

17. **Can this condition be managed once the retina has detached?**
    Vitreoretinal surgery may, in some cases, help to reattach the retina. At the time of surgery, it is necessary to treat the abnormal vessels by laser photocoagulation or cryotherapy. The vision in these eyes, however, is usually quite limited, and sometimes, despite reattachment of the retina, there is no light perception.

18. **If left untreated, what is the outcome?**
    Untreated Coats' disease does not invariably lead to intractable glaucoma. However, retinal detachment and neovascular glaucoma are the ultimate complications that may precede phthisis and loss of the globe.

19. **When should an eye with Coats' disease be enucleated?**
    When retinoblastoma cannot be ruled out or when neovascular glaucoma is present in blind, painful eyes, enucleation is the best option.

20. **Can Coats' disease occur with any other retinal conditions?**
    Coats' disease may occur in conjunction with retinitis pigmentosa. Retinal antigen autoimmune reactivity may play a role in specific types of retinitis pigmentosa. In addition, retinitis pigmentosa has been noted to be associated with muscular dystrophy, and the son of a mother with retinal telangiectasis had Norrie disease.

KEY POINTS OF COATS' DISEASE

1. Affected patients are predominantly male of ages 8 to 12, but it may present in infancy.
2. Exudate often accumulates in the macular area owing to abnormal peripheral telangiectatic and aneurysmal changes.
3. Retinoblastoma is important to rule out noninvasively with ultrasound and sometimes CT scan because of its malignant nature.
4. Primary treatment is usually laser or cryotherapy. Anti-VEGF treatment can be helpful.
5. It is a lifetime disease because multiple recurrences may occur in about one of three patients, 3 to 4 years or more after what appears to be successful resolution of the disease.

BIBLIOGRAPHY

Char DH: Coats' syndrome: long-term follow up, Br J Ophthalmol 84:37–39, 2000.
Coats G: Forms of retinal disease with massive exudation, R Lond Ophthalmol Hosp Rep 17:440–525, 1908.
Egerer I, Tasman W, Tomer TL: Coats disease, Arch Ophthalmol 92:109–112, 1974.
Fogle JA, Welch RB, Green WR: Retinitis pigmentosa and exudative vasculopathy, Arch Ophthalmol 96(4):696–702, 1978.
He YG, Wang H, Zhao B, Lee J, Bahl D, McCluskey J: Elevated vascular endothelial growth factor level in Coats' disease and possible therapeutic role of bevacizumab, Graefes Arch Clin Exp Ophthalmol 248(10):1519–1521, 2010). doi:10.1007/s00417-010-1366-1.
Haik BG, Saint Louis L, Smith ME, et al.: Computed tomography of the nonrhegmatogenous retinal detachment in the pediatric patient, Ophthalmology 92:1133–1142, 1985.
Howard GM, Ellsworth RM: Differential diagnosis of retinoblastoma: a statistical survey of 500 children: I. Relative frequency of the lesions which simulate retinoblastoma, Am J Ophthalmol 60:610–617, 1965.
Kodama A, Sugioka K, Kusaka S, Matsumoto C, Shimomura Y: Combined treatment for Coats' disease: retinal laser photocoagulation combined with intravitreal bevacizumab injection was effective in two cases, BMC Ophthalmol 14(1):36, 2014.
Leber T: Über eine durch Vorkommen multipler Miliaraneurysmen charakterisierte Form von Retinaldegeneration, Arch Ophthalmol 81:1–14, 1912.

Lin CJ, Hwang JF, Chen YT, Chen SN: The effect of intravitreal bevacizumab in the treatment of Coats' disease in children, Retina 30(4):617–622, 2010. doi:10.1097/IAE.0b013e3181c2e0b7.

Muftuoglu G, Gulkilik G: Pars plana vitrectomy in advanced Coats' disease, Case Rep Ophthalmol 2(1):15–22, 2011. doi:10.1159/000323616.

Saatci AO, Doruk HC, Yaman A: Intravitreal dexamethasone implant (Ozurdex) in Coats' disease, Case Rep Ophthalmol 4(3):122–128, 2013. doi:10.1159/000355363. eCollection 2013.

Shienbaum G, Tasman W: Coats disease a lifetime disease, J Retinal Vitreous Dis 26:422–424, 2006.

Shields JA, Shields CL, Honavar SG, Demirci H: Clinical variations and complications of Coats disease in 150 cases: the 2000 Sanford Gifford memorial lecture, Am J Ophthalmol 131:561–571, 2001.

Tarkkanen A, Laatikainen L. Coats disease: clinical, angiographic, histopathological findings and clinical management, Br J Ophthalmol 67:766–776, 1983.

Zheng XX, Jiang YR: The effect of intravitreal bevacizumab injection as the initial treatment for Coats' disease, Graefes Arch Clin Exp Ophthalmol 252(1):35–42, 2014. doi:10.1007/s00417-013-2409-1.

CHAPTER 42

FUNDUS TRAUMA

Jeffrey P. Blice

1. **What are the mechanisms of injury to the fundus in blunt trauma?**
   Blunt trauma to the sclera can produce a direct effect on the underlying choroid and retina. In addition, a concussive effect from force transmitted through the vitreous may be seen away from the initial point of impact. The sudden deformation of the globe may cause stretching of the retina and retinal pigment epithelium (RPE) and traction on the vitreous base. The shearing forces generated by this traction may tear the retina in the area of the vitreous base or result in avulsion of the vitreous base. Forces can be severe enough to avulse the optic nerve (Fig. 42.1).[1]

2. **What clinical entity is caused by the contrecoup mechanism?**
   Indirect damage from the concussive effect of an injury tends to occur at the interfaces of tissue with the greatest differences in density, most commonly, the lens–vitreous interface and the posterior vitreoretinal interface. The transmitted force may cause fragmentation of photoreceptor outer segments and damage to the receptor cell bodies. Clinically, these areas appear as opacified retina and are termed *commotio retinae*. Although the retinal whitening is only temporary, resolving over 3 to 4 weeks, permanent damage may occur. Loss of vision depends on the amount and location of early photoreceptor loss. The RPE underlying an area of commotio may develop a granular hyperpigmentation or atrophic appearance and lead to decreased vision. The eponym associated with this entity is Berlin's edema; however, there is no true intracellular or extracellular edema, and no fluorescein leakage is seen.

3. **Name the five types of retinal breaks seen in fundus trauma.**
   - Retinal dialyses
   - Horseshoe tears
   - Operculated holes
   - Macular holes
   - Retinal dissolution (necrosis)[2]

4. **Where are retinal dialyses most commonly seen?**
   Retinal dialyses are usually located in the superonasal or inferotemporal quadrants (Figs. 42.2 and 42.3). Trauma is more clearly related to superonasal than to inferotemporal dialyses. Dialyses may be associated with avulsion of the vitreous base. Because they can lead to retinal detachment, a careful depressed exam of all patients with a history of blunt trauma is essential. Prophylactic treatment of all dialyses with cryopexy or laser photocoagulation is recommended in the hope of decreasing the likelihood of future retinal detachments.[3]

5. **When do retinal detachments occur with dialyses?**
   Retinal detachments present at variable intervals after injury; however, the dialysis is usually detectable early or immediately at the time of injury. Approximately 10% of dialysis-related detachments present immediately; 30%, within 1 month; 50%, within 8 months; and 80%, within 2 years. Most trauma victims are young, with a formed vitreous that tamponades a break or dialysis, but as the vitreous eventually liquefies, fluid passes through retinal breaks causing detachments. The nature of the vitreous in such cases may explain the delay in presentation of the detachments.[4]

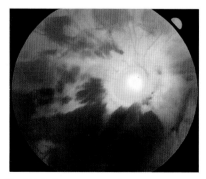

Fig. 42.1 Optic nerve avulsion after severe blunt trauma.

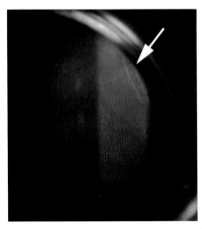

Fig. 42.2 Retinal dialysis *(arrow)* with associated chronic retinal detachment through contact lens.

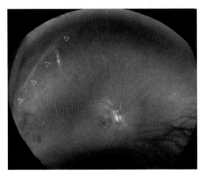

Fig. 42.3 Wide-angle photograph of a retinal dialysis *(arrows)* from bungee cord injury in a 15-year-old.

6. In addition to retinal dialyses, do other trauma-related breaks need to be treated prophylactically?
   Horseshoe tears and operculated holes in the setting of acute trauma are usually treated by cryopexy or laser photocoagulation. Macular holes require pars plana vitrectomy with gas exchange if closure of the hole is attempted; however, macular holes usually do not progress to retinal detachments. Surgery is not performed for the purposes of prophylactic closure. Direct injury with necrosis of the retina is usually associated with underlying choroidal injury so that a chorioretinal adhesion may be formed spontaneously. However, any accumulation of subretinal fluid or persistent traction on damaged retina makes prophylactic treatment reasonable.

7. What is the prognosis for repair of a retinal detachment associated with a dialysis?
   Dialysis-related detachments are usually smooth, thin, and transparent. Intraretinal cysts are common, and half have demarcation lines. In addition, proliferative vitreoretinopathy is rare. The characteristics of the detachment are suggestive of its chronic nature and insidious onset; however, the prognosis for repair with conventional scleral buckling techniques is good. A more acute presentation will resemble an acute rhegmatogenous detachment (Fig. 42.4).

8. Are traumatic macular holes the same as typical macular holes?
   Traumatic macular holes often behave differently compared to a typical macular hole formed as a result of vitreoretinal interface disease. Traumatic macular holes that form immediately at the time of initial injury may close spontaneously. Those that fail to close after a few months of observation can be anatomically improved by surgical intervention. However, the improvement in vision may be disappointing. Developing techniques using an inverted internal limiting membrane flap is promising. However, the initial trauma can result in retinal damage that is incompatible with good vision. Careful consideration by the surgeon in discussions with the patient is required before considering surgical intervention[5,6] (Figs. 42.5 and 42.6).

9. Describe the clinical features of a choroidal rupture.
   The retina is relatively elastic, and the sclera is mechanically strong. The Bruch's membrane, the structure between the RPE and the choriocapillaris, is neither elastic nor strong. Consequently, it is susceptible to the stretching forces

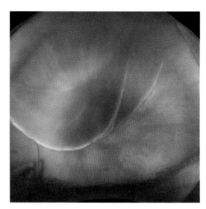

Fig. 42.4 Wide-angle photograph of a retinal detachment from a traumatic retinal dialysis in a 50-year-old assault victim.

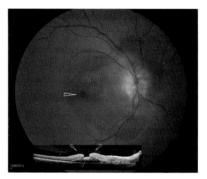

Fig. 42.5 Fundus photograph of a traumatic macular hole *(arrow)* with peripapillary subretinal hemorrhage. Corresponding optical coherence tomography with subfoveal hemorrhage and edges of macular hole *(arrows)*.

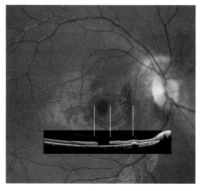

Fig. 42.6 Fundus photograph 12 months later of same patient in Fig. 42.5. Resolution of hemorrhage and traumatic macular hole. Corresponding optical coherence tomography with edges of macular hole noted with two *white lines* on the left. The *white line* on the right notes disruption of outer retina peripapillary fibrosis at rupture of choroid.

exerted on the globe in blunt trauma. The Bruch's membrane usually tears along with the choriocapillaris and RPE. Choroidal ruptures may be found at the point of contact with the globe or in the posterior pole as a result of indirect forces. Clinically, choroidal rupture appears as a single area or multiple areas of subretinal hemorrhage, usually concentric and temporal to the optic nerve (Fig. 42.7). The hemorrhage may dissect into the vitreous. As the blood resolves, a crescent-shaped or linear white area is seen where the rupture occurred. With time, surrounding RPE hyperplasia or atrophy may be seen. Linear white areas are most consistent with a fibrotic response following the resolution of the hemorrhage. This can be seen on optical coherence tomography (OCT) (Figs. 42.8 and 42.9).[7]

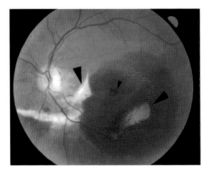

Fig. 42.7 Choroidal ruptures *(large arrowheads)* located concentric to the optic nerve. The *small arrowhead* indicates the center of the associated subretinal hemorrhage.

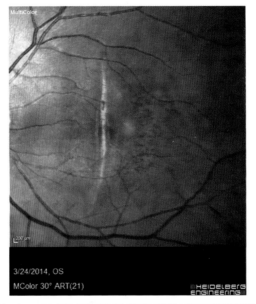

Fig. 42.8 Choroidal rupture color photograph corresponding to optical coherence tomography scan in Fig. 42.9.

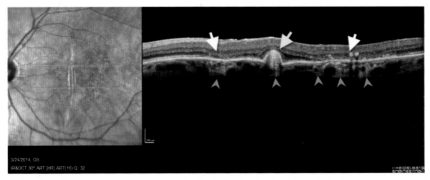

Fig. 42.9 An optical coherence tomography scan through the choroidal rupture in color photograph Fig. 42.8. There is an elevated mound of fibrosis visible at the level of the choroid *(yellow arrow)* with an absence of normal retinal architecture. Areas of disrupted outer retinal anatomy with absence of the ellipsoid line are shown by the *white arrows*. The *orange arrowheads* indicate increased transmission through the damaged retinal pigment epithelium.

10. **Are there any long-term complications of choroidal ruptures?**

The visual consequences of a choroidal rupture depend on its location with respect to the fovea. A patient with a choroidal rupture near the fovea may have good vision; however, the break in the Bruch's membrane predisposes him or her to the development of a choroidal neovascular membrane, which may threaten vision long after the initial injury (Figs. 42.10 and 42.11). Therefore, patients at risk should be followed regularly and advised of the potential complication. Anti-VEGF treatment seems to be an effective treatment to control subretinal fluid (Figs. 42.12 and 42.13), although high-quality large studies are not available.[8]

11. **Can orbital adnexal trauma result in fundus abnormalities?**

High-velocity missile injuries may cause an indirect concussive injury to the globe, resulting in retinal breaks and ruptures in the Bruch's membrane that resemble a claw. A fibroglial scar with pigment proliferation forms, but retinal detachment is rare, possibly because a firm adhesion develops, acting as a retinopexy. Chorioretinitis sclopetaria is the name given to this clinical entity.

KEY POINTS: RETINAL BREAKS IN BLUNT TRAUMA

1. The five types of breaks are horseshoe tears, operculated tears, dialyses, retinal dissolution, and macular holes.
2. Retinal dialyses usually occur superonasally in trauma.
3. A total of 50% of dialysis-related detachments present within 8 months.
4. A dialysis-related detachment has a very high success rate with treatment by scleral buckling.

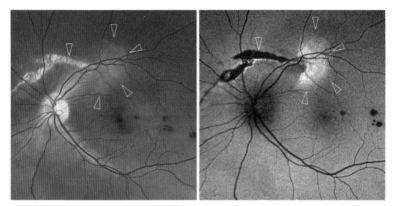

Fig. 42.10 Fundus photograph and corresponding autofluoresence demonstrating choroidal rupture *(white arrow)* and neovascular membrane at tip of rupture near fovea *(yellow arrows).*

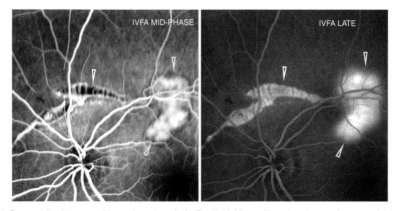

Fig. 42.11 Corresponding intravenous fluorescein angiography for Fig. 42.10. Mid- and late-phase images of rupture *(white arrows)* showing initial hypofluorescence except for remaining large choroidal vessels and late staining. *Yellow arrows* demonstrate marked hyperfluoresence in mid-phase with late leakage.

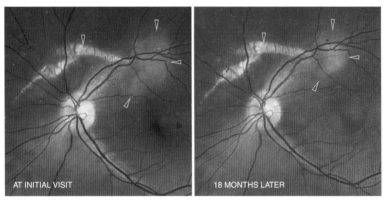

Fig. 42.12 Comparison fundus photos of patient in Fig. 42.10 at initial visit and 18 months following one bevacizumab injection. *White arrows* demonstrate regression of the neovascular membrane.

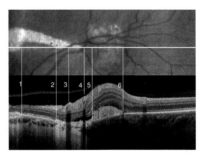

Fig. 42.13 Corresponding optical coherence tomography to the 18-month follow-up image of Fig. 42.12. Lines 1 and 2 demonstrate edges of preserved retina bordering choroidal rupture. Lines 3 and 4 are superficial retinal vessels. Lines 5 and 6 border the regressed neovascular complex *(red arrow)*. A trace amount of subretinal fluid is visible at the *blue arrow*.

12. What are the signs of a scleral rupture?

When a laceration or obvious deformation of the globe is not visible, other findings raise the index of suspicion that an injury may be more serious than initially thought. The presence of an afferent pupillary defect (APD), poor motility, marked chemosis, and vitreous hemorrhage raise the suspicion of an open globe. Other findings that may be helpful include a deeper than normal anterior chamber and a low intraocular pressure; however, in an eye with a posterior rupture and incarcerated uvea, the intraocular pressure may be normal.

13. Why is the initial exam of a severely traumatized eye important?

A poor outcome is associated with initially poor visual acuity, presence of an APD, large wounds (>10 mm) or wounds extending posteriorly to the rectus muscles, and vitreous hemorrhage. The first person to evaluate the traumatized eye may have the only opportunity to assess the best visual acuity. The delay often associated with referral to other institutions or dealing with life-threatening complications may result in diffusion of vitreous hemorrhage and corneal or other anterior segment abnormalities that preclude an adequate view of the posterior segment. The first look may be the best look at a traumatized eye.[9]

14. Where is the most likely place for a globe to rupture?

The globe may rupture anywhere, depending on the nature of the injury. However, the globe most often ruptures at the limbus, beneath the rectus muscles, or at a surgical scar. The sclera is thinnest and therefore weakest behind the insertions of the rectus muscles. The site of a previous cataract extraction or glaucoma procedure is weaker than normal sclera.

15. Outline the goals of managing a ruptured globe.

1. Identify the extent of the injury. Perform a 360-degree peritomy, inspecting all quadrants. If necessary, disinsert a muscle to determine the extent of a laceration.
2. Rule out a retained foreign body. In any case of projectile injury, sharp lacerations, uncertain history, or questionable mechanism of injury, consider a computed tomography (CT) scan to detect a foreign body.

3. Close the wound, and limit reconstruction as much as possible. Close the sclera with a relatively large suture (e.g., 8-0 or 9-0 nylon), and reposit any protruding uvea. If vitreous is protruding, cut it flush with the choroidal tissues, using fine scissors and a cellulose sponge or automated vitreous cutter.
4. Guard against infection. Start prophylactic systemic antibiotic treatment. An intravenous (IV) aminoglycoside or third-generation cephalosporin in combination with vancomycin (e.g., ceftriaxone, 1–2 mg every 12 hours, and vancomycin, 1 mg every 12 hours) is acceptable. Alternatively, a systemic fluoroquinolone may be used initially IV with an oral regimen at discharge for outpatient care (e.g., levofloxacin 500 or 750 mg daily). Clindamycin can be added if coverage for *Bacillus* spp. is desired.
5. Protect the remaining eye. Place a shield over the fellow eye during the repair procedure to prevent accidental injury. Counsel the patient at the earliest opportunity about the need for protective eyewear to prevent future injury to the "good" eye.

KEY POINTS: GLOBE RUPTURES

1. Vitreous hemorrhage, poor vision, APD, and massive chemosis/subconjunctival hemorrhage are the hallmarks of a ruptured globe.
2. The globe is most likely to rupture at the limbus, underneath a rectus muscle, or at a previous surgical site.
3. Large ruptures (>10 mm) are associated with a poor prognosis.
4. Sympathetic ophthalmia is an exceedingly rare complication.
5. Remember to protect the remaining eye during repair and afterward.

16. Discuss the role of computed tomography and magnetic resonance imaging in the detection of intraocular foreign bodies.
    The best method of detecting intraocular foreign bodies is indirect ophthalmoscopy (Fig. 42.14). Patients with delayed presentation may have pigment reaction at the site of impact (Fig. 42.15). If a view of the posterior

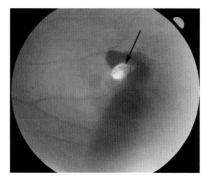

Fig. 42.14 Fundus photograph of intraocular foreign body *(arrow)* resting on the surface of the retina.

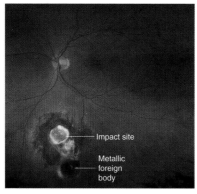

Fig. 42.15 Wide-angle fundus photograph of intraocular foreign body embedded in the retina with impact point and surrounding pigment changes.

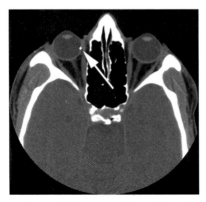

Fig. 42.16 Computed tomography scan demonstrating the presence of a small intraocular foreign body *(arrow)* located nasally.

segment is impossible, CT is the next best alternative. A CT scan is excellent for the detection of metallic foreign bodies but also detects glass or even plastic foreign bodies in some instances (Fig. 42.16). When an organic foreign body is suspected, magnetic resonance imaging (MRI) offers the advantage of better soft-tissue discrimination and is an excellent supplement to CT. However, any suspicion of a metallic foreign body prevents the use of MRI. Ultrasonography also supplements the information provided by a CT, possibly detecting a radiolucent foreign body as well as providing information about the status of the retina and vitreous. Plain films of the orbit are still useful for the detection of a foreign body if a CT scanner is not available; however, the ability to localize and detect nonmetallic foreign bodies is more limited.

17. **What ultrasound artifacts are important to recognize in the evaluation of a traumatized globe?**
    The appearances of intraocular foreign bodies on ultrasonography are related to the nature, shape, and size of the foreign body, in addition to the angle of incidence of the sound waves. Reverberations and shadowing are characteristic ultrasound artifacts seen with intraocular foreign bodies. Reverberations are the multiple echoes that appear behind the initial reflection from a foreign body. Shadowing is the absence of echoes seen behind the initial reflection from a foreign body. Both of these artifacts may be demonstrable on the same patient by altering the angle of incidence of the ultrasound.

18. **Do all intraocular foreign bodies need to be removed immediately? Which ones require early vitrectomy for removal?**
    Not all foreign bodies require immediate removal. The decision to remove a foreign body at the time of initial repair is complex and depends somewhat on the preferences of the surgeon and the specific situation. However, in a patient with acute traumatic endophthalmitis or a known toxic or reactive foreign body, vitrectomy with removal of any intraocular foreign bodies at the time of initial repair, or soon after, is a reasonable option.[10]

19. **Which metals are toxic to the eye?**
    The toxicity of a metal is related to the reduction–oxidation potential (redox potential). Metals such as copper and iron have a low redox potential and tend to dissociate into their respective ionic forms, which makes them more toxic. Pure forms are more reactive than alloys. The ocular toxicity from an iron foreign body is called *siderosis*. When copper is the offending agent, the condition is *chalcosis*. Other metals such as gold, platinum, silver, and aluminum are relatively inert. Nonmetallic substances such as glass, plastic, porcelain, and rubber are also relatively inert and pose no threat of toxicity on the basis of their chemical composition.

20. **List the clinical findings in siderosis bulbi.**
    Iron tends to be deposited in epithelial tissues. An affected eye has hyperchromic heterochromia of the iris and a mid-dilated, minimally reactive pupil. Brownish dots are visible in the lens from iron deposition in the lens epithelium, along with generalized yellowing of the lens from involvement of the cortex. The retinal effects of iron toxicity can be detected and followed by electroretinography (ERG). Pure iron particles may cause a flat ERG in 100 days. Clinically, a pigmentary degeneration with sclerosis of vessels, retinal thinning, and, later, atrophy develops in the periphery and progresses posteriorly. If not removed initially, the potential toxic effects of a foreign body can be monitored by clinical exam and serial ERG. However, siderosis generally causes progressive gradual permanent visual loss unless the foreign body is removed.

21. **Do all copper foreign bodies cause chalcosis?**
    Foreign bodies composed of less than 85% pure copper cause chalcosis; greater than 85% pure copper foreign bodies cause sterile endophthalmitis. Copper ions are deposited in basement membranes. In the peripheral cornea, a Kaiser Fleischer ring is a brownish discoloration of the Descemet's membrane. The iris may be

sluggishly reactive to light and have a greenish color. Deposition of copper in the anterior capsule results in a "sunflower" cataract, and the vitreous may become opacified. ERG findings are similar to those found in siderosis but may improve if the foreign body is removed.

KEY POINTS: INTRAOCULAR FOREIGN BODIES

1. The best method of detection is indirect ophthalmoscopy whenever possible.
2. An intraocular foreign body does not usually require immediate removal.
3. Topical and systemic antibiotics are required as prophylaxis against endophthalmitis.
4. MRI is contraindicated in any patient with a suspected metallic intraocular foreign body.
5. Iron can cause siderosis and copper can cause chalcosis or sterile endophthalmitis.

22. **Which organisms most commonly cause posttraumatic endophthalmitis?**
    The most common organism associated with endophthalmitis in the setting of acute trauma is *Staphylococcus aureus*. Skin flora are the most likely source of contamination of a traumatic ocular wound. Infections caused by *Bacillus cereus*, although much less common (estimates range from 8% to 25%), are important because of the severity and damage caused by the infection. In any ocular injury contaminated by soil, the possibility of infection with *B. cereus* needs to be considered and the regimen of prophylactic antibiotics adjusted accordingly.

23. **Outline the role of prophylactic antibiotics.**
    Posttraumatic endophthalmitis is a relatively rare complication of penetrating ocular trauma, occurring in only 7% of cases; however, the potential for devastation to the eye warrants prophylactic treatment. In cases of obvious endophthalmitis, a grossly contaminated wound, or contaminated foreign body, initial intravitreal antibiotic injection may be considered. Although no definitive evidence exists for a clinical benefit, all ruptured or lacerated globes are usually treated with prophylactic topical and systemic antibiotics for 3 to 5 days postoperatively. Although the Endophthalmitis Vitrectomy Study showed no benefit to systemic antibiotic treatment in postoperative endophthalmitis, the issue of prophylaxis in trauma was not specifically addressed.
    Recent experiences of U.S. military physicians with severely injured and grossly contaminated ocular wounds have seen almost no endophthalmitis with timely antibiotics prophylaxis, usually with an oral fluoroquinolone.[11–13]

24. **What regimen of antibiotics is used to treat posttraumatic endophthalmitis?**
    The choice of intravitreal injections is directed at covering a broad spectrum of organisms. Although a number of combinations are possible, a regimen with coverage for typical pathogens is vancomycin, 1 mg/0.1 mL, in combination with amikacin, 0.2 to 0.4 mg/0.1 mL. Concerns for aminoglycoside toxicity often drive a choice to substitute ceftazadime 2.25 mg/0.1 mL for amikacin. Clindamycin, 1 mg/0.1 mL, is considered an additional agent for any suspicion of *Bacillus* species. Frequently applied topical treatment with a fluoroquinolone should be initiated postoperatively in addition to systemic antibiotics for 7 to 10 days.

25. **Does injury to one eye place the other eye at risk for visual loss?**
    Granulomatous inflammation may affect both the uninjured and the injured eye weeks to years after a penetrating injury. Sympathetic ophthalmia (SO) is a bilateral granulomatous uveitis manifested by anterior segment inflammation and multiple yellow-white lesions in the peripheral fundus. Complications include cataract, glaucoma, optic atrophy, exudative retinal detachments, and subretinal fibrosis. Exposure of the immune system to a previously immunologically isolated antigen in the uvea probably triggers the response. Eighty percent of cases develop within 3 months of injury, and 90% develop within 1 year. Rare cases of SO have occurred after ocular surgery. Therapy is directed at immunosuppression with steroids, cyclosporine, and/or cytotoxic agents. Most patients retain 20/60 vision or better at 10-year follow-up, but complications limit vision in many patients.

26. **How can the uninjured eye be protected from the long-term sequelae of penetrating ocular injury?**
    The incidence of SO is extremely rare (<0.5% of penetrating trauma). The only known way to absolutely prevent the disease is enucleation of the injured eye 10 to 14 days after the injury. With modern repair techniques, the potential for vision in severely injured eyes has improved; therefore, enucleation as a prophylactic treatment for SO should be reserved only *for eyes confirmed to have no visual potential.* Removal of the inciting eye after inflammation has developed may improve the final acuity of the uninjured eye, but the inciting eye may eventually retain the best visual acuity. Enucleation as a treatment is reserved for inciting eyes with *no visual potential.*[14]

27. **Can trauma elsewhere in the body cause fundus abnormalities?**
    Cotton-wool spots, usually in the peripapillary distribution, retinal hemorrhages, and optic disc edema have been described after severe head injury or compressive chest trauma. Purtscher's retinopathy, the name given to this entity, is a result of microvascular occlusion presumed to be embolic in nature and related to complement activation; however, the true pathogenesis is unknown. A similar appearance in other conditions, such as acute pancreatitis, collagen vascular disease, renal dialysis, and eclampsia, suggests a systemic process with

secondary retinal capillary occlusion. The fundus manifestations in severe trauma may be related to the generally poor condition of patients who sustained such trauma rather than the trauma itself. Vitreous, preretinal, and retinal hemorrhages may be seen in birth trauma; however, if seen in the absence of such trauma or other causes (leukemia or bleeding diathesis), nonaccidental trauma should be suspected. Ocular manifestations are present in 40% of abused children, and the ophthalmologist is first to recognize the abuse in 6% of cases. Suspicious injuries need to be reported to protect children from further abuse.

REFERENCES

1. Delori F, Pomerantzeff O, Cox MS: Deformation of the globe under high-speed impact: its relation to contusion injuries, Invest Ophthalmol 8:290–301, 1969.
2. Cox MS, Schepens CL, Freeman HM: Retinal detachment due to ocular contusion, Arch Ophthalmol 76:678–685, 1966.
3. Hollander DA, Irvine AR, Poothullil AM, Bhisitkul RB: Distinguishing features of nontraumatic and traumatic retinal dialyses, Retina 24:669–675, 2004.
4. Tasman W: Peripheral retinal changes following blunt trauma, Trans Am Ophthalmol Soc 70:190–198, 1972.
5. Tang YF, Chang A, Campbell WG, et al.: Surgical management of traumatic macular hole: optical coherence tomography features and outcomes, Retina 40(2):290–298, 2020.
6. Miller JB, Yonekawa Y, Eliott D, et al.: Long-term follow-up and outcomes in traumatic macular holes, Am J Ophthalmol 160(6):1255–1258, 2015.
7. Kelley JS, Dhaliwal RS: Traumatic choroidopathies. In Ryan SJ, editor: Retina, vol. 2, St. Louis, 1994, Mosby, pp 1783–1796.
8. Barth T, Zeman F, Helbig H, Gamulescu MA: Intravitreal anti-VEGF treatment for choroidal neovascularization secondary to traumatic choroidal rupture, BMC Ophthalmol 19(1):239, 2019. doi:10.1186/s12886-019-1242-7.
9. Pieramici DJ, MacCumber MW, Humayun MU, et al.: Open-globe injury. Update on types of injuries and visual results, Ophthalmology 103:1798–1803, 1996.
10. Wani VB, Al-Ajmi M, Thalib L, et al.: Vitrectomy for posterior segment intraocular foreign bodies: visual results and prognostic factors, Retina 23:654–660, 2003.
11. Meredith TA: Posttraumatic endophthalmitis, Arch Ophthalmol 117:520–521, 1999.
12. Colyer MH, Weber ED, Weichel ED, et al.: Delayed intraocular foreign body removal without endophthalmitis during operations Iraqi Freedom and Enduring Freedom, Ophthalmology 114(8):1439–1447, 2007.
13. Colyer MH, Chun DW, Bower KS, Dick JS, Weichel ED: Perforating globe injuries during operation Iraqi Freedom, Ophthalmology 115(11):2087–2093, 2008.
14. Chu DS, Foster CS: Sympathetic ophthalmia, Int Ophthalmol Clin 42:179–185, 2002.

CHAPTER 43

AGE-RELATED MACULAR DEGENERATION

James F. Vander and Joseph I. Maguire II

1. **What is age-related macular degeneration?**
   Age-related macular degeneration (ARMD) is the leading cause of significant, irreversible central visual loss in the Western world. It is characterized by age-dependent alterations in the sensory retina, retinal pigment epithelium (RPE), and choriocapillaris complex in the central retina (macula). The macula is defined clinically by the area within the major temporal vascular arcades and provides the sharpest, most discriminating vision (Fig. 43.1). The incidence of this disease is age dependent, and prevalence steadily increases past age 55. A common international classification exists, but most clinicians still divide ARMD into exudative (wet) and nonexudative (dry) forms.

2. **Who develops age-related macular degeneration?**
   Macular degeneration development is a condition of aging. All long-term epidemiologic studies indicate an increasing prevalence of exudative and nonexudative macular changes, as well as visual loss, with increasing age. Most reports point to a greater incidence of disease in women over men. In addition, skin pigmentation plays an important role in exudative disease; Black Americans have a significantly lower incidence of choroidal neovascularization compared with White.[1]

3. **Why is age-related macular degeneration such an enormous challenge?**
   The number of Americans age 65 and over continues to increase. The visual morbidity and mortality associated with ARMD affects a large number of elderly Americans socially, emotionally, and economically. The loss of reading and driving vision, the increased need for social and familial support, the cost of treatment, and the resultant emotional consequences have a significant impact on increasingly limited resources.

4. **Describe the etiologic factors involved in the development of age-related macular degeneration.**
   The exact cause of ARMD is unknown, but multifactorial. In addition to increasing age, smoking is a consistent risk predictor. Individuals with a family history of ARMD have a fivefold increased risk of developing macular degeneration themselves. Genetic predisposition is an increasingly active area of research. The genetics of ARMD is complex, although one consistent factor seems to be a link to the complement factor H (*CFH*) gene. This supports theories that ARMD is an inflammatory disease.

   Female gender, white race, smoking, poor nutrition, scleral rigidity, photic exposure, previous cataract surgery, and hypertension have been implicated as well.[2–5]

5. **Name common visual symptoms in age-related macular degeneration patients.**
   - Visual blur
   - Central scotoma
   - Metamorphopsia

   Metamorphopsia is visual distortion. Images may appear smaller (micropsia) or larger (macropsia) than they really are. Patients frequently comment that straight lines appear curved. Special graphs, *Amsler grids*, test the central 20 degrees of vision and are effective home-testing devices for eyes at higher risk for development of exudative ARMD. Recent results from hyperacuity home monitoring devices have shown increased sensitivity in early exudative macular disease detection.[6] These are not widely used presently.

6. **What is dry or nonexudative age-related macular degeneration?**
   Nonexudative ARMD is characterized by drusen, pigmentary changes, and atrophy. Drusen are the most common and earliest dry ARMD changes (Fig. 43.2). Drusen represent metabolic byproducts of retinal pigment epithelial cell metabolism. They vary in shape, size, and color. Hard drusen are small, discrete, yellow-to-white nodules, whereas soft drusen tend to be larger and more amorphous. Soft drusen may coalesce with neighboring drusen and are frequently associated with overlying pigmentary changes either from photoreceptor dysfunction or from retinal pigment epithelial demise. Progressive retinal pigment epithelial disruption eventually causes loss of overlying sensory retina and underlying choriocapillaris. Such developments result in localized atrophic regions that extend and coalesce around the fovea, eventually involving the fovea itself.

7. **What is wet or exudative age-related macular degeneration?**
   Exudative ARMD is characterized by the development of neovascular changes and fluid in and under the sensory retina and RPE. Choroidal neovascular membranes progressing to end-stage disciform macular scarring are the

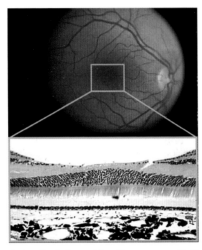

Fig. 43.1 The clinical macula describes that area of the retina encompassed by the temporal arcade vessels.

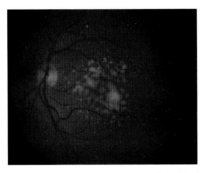

Fig. 43.2 Drusen are the by-product of retinal metabolism and manifest as focal yellow-white deposits deep to the retinal pigment epithelium. They serve as markers of nonexudative age-related macular degeneration.

typical outcome of untreated exudative ARMD. Variations in age-related neovascular disease include type 1 (occult), type 2 (classic), and type 3 (retinal angiomatous proliferation). All can be associated with pigment epithelial detachments. Clinically, choroidal neovascular membranes are slate green-hued subretinal lesions associated with hard exudates, hemorrhage, or fluid. These vessels commonly originate from the normal choriocapillaris and enter the subretinal space through defects in the Bruch's membrane, a collagenous layer separating the choroidal circulation from the retina (Fig. 43.3). Pigment epithelial detachments are dome-shaped clear, turbid, or blood-filled elevations of the RPE; they may or may not be associated with choroidal neovascular ingrowth.[7,8]

KEY POINTS: CLINICAL FINDINGS ASSOCIATED WITH ARMD

1. Nonexudative changes
   - Drusen
   - Pigmentary alterations
   - Atrophy: Incipient, geographic
2. Exudative changes
   - Hemorrhage
   - Hard exudate
   - Subretinal, sub-RPE, and intraretinal fluid

8. Name the three processes necessary for choroidal neovascular membrane development.
   - Increased vascular permeability
   - Extracellular matrix breakdown
   - Endothelial budding and vascular proliferation

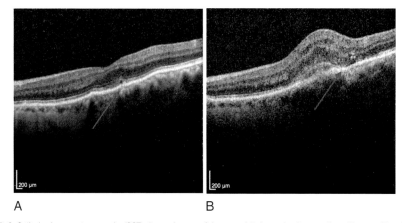

A   B

Fig. 43.3 A, Optical coherence tomography (OCT) shows changes of dry age-related macular degeneration with a possible subtle defect in Bruch's membrane *(arrow).* **B,** Follow-up OCT of the same eye 3 months later shows development of choroidal neovascularization (CNV) with overlying macular edema. The arrow points to the same defect in Bruch's membrane with adjacent thickening of the retinal pigment epithelium caused by the CNV.

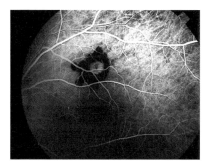

Fig. 43.4 Angiographically, classic neovascular membranes appear as focal hyperfluorescent lesions deep to the retina. This example shows a corona of hypofluorescence, which is associated with hemorrhage.

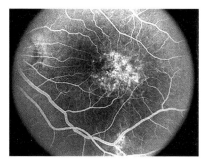

Fig. 43.5 The majority of choroidal neovascularization is nondiscrete or occult in character. This presentation is often not fully localized with fluorescein angiography. It has a punctate hyperfluorescent pattern with nondiscrete borders.

9. Describe the difference between occult and classic choroidal neovascularization.
   Classic choroidal neovascularization is clinically well defined. Fluorescein angiography demonstrates a discrete hyperfluorescent lesion with a cartwheel configuration that increases in intensity over the course of the study (Fig. 43.4). Occult neovascularization usually demonstrates a poorly defined, stippled, pigmented appearance with associated retinal thickening. It is not well localized with fluorescein angiography, exhibiting diffuse punctate hyperfluorescence (Fig. 43.5).

10. **How does age-related macular degeneration cause visual loss?**
    ARMD ultimately leads to visual loss via permanent alterations in the sensory retina, RPE, and choroid within the macula. These changes may arise from the development of disciform scarring secondary to choroidal neovascularization or atrophy in which areas of retina cease to exist.

11. **What is fluorescein angiography?**
    Fluorescein angiography is a photographic test used in the diagnosis and treatment management decisions of ARMD. Fluorescein dye is injected via an antecubital vein while simultaneous photographs of the macula are taken with a fundus camera. Fluorescein dye demonstrates fluorescence when stimulated with visible light in the blue frequency range. This property, along with anatomic constraints in the retinal and choroidal circulations, allows the identification and localization of abnormal vascular processes, such as choroidal neovascularization, that are found frequently in ARMD.

12. **What is indocyanine green video-angiography?**
    Indocyanine green (ICG) videoangiography is a photographic technique similar to fluorescein angiography. The major difference is the use of ICG dye, which has a peak absorption and emission in the infrared range, whereas the spectral qualities of fluorescein dye are in the visible range. ICG angiography's advantage is allowing visualization through pigment and thin blood, which facilitates viewing of the choroid.[9] ICG is an iodine-based dye and should not be used for patients allergic to iodine or shellfish.

13. **What is optical coherence tomography?**
    Optical coherence tomography (OCT) uses the property of optical coherence to give a cross-sectional representation of the macula. Its high resolution allows localization of choroidal neovascular processes and secondary effects such as retinal edema, sensory retinal detachment, and atrophy. Its articulation of retinal edema may make it an equal or even a superior diagnostic test in eliciting and following choroidal neovascular membrane activity.[10] It is noninvasive and does not require the injection of any dye.

14. **What is optical coherence tomography angiography?**
    The intravascular movement of red blood cells creates fluctuating signals that adjacent tissues do not demonstrate. Using the same imaging technology as OCT and taking advantage of this property, OCT angiography (OCT-A) allows for noncontrast imaging of retinal and choroidal vessels. Image acquisition is quick and the absence of intravenous contrast injection makes the test much easier and safer than fluorescein or ICG angiography. Choroidal neovascularization is generally easily recognized with OCT-A.

15. **Name proven therapies for exudative age-related macular degeneration.**
    Current proven therapies for ARMD involve thermal laser photocoagulation, photodynamic therapy (PDT), and intravitreal injection of vascular endothelial growth factor (VEGF) inhibitors. Intravitreal anti-VEGF injections are currently the preeminent treatment for exudative ARMD.[11]

16. **What is the role of pharmacologic management in age-related macular degeneration?**
    Currently, medical management involves the inhibition of angiogenic growth factors and associated modulators. Inhibition of VEGF has assumed primary importance. These agents can cause successful regression or inhibition of neovascular membranes in selected vascular neoplasms and animal models of neovascularization. Several vascular inhibitors and their delivery systems are available.
    Although Food and Drug Administration (FDA)–approved and off-label intravitreal anti-VEGF injections have assumed primary importance in the treatment of exudative ARMD, the aging of our population has increased the incidence of visual loss from nonexudative ARMD. Although AREDS2 vitamin supplements are the only available form of prophylaxis, multiple investigational protocols attacking other mechanisms of atrophic macular disease evolution are undergoing trials. These include complement inhibition, vitamin A analogs, interdiction of other inflammatory pathways, and addition of neurotrophic factors.[12,13] More recently, cellular replacement using a variety of stem cell strategies is being studied.

17. **Describe vascular endothelial growth factor and its role in ocular neovascularization.**
    VEGF is a homodimeric glycoprotein with multiple isomers, split products, and receptor sites. It is essential in the development and proper maintenance of normal vasculature. It is influenced by multiple growth factors, cofactors, and environmental influences such as ischemia. Loss of normal VEGF homeostasis can result in its upregulation with resultant neovascularization.[14]

18. **What are the advantages of current anti-vascular endothelial growth factor therapy in the treatment of exudative age-related macular degeneration compared to previous therapies such as thermal laser and photodynamic therapy?**
    Previous laser-based therapies created thermal or photodynamic tissue damage. This treatment for exudative ARMD lesions is based on either location or type. Although these treatments might slow the process, most patients progress to end-stage foveal involvement and visual decline is the rule. Anti-VEGF therapies have the advantage of being effective on nearly all subtypes of wet ARMD especially in subfoveal lesions. Their track record for visual stability and improvement is extremely good over time and their mechanism of effect is physiologic, not tissue destructive.

19. What are disadvantages of current anti–vascular endothelial growth factor therapy for exudative age-related macular degeneration?

Unfortunately, anti-VEGF agents must currently be delivered intravitreally via pars plana injection. They are effective for approximately 1 month after injection; thus, recurrence is noted in nearly all eyes over time. This necessitates the need for multiple visits both for active treatment and for surveillance. Patients are seen every 4 to 8 weeks. Intravitreal injections have secondary risks, including endophthalmitis, intraocular pressure elevation, and possible progression of atrophic macular disease.[15]

20. Describe the role of vitamins in the treatment and prophylaxis of age-related macular degeneration.

The Age-Related Eye Disease Study (AREDS) was sponsored jointly by the National Institutes of Health and the National Eye Institute and has proved the benefit of high-dose vitamins in the prophylaxis of ARMD. Individuals with intermediate or high risk of developing ARMD had a 25% reduction in developing visual loss from either exudative or nonexudative forms of ARMD. Theoretically, the intake of certain vitamins and trace elements acts directly or indirectly through association with certain enzymes in free radical scavenging, thereby modulating the aging process.

AREDS vitamins include high concentrations of vitamins C and E, lutein/zeoxanthine, zinc, and copper. Release of the AREDS2 study demonstrated no benefit from ω-3 fatty acids and potential increased risk of lung cancer in previous smokers taking β-carotene, prompting elimination of β-carotene from current AREDS2 formulations and replacement with lutein/zeoxanthine.[16]

AREDS summary: www.nei.nih.gov/amd/summary.asp.

21. What is polypoidal choroidal maculopathy?

This form of exudative maculopathy, which is sometimes confused with typical ARMD and generally develops in older individuals, occurs most often in patients of African and Asian descent. It presents with serosanguinous detachments in the macula. There is usually prominent hemorrhage often associated with exudate and fluid. RPE changes and fibrosis from prior episodes of bleeding are frequently present. Fluorescein angiography may show ill-defined leakage. ICG shows characteristic saccular enlargement of choroidal vessels with late leakage.

22. What is photodynamic therapy? How does it differ from laser photocoagulation?

PDT is an FDA-approved intervention for predominantly discrete subfoveal choroidal neovascular membranes secondary to ARMD. It involves the intravenous administration of a porphyrin-based medication that is absorbed by abnormal subretinal vessels. The drug is activated by wavelength-specific, low-energy, nonthermal infrared laser exposure. Activation of the photosensitizing compounds produces localized vascular damage via generation of free radicals. Because its action is local, the overlying sensory retina is spared while abnormal neovascularization is destroyed. The primary use of PDT in ARMD is either as monotherapy or in combination with anti-VEGF injections for the polypoidal variant of wet ARMD.[17]

23. What are low-vision aids?

Low-vision support involves the use of devices that maximize a visually deficient eye's visual function through magnification, lighting, and training. It allows patients to take advantage of near peripheral vision. Such aids take many forms, including special spectacles, magnifiers, closed-circuit television devices, digitally enhanced cameras, and overhead viewers. People often can read print and carry out important functions not possible without such support. In patients with untreatable bilateral visual loss, evaluation for low-vision support is critical.

REFERENCES

1. Leibowitz HM, Krueger DE, Maunder LR, The Framingham Eye Study monograph: An ophthalmological and epidemiological study of cataract, glaucoma, diabetic retinopathy, macular degeneration, and visual acuity in a general population of 2631 adults, 1973–1975, Surv Ophthalmol 24(Suppl):335–610, 1980.
2. Age-Related Eye Disease Study Research Group: Risk factors for the incidence of advanced age-related macular degeneration in the age-related eye disease study (AREDS). AREDS report no. 19, Ophthalmology 112:533–539, 2005.
3. Edwards AO, Ritter R, Abel KJ, et al.: Complement factor H polymorphism and age-related macular degeneration, Science 308: 421–424, 2005.
4. Neale BM, Fagerness J, Reynolds R, et al.: Genome-wide association study of advanced age-related macular degeneration identifies a role of the hepatic lipase gene (LIPC), Proc Natl Acad Sci U S A 107(16):7395–7400, 2010.
5. Young R: Pathophysiology of age-related macular degeneration, Surv Ophthalmol 31:291–306, 1987.
6. AREDS2-HOME Study Research Group, Chew EY, Clemons TE, Bressler SB, et al.: Randomized trial of a home monitoring system for early detection of choroidal neovascularization home monitoring of the Eye (HOME) study, Ophthalmology 121(2): 535–544, 2014.
7. Gass JDM: Drusen and disciform macular detachment and degeneration, Arch Ophthalmol 90:206–217, 1973.
8. Querques G, Souied EH, Freund KB: Multimodal imaging of early stage 1 type 3 neovascularization with simultaneous eye-tracked spectral domain optical coherence tomography and high speed real-time angiography, Retina 33:1881–1887, 2013.
9. Yannuzzi LA, Slakter JS, Sorenson JA, et al.: Digital indocyanine green videoangiography and choroidal neovascularization, Retina 12:191–223, 1992.
10. Voo I, Mavrofrides EC, Puliafito CA: Clinical applications of optical coherence tomography for the diagnosis and management of macular disease, Ophthalmol Clin North Am 17:21–31, 2004.

11. Brown DM, Kaiser PK, Michels M, et al., ANCHOR Study Group: Ranibizumab versus verteporfin for neovascular age-related macular degeneration, N Engl J Med 355(14):1432–1444, 2006.
12. Ferris FL: A new treatment for ocular neovascularization, N Engl J Med 351:2863–2865, 2004.
13. Zarbin MA, Rosenfeld PJ: Pathway-based therapies for age-related macular degeneration: an integrated survey of emerging treatment alternatives, Retina 30:1350–1367, 2010.
14. D'Amato RJ, Adamis AP: Angiogenesis inhibition in age-related macular degeneration, Ophthalmology 102:1261–1262, 1995.
15. Fung AE, Rosenfeld PJ, Reichel E: The International Intravitreal Bevacizumab Safety Survey: using the internet to assess drug safety worldwide, Br J Ophthalmol 90(11):1344–1349, 2006.
16. AREDS2 Research Group: Lutein/zeaxanthin and omega-3 fatty acids for age-related macular degeneration. The Age-Related Eye Disease Study 2 (AREDS2) controlled randomized clinical trial, JAMA 309(19):2005–2015, 2013.
17. Yannuzzi LA, Sorenson J, Spaide RF, Lipson B: Idiopathic polypoidal choroidal vasculopathy (IPCV), Retina 10:1–8, 1990.

CHAPTER 44

RETINOPATHY OF PREMATURITY

James F. Vander

1. **What is retinopathy of prematurity?**
   Retinopathy of prematurity (ROP) is a vasoproliferative retinal disease that affects infants born prematurely. It has two phases. In the acute phase, normal vascular development goes awry with the development of abnormal vessels that proliferate, occasionally with associated fibrous proliferation. In the chronic or late proliferation phase, retinal detachment, macular ectopia, and severe visual loss may occur. More than 90% of cases of acute ROP go on to spontaneous regression.

2. **Who is at risk for retinopathy of prematurity?**
   Infants weighing less than 1500 g at birth and those born at a gestational age of 32 weeks or less are at risk for developing ROP. The disease is more likely to affect the smallest and most premature of infants. The incidence of acute ROP in infants weighing less than 1 kg at birth is three times greater than that of infants weighing between 1 and 1.5 kg. Infants born at 23 to 27 weeks of gestation have a particularly high chance of developing ROP.

3. **Who should be screened for retinopathy of prematurity?**
   Guidelines published by the American Academy of Pediatrics, Section on Ophthalmology; the American Association of Pediatric Ophthalmology and Strabismus; and the American Academy of Ophthalmology recommend that all infants weighing less than 1500 g at birth or those with a gestational age of 28 weeks or less should be examined. Selected infants with a birth weight between 1500 and 2000 g with an unstable clinical course should also be examined.

4. **Which infants are at highest risk for retinopathy of prematurity?**
   Infants at particularly high risk are those who weigh less than 1000 g at birth and those born at less than 27 weeks' gestation. The first exam should take place 4 to 6 weeks after birth or between 31 and 33 weeks of postconceptional or postmenstrual age.

5. **When should follow-up exams be done when screening for retinopathy of prematurity?**
   The frequency of follow-up examinations is based on the retinal status at the time of the first exam. Exams should be done every 1 to 2 weeks, either until there is complete retinal vascularization or until two successive 2-week examinations show stage 2 ROP in zone III (more on staging is discussed later in this chapter). Infants should then be examined every 4 to 6 weeks until the retina is fully vascularized. If there is prethreshold disease (see further discussion), treatment may be indicated. If not, examinations should be done at least every week until treatment is indicated or until the disease regresses.

KEY POINTS: INDICATIONS FOR SCREENING INFANTS FOR ROP

1. All infants weighing less than 1500 g at birth
2. All infants with a gestational age of 28 weeks
3. Infants with a birth weight between 1500 and 2000 g with an unstable clinical course
4. Any infant that the neonatologist considers at risk because of an unstable clinical course

6. **How is retinopathy of prematurity classified?**
   The International Classification of Retinopathy of Prematurity (ICROP) is the system used for describing the findings in ROP. ICROP defines the location of disease in the retina and the extent of involvement of the developing vasculature. It also specifies the stage of involvement with levels of severity ranging from 1 (least affected) to 5 (severe disease).

7. **What are the zones of retinopathy of prematurity?**
   For the purpose of defining location, the retina is divided into three zones, with the optic nerve as the center because vascularization starts from the optic nerve and progresses peripherally (Fig. 44.1). Zone I consists of a circle, the radius of which subtends an angle of 30 degrees and extends from the disc to twice the distance from the disc to the center of the macula (twice the disc-to-fovea distance in all directions from the optic disc). Zone II extends from the edge of zone I peripherally to a point tangential to the nasal ora serrata and around to an area near the temporal anatomic equator. Zone III is the residual temporal crescent of retina anterior to zone II.

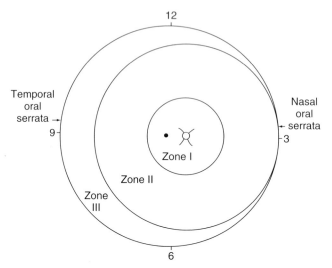

Fig. 44.1 The zones of retinopathy of prematurity are shown schematically.

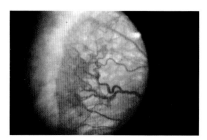

Fig. 44.2 Stage 3 retinopathy of prematurity.

8. **Describe the stages of retinopathy of prematurity.**
   Staging pertains to the degree of abnormal vascular response observed. Staging of the eye as a whole receives the stage of the most severe manifestation present.
   Stage 1 is a demarcation line. It is a thin, but definite, structure that separates avascular retina anteriorly from the vascularized retina posteriorly. Abnormal branching of vessels can be seen leading up to the line. It is flat and white and is in the plane of the retina.
   Stage 2 is a ridge. The line of stage 1 has height and width and occupies a volume extending out of the plane of the retina. The ridge may be pink or white. Vessels may leave the plane of the retina to enter it. Small tufts of new vessels may be seen on the surface of the retina posterior to the ridge. These vessels do not constitute fibrovascular growth.
   Stage 3 is the ridge of stage 2 with extraretinal fibrovascular proliferation (ERFP) (Fig. 44.2). Stage 4 ROP is a subtotal retinal detachment. Retinal detachments in ROP are concave, tractional retinal detachments. Stage 4A ROP is a subtotal retinal detachment that does not involve the central macula. Typically, it is present in the temporal region of zones II and III. Stage 4B ROP is a subtotal retinal detachment that involves the central macula.
   Last, stage 5 ROP is a total retinal detachment. These retinal detachments are funnel shaped but may have an open or closed configuration in their anterior and posterior areas.

9. **What is plus disease?**
   Plus disease is indicative of progressive vascular incompetence and is a strong risk factor for the development of more severe ROP. Anteriorly, plus disease is iris vascular engorgement and pupillary rigidity. Posteriorly, plus disease was originally defined as retinal venous dilation and arterial tortuosity in the posterior pole, involving all four quadrants (Fig. 44.3). More recently, if at least two quadrants are involved, plus disease is considered present. If plus disease is present in the posterior pole, a plus sign (i.e., +) is added to the number stage of the disease, that is, stage 3+. Before the appearance of plus disease, increasing dilation and tortuosity of the

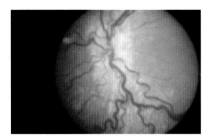

Fig. 44.3 Moderately severe plus disease.

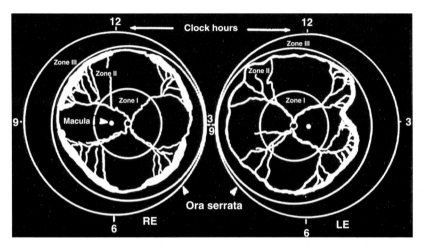

Fig. 44.4 The Cryo-Retinopathy of Prematurity definition of threshold disease is shown schematically.

posterior vessels signify increased activity of ROP. Pre-plus disease is present when there are vascular abnormalities of the posterior pole that are insufficient for the diagnosis of plus disease, but that demonstrate more venous dilation and arterial tortuosity than normal.

10. **What is the worst form of acute retinopathy of prematurity?**
    There is a more virulent retinopathy usually observed in the lowest-birth-weight infants that is called aggressive posterior ROP (AP-ROP). This form of ROP is posteriorly located and has prominent plus disease with ill-defined retinopathy. The plus disease is out of proportion to the peripheral retinopathy and usually progresses rapidly to stage 5 disease. AP-ROP typically extends circumferentially and is associated with a circumferential vessel.

11. **What is the rationale for treating acute retinopathy of prematurity?**
    Because ROP can lead to blindness from retinal detachment, treatment to prevent progression to retinal detachment is indicated. However, 90% of infants who develop acute ROP undergo spontaneous regression. Treatment should therefore be performed only for those infants who have a high risk of developing retinal detachment.

12. **What did the Cryotherapy for Retinopathy of Prematurity study teach us?**
    The Cryotherapy for Retinopathy of Prematurity (Cryo-ROP) study set out to determine whether treatment for ROP would prevent poor outcomes. For the purposes of that study, a level of disease (called *threshold disease*) was chosen at which 50% of infants were predicted to go blind without treatment. Threshold disease is defined as the presence of at least five contiguous or eight cumulative 30-degree sectors (clock hours) of stage 3 ROP in zone I or II, in the presence of plus disease (Fig. 44.4).

13. **Do all treated infants do well?**
    Analysis of natural history data from the Cryo-ROP study indicated that certain infants are at high risk for an unfavorable outcome. Infants with zone I ROP are included as infants at high risk for an unfavorable outcome. The Early Treatment for Retinopathy of Prematurity (ETROP) study used a risk model (RM-ROP2) based on the natural history data from the Cryo-ROP study to identify infants at high risk for an unfavorable outcome. The model used demographic characteristics of the infants and clinical features of ROP to classify eyes with prethreshold ROP at

high or low risk. High-risk prethreshold eyes that received conventional management had a higher likelihood of unfavorable structural outcome at 12 months.

14. **What did the Early Treatment for Retinopathy of Prematurity study teach us?**
The ETROP study described a clinical algorithm for which eyes should be treated. High-risk eyes (termed *type 1 ROP*) were those with the following findings: zone I, any stage ROP with plus disease; zone I, stage 3 ROP with or without plus disease; and zone II, stage 2 or 3 ROP with plus disease. Based on these criteria applying laser treatment to the anterior avascular zone of affected high-risk prethreshold eyes, there was a reduction from 19.5% to 14.5% in an unfavorable grating visual acuity measurement and from 15.6% to 9.1% in an unfavorable structural outcome at 9 months compared to the control group, which was not treated until threshold was reached. Less severely advanced, low-risk prethreshold eyes (termed *type 2 ROP*) included the following: zone I, stage 1 or 2 ROP without plus disease, and zone II, stage 3 ROP without plus disease. It was recommended that infants with type 2 ROP should be monitored closely and treated if they progressed to type 1 ROP or to threshold disease. The recommendation to treat type 1 eyes and adopt a "wait-and-watch" approach for type 2 eyes (treat if the eyes progress to type 1 or threshold) was supported by the final results of the ETROP study and is the strategy generally applied unless extenuating circumstances are present.

15. **How do you treat acute retinopathy of prematurity?**
Cryotherapy was the standard of care for treating acute ROP. More recently, multiple studies have reported on the efficacy of treating ROP with laser photocoagulation delivered by the indirect ophthalmoscope. Indirect laser has become the most common form of treatment for acute ROP.
    Indirect laser can be delivered in the intensive care nursery or in an operating room. Intravenous sedation with topical anesthesia or general anesthesia is administered. Laser is applied to the entire peripheral avascular zone, with the use of a laser indirect ophthalmoscope. The laser spot desired is a dull white or gray spot, and the spots are placed approximately 1 to 1.25 lesion-widths apart (Fig. 44.5). Critical focus on the retina is essential.

16. **How is cryotherapy applied?**
Cryotherapy is still occasionally performed for managing acute ROP. Some ophthalmologists prefer general anesthesia because of the greater stress on the infant and the greater risk of cardiopulmonary complications with cryotherapy than with laser photocoagulation. Cryotherapy is applied to the entire peripheral avascular zone using a handheld cryo-pencil. The peripheral retina is brought into view using the cryo-pencil as a scleral depressor. A white freeze spot seen for 1 to 2 seconds is the desired endpoint. The lesions are placed contiguously.

17. **Does posterior retinopathy of prematurity respond to treatment?**
Zone I and posterior zone II disease have a worse prognosis than more anterior ROP. Cryotherapy is often ineffective in posterior ROP. Investigations have shown that laser photocoagulation for posterior disease can limit the likelihood of an unfavorable anatomic outcome to 20% or less. Applying the criteria of the ETROP noted previously will generally result in a better prognosis for zone I disease.

18. **What is the expected result after laser treatment for retinopathy of prematurity?**
Various reports have quoted a regression rate of approximately 90% or higher after laser photocoagulation for prethreshold ROP. If regression is to occur, plus disease is usually less on the first week's follow-up visit. There may not be much change in the ERFP. By 2 weeks, one should start to see a reduction in the ERFP.

19. **When should you consider retreatment for retinopathy of prematurity?**
Occasionally, supplemental treatment after the initial session is necessary to induce regression. Retreatment should be considered if there is worse disease (worse plus disease and increased extraretinal fibrovascular proliferation) at the 1-week visit or persistently active disease (ERFP with plus disease) and the presence of "skip lesions" (areas of apparently missed treatment) or widely spaced laser lesions at the 2-week follow-up visit. Additional treatment should be applied to previously untreated areas rather than treating over old laser spots. In a similar fashion, supplemental cryotherapy can be applied to "skip areas" if there has not been an adequate response to initial cryotherapy treatment.

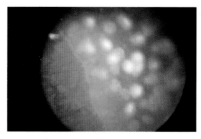

Fig. 44.5 Appearance of the peripheral fundus immediately after laser treatment.

KEY POINTS: INDICATIONS FOR LASER TREATMENT OF ROP PER ETROP

1. Zone I, any stage ROP with plus disease
2. Zone I, stage 3 ROP without plus disease
3. Zone II, stage 2 or 3 ROP with plus disease
4. Eyes with threshold ROP: At least five contiguous or eight cumulative 30-degree sectors (clock hours) of stage 3 ROP in zone I or II, in the presence of plus disease

20 Are there any options other than laser for acute retinopathy of prematurity?
   Many ophthalmologists are now using an intravitreal anti-vascular endothelial growth factor injection (usually bevacizumab) to induce regression of plus disease and ERFP. There is evidence that this treatment may be particularly helpful with posterior ROP. To date, no large randomized studies have been able to demonstrate systemic safety with this treatment, which is concerning with fragile, growing infants. These injections may reduce or eliminate the need for destructive retinal ablation and further evaluation is warranted.

21. What can be done for more advanced stages of retinopathy of prematurity?
   Stage 4B and progressive stage 4A retinal detachments may be managed with lens-sparing vitrectomy. There is a 70% to 85% rate of retinal reattachment. Vitrectomy surgery may be tried for more advanced stage 5 ROP. However, the anatomic and visual success rates are extremely poor.

22. What are some of the late complications of retinopathy of prematurity?
   The late complications of ROP include myopia, retinal pigmentation, dragging of the retina (Fig. 44.6), lattice-like vitreoretinal degeneration, retinal holes, retinal detachment, and angle-closure glaucoma. Obviously, these children need long-term follow-up by both a retina specialist and a pediatric ophthalmologist. Amblyopia and strabismus are also common.

23. What is the differential diagnosis for retinopathy of prematurity?
   The differential diagnosis differs depending on the extent of the disease (Table 44.1). In less severe ROP, conditions that lead to peripheral retinal vascular changes and retinal dragging should be considered. In more severe disease, the differential diagnosis of a white pupillary reflex must be considered.

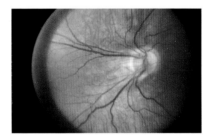

Fig. 44.6 Moderate temporal dragging of the macula caused by regressed retinopathy of prematurity.

Table 44.1 Differential Diagnosis of Retinopathy of Prematurity

LESS SEVERE DISEASE	MORE SEVERE DISEASE
Familial exudative vitreoretinopathy	Congenital cataract
Incontinentia pigmenti (Bloch-Sulzberger syndrome)	Persistent hyperplastic primary vitreous/persistent fetal vasculature
X-linked retinoschisis	Retinoblastoma
	Ocular toxocariasis
	Intermediate uveitis
	Coats disease
	Advanced X-linked retinoschisis
	Vitreous hemorrhage

BIBLIOGRAPHY

American Academy of Pediatrics: Screening examination of premature infants for retinopathy of prematurity, Pediatrics 108:809–811, 2001.

An International Committee for the Classification of Retinopathy of Prematurity: The International Classification of Retinopathy of Prematurity revisited, Arch Ophthalmol 123:991–999, 2005.

Committee for the Classification of Retinopathy of Prematurity: An international classification of retinopathy of prematurity, Arch Ophthalmol 102:1130–1134, 1984.

Cryotherapy for Retinopathy of Prematurity Cooperative Group: Multicenter trial of cryotherapy for retinopathy of prematurity: Snellen visual acuity and structural outcome at 51/2 years after randomization, Arch Ophthalmol 114:417–424, 1996.

Early Treatment for Retinopathy of Prematurity Cooperative Group: Revised indications for the treatment of retinopathy of prematurity: results of the early treatment of retinopathy of prematurity randomized trial, Arch Ophthalmol 121:1684–1694, 2003.

Hartnett M, Maguluri S, Thompson HW, McColm JR: Comparison of retinal outcomes after scleral buckling or lens-sparing vitrectomy for stage 4 retinopathy of prematurity, Retina 24:753–757, 2004.

International Committee for the Classification of the Late Stages of Retinopathy of Prematurity: An international classification of retinopathy of prematurity. II: The classification of retinal detachment, Arch Ophthalmol 105:906–912, 1987.

Lakhanpal RR, Sun RL, Albini TA, Holz ER: Anatomic success rate after 3-port lens-sparing vitrectomy in stage 4A or 4B retinopathy of prematurity, Ophthalmology 112:1569–1573, 2005.

McNamara J, Tasman W, Brown G, Federman J: Laser photocoagulation for stage 3+ retinopathy of prematurity, Ophthalmology 98:576–580, 1991.

McNamara J, Tasman W, Vander J, Brown G: Diode laser photocoagulation for retinopathy of prematurity preliminary results, Arch Ophthalmol 110:1714–1716, 1992.

Quinn G, Dobson V, Barr C, et al.: Visual acuity in infants after vitrectomy for severe retinopathy of prematurity, Ophthalmology 98:5–13, 1991.

Vander J, Handa J, McNamara J, et al.: Early laser photocoagulation for posterior retinopathy of prematurity: randomized controlled clinical trial, Ophthalmology 104:1731–1734, 1997.

CHAPTER 45

DIABETIC RETINOPATHY

James F. Vander

1. How is diabetic retinopathy classified? What fundus features are characteristic of each category?
   - **Nonproliferative diabetic retinopathy (NPDR):** This form is arbitrarily divided into three categories based on severity: mild, moderate, and severe. Features of mild and moderate nonproliferative retinopathy result predominantly from loss of capillary integrity (i.e., microaneurysms, dot-and-blot hemorrhages, hard yellow exudates, and macular edema) (Fig. 45.1). Cotton-wool spots are found. Features of more severe NPDR are related to early signs of ischemia. In addition to the features found in mild nonproliferative disease, the fundus shows venous beading and intraretinal microvascular abnormalities (IRMAs) as well as more extensive intraretinal hemorrhages (Fig. 45.2).
   - **Proliferative diabetic retinopathy (PDR):** Typical features are related to the consequences of extensive retinal capillary nonperfusion. Fundus findings include those of NPDR as well as the development of neovascularization of the disc (NVD; Fig. 45.3), neovascularization elsewhere in the retina (NVE), preretinal and/or vitreous hemorrhage, and vitreoretinal traction with tractional retinal detachment.

2. What is the most common cause of vision loss in diabetic retinopathy?
   The most common cause of vision loss in diabetic retinopathy is macular edema (DME).

3. Who is at risk for the development of diabetic retinopathy?
   All patients with diabetes mellitus are at risk for diabetic retinopathy. Relative risk factors include the following:
   - **Duration of diabetes:** The longer diabetes has been present, the greater the risk of some manifestation of diabetic retinopathy. After 10 to 15 years, more than 75% of patients show some signs of retinopathy.
   - **Age:** Diabetic retinopathy is uncommon before puberty even in patients who were diagnosed shortly after birth. NPDR appears sooner in patients diagnosed with diabetes after the age of 40. This may be related to duration of disease before diagnosis.
   - **Diabetic control:** The Diabetic Control and Complications Trial (DCCT) clearly demonstrated a correlation between poor long-term glucose control and subsequent development of diabetic retinopathy as well as other complications of diabetes.
   - **Renal disease:** Proteinuria is a particularly good marker for the development of diabetic retinopathy. This association may not be causal, but a patient with renal dysfunction should be followed more closely.
   - **Systemic hypertension:** Again, the causal nature of the relationship is not certain.
   - **Pregnancy:** Diabetic retinopathy may progress rapidly in patients who are pregnant. Patients with preexisting retinopathy are at particular risk.

KEY POINTS: MECHANISMS OF VISION LOSS IN DIABETES

1. Macular edema
2. Macular ischemia
3. Vitreous hemorrhage
4. Macular traction detachment
5. Combined rhegmatogenous/tractional retinal detachment

4. What is the significance of the hemoglobin A_1C? What is its correlation with the development of diabetic retinopathy?
   Hemoglobin A_1C is serum glycosylated hemoglobin. It is an indicator of the average level of serum glucose for the preceding 3 months. Thus, it provides a report card of the adequacy of glucose control for the preceding 3 months without identifying peaks, valleys, or timing of glucose fluctuation. Hemoglobin A_1C has been found to correlate most closely with the development of diabetic retinopathy. Nondiabetic patients typically have a level of 6 or less. The DCCT demonstrated that hemoglobin A_1C of less than 8 was associated with a significantly reduced risk of retinopathy compared with a value greater than 8.

5. What is the recommendation for screening patients with diabetes?
   Patients with juvenile insulin-dependent diabetes should have a dilated ophthalmologic examination 5 years after diagnosis. Patients with type II adult-onset diabetes should be examined at diagnosis. All diabetic patients should have an annual dilated funduscopic examination; more frequent examinations depend on the findings.

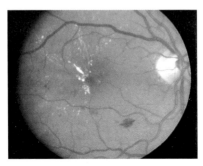

Fig. 45.1 Nonproliferative diabetic retinopathy with exudates, hemorrhages, and edema.

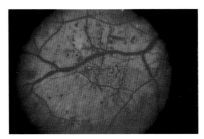

Fig. 45.2 Severe nonproliferative retinopathy with venous beading and intraretinal microvascular abnormalities.

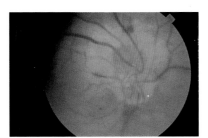

Fig. 45.3 Neovascularization of the disc in proliferative retinopathy.

6. What are the fluorescein angiographic features of nonproliferative and proliferative diabetic retinopathy?
   - In **mild to moderate NPDR,** the large vessels fill normally. Pinpoint areas of early hyperfluorescence correspond to microaneurysms, whereas dot-and-blot hemorrhages are hypofluorescent. Microaneurysms leak in the later frames with blurring of margins and diffusion of fluorescein dye, whereas hemorrhages remain hypofluorescent throughout the study. Telangiectasis hyperfluoresces with late leakage. Hard yellow exudate generally does not appear on a fluorescein angiogram unless it is extremely thick, in which case it is hypofluorescent. Macular edema is apparent as fluorescein leaks into the retina as the angiogram progresses (Figs. 45.4 and 45.5).
   - More **severe NPDR** has the features noted earlier as well as evidence of retinal capillary loss. Cotton-wool spots are usually hypofluorescent, sometimes with late hyperfluorescence along the margins. Areas of capillary dropout appear as smooth, hypofluorescent "ground-glass" patches, with staining at the margins in the later frames of the angiogram. IRMAs fill in the arterial phase of the angiogram and does not leak significantly in the later frames (Fig. 45.6).
   - **PDR.** Extensive retinal capillary loss is seen early in the angiogram with diffuse leakage at the edges of the ischemic areas in the later frames. NVD and NVE show intense early hyperfluorescence with marked leakage developing rapidly (Fig. 45.7).

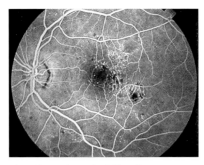

Fig. 45.4 Early-phase fluorescein angiogram shows pinpoint hyperfluorescence corresponding to microaneurysms.

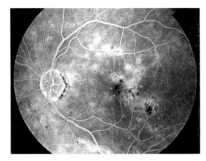

Fig. 45.5 Later-phase fluorescein angiogram shows leakage with diffusion of dye and blurring of the microaneurysms.

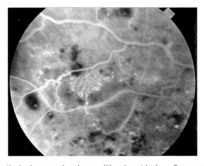

Fig. 45.6 Intraretinal microvascular abnormalities do not leak on fluorescein angiography.

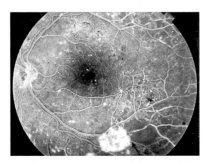

Fig. 45.7 Neovascularization *(arrow)* is markedly hyperfluorescent early and develops at the border of perfused and nonperfused retina.

7. What are the uses of optical coherence tomography in the management of diabetic retinopathy?

Optical coherence tomography (OCT) provides a noninvasive, photographic method for obtaining a cross-sectional view of the macula. Macular thickness and volume may be quantified, providing an objective measurement that is especially useful when serial studies are available and progression or response to treatment can be evaluated. The studies are helpful to show patients their condition. Significant vitreomacular traction, if present, lends insight into a possible mechanism for the presence of macular edema and points toward vitrectomy as a therapeutic option. OCT may also show significant macular thinning as can sometimes occur after treatment of macular edema. This may explain a poor visual result in an eye after resolution of intraretinal fluid.

8. What treatment options are there for the management of diabetic macular edema?

Although thermal laser was the standard of care for many years, it has been supplanted by the use of intravitreal injections for most cases of diabetic macular edema

9. What does the term *center-involving edema* mean?

This is an anatomic term, as measured by OCT, that represents the minimum level of central macular edema necessary for enrollment in clinical trials and, by extension, as a level of disease at which point one should consider treatment based on a number of trials performed over several years. The exact thickness may vary depending on the specific trial, but a widely used threshold is 250 microns central subfield thickness as measured using spectral domain OCT. Clinical decision making for the use of intravitreal injections for DME is largely based on the presence or absence of center-involving edema.

10. How are intravitreal injections used in managing diabetic macular edema?

Corticosteroids were the first agents widely used for treating DME. Injection of triamcinolone and other agents will usually produce a rapid reduction in edema and often dramatic visual improvement. A sustained-release dexamethasone implant is Food and Drug Administration (FDA) approved for the treatment of DME. The effect typically lasts months and then edema usually recurs. Repeated injections are required. Common complications include variable elevation of intraocular pressure, sometimes substantial requiring medications and/or surgery, and cataract progression, frequently requiring cataract removal to improve visual acuity and allow better visualization for the treating physician. Rarely, a patient may develop endophthalmitis.

Anti-vascular endothelial growth factor (VEGF) agents are now used as first-line treatment for DME in most cases. Numerous controlled clinical trials have shown that repeated intravitreal injections reduce or eliminate DME and with stable or improved vision. Ranibizumab and, more recently, aflibercept are FDA approved for center involving DME. Treatment is usually begun with monthly injections until edema is resolved or at least stabilized. Various strategies for ongoing treatment include scheduled monthly injections, gradually extending treatment intervals or treatment only with recurrence of edema (PRN). Treatment may need to continue for years, although not always. Off-label bevacizumab is also widely used. Given that glaucoma and cataract formation are not expected side effects, anti-VEGF drugs are preferred over steroid use for most cases.

11. What is the definition of clinically significant macular edema?

Clinically significant macular edema (CSME), as defined in the Early Treatment Diabetic Retinopathy Study (ETDRS), is present in patients with any one of the following:
- Retinal thickening within 500 microns of the center of the fovea (Fig. 45.8)
- Hard yellow exudate within 500 microns of the center of the fovea with adjacent retinal thickening

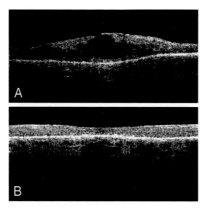

Fig. 45.8 A, Optical coherence tomography (OCT) shows marked macular edema with cystic spaces. **B,** Repeat OCT taken 3 weeks after injection of intravitreal steroids shows resolution of edema.

- At least one disc area of retinal thickening, any part of which is within one disc diameter of the center of the fovea

    CSME describes the fundus features as seen on stereoscopic high-magnification viewing of the macula. Visual acuity is not relevant; a patient with 20/20 vision may still have CSME. The fluorescein angiographic appearance is not relevant for the definition of CSME. Monocular viewing of the macula with a direct ophthalmoscope or a solitary color photograph is not adequate for diagnosing CSME, nor is the low-magnification view provided by the indirect ophthalmoscope.

12. **What are the results of the Early Treatment Diabetic Retinopathy Study concerning treatment of diabetic macular edema?**
    The ETDRS showed that macular laser treatment for patients with CSME reduced the risk of doubling of the visual angle over a 3-year period. Significant visual improvement is uncommon after macular laser treatment. The goal is to prevent vision from worsening in the future. Treatment is directed at areas of diffuse leakage by using a grid pattern and at areas of focal leakage by direct treatment of the leaking abnormality (Fig. 45.9). Resolution of macular edema may take several months, and retreatment is occasionally necessary.

13. **What other findings did the Early Treatment Diabetic Retinopathy Study report?**
    The ETDRS also was designed to determine whether aspirin use was helpful or harmful in patients with diabetic retinopathy; the study concluded that it was neither. The study also assessed the role of early panretinal laser treatment for proliferative disease (see further discussion).

14. **What is the definition of high-risk characteristics?**
    High-risk characteristics (HRC) was used by the Diabetic Retinopathy Study (DRS) to describe patients at a high risk of severe vision loss from PDR. The study found that patients with (1) NVE and vitreous hemorrhage, (2) mild NVD and vitreous hemorrhage, and (3) moderate or severe NVD with or without vitreous hemorrhage are at high risk for severe vision loss over the ensuing 3 years. Initiation of full-scatter panretinal photocoagulation (PRP) greatly reduced the risk of severe vision loss in patients with HRC (Fig. 45.10). Subsequently, the ETDRS found that for patients with severe nonproliferative retinopathy and/or early proliferative retinopathy without HRC, there was no clear-cut benefit to initiation of full-scatter PRP. As long as careful follow-up can be ensured, PRP may be safely withheld in such cases.

KEY POINTS: DRS HIGH-RISK CHARACTERISTICS

1. NVD of ¼ to ⅓ of the disc area
2. NVD of <¼ of the disc area with any vitreous hemorrhage
3. NVE with any vitreous hemorrhage

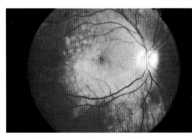

Fig. 45.9 Clinically significant macular edema with thickening and exudate within 500 microns of the center of the fovea.

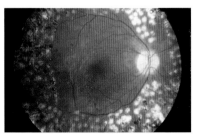

Fig. 45.10 Panretinal photocoagulation several months after treatment.

15. What are the side effects of panretinal photocoagulation?

PRP does not improve vision but is performed to prevent the blinding complication of proliferative retinopathy. However, it does cause a loss of peripheral vision and night vision. Loss of central vision may result from exacerbation of macular edema. Thus, if possible, macular focal laser should be performed before PRP when both are indicated. Other complications include impaired accommodation, pupillary dilation, and inadvertent macular burns.

16. Do all patients treated with panretinal photocoagulation show resolution of high-risk characteristics?

No. As many as one-third of patients do not show resolution of NVD or NVE, and in some cases, there will be no apparent regression.

17. Are there alternatives to panretinal photocoagulation for proliferative diabetic retinopathy?

Anti-VEGF agents are often used for managing the proliferative complications of diabetes as well as DME. Ranibizumab is FDA approved for the treatment of PDR. The role of anti-VEGF drugs as primary treatment or in conjunction with PRP is evolving. An anti-VEGF injection may also be helpful as a preoperative adjunct for certain patients undergoing vitrectomy for more advanced retinopathy.

18. What is the differential diagnosis of diabetic retinopathy?

The differential diagnosis includes branch or central retinal vein obstruction, ocular ischemic syndrome, radiation retinopathy, hypertensive retinopathy, and miscellaneous proliferative retinopathies such as sarcoidosis, sickle cell hemoglobinopathy, and other less common causes. In patients with typical macular features of nonproliferative retinopathy such as microaneurysms and macular edema, but no evidence of diabetes mellitus, the disease usually is categorized as idiopathic juxtafoveal telangiectasia.

19. What is the significance of neovascularization of the iris in diabetes?

Neovascularization of the iris (NVI) is an ominous sign of severe PDR and generally requires urgent treatment. NVI may progress to occlude the trabecular meshwork in a relatively short period, leading to severe neovascular glaucoma. This dreaded complication of proliferative disease usually can be avoided by injecting anti-VEGF drugs or performing PRP before the angle has become occluded.

20. What are the indications for vitrectomy in diabetic retinopathy?

- **Vitreous hemorrhage:** Vitreous hemorrhage obscuring the visual axis causes severe vision loss. Although it generally clears spontaneously, for patients with more extensive hemorrhage, vitrectomy may be indicated. As vitrectomy techniques have improved, earlier surgery has been the trend.
- **Tractional retinal detachment:** Most surgeons agree that tractional retinal detachment involving the macula is an indication for diabetic vitrectomy. If the vitreoretinal traction can be relieved within weeks or a few months of onset, visual results are excellent. Long-standing tractional retinal detachments generally do not respond favorably in terms of visual recovery. Progressive extramacular tractional retinal detachment moving toward the fovea is occasionally an indication for surgery, although this is controversial.
- **Combined tractional–rhegmatogenous retinal detachment:** The development of combined retinal detachment with an open retinal break is an indication for vitrectomy. Such detachments are notoriously difficult to fix, and patients are usually taken to surgery shortly after diagnosis.
- **Refractory macular edema:** Patients with a taut posterior hyaloid face producing chronic macular edema that is not responsive to focal laser therapy can undergo surgery, sometimes with significant visual improvement. It is believed that the chronic traction of the vitreous face on the macula produces persistent leakage and that the edema can resolve only after traction is released.

21. What are the complications of vitrectomy for diabetes?

- **Progression of cataract:** Progressive nuclear sclerotic or posterior subcapsular cataracts occur frequently after vitrectomy.
- **Nonhealing corneal epithelial defects:** The cornea may swell, and the surface may break down during vitrectomy. Diabetic patients are prone to poor healing of corneal epithelial defects.
- **Retinal detachment:** Retinal detachment may be related to a peripheral tear near one of the sclerotomy sites or posteriorly as a result of persistent or recurrent vitreoretinal traction.
- **Vitreous hemorrhage:** Some degree of vitreous hemorrhage is frequently present postoperatively. It generally clears quickly.

BIBLIOGRAPHY

Diabetic Control and Complications Trial Research Group: The effect of intensive diabetes treatment on the progression of diabetic retinopathy in insulin-dependent diabetes mellitus, Arch Ophthalmol 113:36–51, 1995.

Diabetic Retinopathy Clinical Research Network: Expanded 2-year follow-up of ranibizumab plus prompt or deferred laser or triamcinolone plus prompt laser for diabetic macular edema, Ophthalmology 118:609–614, 2011.

Diabetic Retinopathy Clinical Research Network, Wells JA, Glassman AR, Ayala AR, et al.: Aflibercept, bevacizumab, or ranibizumab for diabetic macular edema, N Engl J Med 372(13):1193–1203, 2015.

Diabetic Retinopathy Study Research Group: Photocoagulation treatment of proliferative diabetic retinopathy. Clinical application of Diabetic Retinopathy Study (DRS) findings, DRS report number 8, Ophthalmology 88:583–600, 1981.

Early Treatment for Diabetic Retinopathy Study Research Group: Photocoagulation for diabetic macular edema: Early Treatment for Diabetic Retinopathy Study report number 1, Arch Ophthalmol 103:1796–1806, 1985.

Martidis A, Duker JS, Greenberg PB, et al.: Intravitreal triamcinolone for refractory diabetic macular edema, Ophthalmology 109:920–927, 2002.

Pendergast SD, Hassan TS, Williams GA: Vitrectomy for diffuse diabetic macular edema associated with a taut premacular posterior hyaloid, Am J Ophthalmol 130:178–186, 2000.

CHAPTER 46

RETINAL ARTERIAL OBSTRUCTION

Jacob Duker

1. **What types of retinal arterial obstructions can occur?**

   Retinal arterial obstructions are generally divided into branch retinal arterial obstructions (BRAOs) and central retinal arterial obstructions (CRAOs), depending on the precise site of obstruction:

   - A BRAO occurs when the blockage is distal to the lamina cribrosa of the optic nerve; in other words, within the visible vasculature of the retina. A BRAO can involve an area as large as three-quarters of the retina or as small as just a few micrometers.
   - A CRAO occurs when the blockage is within the optic nerve substance itself. The site of obstruction is therefore not generally visible on ophthalmoscopy. In a CRAO, most, if not all, of the retina is affected.

     Obstructions more proximal to the central retinal artery, in the ophthalmic artery, or even in the internal carotid artery can cause visual loss as well. Ophthalmic arterial obstructions can be difficult to differentiate from CRAO on a clinical basis.

2. **What causes a retinal artery to become blocked?**

   The typical causes differ for CRAO and BRAO. Because the site of obstruction is not visible on clinical examination and, in general, the central retinal artery is too small to image with most techniques, the precise cause of most CRAOs cannot be definitely determined. It is currently believed that most CRAOs are caused by thrombus formation. Localized intimal damage from atherosclerosis probably incites the thrombus in most cases. In approximately 20% of cases, an embolus is visible in the central retinal artery or one of its branches, suggesting an embolic cause (Fig. 46.1). Emboli are the cause of more than 90% of BRAOs. Cholesterol, calcium, fibrin, and platelets have all been implicated individually or together. Emboli are usually visible in the retinal arterial tree. Rarely, extrinsic mechanical compression is caused by an orbital or an optic nerve tumor, hemorrhage, or inflammation. Inflammation due to vasculitis, optic neuritis, or even orbital disease (e.g., mucormycosis) can cause a CRAO as well. Trauma with direct damage to the optic nerve or blood vessels can lead to CRAO. In addition, systemic coagulopathies can also be associated with both CRAO and BRAO.

3. **Describe the typical symptoms of a retinal arterial obstruction.**

   The hallmark symptom of an acute retinal arterial obstruction is abrupt, painless loss of sight in the visual field that corresponds to the territory of the obstructed artery. In a CRAO, this would be most, if not all, of the visual field. In some patients, an artery derived from the choroidal circulation, called a *cilioretinal artery*, may perfuse a small amount of the central retina. The cilioretinal artery, which is present in up to 20% of individuals, remains patent when the site of obstruction is the central retinal artery. Some of the visual field corresponding to the territory of the patent cilioretinal vessel can be spared in select individuals. Rarely, cilioretinal artery sparing can leave a patient with 20/20 (normal) central vision, albeit with a very constricted visual field (Fig. 46.2).

   Occasionally, patients report stuttering visual loss or episodes of amaurosis fugax before arterial obstruction. Pain is not generally a part of retinal arterial obstruction unless some other underlying disease is present (e.g., giant cell arteritis, ocular ischemia).

   In a BRAO, the visual field loss can vary from up to three-quarters of the visual field to as little as a few degrees, depending on the territory of the obstructed vessel. Often, the central vision will be 20/20, thus sparing the macular area.

4. **What do you see on examination when a retinal arterial obstruction has occurred?**

   The decreased blood flow results in ischemic whitening of the retina in the territory of the obstructed artery. Because the retinal vasculature supplies circulation only to the inner retina (the outer retina gets its circulation from the choroid), the ischemia is limited to the inner retina. The retinal whitening is most pronounced in the posterior pole where the nerve fiber layer (NFL) is thickest.

   In an arterial obstruction, the retinal arteries distal to the blockage appear thin and attenuated. The blood column may be interrupted in both the distal arteries and the corresponding draining veins. This phenomenon has been labeled "boxcarring." Splinter retinal hemorrhages on the disc are common. Embolic material may be visible in the central retinal artery, where it exits the disc, or in one of the branches of the central retinal artery. In most instances, a cherry-red spot will be visible in the macular area. The most common sites of obstruction in a BRAO are the retinal arterial bifurcations.

   In a CRAO, the visual acuity is usually quite poor. The patient typically can only discern motion or, perhaps, count fingers from a distance of several feet. Many episodes of BRAO result in only peripheral visual loss with intact central acuity.

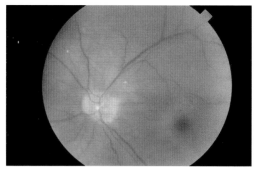

Fig. 46.1 A central retinal arterial obstruction caused emboli in this patient. Note the refractile particles in the central retinal artery in the center of the optic disc, as well as in two branch retinal arteries superior to the optic disc.

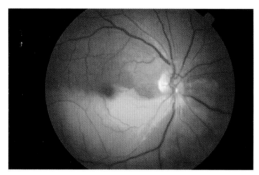

Fig. 46.2 Typical inferior hemispheric branch retinal arterial obstruction. The visual acuity was 20/20, but there was a marked superior visual field defect.

5. **What is a cherry-red spot?**
   A cherry-red spot represents a pathologic appearance of the macula, the center of the retina. There are two main causes: ischemia and abnormal NFL deposits. A cherry-red spot occurs in CRAO because of the retinal whitening of the surrounding NFL. The fovea itself has no nerve fibers, so its appearance does not change significantly from normal. The retinal whitening surrounding the normal reddish tint of the macular area produces the cherry-red spot.

6. **What other conditions result in a cherry-red spot of the retina?**
   In addition to CRAO, a cherry-red spot may be seen in conditions in which abnormal deposits accumulate in cells of the retinal NFL. The classic example is Tay-Sachs disease, a sphingolipidosis. A cherry-red spot has been reported in other sphingolipidoses, as well as β-galactosidase deficiency (MPS VII), Hallervorden-Spatz disease, and Batten-Mayou (Vogt-Spielmeyer) disease.
   An ischemic cherry-red spot can be differentiated from these other entities by a history of visual loss, concurrent systemic disease, the age of the patient, and the appearance of the surrounding retinal blood vessels and retina.

7. **Is there any ancillary testing that can be done to confirm the diagnosis?**
   In most cases, an experienced observer can accurately diagnose CRAO and BRAO. In cases in which the diagnosis is in doubt, an intravenous fluorescein angiogram can be performed. This will show a significant diminution in dye flow through the obstructed vessels. A color Doppler ultrasound evaluation of the orbital circulation can also be used to determine the degree of obstruction and to differentiate an ophthalmic artery obstruction from CRAO. Optical coherence tomography (OCT) angiography of a retinal artery obstruction will reveal decreased flow in the superficial retinal plexus, deep retinal plexus, outer retina, and choroidal slab.

8. **Which systemic diseases are associated with retinal arterial obstruction?**
   Although many systemic diseases are associated with retinal arterial obstruction, more than 50% of all affected patients will manifest no apparent systemic or local cause for their retinal disease. The most common association is ipsilateral carotid artery disease, which is present in approximately one-third of affected patients. Approximately

10% of arterial obstructions in patients over 50 years of age are associated with giant cell arteritis. This is a critical association because visual loss can occur rapidly in the fellow eye in these patients. Prompt administration of high doses of corticosteroids may prevent the contralateral visual loss and a cerebrovascular accident.

In both CRAO and BRAO, all patients should be evaluated for embolic sources from the carotid artery system and the heart with carotid noninvasive testing and echocardiogram.

9. **Do you always have to test for giant cell arteritis?**
It is of paramount importance that giant cell arteritis be ruled out in all patients older than age 50 with a CRAO. A stat erythrocyte sedimentation rate, C-reactive protein, and platelet count should be ordered and, if the results are high, or if there is a strong clinical suspicion of giant cell arteritis, a temporal artery biopsy should be considered along with high-dose corticosteroids until definitive biopsy results are known. BRAO associated with giant cell arteritis is exceedingly uncommon.

KEY POINTS: GIANT CELL ARTERITIS

1. Must be considered in all patients over age 50 with amaurosis fugax.
2. Order a stat erythrocyte sedimentation rate, C-reactive protein, and platelet count.
3. Temporal arteritis may occur in patients with normal blood tests. Clinical suspicion is important.
4. High-dose steroids must be started immediately. A temporary artery biopsy should be done within 2 weeks, but may be positive up to a month after steroids are initiated.

10. **Which patients are at risk to get a retinal arterial obstruction?**
The incidence of all nonarteritic forms of CRAO is approximately 1 to 2 in 100,000 and CRAO accounts for approximately 1 in 10,000 ophthalmology visits. The incidence of CRAO increases with age and may be as high as 10 in 100,000 in patients 80 years and older, likely due to higher prevalence of cardiovascular disease in this age group. Patients who have suffered an arterial obstruction in one eye are at a higher risk for developing an obstruction in the contralateral eye. Patients with known carotid artery disease, diseased heart valves, or cardiac arrhythmias are also at increased risk. In the patient population included in the European Assessment Group for Lysis in the Eye (EAGLE) trial, 73% of 77 patients with CRAO had arterial hypertension, 40% had at least a 70% stenosis of a carotid artery (with most having ipsilateral carotid artery stenosis), 22% had coronary artery disease, 20% had atrial fibrillation, and 17% had valvular heart disease. In addition, conditions that result in abnormal rheologic parameters such as pancreatitis, lupus, pregnancy, and amniotic fluid emboli can result in artery obstructions.

11. **Can any prophylactic treatment be given?**
With the exception of corticosteroid treatment for giant cell arteritis, prophylaxis against arterial obstructions is not generally given. The utility of anticoagulation to prevent retinal arterial obstructions in the setting of known carotid disease is not definitively proven. Extrapolation from studies showing a benefit of lowering the risk of subsequent stroke in this situation suggests that anticoagulation is useful to lower the risk of arterial obstruction as well. The same conclusion may be extrapolated from the studies proving a benefit for carotid endarterectomy for appropriate patients with carotid arterial disease.

12. **What is the incidence of bilateral retinal arterial obstructions?**
Ten percent.

13. **Is there any proven treatment for retinal arterial obstruction?**
There is no proven treatment for either CRAO or BRAO. Some investigators feel that none of the currently recommended treatments have any value. Because the inner retina is highly sensitive to loss of perfusion, intervention is rarely, if ever, attempted in anyone with an obstruction more than 72 hours old. Proposed therapies for retinal arterial obstructions are as follows:
- Dislodging emboli to a more distal location
- Dissolving thrombi
- Increasing oxygenation to the retina
- Protecting surviving retinal cells from ischemic damage

The traditional approach to CRAO includes paracentesis, ocular massage, and medications to lower the intraocular pressure. All three of these interventions are an attempt to dislodge any embolus that may be present. A paracentesis is the removal of a small amount of aqueous humor via a small needle (30 or 27 gauge). This can be done in an office setting.

Increasing oxygenation to the retina is attempted by having patients inhale a mixture of 95% oxygen and 5% carbon dioxide (carbogen) for 10 minutes every 2 hours for 24 to 48 hours after the blockage. Carbon dioxide counteracts the normal retinal arterial vasoconstriction that occurs when pure oxygen is inhaled. However, there is no clinical evidence of any beneficial effect. Hyperbaric oxygen therapy is another approach intended to increase oxygenation to the ischemic inner retina.

More recently, both systemic (via intravenous infusion) and local (directly into the ophthalmic artery via an arterial catheter) infusions of clot-dissolving medications (streptokinase, tissue plasminogen activator, urokinase, heparin) have been tried for retinal arterial obstruction. However, a randomized clinical trial found no difference in visual outcome between intra-arterial thrombolysis (IAT) via local infusion of tissue plasminogen activator and traditional CRAO treatments at 1-month follow-up, although IAT was associated with more adverse reactions. The long-term procedural results and potential favorable anatomic outcomes of IAT, such as central retinal artery reperfusion, have not yet been determined. IAT is not without risk and should be contemplated only for obstructions less than 48 hours old. Because BRAOs do not usually affect central vision, such invasive procedures probably should not be attempted in these cases.

At present, there are no means to "rescue" ischemic retinal tissue. This is an area of active research and it may be possible in the future.

KEY POINTS: RETINAL ARTERIAL OBSTRUCTION

1. Systemic disease must be ruled out in any retinal artery obstruction.
2. Giant cell arteritis should be considered and ruled out in any patient older than age 60 with a central retinal artery obstruction.
3. No proven treatment exists for retinal artery obstruction.

14. **Why is the retina so sensitive to arterial inflow problems?**
The retina is a highly metabolic organ and is therefore sensitive to ischemia. The central retinal artery is an end artery with no true normal anastomosis. As part of the central nervous system, the retina is unable to regenerate if damaged.

15. **How do you tell a retinal arterial obstruction from a retinal venous obstruction?**
It is simple—white versus red. The hallmark of retinal arterial obstructions is ischemic retinal whitening. The hallmark of retinal venous obstruction is retinal hemorrhage in the territory of the obstructed vessel. In addition, the retinal veins will appear dilated and tortuous as opposed to thin and attenuated. Rarely, a patient may present with a combined obstruction, which produces a combined fundus picture (i.e., whitening from ischemia with red from retinal hemorrhage).

16. **Is acute obstruction of a retinal artery an emergency?**
CRAO is considered a true ophthalmic emergency, even though there is no proven treatment. Because the retina is highly sensitive to ischemia, treatment should be initiated as quickly as possible if contemplated. Although animal studies indicate that more than 90 minutes of ischemia produces irreversible retinal cell death, clinical experience suggests that some eyes can tolerate ischemia for up to 72 hours and still recover. If a potentially risky intervention such as anticoagulation is contemplated, the visual loss should be no more than 48 hours old to maximize the possibility of recovery and the overall risk-to-benefit ratio. Optimal timing for anticoagulation is within 6 to 8 hours of visual loss. CRAO is a stroke equivalent and should prompt immediate referral to the nearest stroke center to minimize further ischemic complications.

17. **What does the retina look like months or years after an arterial obstruction?**
The retinal vessels look attenuated and the optic disc is often pale, owing to the loss of the retinal NFL. Because the retina itself is transparent and the underlying retinal pigment epithelium and choroid are unaffected by a pure CRAO or BRAO, the retina appears normal.

18. **Are there any other late complications after retinal arterial obstructions?**
Neovascularization of the iris (NVI) occurs in approximately 15% of patients with CRAO. It is usually seen within 3 months of the CRAO and can result in a severe type of glaucoma called *neovascular glaucoma*. If NVI is detected, a laser treatment to the ischemic retina, panretinal photocoagulation, is usually performed. Intravitreal injections of antiangiogenic (vascular endothelial growth factor [VEGF]) medications may also be used. Neovascularization is extremely rare after BRAO.

ACKNOWLEDGMENT

The author would like to thank Jay Duker for his work on the prior edition of this chapter.

BIBLIOGRAPHY

Ahn SJ, Kim JM, Hong J-H, et al.: Efficacy and safety of intra-arterial thrombolysis in central retinal artery occlusion, Invest Ophthalmol Vis Sci 54:7746–7755, 2013.

Arruga J, Sanders MD: Ophthalmologic findings in 70 patients with evidence of retinal embolism, Ophthalmology 89:1336–1347, 1982.

Atebara NH, Brown GC, Cater J: Efficacy of anterior chamber paracentesis and carbogen in treating acute nonarteritic central retinal artery obstruction, Ophthalmology 102:2029–2035, 1995.

Atkins EJ, Bruce BB, Newman NJ, Biousse V. Translation of clinical studies to clinical practice: survey on the treatment of central retinal artery occlusion. Am J Ophthalmol 148:172–173, 2009.

Brown GC, Magargal LE: Central retinal artery obstruction and visual acuity, Ophthalmology 89:14–19, 1982.

Brown GC, Magargal LE, Sergott R: Acute obstruction of the retinal and choroidal circulations, Ophthalmology 93:1373–1382, 1986.

Callizo J, Feltgen N, Pantenburg S, et al., European Assessment Group for Lysis in the Eye: Cardiovascular risk factors in central retinal artery occlusion: results of a prospective and standardized medical examination, Ophthalmology 122:1881–1888, 2015.

Duker JS, Brown GC: Recovery following acute obstruction of the retinal and choroidal circulations, Retina 8:257–260, 1988.

Duker JS, Sivalingham A, Brown GC, Reber R: A prospective study of acute central retinal artery obstruction, Arch Ophthalmol 109: 339–342, 1991.

Duker JS: Retinal arterial obstruction. In Yanoff M, Duker JS, editors: Ophthalmology, St. Louis, Mosby, pp 856–863.

Greven CM, Slusher MM, Weaver RG: Retinal arterial occlusions in young adults, Am J Ophthalmol 120:776–783, 1995.

Hayreh SS, Podhajsky P: Ocular neovascularization with retinal vascular occlusion. II. Occurrence in central and branch retinal artery obstruction, Arch Ophthalmol 100:1585–1596, 1982.

Menzel-Severing J, Siekmann U, Weinberger A, et al.: Early hyperbaric oxygen treatment for nonarteritic central retinal artery obstruction, Am J Ophthalmol 153:454–459, 2012.

Park SJ, Choi NK, Seo KH, Park KH, Woo SJ: Nationwide incidence of clinically diagnosed central retinal artery occlusion in Korea, 2008 to 2011, Ophthalmology 121:1933–1938, 2014.

Schmidt D, Schumaker M, Wakhloo AK: Microcatheter urokinase infusion in central retinal artery occlusion, Am J Ophthalmol 113: 429–434, 1992.

Schumacher M, Schmidt D, Jurklies B, et al.: Central retinal artery occlusion: local intra-arterial fibrinolysis versus conservative treatment, a multicenter randomized trial, Ophthalmology 117:1367–1375, 2010.

CHAPTER 47

RETINAL VENOUS OCCLUSIVE DISEASE

Ehsan Rahimy

BRANCH RETINAL VEIN OCCLUSION

1. What are the symptoms of a branch retinal vein occlusion?

   Patients may notice an acute, painless loss of vision if there is macular edema, ischemic maculopathy, or intraretinal hemorrhage involving the fovea. A branch retinal vein occlusion (BRVO) in a nasal quadrant may be asymptomatic. A long-standing BRVO can present with floaters or an abrupt decrease in vision from vitreous hemorrhage (VH) secondary to retinal neovascularization.

2. What are the clinical signs of a branch retinal vein occlusion?

   The acute funduscopic findings of BRVO include a wedge-shaped segmental pattern of intraretinal hemorrhages with its apex near the site of occlusion, tortuous and dilated veins, cotton-wool spots, and macular edema (Fig. 47.1). In a chronic BRVO, collateral vessels on the disc or bridging the horizontal raphe, macular retinal pigment epithelium changes, or neovascularization of the retina (NVE) or disc can develop.

3. Are there systemic associations in patients with a branch retinal vein occlusion?

   The Eye Disease Case–Control Study Group identified a number of risk factors for BRVO: hypertension, cardiovascular disease, increased body mass index, and glaucoma. Interestingly, diabetes mellitus was not found to be a major independent risk factor for BRVO. Bilaterality, young age, or other atypical features should prompt further investigation for an underlying systemic disease (hypercoagulable state, autoimmune/inflammatory condition, or infectious disease).[1]

4. Where does a branch retinal vein occlusion most commonly occur?

   The superotemporal quadrant is the most common location for a BRVO, representing approximately 60% of observed cases. Inferotemporal BRVOs account for an additional 30% of cases, while nasally distributed ones represent the remaining 10%. However, these numbers may be misrepresented because most patients with nasal BRVOs do not have visual complaints and are often found only incidentally. Approximately 10% of patients with a BRVO will develop a retinal vein occlusion in the fellow eye.

KEY POINTS: COMMON CHARACTERISTICS OF A BRANCH RETINAL VEIN OCCLUSION

1. Occurs at arteriovenous crossing
2. Segmental pattern of intraretinal hemorrhages
3. Macular edema
4. Majority occur in the superotemporal quadrant

5. How is a branch retinal vein occlusion categorized?

   A BRVO is classified as either ischemic or nonischemic. A nonischemic BRVO is defined as having fewer than five disc areas of retinal capillary nonperfusion, as documented by fluorescein angiography. An ischemic BRVO is defined as having more than five disc areas of retinal capillary nonperfusion.

6. What are the complications of a branch retinal vein occlusion?

   Patients with a nonischemic BRVO may lose vision secondary to macular edema, which may be appreciated clinically and confirmed with ancillary imaging studies, such as fluorescein angiography or, more commonly, optical coherence tomography. Patients with an ischemic BRVO most commonly lose vision from macular edema, ischemic maculopathy, or VH. Fluorescein angiography is useful in detecting macular ischemia, revealing an enlarged and irregular foveal avascular zone. Depending on the degree of macular ischemia present, permanent visual loss is common. Additional sequelae of BRVO include retinal neovascularization (25%), which can result in VH from traction on the neovascular fronds, and epiretinal membrane formation (20%).

7. What is the treatment for an uncomplicated branch retinal vein occlusion?

   Patients with a nonischemic BRVO without macular edema are followed clinically for the development of macular edema and for potential progression into an ischemic BRVO and its complications, which include ischemic maculopathy, NVE, and VH.

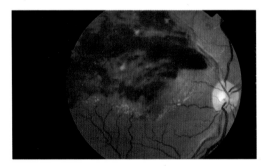

Fig. 47.1 Superotemporal branch retinal vein occlusion with intraretinal hemorrhages, cotton-wool spots, hard exudates, and macular edema.

8. **What is the first-line treatment for macular edema secondary to branch retinal vein occlusion?**
   The introduction of anti-vascular endothelial growth factor (VEGF) therapy has revolutionized the management of macular edema associated with retinal vascular disease. The BRAVO study is a large, multicenter, phase 3, randomized study that evaluated monthly ranibizumab (Lucentis, Genentech, South San Francisco, CA, USA) versus sham injections in treating acute macular edema secondary to BRVO. After 6 months, patients who received 0.3 mg ranibizumab had a mean gain from baseline of 16.6 letters, those who received 0.5 mg ranibizumab gained 18.3 letters, and the sham group gained 7.3 letters. Similar gains were observed in the VIBRANT trial, a phase 3, randomized study that evaluated monthly 2.0 mg aflibercept (Eylea, Regeneron, Tarrytown, NY, USA) compared to focal laser. After 6 months, the aflibercept group experienced a mean gain of 17.0 letters from baseline, compared to 6.9 letters in the laser group. Many clinicians have extrapolated these results to bevacizumab (Avastin, Genentech), a cheaper off-label alternative, which has been shown to substantially reduce macular edema in a number of smaller uncontrolled studies.[2]

9. **What is the role of intravitreal steroids in the treatment of macular edema secondary to branch retinal vein occlusion?**
   The Standard Care versus Corticosteroid for Retinal Vein Occlusion (SCORE) BRVO study compared the safety and efficacy of macular grid laser treatment versus intravitreal triamcinolone corticosteroid injections (1 and 4 mg doses) to treat vision loss from macular edema associated with BRVO. After 1 year, a comparable percentage of patients experienced a substantial gain of three or more lines of vision across all three groups (29% in the laser group, 26% in the 1 mg triamcinolone group, and 27% in the 4 mg triamcinolone group). However, patients who received either dose of steroid were more likely to develop a cataract or elevated intraocular pressure than those who received laser treatment. In the GENEVA study, a biodegradable dexamethasone intravitreal implant (Ozurdex, Allergan, Irvine, CA, USA) demonstrated efficacy in treating macular edema from BRVO with much less intraocular pressure elevation or cataract progression than was reported with triamcinolone.[3,4]

10. **What is the role of macular grid laser in the treatment of macular edema secondary to branch retinal vein occlusion?**
    The Branch Vein Occlusion Study is a historic multicenter, randomized, controlled clinical trial designed to answer whether argon macular grid laser photocoagulation is useful in improving visual acuity in eyes with a BRVO and macular edema that reduced vision to 20/40 or worse. The study found that 65% of eyes treated with macular grid laser compared to 37% of control eyes gained two or more lines of vision. The investigators recommended macular grid laser for patients with a BRVO of at least 3 months' duration and vision 20/40 or worse secondary to macular edema. Although the results of this study may seem outdated in the modern era of anti-VEGF pharmacotherapy, there is still a distinct role for macular grid laser treatment, either alone or as an adjunct to intravitreal therapy.[3,5]

11. **What is the treatment for a patient with an ischemic branch retinal vein occlusion before the development of neovascularization?**
    A second arm of the Branch Vein Occlusion Study was designed to determine whether peripheral sectoral scatter argon laser photocoagulation in the distribution of the vein occlusion can prevent the development of retinal neovascularization and VH. Significantly less neovascularization developed in patients treated with laser (19%) than in control patients (31%). Although the Branch Vein Occlusion Study was not designed to determine whether peripheral scatter laser treatment should be applied before rather than after the development of neovascularization, data accumulated in the study suggested that there was minimal risk for severe vision loss if laser treatment was performed after the development of neovascularization. Thus, the authors did not advocate for prophylactic laser.[6]

12. **What is the treatment for a patient with an ischemic branch retinal vein occlusion after the development of neovascularization?**

    The Branch Vein Occlusion Study determined that peripheral sectoral scatter argon laser photocoagulation in the distribution of the vein occlusion can prevent VH in patients who have already developed neovascularization. Patients treated with laser developed VH significantly less often (29%) compared to the control patients (61%).[6]

KEY POINTS: WORKUP TO CONSIDER IN PATIENTS WITH BRVO

1. Blood pressure
2. Hemoglobin A_1C, fasting blood glucose
3. Lipid profile
4. Prothrombin time/partial thromboplastin time
5. Hypercoagulable panel (e.g., protein C activity, protein S activity, homocysteine, antiphospholipid antibody, antithrombin III, factor V Leiden)

CENTRAL RETINAL VEIN OCCLUSION

1. **What are the symptoms of a central retinal vein occlusion?**

    Patients may complain of sudden, painless loss of vision. A patient who has developed neovascular glaucoma (NVG) secondary to ischemic central retinal vein occlusion (CRVO) may present with complaints of a painful red eye.

2. **What are the clinical signs of a central retinal vein occlusion?**

    In an acute CRVO, dilated fundus examination reveals certain characteristic findings: tortuosity and dilation of the central retinal vein, intraretinal hemorrhages throughout all four quadrants, cotton-wool spots, optic disc edema, and/or macular edema (Figs 47.2 and 47.3). Increased intraocular pressure or even frank open-angle glaucoma

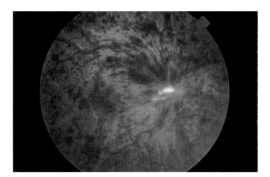

Fig. 47.2 Nonischemic central retinal vein occlusion with dilated tortuous veins, prominent disc edema, intraretinal hemorrhages in four quadrants, and macular edema.

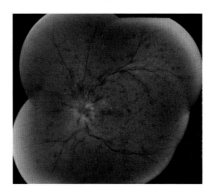

Fig. 47.3 Ischemic central retinal vein occlusion with dilated tortuous veins, extensive intraretinal hemorrhages in four quadrants, and macular edema.

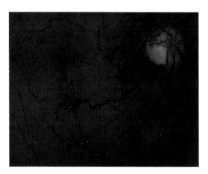

Fig. 47.4 Disc and retinal collaterals that have formed in the setting of a long-standing central retinal vein occlusion.

may be noted in a patient presenting with an acute CRVO. Cases of ischemic CRVO can develop anterior-segment or posterior-segment neovascularization, which manifests as proliferating new vessels on the iris, angle, disc, or retina. In a long-standing CRVO, patients may develop disc or retinal venous collaterals (Fig. 47.4).

KEY POINTS: COMMON CHARACTERISTICS OF A CRVO

1. Intraretinal hemorrhages in all four quadrants
2. Dilated tortuous retinal veins
3. Cotton-wool spots
4. Disc edema
5. Macular edema

3. **What are the risk factors for a central retinal vein occlusion?**
   The Eye Disease Case–Control Study Group identified a number of risk factors for CRVO: hypertension, diabetes mellitus, and glaucoma. Oral contraceptives and diuretics have also been implicated in causing CRVO. Other systemic conditions that affect the retinal vasculature or clotting mechanisms may also be associated with CRVO: blood dyscrasias (i.e., polycythemia vera), hypercoagulable states (i.e., protein C/S deficiencies), or autoimmune/inflammatory diseases. Notably, hyperviscosity retinopathy is a bilateral condition that can mimic CRVO; however, it is due to an underlying systemic dysproteinemia, such as Waldenstrom macroglobulinemia or multiple myeloma.[7]

4. **How is a central retinal vein occlusion categorized?**
   A CRVO is classified as either ischemic or nonischemic. A nonischemic CRVO is defined as having fewer than 10 disc areas of capillary nonperfusion as demonstrated by fluorescein angiography, whereas an ischemic CRVO is defined as having more than 10 disc areas of capillary nonperfusion (Fig. 47.5). Clinically, ischemic CRVO tends to be associated with poor vision, an afferent pupillary defect, and dense central scotoma.[8] Clinically, it is nearly impossible to determine if a CRVO is ischemic or nonischemic. A fluorescein angiogram is necessary to classify and thus determine prognosis and treatment.

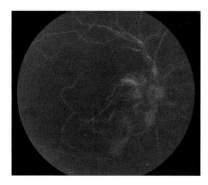

Fig. 47.5 Fluorescein angiogram of an ischemic central retinal vein occlusion demonstrating extensive retinal nonperfusion involving the macula.

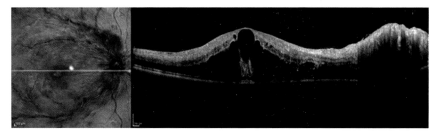

Fig. 47.6 Spectral-domain optical coherence tomography scan demonstrating macular and disc edema associated with central retinal vein occlusion.

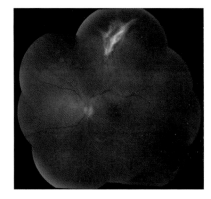

Fig. 47.7 Ischemic central retinal vein occlusion that has developed secondary neovascular membranes superiorly with associated traction and early vitreous hemorrhage.

5. **What are the complications of a central retinal vein occlusion?**
   Patients with a nonischemic CRVO can lose vision due to macular edema (Fig. 47.6). Patients with an ischemic CRVO can lose vision from macular edema, ischemic maculopathy, NVG, and VH. If ischemia occurs in the macula, the patient complains of central vision loss, and a fluorescein angiogram will demonstrate an enlarged and irregular foveal avascular zone. The most feared complication of an ischemic CRVO is anterior-segment neovascularization, which can lead to NVG. Approximately 15% of patients with an ischemic CRVO develop NVE or disc. Traction from the vitreous may cause these new vessels to bleed, leading to VH and decreased vision (Fig. 47.7).[9]

6. **What is the most important risk factor for development of iris neovascularization in central retinal vein occlusion?**
   The Central Vein Occlusion Study (CVOS) determined that poor presenting visual acuity is the most important risk factor predictive of iris neovascularization.[10]

7. **What is the proposed pathophysiologic basis for development of a combined cilioretinal artery occlusion and central retinal vein occlusion?**
   In an acute CRVO, increased venous intraluminal pressure is transmitted upstream to the feeding capillary bed. This increase in pressure carries over to the typically low-pressure cilioretinal artery system (which is unable to autoregulate), resulting in a transient blockage and, thus, a cilioretinal artery occlusion (Fig. 47.8).

8. **What is the treatment for an uncomplicated central retinal vein occlusion?**
   Patients with a nonischemic CRVO without macular edema are followed clinically for the development of macular edema and for progression into an ischemic CRVO and its complications, including ischemic maculopathy, NVG, and VH. These patients should be monitored at monthly intervals for potential progression and for at least 6 months for the development of anterior-segment neovascularization/NVG.

9. **What is the first-line treatment for a patient with a central retinal vein occlusion and macular edema?**
   As with BRVO, intravitreal anti-VEGF injections are the mainstay treatment for macular edema secondary to CRVO. In the CRUISE study (counterpart to the BRAVO study), patients were randomized to receive monthly injections of either 0.3 or 0.5 mg ranibizumab for 6 months versus sham injections. After 6 months, patients

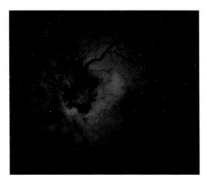

Fig. 47.8 Combined central retinal vein occlusion and cilioretinal artery occlusion.

who received 0.3 mg ranibizumab had a mean gain from baseline of 12.7 letters, those who received 0.5 mg ranibizumab gained 14.9 letters, and the sham group gained 0.8 letters. Ophthalmologists have extrapolated these results to bevacizumab (Avastin, Genentech), a cheaper off-label alternative, which has been demonstrated to reduce macular edema in a number of smaller uncontrolled studies. More recently, a third anti-VEGF drug, aflibercept (Eylea, Regeneron, Tarrytown, NY, USA), has been approved for the indication of macular edema secondary to CRVO. In the nearly identical COPERNICUS and GALILEO studies, patients received 6-monthly injections of aflibercept at a dose of 2 mg versus sham injections. In the COPERNICUS trial, 56.1% of patients receiving aflibercept gained at least 15 letters of vision from baseline, compared with 12.3% of patients receiving sham injections. In the GALILEO study, 60.2% of patients receiving aflibercept gained at least 15 letters of vision from baseline, compared with 22.1% of patients receiving sham injections.[11–13] Use of intravitreal bevacizumab was shown to be noninferior to aflibercept in terms of visual acuity outcomes in the head-to-head SCORE2 comparison trial. In this study, patients were randomized 1:1 to receive either 1.25 mg bevacizumab or 2.0 mg aflibercept every 4 weeks through 6 months. At month 6, there was a mean vision improvement from baseline of 18.9 letters in the aflibercept group compared to 18.6 letters in the bevacizumab group, which met the criteria for noninferiority between both treatments. Both treatment arms additionally showed significant reductions in OCT subfield thickness measurements from baseline by month 6 (mean decrease of 425 microns with aflibercept compared to 387 microns with bevacizumab).[14]

10. What is the role of intravitreal steroids in the treatment of macular edema secondary to central retinal vein occlusion?
In the SCORE-CRVO study, more patients experienced an improvement of 15 ETDRS letters or more after 1 year in the 1 mg triamcinolone (27% of patients) and 4 mg triamcinolone (26%) groups compared to only 7% of patients in the observation group. In the GENEVA study, a biodegradable dexamethasone intravitreal implant (Ozurdex, Allergan) demonstrated efficacy in improving visual acuity outcomes and reducing macular edema from CRVO, with a lower incidence of elevated intraocular pressure or cataract progression than was previously reported with triamcinolone.[4,15]

11. What is the role of macular grid laser in the treatment of macular edema secondary to central retinal vein occlusion?
The CVOS was a multicentered, randomized, controlled clinical trial designed to answer whether argon macular grid laser photocoagulation was useful in improving visual acuity in eyes with a CRVO and macular edema that reduced vision to 20/50 or worse. Patients were randomized to macular grid photocoagulation or no treatment. Although the grid laser treatment reduced angiographic evidence of macular edema, there was no improvement in final visual acuity compared to untreated eyes. However, a trend was observed that revealed that grid laser treatment may be beneficial in younger patients. Taking the results together, the study investigators did not recommend routine macular grid photocoagulation for patients with macular edema secondary to CRVO.[16]

KEY POINTS: WORKUP TO CONSIDER IN PATIENTS WITH CRVO

1. Blood pressure
2. Hemoglobin A_1C, fasting blood glucose
3. Lipid profile
4. Prothrombin time/partial thromboplastin time
5. Hypercoagulable panel (e.g., protein C activity, protein S activity, homocysteine, antiphospholipid antibody, lupus anticoagulant, antithrombin III, factor V Leiden)
6. Consider hemoglobin electrophoresis, cryoglobulins, and serum protein electrophoresis if clinically indicated

12. What is the treatment for a patient with an ischemic central retinal vein occlusion?

The CVOS was also designed to answer whether scatter panretinal argon laser photocoagulation could prevent the development of anterior-segment neovascularization and NVG. Although prophylactic laser decreased the incidence of anterior-segment neovascularization, 20% of study participants still developed neovascularization despite the prophylactic treatment. Additionally, waiting to perform laser until the time of development of anterior-segment neovascularization was shown to be effective in preventing subsequent NVG. Thus, the study investigators recommended careful follow-up of patients with an ischemic CRVO and panretinal photocoagulation only once a patient develops 2 clock hours of iris neovascularization or any angle neovascularization. In modern clinical practice, however, panretinal photocoagulation is often performed at the first sign of iris neovascularization.[9,17]

ACKNOWLEDGMENTS

We acknowledge Vernon K.W. Wong, chapter author from the previous edition.

REFERENCES

1. The Eye Disease Case-Control Study Group: Risk factors for branch retinal vein occlusion, Arch Ophthalmol 116:286–296, 1993.
2. BRAVO Investigators: Ranibizumab for macular edema following branch retinal vein occlusion: six-month primary end point results of a phase III study, Ophthalmology 117:1102–1112.e1, 2010.
3. SCORE Study Research Group: A randomized trial comparing the efficacy and safety of intravitreal triamcinolone with standard care to treat vision loss associated with macular Edema secondary to branch retinal vein occlusion: the Standard Care vs Corticosteroid for Retinal Vein Occlusion (SCORE) study report 6, Arch Ophthalmol 127:1115–1128, 2009.
4. Ozurdex GENEVA Study Group: Randomized, sham-controlled trial of dexamethasone intravitreal implant in patients with macular edema due to retinal vein occlusion, Ophthalmology 117:1134–1146, 2010.
5. Branch Vein Occlusion Study Group: Argon laser photocoagulation for macular edema in branch vein occlusion, Am J Ophthalmol 98:271–282, 1984.
6. Branch Vein Occlusion Study Group: Argon laser scatter photocoagulation for prevention of neovascularization and vitreous hemorrhage in branch vein occlusion, Arch Ophthalmol 104:34–41, 1996.
7. The Eye Disease Case-Control Study Group: Risk factors for central retinal vein occlusion, Arch Ophthalmol 114:545–554, 1996.
8. Central Vein Occlusion Study Group: Baseline and early natural history report: the central vein occlusion study, Arch Ophthalmol 111:1087–1095, 1993.
9. Central Vein Occlusion Study Group: A randomized clinical trial of early panretinal photocoagulation for ischemic central vein occlusion: the central vein occlusion study group N report, Ophthalmology 102:1434–1444, 1995.
10. The Central Vein Occlusion Study: Baseline and early natural history report, Arch Ophthalmol 111:1087–1095, 1993.
11. CRUISE Investigators: Ranibizumab for macular edema following central retinal vein occlusion: six-month primary end point results of a phase III study, Ophthalmology 117:1124–1133, 2010.
12. COPERNICUS Study. Vascular endothelial growth factor trap-eye for macular edema secondary to central retinal vein occlusion: six-month results of the phase 3 COPERNICUS study, Ophthalmology 119:1024–1032, 2012.
13. GALILEO Study. VEGF trap-eye for macular oedema secondary to central retinal vein occlusion: 6-month results of the phase III GALILEO study, Br J Ophthalmol 97:278–284, 2013.
14. SCORE2 Investigator Group: Effect of bevacizumab vs aflibercept on visual acuity among patients with macular edema due to central retinal vein occlusion. The SCORE2 randomized clinical trial, JAMA 317:2072–2087, 2017.
15. SCORE Study Research Group: A randomized trial comparing the efficacy and safety of intravitreal triamcinolone with observation to treat vision loss associated with macular edema secondary to central retinal vein occlusion: the standard care vs corticosteroid for retinal vein occlusion (SCORE) study report 5, Arch Ophthalmol 127:1101–1114, 2009.
16. Central Vein Occlusion Study Group: Evaluation of grid pattern photocoagulation for macular edema in central vein occlusion: the central vein occlusion study group M report, Ophthalmology 102:1425–1433, 1995.
17. Clarkson JG, Coscas G, Finkelstein D, et al.: The CVOS group M and N reports [letter], Ophthalmology 103:350–354, 1996.

CHAPTER 48

RETINAL DETACHMENT

James F. Vander and Michael J. Borne

1. **What is retinal detachment?**
   Retinal detachment (RD) is separation of the neurosensory retina from the underlying retinal pigment epithelium with accumulation of fluid in the potential space between the two layers. The types of RD include rhegmatogenous, tractional, and exudative.
   - In **rhegmatogenous retinal detachment (RRD)**, a break in the retina allows fluid from the vitreous cavity access to the potential space between the retina and the retinal pigment epithelium.
   - **Tractional retinal detachment** occurs when epiretinal tissue forms and contracts, pulling the retina away from the pigment epithelial layer. Occasionally, the severe traction caused by epiretinal membranes may cause a tear in the retina, creating a combined rhegmatogenous–tractional detachment.
   - **Exudative retinal detachment** is produced by retinal and choroidal conditions that damage the blood–retina barrier and allow fluid to accumulate in the subretinal space (the potential space between the retina and the retinal pigment epithelium).

2. **What are the major characteristics of each type of retinal detachment?**
   - **Rhegmatogenous retinal detachments** typically have a corrugated appearance caused by intraretinal edema (Fig. 48.1). Obviously, they are associated with a retinal break, although in a small percentage of cases, the break is not easily identifiable. Decreased intraocular pressure, pigmented cells in the vitreous cavity, and vitreous hemorrhage are also associated with RRDs. Fixed folds and other signs of proliferative vitreoretinopathy (PVR) strongly suggest an RRD. Extension of fluid through the macula is a poor prognostic sign. The intraocular pressure is usually low.
   - **Tractional retinal detachments** are characterized by a stiff-appearing retinal surface. In most cases, the epiretinal membranes that cause the traction may be ophthalmoscopically observed. The detachment is usually concave toward the front of the eye. The most common location of the tractional membranes is in the postequatorial region; the traction detachment rarely extends to the ora serrata.
   - **Exudative retinal detachments** are characterized by shifting subretinal fluid. The subretinal fluid accumulates according to gravitational forces and detaches the retina in the area, where it accumulates. Thus, the fluid is noted to shift when the patient is viewed in an upright compared with a supine position. The surface of the retina is usually smooth in exudative detachments, compared with the corrugated appearance of an RRD. Occasionally, the retina may be seen directly behind the lens in exudative detachments. This rarely occurs in RRDs, unless severe vitreoretinal traction is present.

3. **What are the major causes of exudative retinal detachments?**
   The major causes of exudative RDs are intraocular tumors, intraocular inflammatory diseases, and congenital abnormalities. Intraocular neoplasms, such as choroidal melanomas, choroidal hemangiomas, and metastatic choroidal tumors, are most likely to produce serous RDs. Intraocular inflammation, such as posterior scleritis, Harada's disease, severe posterior uveitis, and central serous chorioretinopathy, occasionally produce shifting subretinal fluid. The most common congenital abnormalities known to produce exudative RDs are optic pits, nanophthalmos, and the morning glory disc syndrome.

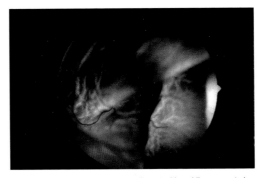

Fig. 48.1 Bullous rhegmatogenous retinal detachment with mobile, corrugated appearance.

4. **How does the retina remain attached?**
The retinal photoreceptors and retinal pigment epithelial (RPE) cells are oriented with the apices of the cells in apposition. An interphotoreceptor matrix between the cells forms a "glue" that helps maintain cellular apposition. It also has been postulated that the RPE functions as a cellular pump to remove ions and water from the interphotoreceptor matrix, providing a "suction force" that helps to keep the retina attached.

5. **What are the major predisposing factors for rhegmatogenous retinal detachments?**
The main predisposing factors for RRDs are previous cataract surgery, lattice degeneration, and myopia. The incidence of RRD after cataract surgery is approximately 2 in 1000. The incidence becomes much higher after complicated cataract surgery, including posterior capsule rupture, vitreous loss, and retained lens fragments. Some studies have shown an incidence of RRD after complicated cataract surgery as high as 15%. Approximately half of all primary RRDs occur in patients with a history of cataract surgery.
    Lattice degeneration (Fig. 48.2) is a peripheral retinal degeneration characterized by thinning of the retina with liquefaction of the overlying vitreous, which results in a high risk for retinal tears and breaks. Lattice degeneration is found in 6% to 7% of the population and is often bilateral. Lattice degeneration is the direct cause of primary RRD in approximately 25% of eyes.
    High myopes have a high risk of RD for several reasons. First, the incidence of lattice degeneration is higher in myopes. Second, myopes tend to have a higher rate of posterior vitreous detachment. Of greater importance, myopic eyes have a higher rate of retinal breaks because of the thin peripheral retina. The rate of retinal breaks tends to be higher with increasing myopia.

6. **What are the signs and symptoms of a retinal break?**
Flashes and floaters are the classic symptoms. Pigmented cells or blood in the vitreous strongly suggests the possibility of a retinal break.

7. **What are the types of retinal breaks?**
- **Horseshoe tear:** A flap of retina created by vitreous traction gives the appearance of a horseshoe. The open end of the horseshoe is anterior. A retinal vessel may bridge the gap of the tear (Figs. 48.3 and 48.4). The risk of subsequent RD is high, especially with acute tears.

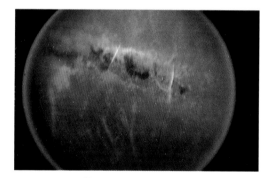

Fig. 48.2 Lattice degeneration.

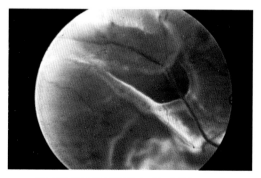

Fig. 48.3 Horseshoe retinal tear with a bridging vessel.

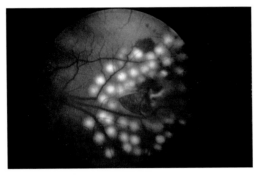

Fig. 48.4 Horseshoe retinal tear after laser photocoagulation.

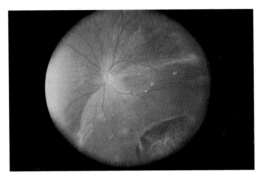

Fig. 48.5 Retinal detachment resulting from inferotemporal dialysis.

- **Operculated tear:** When a piece of retina is completely torn away by vitreous traction, the fragment is seen floating over the retinal defect. The risk of RD is lower than with a horseshoe tear.
- **Atrophic hole:** A round hole without evidence of retinal traction is often associated with lattice degeneration. The risk of RD is low.
- **Dialysis** (Fig. 48.5): A disinsertion of the retina at the ora serrata, which is most common in the inferotemporal quadrant. The second most common site is superonasal. A frequent cause is trauma.

KEY POINTS: SYMPTOMS AND SIGNS OF RRD

1. Flashes
2. Floaters
3. Pigment in the vitreous
4. Posterior vitreous detachment (usually)
5. Elevated mobile retina
6. Corrugations
7. Loss of retinal transparency
8. Presence of a retinal break
9. RPE alterations under detachment, i.e., a demarcation line
10. Fixed folds
11. Peripheral visual field loss
12. Loss of central vision (with macular involvement)

8. **What are the signs of a chronic rhegmatogenous retinal detachment?**
   The retina is more transparent than in an acute RD, and the corrugations are minimal or absent. Pigmentary alterations are more prominent, including hyperpigmented demarcation lines (indicative of progression if multiple), RPE atrophy in the bed of the detachment, and abundant pigment in the vitreous. Retinal cysts, sometimes very large, may develop. The causative retinal break may be difficult to identify. PVR may also be present. The intraocular pressure may be low, normal, or high.

9. What is degenerative retinoschisis?

Sometimes called senile retinoschisis, this is a dome-shaped elevation of the inner retina caused by a splitting within the outer plexiform layer. In contrast to an RRD, this rarely progresses and is usually observed. Occasionally, outer wall holes will form and create a progressive retinoschisis-related RRD. The inferotemporal quadrant is most commonly affected, and 80% are bilateral.

KEY POINTS: SIGNS OF CHRONIC RD VERSUS RETINOSCHISIS

1. Presence of retinal break is the most reliable method to distinguish the two but is often difficult to find
2. Pigment in the vitreous
3. Pigment alterations in the retinal pigment epithelium
4. Retinal folds
5. Absence of schisis in the fellow eye

10. What are the options for repair of retinal detachment?

First, determining the type of RD is important before identifying the modality of treatment. Exudative RDs are approached differently compared with rhegmatogenous or traction detachments. Exudative detachments are repaired by treating the primary cause of the fluid extravasation into the subretinal space. For example, an RD associated with choroidal melanoma is addressed by treating the tumor with radiation, thermotherapy, or resection. Exudative RDs related to intraocular inflammatory conditions are generally treated by aggressive anti-inflammatory regimens. Rarely does an exudative detachment require primary surgical repair.

On the other hand, treatment of rhegmatogenous and tractional RD is primarily surgical. Tractional RDs caused by diabetes or PVR require relief of all traction membranes before the retina will reattach.

Small, localized RRDs are usually treated by cryotherapy or barrier laser photocoagulation. Rarely, an asymptomatic localized detachment may be treated with close observation only. More definitive treatment is usually indicated if significant vitreous traction is present on the retinal tear, especially if the tear is superior in location, or if a large amount of subretinal fluid is found. Options include pneumatic retinopexy, Lincoff balloon, scleral buckling, and pars plana vitrectomy. Scleral buckling surgery is the time-honored approach and has been applied routinely since the 1950s. Pars plana vitrectomy was first performed in the late 1960s and has become the operation of choice for some surgeons. Pneumatic retinopexy has gained popularity since the early 1980s.

11. What is pneumatic retinopexy?

To perform a pneumatic retinopexy, inert gas or sterile air is injected into the vitreous cavity. Strict positioning is required to place the gas bubble in contact with the retinal break. If the break is closed by the surface tension from the gas bubble, the retinal pigment epithelium can pump the subretinal fluid back into the choroid and allow the retina to reattach. The break is sealed either with cryotherapy at the time of gas injection or with laser photocoagulation after the retina is flattened.

12. Which patients are the best candidates for pneumatic retinopexy?

The ideal candidates are patients with a detachment caused by a single retinal break in the superior eight clock hours or multiple breaks if all of the tears are within one to two clock hours of one another. Obviously the patient must not have a systemic disease or mechanical problem that precludes the positioning requirements. Phakic patients tend to fare slightly better than patients with a history of cataract surgery.

13. Which patients are poor candidates for pneumatic retinopexy?

Patients with RDs caused by multiple tears in several locations are generally not good candidates. PVR, especially if fixed folds are present, lessens the chances for reattachment with pneumatic retinopexy. And, as previously stated, patients who are unable to obey the strict postoperative positioning requirements are poor candidates.

KEY POINTS: FACTORS THAT INFLUENCE THE DECISION TO TREAT RETINAL BREAKS PROPHYLACTICALLY

1. Type of break
2. Presence of symptoms of vitreoretinal traction
3. Horseshoe tears are usually treated, especially if symptomatic
4. Operculated tears are generally not treated unless symptomatic
5. History of RD in the fellow eye
6. Family history of RD
7. Anticipated prolonged inaccessibility to care

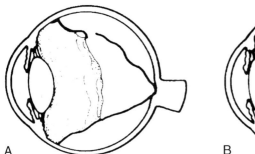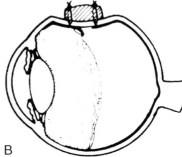

A   B

Fig. 48.6 Placement of a scleral buckle. **A,** Rhegmatogenous retinal detachment. **B,** The retina is attached after placement of a scleral buckle superiorly.

14. **What are the advantages of scleral buckling and pars plana vitrectomy?**
    Scleral buckling and pars plana vitrectomy reduce vitreous traction mechanically. Scleral buckling involves the surgical placement of a silicone band or sponge, either sewn to the sclera as an exoplant or implanted in the sclera after a partial-thickness scleral bed is surgically created (Fig. 48.6). Scleral buckles provide smooth, broad relief of vitreous traction. Subretinal fluid may be drained at the time of placement of the scleral buckle via an external sclerostomy, and intraocular gas may be injected into the vitreous cavity as an adjunct to aid in retinal reattachment. Scleral buckles are especially effective in anterior retinal breaks. This is the most common site for postcataract retinal breaks. Another advantage of scleral buckling is the opportunity to repair the RD from a purely external approach with no intraocular invasion.
    With vitrectomy, it is possible to relieve vitreous traction directly with the vitrectomy cutter. This technique is especially useful in cases with very posterior breaks. Vitrectomy is advantageous in cases of RD with vitreous hemorrhage or vitreous opacities that obscure a view of the retinal breaks. Vitrectomy also allows the surgeon to remove epiretinal membranes when PVR is present. When vitrectomy is performed, the vitreous cavity must be filled with gas, or silicone oil, to keep the retina attached. The presence of intravitreal gas hastens the development of cataract in phakic patients.

15. **What are the major risks and complications with scleral buckling and pars plana vitrectomy?**
    Risks of infection and hemorrhage are found with any invasive ocular procedure. The risk of an infection with a scleral buckle is less than 3%. Other risks and complications from scleral buckles include angle-closure glaucoma, acute glaucoma from intraocular gas injection, intraocular hemorrhage from perforation during drainage of subretinal fluid, and anterior-segment ischemia and necrosis. The surgically placed buckles may cause extrusion or intrusion over time, and, if the buckle is placed under an extraocular muscle, strabismus may result.
    Vitrectomy involves the risks of endophthalmitis, iatrogenic retinal breaks, retinal or vitreous incarceration in the sclerostomy sites, and glaucoma from the use of intraocular gases.

16. **What intraoperative findings should be confirmed at the time of scleral buckle placement?**
    The most important intraoperative decisions at the time of scleral buckling procedures are to find and treat all retinal tears and place the scleral buckle in a position to support all retinal breaks. After the buckle has been temporarily placed, the surgeon should confirm that the tears are flat on the buckle or will be once subretinal is reabsorbed or drained. If the buckle is in the appropriate position but fluid still exists between the retina and the buckle, the decision to drain subretinal fluid or to inject an intravitreal gas bubble should be made. If the detachment is primarily inferior in location, most surgeons prefer to have the retina completely attached before leaving the operating room. Superior detachments may flatten with gas injection and postoperative positioning; the decision to drain subretinal fluid adds potential complications.

17. **What three factors should be confirmed with indirect ophthalmoscopy at the conclusion of scleral buckling surgery?**
    Proper placement of the scleral buckle relative to the retinal breaks, absence of complications at the drainage site, and absence of central retinal artery pulsations should be confirmed before final closure. If pulsations are present, the intraocular pressure is high enough to cause a central retinal artery obstruction. The pressure should be lowered by loosening the buckle and/or removing intraocular fluid or gas until pulsations are no longer seen.

18. **How should cases of rhegmatogenous retinal detachment be approached if pars plana vitrectomy is the chosen treatment?**
    Relieve vitreous traction on all retinal breaks if possible. Take care to avoid damaging retinal blood vessels, if they are coursing across the retinal tears. Use wide-field illumination to ensure a complete posterior vitreous detachment and meticulous removal of peripheral vitreous. Treat all retinal tears completely with laser.

19. **Which gases may be used inside the eye? In what concentrations?**
    The inert gases sulfur hexafluoride (SF_6) and perfluoropropane (C_3F_8), along with sterile air, are the most commonly used intraocular gases. Nonexpansile mixtures are composed of approximately 20% sulfur hexafluoride and 14% perfluoropropane. These are the most commonly used mixtures when the vitreous cavity is filled with gas, as in vitrectomy. Pure 100% gas injection allows a larger bubble to form with a smaller volume of injection. This technique is advantageous in patients with pneumatic retinopexy and scleral buckles. Typically, sulfur hexafluoride expands to two to three times its initial volume, and perfluoropropane expands to approximately four times its initial volume. Thus, injection of 0.4 mL of each gas produces a 20% to 40% intravitreal gas bubble when they are injected as a pure concentration.

20. **What are the primary causes of failure of initial retinal detachment repair?**
    Except for cases of severe PVR, in which epiretinal membranes cause traction RDs (Fig. 48.7), failures of RD repair are caused by an open retinal break. With pneumatic retinopexy, the most common reasons for failure include poor patient compliance with positioning requirements, inadequate identification of all retinal breaks, and development of new retinal tears from ongoing vitreous traction. After scleral buckling surgery, failure to flatten the retina or to keep it attached results most often from undetected retinal breaks; continued vitreous traction with new, extended, or reopened retinal breaks; or a misplaced scleral buckle. The most common reasons for failure after a pars plana vitrectomy are inadequate photocoagulation, continued vitreous traction, and new or missed breaks. Ten percent of retinal reattachments have evidence of PVR. However, only 10% to 25% of these progress to require treatment for detachment.

21. **What are the major objectives in repair of tractional retinal detachment?**
    When tractional RDs are caused by proliferative diabetic retinopathy (Fig. 48.8), one of the major aims is to relieve all anteroposterior traction. Create a complete posterior vitreous separation to remove or segment all retinal traction. Segmentation of diabetic tractional membranes is effective if no anterior traction remains (Fig. 48.9). Delamination of traction membranes is accomplished by carefully identifying the plane between the epiretinal tissue and the retina and by lysing all adhesions. In advanced PVR, retinal traction may be so severe that the retina must be cut to relieve all retinal traction. In cases with such severe traction, especially when a retinotomy must be created, silicone oil is often useful as a long-acting tamponade. The silicone oil is usually removed after 3 to 6 months but may be left in place longer if the retina appears unstable.

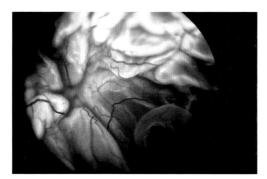

Fig. 48.7 Severe proliferative vitreoretinopathy with total retinal detachment.

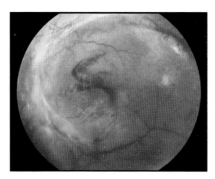

Fig. 48.8 Proliferative diabetic retinopathy causing tractional retinal detachment.

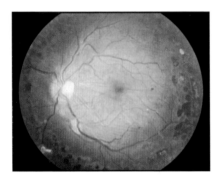

Fig. 48.9 Postoperative appearance of the patient shown in Fig. 48.8 after repair of traction retinal detachment.

BIBLIOGRAPHY

Benson WE: Retinal detachment: diagnosis and management, ed 2, Philadelphia, J.B. Lippincott.

Davis MD: Natural history of retinal breaks without detachment, Arch Ophthalmol 92:183–194, 1974.

Hilton GF, McLean EB, Chuang EL: Retinal detachment: ophthalmology monograph series, San Francisco, American Academy of Ophthalmology.

Kramer SG, Benson WE: Prophylactic therapy of retinal breaks, Surv Ophthalmol 22:41–47, 1977.

CHAPTER 49

RETINOBLASTOMA

Carol L. Shields

1. What is retinoblastoma?

   Retinoblastoma (Rb) is the most common eye cancer in children. This malignancy arises from primitive cells destined to be retinal tissue. Generally, Rb is found in babies from birth to approximately 3 years old. Only 5% are detected in patients over 5 years old.

2. How common is retinoblastoma?

   Rb occurs with a frequency of about 1 in 14,000 live births. Approximately 250 to 300 children in the United States each year are diagnosed with Rb. Worldwide, it is estimated that there are approximately 7000 children with this cancer yearly.

3. What causes retinoblastoma?

   Rb is a result of a genetic mutation on chromosome 13q14 locus. If the mutation is somatic, then the child can develop one tumor in one eye. If the mutation is germline, then the child is at risk for multifocal tumors in both eyes, with an average total of five retinoblastomas. In addition, germline mutation predisposes the child for brain pinealoblastoma and long-term second cancers. There are no specific exposures that lead to this mutation, but research has identified advanced paternal age or possible paternal radiotherapy exposure as risks.

4. On what chromosome is the genetic mutation associated with retinoblastoma?

   The genetic mutation associated with Rb is found on chromosome 13 in the region 13q14. It is believed that this single locus exists for most forms of Rb. Genetic testing can identify 96% of mutations, whereas 4% remain undetected. A minority of patients who carry germline mutation do not manifest Rb, and this is called "low penetrant" Rb.

5. What syndrome is associated with retinoblastoma?

   Retinoblastoma is a manifestation of the 13q deletion syndrome. The characteristic findings include
   - microcephaly
   - broad prominent nasal bridge
   - hypertelorism
   - microphthalmos
   - epicanthus
   - ptosis
   - protruding upper incisors
   - micrognathia
   - short neck with lateral folds
   - large low-set ears
   - facial asymmetry
   - imperforate anus
   - genital malformations
   - perineal fistula
   - hypoplastic or absent thumbs
   - toe abnormalities
   - psychomotor delay
   - mental delay

6. What is the laterality of retinoblastoma?

   Rb is unilateral in approximately 67% of cases and bilateral in 33% of cases. All bilateral cases have germline mutation. Approximately 15% of unilateral cases have germline mutation, whereas 85% have somatic mutation.

7. What is germline mutation retinoblastoma?

   Germline mutation Rb is the occurrence of the Rb mutation on all cells in the body including the retina and systemic sites. These patients typically develop bilateral Rb and are at risk for pinealoblastoma and second cancers.

8. Who manifests germline mutation retinoblastoma?

   All bilateral and all familial Rb by definition have germline mutation. About 10% to 15% of unilateral sporadic Rb have germline mutation.

9. What is somatic mutation retinoblastoma?
   Somatic mutation Rb is the occurrence of the Rb mutation only in the retina in one clone of cells. Hence, these patients typically develop unilateral sporadic Rb. These patients are generally not at increased risk for pinealoblastoma or second cancers.

10. Who manifests somatic mutation retinoblastoma?
    Only unilateral sporadic retinoblastoma patients carry somatic mutation.

11. What are the most common presenting findings of retinoblastoma? (Fig. 49.1)
    In the United States, leukocoria is the presenting feature in nearly 50% of cases and strabismus in 20%. Other less common presenting features include poor vision, red eye, glaucoma, and orbital mass or pseudocellulitis. In less developed nations, Rb often presents with proptosis from tumor extension into the orbit.

12. What are the most common lesions simulating retinoblastoma?
    Of all patients referred to an experienced ocular oncology center with the diagnosis of possible Rb, about 80% prove to have Rb and 20% have pseudoretinoblastoma. The most common pseudoretinoblastomas include Coats disease (40%), persistent hyperplastic primary vitreous (more commonly called persistent fetal vasculature now) (28%), and vitreous hemorrhage of infancy (16%).

13. At what age does retinoblastoma typically present?
    Rb is diagnosed typically in the first 1 to 2 years of life. Bilateral cases are recognized at an earlier average age of 1 year, whereas unilateral cases are typically older at 2 years. In 5% of cases, the tumor is first diagnosed over age 5 years.

14. What is trilateral retinoblastoma?
    Trilateral Rb is the association of bilateral Rb with midline brain tumors, especially pinealoblastoma. Trilateral disease represents 3% of all Rb cases and typically occurs before the age of 5 years. Trilateral Rb is much less common in this era of systemic chemotherapy for treatment of Rb.

15. When is pinealoblastoma diagnosed?
    Pinealoblastoma is generally diagnosed within 1 year of Rb diagnosis. In fact, most cases are found before the age of 5 years. Keep in mind that benign pineal cyst can resemble malignant pinealoblastoma and magnetic resonance imaging (MRI) is necessary to differentiate these two conditions.

16. What second cancers are associated with retinoblastoma?
    The most common second cancers associated with Rb include osteosarcoma (especially of the femur), cutaneous melanoma, and other sarcomas. Second cancers are believed to be related to germline mutation of

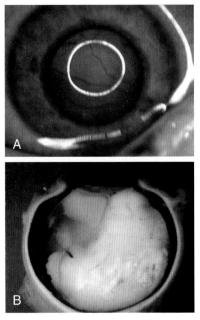

Fig. 49.1 A, Leukocoria from retinoblastoma. **B,** Enucleated globe showing large white retinoblastoma within the eye.

chromosome 13. Second cancers present in approximately 20% of germline-mutation patients by 20 years and 50% by 50 years. There is some evidence that second cancers may be less frequent in this era of intravenous chemotherapy.

17. **How often do eyes with retinoblastoma present with glaucoma?**
    From a clinical standpoint, about 17% of eyes with Rb have glaucoma, most often neovascular or angle-closure glaucoma. From a pathology standpoint, glaucoma is present in 40% of eyes that come to enucleation.

18. **How often does retinoblastoma invade the optic nerve?**
    In the United States, optic nerve invasion by Rb occurs in 29% of eyes that come to enucleation and usually it occurs in the prelaminar area and does not require systemic chemotherapy. If invasion is postlaminar in the optic nerve, then systemic chemotherapy is necessary. Risks for optic nerve invasion by Rb include a large exophytic tumor measuring greater than 15 mm and secondary glaucoma.

19. **What is high-risk retinoblastoma?**
    High-risk Rb is Rb that has invaded
    - the optic nerve beyond the lamina cribrosa
    - the uvea with greatest dimension of 3 mm or greater
    - any combination of optic nerve or uveal invasion
        High-risk Rb requires systemic chemotherapy.

20. **What is the survival rate with retinoblastoma?**
    Currently in the United States, Europe, and Japan, nearly 98% of children with Rb survive this cancer. Less developed nations carry relatively high risk for metastasis and death. The rate for death in South America is approximately 40% and in Africa is 70%. Risks for metastatic disease include substantial optic nerve, choroidal, or orbital invasion by the tumor.

21. **What are the clinical growth patterns of retinoblastoma?**
    The growth patterns of Rb include endophytic and exophytic types. Endophytic Rb invades the inner retina and seeds the vitreous. Exophytic Rb invades the outer retinal layers and extends into the subretinal space, producing retinal detachment. A variant of endophytic Rb is the diffuse infiltrating Rb. These patterns impart no difference to the patient's life prognosis.

22. **What is the differential diagnosis of endophytic retinoblastoma?**
    The differential diagnosis of endophytic Rb includes various inflammatory or infectious processes of the eye in children such as toxocariasis, endophthalmitis, or advanced uveitis.

23. **What is the differential diagnosis of exophytic retinoblastoma?**
    The differential diagnosis of exophytic Rb includes Coats disease, retinal capillary hemangioma, familial exudative vitreoretinopathy, and other causes of rhegmatogenous or nonrhegmatogenous retinal detachment in children.

KEY POINTS: RETINOBLASTOMA

1. Retinoblastoma is an ocular cancer of childhood, usually detected before age 3 years. However, about 5% of newly diagnosed cases are in children over 5 years old.
2. The diagnosis of retinoblastoma must be excluded in any child, even a teenager or young adult, who manifests atypical uveitis, vitreous hemorrhage, or nonrhegmatogenous retinal detachment.
3. Do not perform a vitrectomy or intraocular needle aspiration biopsy on an eye with retinoblastoma. This could seed the tumor into the orbit and lead to metastases.
4. Any child with spontaneous hyphema or vitreous hemorrhage should be evaluated for trauma, retinoblastoma, and other intraocular tumors and inflammations.
5. The best way to diagnose retinoblastoma is with indirect ophthalmoscopy by an experienced observer. If uncertain, ultrasonography, fluorescein angiography, and computed tomography can be useful tests. MRI is most useful for evaluation of tumor invasion into the optic nerve or orbit, as well as assessment of the brain for related intracranial neuroblastic malignancy (trilateral retinoblastoma; pinealoblastoma).

24. **Can retinoblastoma spontaneously regress?**
    Yes, it is estimated that 3% of all cases of Rb are classified as spontaneously regressed or arrested. They are also termed *retinocytoma* and *retinoma*. These tumors do carry 5% risk for demonstrating growth, requiring therapy.

25. **When is genetic testing appropriate?**
    All children with Rb are offered genetic testing to ascertain whether they carry germline or somatic mutation. This affects their follow-up, as germline mutation children are at risk for pinealoblastoma and second cancers, unlike somatic mutation children.

26. How do we classify retinoblastoma?

In the past, the Reese Ellsworth classification scheme was used, but it is now outdated. Currently, the International Classification of Retinoblastoma is used worldwide (Table 49.1). This classification is simple, practical, and pertinent for current therapies.

27. How does retinoblastoma appear on ultrasound?

On ultrasound, Rb appears as a mass originating from the retina with acoustic solidity and high internal reflectivity. Foci of calcium can be seen as dense echoes with shadowing.

28. How does retinoblastoma appear on computed tomography?

On computed tomography, Rb appears as a solid mass within the globe with foci of bone density, representing calcium. Often, retinal detachment can be detected.

29. How does retinoblastoma appear on magnetic resonance imaging?

On MRI, Rb shows a hyperintense signal to the vitreous on T1-weighted images and a hypointense signal on T2. The mass demonstrates contrast enhancement with gadolinium. The foci of calcium remain hypointense on both T1 and T2 without enhancement. Areas of necrosis appear similar to calcium except that they can show enhancement.

30. Should pars plana vitrectomy or biopsy be performed to obtain tissue to confirm the diagnosis of retinoblastoma?

No. Biopsy is not indicated and should not be performed in any eye with Rb, because it can potentially seed the tumor into the orbit and could lead to metastasis.

31. What are the pathology features of a well-differentiated retinoblastoma? (Fig. 49.2)

Flexner-Wintersteiner rosettes and fleurettes represent well-differentiated Rb.

32. List the options for management of an eye with intraocular retinoblastoma.

The options for management include
- enucleation
- intravenous chemotherapy (chemoreduction)
- intra-arterial chemotherapy
- intravitreal chemotherapy

Table 49.1 The International Classification of Retinoblastoma

GROUP	QUICK REMEMBER BY LETTER	DETAILS
A	SmAll	Small Rb (≤ 3 mm diameter)
B	Bigger	Bigger Rb (>3 mm diameter) or • Any Rb in the macula (<3 mm to the foveola) • Any Rb in the juxtapapillary area (<1.5 mm from disc) • Any Rb with subretinal fluid
C	Contained seeds	Localized subretinal or vitreous seeds (≤ 3 mm from Rb)
D	Diffuse seeds	Diffuse subretinal or vitreous seeds (≤ 3 mm from Rb)
E	Extensive	Extensive Rb involving over 50% of the fundus • Opaque media • Neovascularization of iris • Suspicion of invasion of optic nerve, choroid, or orbit

Rb, Retinoblastoma.

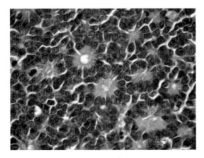

Fig. 49.2 Flexner-Wintersteiner rosettes in well-differentiated retinoblastoma.

- thermotherapy
- cryotherapy
- laser photocoagulation
- plaque radiotherapy
- external beam radiotherapy

33. What are the conservative options for management of a medium-sized retinoblastoma posterior to the equator of the eye?

Intravenous chemotherapy, intra-arterial chemotherapy, or plaque radiotherapy are the most appropriate therapies for this tumor. Occasionally, consolidation with thermotherapy is performed after intravenous chemotherapy. Cryotherapy is generally limited to small tumors anterior to the equator of the eye.

34. What are the conservative options for the management of a medium retinoblastoma anterior to the equator of the eye?

Intravenous chemotherapy with additional thermotherapy or cryotherapy, intra-arterial chemotherapy, or plaque radiotherapy are the most conservative options.

KEY POINTS: MANAGEMENT OF RETINOBLASTOMA

1. The goals in management of retinoblastoma are to first save the patient's life, then save the globe if possible and then preserve or rehabilitate the visual acuity.
2. The most common method for the management of unilateral advanced retinoblastoma (groups D or E) is intra-arterial chemotherapy or enucleation.
3. Most bilateral retinoblastomas can be treated with intravenous chemotherapy. However, enucleation of one eye or intra-arterial chemotherapy is often necessary.
4. Intravitreal chemotherapy is injected directly into the vitreous cavity for active vitreous seeds.
5. Fresh retinoblastoma tissue should be harvested for DNA analysis and family genetic counseling.

35. When do we use intravenous chemotherapy (chemoreduction)? (Fig. 49.3)

Chemoreduction is generally used for patients with bilateral, multifocal Rb to cure the eyes, protect the patient from pinealoblastoma, and minimize long-term second cancers.

36. When do we use intra-arterial chemotherapy? (Fig. 49.4)

Intra-arterial chemotherapy is usually used for unilateral Rb or those that fail intravenous chemotherapy.

37. When do we use intravitreal chemotherapy?

Intravitreal chemotherapy is used for eyes with viable vitreous Rb seeding following failure of standard intravenous or intra-arterial chemotherapy.

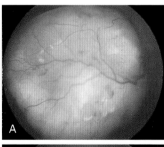

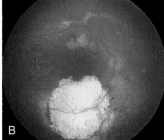

Fig. 49.3 Retinoblastoma **(A)** before and **(B)** after intravenous chemotherapy.

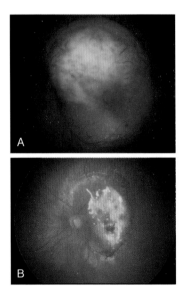

Fig. 49.4 Retinoblastoma **(A)** before and **(B)** after intra-arterial chemotherapy.

38. **When do we use external beam radiotherapy and what are the risks?**
We try to avoid external beam radiotherapy. In the past, it was used for Rb, but now, we avoid this therapy due to its risks for short-term and long-term effects. The short-term effects include
- dry eye
- cilia loss
- cutaneous erythema
    The long-term effects include
- persistent dry eye
- cataract
- retinopathy
- papillopathy
- orbital fat atrophy
- maldevelopment of the orbital bones
- second cancers—which can be fatal

TOP SECRETS

1. Retinoblastoma is the leading eye cancer in children.
2. About 98% of children with retinoblastoma in the United States and developed nations survive due to early detection and proper management.
3. Most children with unilateral retinoblastoma have somatic mutation and are managed with intra-arterial chemotherapy or enucleation.
4. All children with bilateral retinoblastoma have germline mutation and most are managed with intravenous chemotherapy or intra-arterial chemotherapy.

BIBLIOGRAPHY

Kivela T: The epidemiological challenge of the most frequent eye cancer: retinoblastoma, an issue of birth and death, Br J Ophthalmol 93:1129–1131, 2009.
Manjandavida FP, Stathopoulos C, Zhang J, Honavar SG, Shields CL: Intra-arterial chemotherapy in retinoblastoma: a paradigm change, Ind J Ophthalmol 67:740–754,2019.
Ramasubramanian A, Shields CL, editors: Retinoblastoma, New Delhi, India, 2012, Jaypee Brothers Medical Publishers.
Shields CL, Schoenfeld E, Kocher K, et al.: Lesions simulating retinoblastoma (pseudoretinoblastoma) in 604 cases, Ophthalmology 120:311–316, 2013.
Shields JA, Shields CL: Intraocular tumors. An atlas and textbook, ed 3, Philadelphia, 2016, Lippincott Wolters Kluwers.
Shields JA, Shields CL: Intraocular tumors: a text and atlas, Philadelphia, W.B., 1992, Saunders, pp 305–392.

CHAPTER 50

PIGMENTED LESIONS OF THE OCULAR FUNDUS

Carol L. Shields and Jerry A. Shields

1. What are the main differential diagnoses of a relatively flat pigmented ocular fundus lesion?
   - Choroidal nevus
   - Congenital hypertrophy of the retinal pigment epithelium (CHRPE)
   - Choroidal melanoma, diffuse type
   - Subretinal or sub–retinal pigment epithelium (RPE) hemorrhage

2. What ophthalmoscopic and imaging features help to differentiate choroidal nevus, CHRPE, melanoma, and subretinal, sub-RPE hemorrhage?
   Choroidal nevus is typically a slate-gray color, often with overlying drusen or RPE alterations, hypoautofluorescent, and with outer retinal thinning and atrophy on optical coherence tomography (OCT) (Fig. 50.1). CHRPE is usually dark black, with crisply demarcated border, depigmented lacunae, darkly hypoautofluorescent, and flat on OCT (Fig. 50.2). Melanoma tends to show overlying subretinal fluid on OCT and orange pigment on autofluorescence, without drusen (Fig. 50.3). Subretinal/sub-RPE hemorrhage tends to show abrupt margins with layering of red blood and occasionally old yellow de-hemoglobinized blood in the subretinal or sub-RPE space (Fig. 50.4).

3. Do both choroidal nevus and CHRPE have malignant potential?
   Yes, although both lesions are benign and usually stationary, nevus can give rise to melanoma. CHRPE can show slow enlargement in diameter in >80% cases, but this occurs over many years. Additionally, CHRPE can rarely evolve into RPE adenocarcinoma.

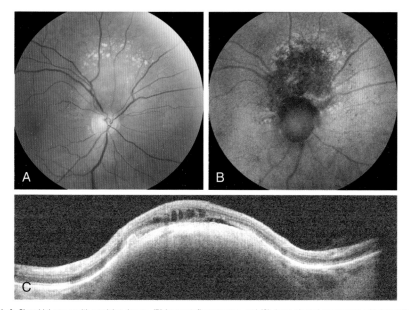

Fig. 50.1 A, Choroidal nevus with overlying drusen, **(B)** hypoautofluorescence, and **(C)** dome-shaped appearance with intraretinal edema and trace subretinal fluid on optical coherence tomography.

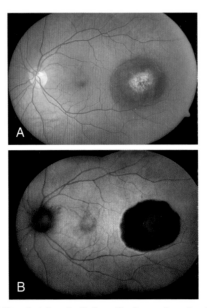

Fig. 50.2 A, Congenital hypertrophy of the retinal pigment epithelium with crisp margins and central lacunae. **B,** Characteristic dark hypoautofluorescence,

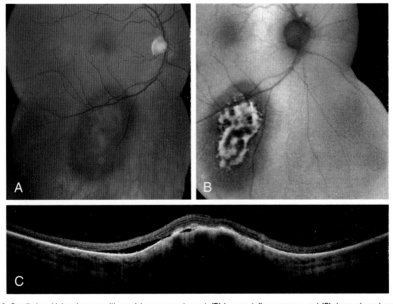

Fig. 50.3 A, Small choroidal melanoma with overlying orange pigment, **(B)** hyperautofluorescence, and **(C)** dome-shaped appearance with subretinal fluid on optical coherence tomography.

4. What are the main differential diagnoses of an elevated pigmented fundus lesion?
   - Choroidal melanoma
   - Subretinal hemorrhage
   - Sub-RPE hemorrhage
   - RPE tumor
   - Uveal effusion

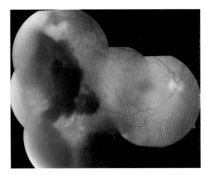

Fig. 50.4 Subretinal hemorrhage from peripheral exudative hemorrhagic chorioretinopathy.

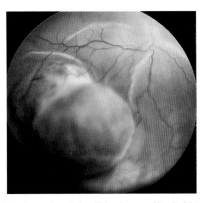

Fig. 50.5 Mushroom-shaped choroidal melanoma with retinal detachment.

5. What ophthalmoscopic features help to differentiate a choroidal melanoma from a subretinal hemorrhage?
   Choroidal melanoma is typically a homogeneous yellow to brown mass with smooth surface and clear subretinal fluid. Subretinal and sub-RPE hemorrhage can occur in the macular area (age-related macular degeneration) or in the peripheral fundus (peripheral exudative hemorrhagic chorioretinopathy) and it initially demonstrates a reddish-blue color, later, as it undergoes resolution hemorrhage, showing a more heterogeneous color with areas of fresh red blood and older yellow blood.

6. What is the most practical ancillary test for differentiating choroidal melanoma from subretinal blood?
   Fluorescein angiography (FA) and OCT. Most melanomas will show hyperfluorescence, and most hemorrhages will show hypofluorescence. By OCT, all melanomas are in the choroid and most hemorrhages are under the RPE or retina, but not in the choroid.

7. What is the significance of a mushroom-shaped fundus lesion?
   A mushroom-shaped fundus lesion is strongly suggestive of choroidal melanoma (Fig. 50.5). Even when the mushroom-shaped lesion is nonpigmented, melanoma is still the most likely diagnosis. It is unusual for other fundus lesion to assume a mushroom shape.

8. What is the best method to diagnose choroidal melanoma?
   The use of binocular indirect ophthalmoscopy by an experienced ophthalmologist who is familiar with the characteristic features of choroidal melanoma and simulating conditions is the best bet to diagnose correctly. Ancillary studies like FA, ultrasonography, OCT, indocyanine green angiography (ICGA), and even magnetic resonance imaging (MRI) can be confirmatory.

9. When the diagnosis is uncertain with ophthalmoscopy, what are the five most helpful ancillary tests in the diagnosis of uveal melanoma?
   1. Transillumination
   2. FA
   3. Ultrasonography
   4. OCT
   5. Fine-needle aspiration biopsy

   Most melanomas cast a shadow with transillumination, are hyperfluorescent with FA, and show low internal reflectivity with ultrasonography. If small, the tumor will be found in the choroid on OCT. Most simulating lesions show different patterns with these modalities. Fine-needle aspiration biopsy is perhaps the most reliable method for establishing the diagnosis, but it is an invasive procedure that requires a skilled clinician and reliable cytopathologist.

10. What clinical and imaging signs suggest that a benign choroidal nevus is likely to grow and eventually evolve into a malignant choroidal melanoma?
    These can be remembered using the mnemonic "To Find Small Ocular Melanoma Doing Imaging" representing (T) thickness more than 2 mm (by ultrasonography), (F) fluid subretinal (by OCT), (S) symptoms of vision loss ($\leq$20/50), (O) orange pigment (by autofluorescence), (M) melanoma hollow (by ultrasonography), and (DIM) diameter (> 5 mm) (by photography). Using these factors, the mean 5-year estimates for transformation are 1% for those with no risk factor, 11% with one factor, 22% with two factors, 34% with three factors, and >50% with four or more factors (Table 50.1). Each 1-mm increase in nevus thickness adds significant risk for future transformation (Table 50.2).

Table 50.1 Risk Factors for Choroidal Nevus Transformation into Melanoma Using Multimodal Imaging

		Findings		Multivariable Analysis	
VARIABLE	**LETTER**	**MNEMONIC**	**TESTING**	**HAZARD RATIO (MEAN)**	**P VALUE**
Thickness tumor >2 mm	T	To	US	3.80	<0.0001
Fluid subretinal	F	Find	OCT	3.56	<0.0001 0.0003
Symptoms visual acuity $\leq$20/50	S	Small	Snellen VA	2.28	0.0050
Orange pigment	O	Ocular	AF	3.07	0.0004
Melanoma acoustic hollowness	M	Melanoma	US	2.10	0.0020
Diameter tumor >5 mm	DIM	Doing IMaging	Photography	1.84	0.0275

AF, Autofluorescence; *OCT,* optical coherence tomography; *US,* ultrasonography; *VA,* visual acuity.

Adapted from Shields CL, Dalvin LA, Ancona-Lezama D, et al.: Choroidal nevus imaging features in 3806 cases and risk factors for transformation into melanoma in 2355 cases. The 2020 Taylor R. Smith and Victor T. Curtin Lecture, *Retina* 39(10):1840–1851, 2019.

Table 50.2 Choroidal Nevus Rate of Transformation into Melanoma per Increasing Millimeter Tumor Thickness

	Kaplan-Meier Estimates per Millimeter Nevus Thickness				
PER YEAR	**THICKNESS $\leq$1.0 mm**	**THICKNESS 1.1–2.0 mm**	**THICKNESS 2.1–3.0 mm**	**THICKNESS >3.0 mm**	**TOTAL**
1	0	0.5%	4.7%	14.4%	1.2%
3	0.3%	1.6%	16.0%	23.6%	3.8%
5	0.8%	2.3%	25.0%	34.5%	5.8%
7	2.2%	6.1%	31.7%	34.5%	9.3%
10	2.2%	10.9%	40.2%	NA	13.9%

*Log-rank test.
NA, Not available.
Adapted from Shields CL, Dalvin LA, Yu MD, et al.: Choroidal nevus transformation into melanoma per millimeter increment in thickness using multimodal imaging in 2355 cases. The 2019 Wendell L. Hughes Lecture, *Retina* 39(10):1852–1860, 2019.

11. How can we estimate prognosis of uveal melanoma clinically?
Studies have shown that prognosis is linearly related to tumor thickness and each 1-mm increase in thickness correlates with a 5% increased risk for metastasis at 10 years. So a 2-mm-thick melanoma carries a (5% × 2) 10% risk for metastasis at 10 years and a 5-mm-thick melanoma has a (5% × 5) 25% risk for metastasis at 10 years (see Table 50.1).

12. What congenital ocular conditions are associated with a higher incidence of uveal melanoma?
Congenital oculo(dermal) melanocytosis (nevus of Ota) can predispose to uveal melanoma. The risk is 1/400 affected patients develop uveal melanoma.

13. Does uveal melanoma have a predilection for age, race, or sex?
Uveal melanoma generally occurs in patients between 40 and 70 years of age and is highly uncommon in individuals ≤20 years of age. Uveal melanoma has a predilection for Caucasians, with >95% of uveal melanoma in Caucasians and <5% in non-Caucasians (African Americans, Hispanics, and Asians). There is no predilection for sex.

14. What external ocular signs suggest the possibility of an underlying ciliary body or peripheral choroidal melanoma?
1. Sentinel vessels—These are one or more dilated, tortuous episcleral blood vessels overlying the affected ciliary body region (Fig. 50.6).
2. Extrascleral extension—This is a dark brown focus of tumor that has grown through an emissary canal onto the episcleral surface (Fig. 50.6).

15. What is the main route of distant spread of uveal melanoma?
Melanoma spreads to extraocular locations primarily by hematogenous metastasis to the liver. Metastatic uveal melanoma to skin, lung, and other organs is less common but often occurs. Because there are no lymphatic channels in the eye, lymphatic metastasis rarely occurs.

16. What is a melanocytoma?
A melanocytoma is a variant of benign nevus that has distinct clinical and histopathologic features. Clinically, it is usually detected on and next to the optic disc as a deeply pigmented lesion that may have a feathery border because of involvement of the nerve fiber layer of the retina (Fig. 50.7). Melanocytoma can also occur as a deeply pigmented lesion in the iris, ciliary body, or choroid. Histopathologically, melanocytoma is composed of round-to-oval cells that have densely packed cytoplasmic melanosomes, small uniform nuclei, and few prominent nucleoli. Like other uveal nevi, it rarely gives rise to uveal melanoma.

17. What is the most acceptable method of treating a choroidal melanoma that occupies more than half of the globe and has produced severe visual loss?
Enucleation, because there is little hope for useful vision and current radiotherapy methods, often cannot successfully treat such a large tumor without extensive damage to the eye, which could be painful.

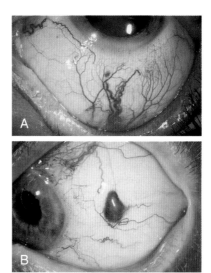

Fig. 50.6 Ciliary body melanoma with overlying **(A)** sentinel vessels and **(B)** extraocular extension.

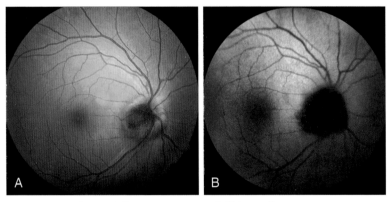

Fig. 50.7 (A) Optic disc melanocytoma with **(B)** hypoautofluorescence.

18. What is the most often used alternative to enucleation for a medium-sized melanoma?
Radiotherapy. Plaque radiotherapy with a radioactive plaque and proton beam radiotherapy with a linear accelerator are the most common alternatives.

19. What is the most common treatment for a melanoma that occupies two clock hours of the ciliary body?
Plaque radiotherapy and surgical resection by iridocyclectomy are reasonable alternatives, depending on the patient's health.

20. What is the most acceptable method of management for an asymptomatic pigmented lesion that measures 3 mm in diameter and 1 mm in thickness and has fine drusen on its surface?
Observation. This is most likely a choroidal nevus. Baseline fundus photography and examination every 6 to 12 months is advised. The risk for transformation into melanoma is <1%.

21. How is BAP-1 tumor predisposition syndrome related to uveal melanoma?
Germline BAP-1 mutation is a tumor predisposition syndrome and affected carriers are predisposed to familial cancers including uveal melanoma, mesothelioma, cutaneous melanoma (CM), renal cell carcinoma (RCC), and others. In one analysis of 507 patients with uveal melanoma, 5% showed polymorphisms in the BAP-1 gene.

22. Name a few syndromes that can spawn uveal melanoma.
There are a few syndromes related to uveal melanoma, including
- Oculo(dermal) melanocytosis
- Phakomatosis pigmentovascularis
- Germline BAP-1 tumor predisposition syndrome
- Neurofibromatosis
- Myotonic dystrophy

23. Can CHRPE lead to uveal melanoma?
No, CHRPE can lead to RPE adenoma/adenocarcinoma, but not uveal melanoma.

24. Does melanoma prognosis vary depending on location in the eye?
Yes, melanoma involving the iris carries the best prognosis, choroid has the second best prognosis, and ciliary body melanoma has the worst prognosis.

25. How can we differentiate uveal melanoma from uveal metastasis?
Uveal melanoma tends to be pigmented and hollow on ultrasound and shows smooth anterior surface on OCT, whereas uveal metastasis tends to be nonpigmented and dense on ultrasound and shows a lumpy-bumpy anterior surface on OCT.

26. What did the Collaborative Ocular Melanoma Study tell us about medium-sized melanoma?
In the medium-sized melanoma trial of 1317 patients comparing mortality after enucleation versus plaque radiotherapy, the 5-year and 12-year melanoma-related mortality were not significantly different. This study justified the use of plaque radiotherapy, rather than enucleation, for most medium-sized melanomas.

27. What did the Collaborative Ocular Melanoma Study tell us about large-sized melanoma?
    In the large melanoma trial of 1003 patients, 5-year melanoma-related mortality was not significantly different at 28% for enucleation alone and 26% for enucleation preceded by external beam radiotherapy, and the 10-year melanoma-related mortality rates showed no difference in therapy with 40% following enucleation and 45% following enucleation preceded by radiotherapy. Thus, preenucleation irradiation has been abandoned.

BIBLIOGRAPHY

Aronow ME, Topham AK, Singh AD: Uveal melanoma: 5-year update on incidence, treatment, and survival (SEER 1973–2013), Ocul Oncol Pathol 4:145–151, 2018.

Dalvin LA, Shields CL, Ancona-Lezama D, et al.: Combination of multimodal imaging features predictive of choroidal nevus transformation into melanoma, Br J Ophthalmol. 103:i-ii, 2019.

Gupta MP, Lane AM, DeAngelis MM, et al.: Clinical characteristics of uveal melanoma in patients with germline BAP1 mutations, JAMA Ophthalmol 133:881–887, 2015.

Kaliki S, Shields CL: Uveal melanoma: relatively rare but deadly cancer, Eye (Lond) 31(2):241–257, 2017.

Masoomian B, Shields JA, Shields CL: Overview of BAP1 cancer predisposition syndrome and the relationship to uveal melanoma, J Curr Ophthalmol 0:102–109, 2018.

Shields CL, Dalvin LA, Ancona-Lezama D, et al.: Choroidal nevus imaging features in 3806 cases and risk factors for transformation into melanoma in 2355 cases. The 2020 Taylor R. Smith and Victor T. Curtin Lecture, Retina 39(10):1840–1851, 2019.

Shields CL, Dalvin LA, Yu MD, et al.: Choroidal nevus transformation into melanoma per millimeter increment in thickness using multimodal imaging in 2355 cases. The 2019 Wendell L. Hughes Lecture, Retina 39(10):1852–1860, 2019.

Shields CL, Furuta M, Thangappan A, et al.: Metastasis of uveal melanoma millimeter by millimeter 8033 consecutive eyes, Arch Ophthalmol 127:989–998, 2009.

Shields JA, Demirci H, Mashayekhi A, Shields CL: Melanocytoma of the optic disc in 115 cases: The 2004 Samuel Johnson Memorial Lecture, Ophthalmology 111:1739–1746, 2004.

Shields CL, Kaliki S, Furuta M, et al.: Clinical spectrum and prognosis of uveal melanoma based on age at presentation in 8033 cases, Retina 32:1363–1372, 2012.

Shields CL, Kaliki S, Furuta M, Shields JA: Diffuse versus nondiffuse small (<3 millimeters thickness) choroidal melanoma: comparative analysis in 1751 cases. The 2012 F. Phinizy Calhoun Lecture 2012, Retina 33:1763–1776, 2013.

Shields CL, Kaliki S, Livesey M, et al.: Association of ocular and oculodermal melanocytosis with rate of uveal melanoma metastasis. Analysis of 7872 consecutive eyes, JAMA Ophthalmol 131:993–1003, 2013.

Shields CL, Lim LAS, Dalvin LA, Shields JA: Small choroidal melanoma: detection with multimodal imaging and management with plaque radiotherapy or AU-011 nanoparticle therapy, Curr Opin Ophthalmol 30:206–214, 2019.

Shields CL, Manalac J, Das C, et al.: Choroidal melanoma. Clinical features, classification, and top 10 pseudomelanomas, Curr Opin Ophthalmol 5:177–185, 2014.

Shields CL, Mashayekhi A, Ho T, et al.: Solitary congenital hypertrophy of the retinal pigment epithelium: clinical features and frequency of enlargement in 330 patients, Ophthalmology 110:1968–1976, 2003.

Shields CL, Salazar P, Mashayekhi A, Shields JA: Peripheral exudative hemorrhagic chorioretinopathy (PEHCR) simulating choroidal melanoma in 173 eyes, Ophthalmology 116:529–535, 2009.

Shields JA, Shields CL: Management of posterior uveal melanoma. Past, present and future. The 2014 Charles L. Schepens Lecture, Ophthalmology 122(2):414–428, 2015.

Shields JA, Shields CL, Ehya H, et al.: Fine needle aspiration biopsy of suspected intraocular tumors. The 1992 Urwick Lecture, Ophthalmology 100:1677–1684, 1993.

Shields JA, Shields CL, Singh AD: Acquired tumors arising from congenital hypertrophy of the retinal pigment epithelium, Arch Ophthalmol 118:637–641, 2000.

Singh AD, De Potter P, Fijal BA, et al.: Lifetime prevalence of uveal melanoma in White patients with ocular (dermal) melanocytosis, Ophthalmology 105:195–198, 1998.

CHAPTER 51

OCULAR TUMORS

Ralph C. Eagle, Jr.

1. What is the most common malignant intraocular neoplasm?

   Uveal metastasis, usually from a distant primary carcinoma, is thought to be the most common malignant intraocular neoplasm. An estimated 66,000 patients develop uveal metastases each year. Most of these tumors occur in terminally ill patients, few of whom are evaluated ophthalmologically or pathologically. In contrast, only 1800 cases of uveal malignant melanoma and 300 cases of retinoblastoma occur in the United States yearly.

   Many textbooks state that uveal malignant melanoma is the most common primary intraocular tumor, but this statement actually applies only to the United States and Europe, because uveal melanoma has a propensity for fair-skinned, blue-eyed persons. Throughout Africa, Asia, and South America, where melanoma is relatively rare, retinoblastoma is the most common primary intraocular tumor. Kivelä has estimated that approximately 1000 more retinoblastomas occur yearly in the world than uveal melanomas.[1,2]

2. What is the characteristic shape of choroidal malignant melanoma?

   Approximately 60% of choroidal malignant melanomas have a mushroom or collar-button configuration (Fig. 51.1). Melanomas have a discoid or almond shape when they initially arise in the choroid. The mushroom or collar-button configuration develops after the tumor ruptures or erodes through Bruch's membrane and invades the subretinal space, where it forms a round or ovoid nodule.

3. Is a mushroom configuration pathognomonic for choroidal melanoma?

   A mushroom or collar-button configuration usually signifies that a choroidal tumor is a malignant melanoma. Few things in medicine are pathognomonic, however. Exceedingly rare mushroom-shaped choroidal metastases, hemangiomas, and schwannomas have been reported.[3,4]

4. What important prognostic features of uveal melanoma can be assessed during routine histopathologic examination?

   Tumor size and cell type are two of the most important prognostic factors assessed during routine histopathological evaluation of uveal melanoma. Larger tumors and tumors that contain epithelioid cells have a poorer prognosis. Tumor size is expressed in millimeters as the largest tumor diameter. Other prognostic features include mitotic activity (expressed as the number of mitoses in 40 high power fields), the presence of extrascleral extension, vasculogenic mimicry patterns called vascular loops and networks, and lymphocytic infiltration.[5–7]

5. What factors does the American Joint Committee on Cancer (AJCC) *Cancer Staging Manual* use to stage uveal melanomas?

   Tumor size, ciliary body involvement, and extrascleral extension are important factors used to prognostically stratify uveal melanomas in the American Joint Committee on Cancer's (AJCC's) TNM classification. TNM stands for Tumor, Node, Metastasis. Uveal melanomas are classified by size using a chart that includes both the largest tumor basal diameter and thickness. Tumors greater than 18 mm in diameter are size category 4. Ciliary body tumors have a poorer prognosis.[8]

6. What is the Callender classification?

   In 1931, Major George Russell Callender reported that there was an association between survival and the histologic characteristics of uveal melanomas cell type. Callender showed that uveal melanomas contain two types of spindle cells (spindle A and spindle B cells), and/or less differentiated epithelioid cells. Dr. Ian McLean modified Callender's classification in 1978. Spindle A and spindle B melanomas were lumped together as spindle melanomas in the modified classification, and necrotic and fascicular variants were deleted.[9,10]

7. What is the most common cell type?

   Most melanomas that are enucleated and examined histopathologically are mixed-cell tumors that contain a mixture of spindle and epithelioid cells. Eighty-nine percent of the melanomas that were enucleated in the Collaborative Ocular Melanoma Study (COMS) were mixed-cell tumors.

8. How are melanoma cell types distinguished histopathologically?

   Melanoma cells are readily differentiated by the characteristics of their nuclei. Spindle A cells have long, tapering cigar-like nuclei, an absent or indistinct nucleolus, and a characteristic longitudinal stripe caused by a fold in the nuclear membrane. Spindle B nuclei are oval and plumper and have less finely dispersed chromatin and a distinct nucleolus (Fig. 51. 2). Epithelioid cell nuclei are typically round and vesicular and have prominent reddish-purple nucleoli (Fig. 51.3). The chromatin is coarse and often clumps along the inside of the nuclear membrane (peripheral margination of chromatin).

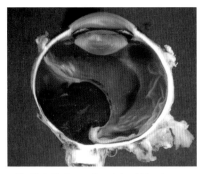

Fig. 51.1 Mushroom-shaped choroidal melanoma.

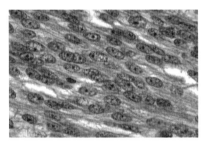

Fig. 51.2 Spindle melanoma cells.

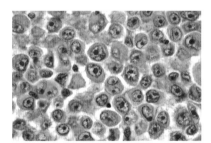

Fig. 51.3 Epithelioid melanoma cells.

Spindle melanoma cells grow as a syncytium, making it difficult to discern the cytoplasmic margins of the bipolar fusiform cells. Epithelioid cells are poorly cohesive and their cytoplasmic margins are readily discernible.[11]

9. Which cell type has the worst prognosis?
   The presence or absence of epithelioid cells in a uveal melanoma has an important effect on prognosis. If no epithelioid cells are present, the expected survival at 15 years is 72%. If epithelioid cells are present (mixed, epithelioid, or necrotic cell type), the survival at 15 years drops to 37%. A tumor composed entirely of spindle A cells is now considered to be a benign nevus incapable of metastasis. Tumors composed entirely of epithelioid cells have the worst prognosis. Overall, approximately 50% of patients with uveal melanoma will die from their tumors.[7]

10. What special tests are powerful prognostic indicators in patients with uveal melanoma?
    Special tests that are powerful prognostic indicators in patients with uveal melanoma include:
    1. Assessment for nonrandom chromosomal abnormalities in the tumor cells
    2. Gene expression profiling (GEP).

Nonrandom chromosomal abnormalities, including loss of chromosome 3 and gains in chromosome 8, are associated with metastatic death. Monosomy 3 is a significant predictor of poor prognosis in uveal melanoma. In one study, 57% of patients with monosomy 3 had developed metastases at 3 years, compared with none of the patients with disomy 3. Chromosomal 3 abnormalities have been identified using a variety of techniques, including fluorescence in situ hybridization (FISH) and DNA amplification and microsatellite assay.

GEP of uveal melanomas by microarray analysis has disclosed three classes of tumors that differ markedly in their potential for metastasis. Class IA melanomas are low-grade tumors with less than 5% risk for metastasis. In contrast, a patient with a class II melanoma has a greater than 90% risk for metastasis. The gene expression profile of class II melanomas resembles primitive neural/ectodermal stem cells. They typically have other high-risk features including epithelioid cells, vasculogenic mimicry patterns, and monosomy 3. Class I B tumors develop late metastases and express the PRAME gene. GEP is available as a proprietary commercial test.[12–15]

KEY POINTS: PROGNOSTIC FACTORS IN UVEAL MELANOMA

1. Size
2. Ciliary body involvement
3. Cell type
4. Extrascleral extension
5. Mitotic activity
6. Lymphocytic infiltration
7. Vasculogenic mimicry patterns
8. Non-random chromosomal abnormalities (monosomy 3)
9. Gene expression profile (class II—poor prognosis)

11. **What is the most common site of metastatic uveal melanoma?**
The liver. Liver metastases occur in 93% of patients who develop metastatic uveal melanoma. Other sites include the lungs (24%) and bone (16%).[16]

12. **Does enucleation of uveal melanoma increase tumor deaths by disseminating tumor cells?**
Probably not. In 1978, Zimmerman, McLean, and Foster hypothesized that enucleation of uveal melanoma increased tumor deaths by disseminating tumor cells. This became known as the Zimmerman hypothesis. It is currently believed that melanomas have already micrometastasized years before they produce symptoms and are treated. This conclusion is based on studies of tumor doubling times and the observation that increased mortality also occurs after plaque brachyradiotherapy and charged particle therapy.[17–19]

13. **What was the Collaborative Ocular Melanoma Study?**
The COMS was a large prospective, randomized, multicentered study funded by the National Eye Institute that investigated the treatment of choroidal malignant melanoma. The arm of the study that focused on medium-sized tumors compared survival after enucleation and radioactive iodine 125 (^{125}I) plaque brachytherapy. The large tumor study compared survival after standard enucleation and enucleation preceded by external beam radiotherapy.[20]

14. **What did the Collaborative Ocular Melanoma Study results reveal?**
The medium-sized tumor arm of the study showed that survival was similar after both enucleation and plaque brachytherapy. The large tumor arm showed that "sterilization" of large melanomas with pre-enucleation external-beam radiotherapy did not improve survival.[21,22]

15. **How are most uveal melanomas treated?**
Today, most posterior uveal melanomas are treated with radioactive plaques. Plaque treatment failures and eyes with larger tumors and/or tumor-related complications, such as secondary glaucoma or extrascleral extension, are still enucleated. Some smaller tumors can be locally resected or treated with transpupillary thermotherapy.[23]

16. **How effective is treatment of posterior uveal melanoma?**
Treatment is relatively ineffective from the standpoint of survival. All forms of treatment seem to have little effect on decreasing subsequent death from metastases. Unfortunately, most tumors have already metastasized before they are treated. Current therapy for metastatic melanoma is also ineffective. Phase II studies of ipilimumab-nivolumab immunotherapy for metastatic uveal melanoma are ongoing. This treatment has been revolutionary in treating metastatic cutaneous melanoma.[18]

17. **What clinical features suggest that a small pigmented choroidal tumor is a melanoma?**
The mnemonic **TFSOM** (**T**o **F**ind **S**mall **O**cular **M**elanoma **U**sing **H**elpful **H**ints **D**aily) lists the clinical factors that suggest that a small, pigmented tumor is a melanoma that is likely to grow, thereby putting the patient at greater risk for metastasis.

T = Thickness greater than 3 mm
F = Subretinal fluid
S = Symptoms
O = Orange pigment
M = Margin touching optic disk
UH = Ultrasound hollow
H = Halo absent
D = Drusen absent

Choroidal melanocytic tumors that display none of these factors have a 3% risk of growth into melanoma at 5 years and most likely represent choroidal nevi. Tumors with two or more factors show growth in more than 50% of cases. Most tumors with two or more risk factors probably represent small choroidal melanomas, and early treatment is generally indicated.[24]

18. **What genes are involved in uveal melanoma?**
Genes involved in uveal melanoma include GNAQ, GNA11, BAP1, EIF1AX, SF3B1, and PRAME. GNAQ/GNA11 mutations have been found in 46% of uveal melanomas. They appear to be an early event, since they are also present in blue nevi and the nevus of Ota. Inactivating mutations in the BAP1 gene play an important role in the metastasis of uveal melanoma. BAP1 mutations are found in 84% of class II melanomas. The BAP1 gene is located on chromosome 3, and the inactivating mutations are thought to be disclosed by loss of chromosome 3 in tumors with monosomy 3. Mutations in EIF1AX or SF3B1 are involved in the class I pathway.[25]

19. **What is the BAP1 syndrome?**
Autosomal dominantly inherited mutations in the BAP1 gene cause a familial cancer syndrome. Patients and families with germline mutations in BAP1 are predisposed to a variety of tumors, including uveal melanoma, mesothelioma, cutaneous melanoma, renal cell carcinoma, and benign atypical melanocytic skin tumors.[26]

KEY POINTS: OVERVIEW OF UVEAL MELANOMA

1. Caucasian patients at risk
2. Mushroom shape
3. Spindle and epithelioid cells
4. Liver metastases
5. A 50% mortality rate

20. **Do melanomas of the iris behave differently?**
The prognosis of iris melanoma generally is excellent (4%–10% mortality). Most pigmented tumors of the iris are benign spindle cell nevi. In one large series, 8% of nevi grew into melanomas in 15 years. Although tumors containing epithelioid cells occasionally are encountered, most iris melanomas are low-grade spindle cell tumors.
An **ABCDEF** guide identifies risk factors for growth that suggest that a pigmented iris tumor is a melanoma. These risk factors include **A**ge (young), **B**lood (hyphema), **C**lock hour (inferior), **D**iffuse configuration, **E**ctropion uveae, and **F**eathery tumor margin. Although they can occur anywhere, melanomas arise most frequently in the inferior sun-exposed part of the iris.[27,28]

21. **What clinical features suggest that a uveal tumor is a metastasis?**
Uveal metastases usually are creamy yellow amelanotic tumors that have a placoid or nummular configuration. Pigment mottling may occur on the tumor apex. Metastases are often multiple but can be solitary. Metastases usually cause a nonrhegmatogenous serous detachment of the retina with shifting subretinal fluid. They typically appear acoustically solid on B-scan ultrasonography and have a "lumpy-bumpy" surface on SD-optical coherence tomography (OCT).[29]

22. **What is the most common site of uveal metastasis?**
Uveal metastases involve the choroid 90% of the time. They typically are found in the region of the macula where the choroidal blood supply is richest.[29]

23. **What primary tumors are responsible for most uveal metastases?**
Breast carcinoma in women and lung carcinoma in men. Breast carcinoma is responsible for 37% of ocular metastases. Nearly one-fourth are caused by lung cancer. Most women with uveal metastases from breast tumors have a history of breast carcinoma. In contrast, uveal metastasis may herald the presence of an occult lung tumor. Other common primary sites include kidney (4%), gastrointestinal (GI) tract (4%), cutaneous melanoma (2%), lung carcinoid (2%), and prostate (2%).[29]

24. **How is immunohistochemistry used to assess uveal metastases?**
Primary uveal melanomas usually can be distinguished from uveal metastases using routine light microscopy. If a metastasis is found in patient with no prior history of cancer, immunohistochemistry (IHC) often can identify the

primary tumor. For example, breast and lung cancers frequently stain positively (i.e., are immunoreactive for) cytokeratin 7 (CK7) and are negative for CK20. In contrast, most GI cancers are CK20 positive. More specific markers that are expressed only by certain cancers help to pinpoint the primary. Examples include the BRST2 marker in breast carcinoma, the TTF1 marker in lung cancer, and PSA and PSAP in prostate cancers.

IHC also is used as a prognostic marker and a guide to therapy. For example, breast carcinomas that express extrogen receptors can be treated with tamoxifen and aromatase inhibitors, whereas tumors that express HER/2neu can be treated with trastuzumab (Herceptin).[30]

25. What type of hemangiomas occurs in the choroid?
Choroidal hemangiomas are classified as capillary, cavernous, or mixed. They are composed of thin-walled vessels and have little stroma (Fig. 51.4). Sporadic hemangiomas tend to be discrete, localized, elevated reddish-orange tumors. The choroidal hemangiomas that occur in patients with Sturge-Weber syndrome are typically diffuse, with indistinct tapering margins. These obscure the underlying choroidal architecture and impart a "tomato ketchup" appearance to the fundus.[31]

26. If choroidal hemangiomas are benign, why are they treated?
Choroidal hemangiomas are treated to save vision or the eye itself. Although they are benign from a systemic standpoint, choroidal hemangiomas cause retinal detachment and secondary glaucoma via iris neovascularization and/or a papillary block mechanism. The latter can lead to eye loss. Hemangiomas are treated with laser photocoagulation or photodynamic therapy (PDT).[32,33]

27. What is the typical clinical presentation of retinoblastoma in the United States?
Retinoblastoma typically presents with leukocoria (a white pupillary reflex) in the United States and Europe. Smaller tumors that involve the macula initially may present with strabismus. All children with strabismus should have a careful fundus examination to exclude retinoblastoma or other significant macular pathology. In developing countries, children may present in an advanced stage of the disease with a large orbital tumor secondary to extraocular extension.[34]

28. How old are patients when diagnosed with retinoblastoma?
The mean age at diagnosis is 18 months. Patients who have the familial form of the disease (i.e., who have germline mutations) are diagnosed earlier (mean age of 12 months), probably because only a solitary "hit" or gene inactivation is required. Sporadic somatic cases occur in slightly older patients; they are diagnosed at a mean age of 24 months.[34]

29. What does retinoblastoma look like grossly?
Grossly, retinoblastoma has a distinctly encephaloid or brain-like appearance. This is not surprising because the tumor arises from the retina, which is a peripheral colony of brain cells. Foci of dystrophic calcification occur in many retinoblastomas. These foci of calcification are evident grossly as lighter flecks.

30. What is an exophytic retinoblastoma?
Retinoblastoma shows several growth patterns. Exophytic retinoblastoma arises from the outer retina and grows in the subretinal space, causing retinal detachment (Fig. 51.5). Endophytic retinoblastoma arises from the inner layers of the retina, which remains attached (Fig. 51.6). Endophytic tumors invade the vitreous and may seed the anterior chamber, forming a pseudohypopyon of tumor cells. Most large retinoblastomas exhibit a combined endophytic/exophytic growth pattern. The diffuse infiltrative growth pattern is relatively rare and occurs in older children. The retina is diffusely thickened without a distinct tumefaction.[34]

31. Why do retinoblastomas appear blue, pink, and purple under low-magnification light microscopy?
The blue, pink, and purple areas evident on low-magnification light microscopy of retinoblastoma represent zones of viable, necrotic, and calcified tumor cells, respectively. Areas of viable tumor are basophilic. Retinoblastoma is

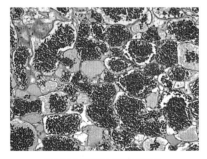

Fig. 51.4 Choroidal hemangioma.

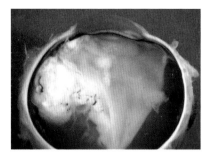

Fig. 51.5 Exophytic retinoblastoma with total retinal detachment.

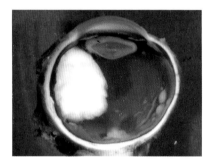

Fig. 51.6 Endophytic retinoblastoma.

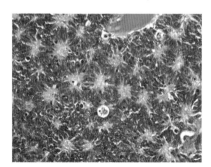

Fig. 51.7 Homer Wright rosettes, retinoblastoma.

composed of poorly differentiated neuroblastic cells that have intensely basophilic nuclei and scanty cytoplasm. Retinoblastoma cells tend to outgrow their blood supply rapidly and undergo spontaneous necrosis. The necrotic parts of the tumor are eosinophilic because the dead cells lose their basophilic nuclear DNA. Dystrophic calcification often occurs in necrotic parts of the tumor. The calcium has a purple hue in sections stained with hematoxylin and eosin.[34,35]

32. What do rosettes signify in retinoblastoma?
Rosettes are histologic markers for tumor differentiation in retinoblastoma. Homer Wright rosettes reflect low-grade neuroblastic differentiation. They are nonspecific and occur in other tumors such as neuroblastoma. Flexner-Wintersteiner rosettes represent early retinal differentiation and are highly characteristic for retinoblastoma, but they are not pathognomonic. They are also found in some medulloepitheliomas.[36]

33. How are Homer Wright and Flexner-Wintersteiner rosettes distinguished histopathologically?
The nuclei of Homer Wright rosettes encircle a central tangle of neural filaments (Fig. 51.7). No lumen is present. Flexner-Wintersteiner rosettes have a central lumen that corresponds to the subretinal space (Fig. 51.8). The cells

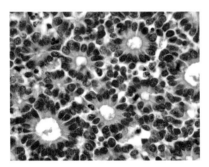

Fig. 51.8 Flexner-Wintersteiner rosettes, retinoblastoma.

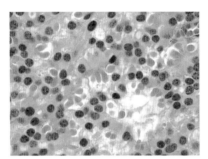

Fig. 51.9 Fleurettes, retinoblastoma.

that enclose the lumen are joined by a girdle of apical intercellular connections analogous to the retinal external limiting membrane. Cilia, the precursors of photoreceptors, project into the lumen of the rosette.[36,37]

34. What are fleurettes?

Fleurettes are aggregates of neoplastic photoreceptors (Fig. 51.9). Photoreceptor differentiation is the highest degree of differentiation found in retinoblastomas. Fleurettes are composed of groups of bulbous eosinophilic cellular processes that correspond to photoreceptor inner segments. They typically are aligned along a segment of neoplastic external limiting membrane in a bouquet-like arrangement.[34,38]

35. What are the most important prognostic features of retinoblastoma?

Important prognostic features of retinoblastoma that can be assessed histopathologically include the presence and degree of optic nerve invasion, extrascleral extension, massive uveal invasion, and possibly, anterior segment involvement. Unlike uveal melanoma, the size of the tumor does not appear to be important. Mortality rises as the depth of tumor invasion into the optic nerve increases. Retrolaminar optic nerve invasion is equivalent to extraocular extension. Although anterior segment involvement is considered to confer poorer prognosis, its significance is uncertain because it tends to be found in eyes with other high-risk features.[39,40]

36. What histopathologic risk factors found in enucleated eyes with retinoblastoma are indications for adjuvant chemotherapy?

Certain histopathologic features detected during the histopathologic examination of eyes with retinoblastoma are indications for adjuvant chemotherapy in most centers. These include:

1. Tumor invasion of the optic nerve behind the lamina cribrosa (retrolaminar optic nerve invasion), or to the surgical margin
2. Massive invasion of the choroid
3. Any amount of concurrent prelaminar optic nerve and non-massive choroidal invasion.

Massive choroidal invasion has been defined as greater than 3 mm in diameter or involving the full-thickness of the choroid.[41,42]

37. How does retinoblastoma become fatal?

Many children who die from retinoblastoma have some degree of intracranial involvement. This is caused by direct extension of tumor cells along the optic nerve, subarachnoid space, or orbital foramina. Distant hematogenous metastases to bone and viscera can develop after the tumor invades the richly vascularized uvea. Anterior extrascleral extension provides access to conjunctival lymphatics and may be associated with regional lymph node metastases.[34]

38. **The retinoblastoma gene is located on what chromosome?**
Chromosome 13, found in the segment of the long, or "q," arm, which is designated the 1 to 4 band (13q1–4).[43]

39. **How is the retinoblastoma gene classified?**
The retinoblastoma (RB1) gene is the paradigmatic example of a recessive oncogene. Both copies of the gene must be lost or inactivated before a tumor can develop. Normal individuals have two functional copies of the RB1 gene, although only one is needed for normal functioning. The gene's protein product, called RB1 protein, is found in the nucleus, where it interacts with other transcription factors to control the cell cycle. The absence of RB1 protein allows continual cell division and lack of terminal differentiation.[43]

40. **If the RB1 gene is recessive, why do cases of familial retinoblastoma appear to be inherited in an autosomal-dominant fashion?**
Patients with hereditary retinoblastoma are heterozygous for the RB1 gene. The genotype of carriers includes a single functional wild-type gene. The second copy of the RB1 gene has been lost or inactivated or produces a defective gene product. A retinoblastoma will develop when a retinal cell loses its single functional copy of the RB1 gene. A mating between a normal individual (RbRb) and a heterozygous carrier (Rb1rb1) gives rise to 50% normal offspring and 50% heterozygous carriers—a 50/50 ratio that perfectly mimics autosomal dominant transmission.

41. **What does bilateral retinoblastoma signify clinically?**
The presence of bilateral retinoblastoma indicates that the affected patient carries a germline mutation in the RB1 gene and is capable of transmitting the tumor to offspring.

42. **Can a child with a unilateral retinoblastoma have hereditary disease?**
Yes. Unfortunately, the presence of a unilateral tumor does not exclude a germline mutation and transmissible disease. Only approximately 60% of patients with familial retinoblastoma actually develop bilateral tumors.

43. **Are most retinoblastomas familial?**
No, most retinoblastomas occur sporadically in infants who have no family history of the disease. Nearly three-fourths of sporadic retinoblastomas are caused by somatic mutations in retinal cells, which cannot be passed on to offspring. Such somatic sporadic tumors are invariably unilateral and unifocal. The remaining fourth of sporadic retinoblastomas are caused by germline mutations (i.e., they are new familial cases). The latter can be bilateral and can be passed on to offspring in what appears to be autosomal dominant transmission. Only 5% to 10% of retinoblastomas occur in patients with a family history of the tumor.

44. **Why are sporadic retinoblastomas caused by somatic mutations always unilateral and unifocal?**
A sporadic somatic retinoblastoma is caused by the inactivation of both RB1 genes in a single retinal cell. The spontaneous mutation rate of the RB1 gene is very low. Hence, the chance of this occurring in more than a single retinal cell is infinitesimally small. Therefore, sporadic somatic retinoblastomas always are unilateral and unifocal. In contrast, it is highly probable that one or more gene inactivations will occur in *both* retinas of a heterozygous carrier, because the mutation rate is substantially smaller than the number of mitoses involved in the development of the retina and genes usually are lost during cellular division. That is why familial cases typically are bilateral and may be multifocal.

45. **Are patients with hereditary retinoblastomas at risk for other nonocular tumors?**
Yes. Between 20% and 50% of patients who have germline mutations in the retinoblastoma gene will develop a second malignant neoplasm within 20 years. One of the most interesting and characteristic secondary tumors is a pineoblastoma, a retinoblastoma-like tumor of the pineal gland. The association of pineoblastoma and hereditary retinoblastoma has been termed *trilateral retinoblastoma*. There also is a 500-fold increase in the incidence of osteogenic sarcoma in retinoblastoma gene carriers. Patients also are at risk to develop radiation-induced orbital sarcomas (e.g., osteogenic sarcomas) after external-beam radiotherapy for retinoblastoma, which is why oncologists currently try to avoid this therapy.

KEY POINTS: RETINOBLASTOMA

1. Tumor suppressor gene on chromosome 13 (13q1–4)
2. Most cases are sporadic (75% somatic, 25% germline)
3. Bilaterality indicates transmissible germline mutation
4. Heritable cases pass disease to 50% of offspring (autosomal dominant pattern)
5. Heritable cases at risk for second tumors

46. **Name the three diseases that are most often confused with retinoblastoma clinically.**
   - Persistent fetal vasculature (PFV) (previously called persistent hyperplastic primary vitreous [PHPV]).
   - Coats disease
   - Ocular toxocariasis[44–47]

47. **How does Coats disease differ from retinoblastoma?**
    Coats disease is characterized by an exudative retinal detachment caused by leaky congenital vascular anomalies in the retina (Fig. 51.10). The subretinal fluid is rich in lipid-laden macrophages and cholesterol crystals, which appear as empty clefts in microscopic sections. Histopathologically, the retina contains abnormal telangiectatic vessels, and its outer layers are massively thickened by hard exudates. A bullous retinal detachment may abut the lens, displacing it anteriorly and causing pupillary block glaucoma. Coats disease usually occurs unilaterally in boys between ages 4 and 10. It usually is confused clinically with exophytic retinoblastoma.[48,49]

48. **What are the characteristic features of persistent fetal vasculature (persistent hyperplastic primary vitreous?**
    Persistent fetal vasculature (PFV), previously called persistent hyperplastic primary vitreous (PHPV), is a congenital disorder that is present at birth. It is usually unilateral and classically is found in a microphthalmic eye. Leukocoria is caused by a plaque of fibrovascular tissue that adheres to the posterior surface of the lens. The ciliary processes typically are disclosed by dilating the pupil because their tips are attached to the edge of the retrolental plaque and drawn centrally. Congenital retroblastomas have been reported but are exceedingly rare. On average, retinoblastomas are diagnosed at age 18 months.[45,50,51]

49. **What is the second most common primary intraocular tumor of childhood?**
    Embryonal medulloepithelioma is the second most common primary intraocular tumor of childhood. Medulloepitheliomas probably are derived from anlagen of the embryonic medullary epithelium, which lines the forebrain and optic vesicle. Most of these rare tumors become symptomatic around age 4 years and are diagnosed at 5 years of age.[52-54]

50. **Where are most medulloepitheliomas located?**
    Most medulloepitheliomas are ciliary body tumors that arise from the neuroepithelial layers on their inner surface. Rare medulloepitheliomas of the optic nerve do occur, however.[55,56]

51. **What is a teratoid medulloepithelioma?**
    In addition to bands, cords, and rosettes of neoplastic neuroepithelium and pools of hyaluronic acid, teratoid medulloepitheliomas contain foci of heteroplastic tissue including hyaline cartilage, rhabdomyoblasts, striated muscle, and/or brain (Fig. 51.11). More than a third of medulloepitheliomas are teratoid. Nonteratoid medulloepitheliomas lack heteroplastic elements. Both benign and malignant variants of teratoid and nonteratoid tumors occur.

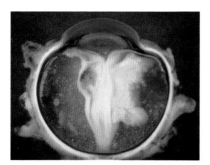

Fig. 51.10 Coats disease.

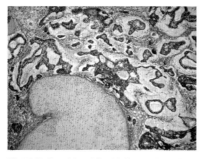

Fig. 51.11 Teratoid medulloepithelioma with cartilage.

REFERENCES

1. Nelson CC, Hertzberg BS, Klintworth GK: A histopathologic study of 716 unselected eyes in patients with cancer at the time of death, Am J Ophthalmol 95:788–793, 1983.
2. Kivelä T: The epidemiological challenge of the most frequent eye cancer: retinoblastoma, an issue of birth and death, Br J Ophthalmol 93:1129–1131, 2009.
3. Shields JA, Shields CL, Brown GC, Eagle RC Jr: Mushroom-shaped choroidal metastasis simulating a choroidal melanoma, Retina 22:810–813, 2002.
4. Spraul CW, Kim D, Fineberg E, Grossniklaus HE: Mushroom-shaped choroidal hemangioma, Am J Ophthalmol 122:434–436, 1996.
5. De la Cruz PO Jr, Specht CS, McLean IW: Lymphocytic infiltration in uveal malignant melanoma, Cancer 65:112–115, 1990.
6. Folberg R, Mehaffey M, Gardner LM, et al: The microcirculation of choroidal and ciliary body melanomas, Eye 11:227–238, 1997.
7. McLean IW, Foster WD, Zimmerman LE: Uveal melanoma: Location, size, cell type, and enucleation as risk factors in metastasis, Hum Pathol 13:123–132, 1982.
8. Amin MB, Edge SB, Greene FL, et al., editors: American Joint Commission on Cancer. AJCC cancer staging manual, ed 8, 2018.
9. Callender G: Malignant melanotic tumors of the eye: A study of histologic types in 111 cases, Trans Am Acad Ophthalmol Otolaryngol 36:131–142, 1931.
10. McLean IW, Foster WD, Zimmerman LE, Gamel JW: Modifications of Callender's classification of uveal melanoma at the Armed Forces Institute of Pathology, Am J Ophthalmol 96:502–509, 1983.
11. Grossniklaus HE, Eagle RC Jr, Albert DM, et al.: Choroidal and ciliary body melanoma. In: Grossniklaus HE, Eberhart CG, Kivelä TT, editors: WHO classification of tumours of the eye, ed 4, Lyon, France, 2018, IARC.
12. Onken MD, Worley LA, Ehlers JP, Harbour JW: Gene expression profiling in uveal melanoma reveals two molecular classes and predicts metastatic death, Cancer Res 64:7205–7209, 2004.
13. Field MG, Decatur CL, Kurtenbach S, et al.: PRAME as an independent biomarker for metastasis in uveal melanoma, Clin Cancer Res 22(5):1234–1242, 2016.
14. Sisley K, Rennie IG, Parsons MA, et al.: Abnormalities of chromosomes 3 and 8 in posterior uveal melanoma correlate with prognosis, Genes Chromosomes Cancer 19:22–28, 1997.
15. White VA, Chambers JD, Courtright PD, et al.: Correlation of cytogenetic abnormalities with the outcome of patients with uveal melanoma, Cancer 83:354–359, 1998.
16. COMS: Assessment of metastatic disease status at death in 435 patients with large choroidal melanoma in the Collaborative Ocular Melanoma Study (COMS). COMS Report No. 15, Arch Ophthalmol 119:670–676, 2001.
17. Eskelin S, Pyrhonen S, Summanen P, et al: Tumor doubling times in metastatic malignant melanoma of the uvea: tumor progression before and after treatment, Ophthalmology 107:1443–1449, 2000.
18. Singh AD, Rennie IG, Kivela T, et al: The Zimmerman-McLean-Foster hypothesis: 25 years later, Br J Ophthalmol 88:962–967, 2004.
19. Zimmerman LE, McLean IW, Foster WD: Does enucleation of the eye containing a malignant melanoma prevent or accelerate the dissemination of tumour cells? Br J Ophthalmol 62:420–425, 1978.
20. COMS: Design and methods of a clinical trial for a rare condition: The Collaborative Ocular Melanoma Study. COMS Report No. 3, Control Clin Trials 14:362–391, 1993.
21. Diener-West M, Earl JD, Fine SL, et al.: The COMS randomized trial of iodine 125 brachytherapy for choroidal melanoma. III: Initial mortality findings. COMS Report No. 18, Arch Ophthalmol 119:969–982, 2001.
22. Hawkins BS: The Collaborative Ocular Melanoma Study (COMS) randomized trial of pre-enucleation radiation of large choroidal melanoma. IV: Ten-year mortality findings and prognostic factors. COMS Report No. 24, Am J Ophthalmol 138:936–951, 2004.
23. Shields CL, Shields JA: Recent developments in the management of choroidal melanoma, Curr Opin Ophthalmol 15:244–251, 2004.
24. Shields CL, Demici H, Materin MA, et al: Clinical factors in the identification of small choroidal melanoma, Can J Ophthalmol 39:351–357, 2004.
25. Helgadottir H, Höiom V: The genetics of uveal melanoma: current insights, Appl Clin Genet 9:147–155, 2016.
26. Masoomian B, Shields JA, Shields CL: Overview of BAP1 cancer predisposition syndrome and the relationship to uveal melanoma, J Curr Ophthalmol 30(2):102–109, 2018.
27. Jakobiec FA, Silbert G: Are most iris "melanomas" really nevi? A clinicopathologic study of 189 lesions, Arch Ophthalmol 99:2117–2132, 1981.
28. Shields CL, Kaliki S, Hutchinson A, et al.: Iris nevus growth into melanoma: analysis of 1611 consecutive eyes: the ABCDEF guide, Ophthalmology 120(4):766–772, 2013.
29. Shields CL, Welch RJ, Malik K, et al.: Uveal metastasis: clinical features and survival outcome of 2214 tumors in 1111 patients based on primary tumor origin, Middle East Afr J Ophthalmol 25(2):81–90, 2018.
30. Eagle RC Jr: Immunohistochemistry in diagnostic ophthalmic pathology: a review, Clin Exp Ophthalmol 36(7):675–688, 2008.
31. Witschel H, Font RL: Hemangioma of the choroid. A clinicopathologic study of 71 cases and a review of the literature, Surv Ophthalmol 20:415–431, 1976.
32. Gunduz K: Transpupillary thermotherapy in the management of circumscribed choroidal hemangioma, Surv Ophthalmol 49:316–327, 2004.
33. Madreperla SA: Choroidal hemangioma treated with photodynamic therapy using verteporfin, Arch Ophthalmol 119:1606–1610, 2001.
34. Eagle RC Jr, Chevez-Barrios P, Li B, et al.: Retinoblastoma. In: Grossniklaus HE, Eberhart CG, Kivelä TT, editors: WHO classification of tumours of the eye, ed 4, Lyon, France, 2018, IARC.
35. Burnier MN, McLean IW, Zimmerman LE, Rosenberg SH: Retinoblastoma. The relationship of proliferating cells to blood vessels, Invest Ophthalmol Vis Sci 31:2037–2040, 1990.
36. Ts'o MO, Fine BS, Zimmerman LE: The Flexner-Wintersteiner rosettes in retinoblastoma, Arch Pathol 88:664–671, 1969.
37. Shields JA, Eagle RC Jr, Shields CL, Potter PD: Congenital neoplasms of the nonpigmented ciliary epithelium (medulloepithelioma), Ophthalmology 103:1998–2006, 1996.
38. Ts'o MO, Zimmerman LE, Fine BS: The nature of retinoblastoma. I. Photoreceptor differentiation: a clinical and histopathologic study, Am J Ophthalmol 69:339–349, 1970.
39. Kopelman JE, McLean IW, Rosenberg SH: Multivariate analysis of risk factors for metastasis in retinoblastoma treated by enucleation, Ophthalmology 94:371–377, 1987.

40. Singh AD, Shields CL, Shields JA: Prognostic factors in retinoblastoma, J Pediatr Ophthalmol Strabismus 37:134–141; quiz, 168–169, 2000.
41. Eagle RC Jr: High-risk features and tumor differentiation in retinoblastoma: a retrospective histopathologic study, Arch Pathol Lab Med 133:1203–1209, 2009.
42. Sastre X, Chantada GL, Doz F, et al.: Proceedings of the consensus meetings from the International Retinoblastoma Staging Working Group on the pathology guidelines for the examination of enucleated eyes and evaluation of prognostic risk factors in retinoblastoma, Arch Pathol Lab Med 33:1199–1202, 2009.
43. Murphree AL: Molecular genetics of retinoblastoma, Ophthalmol Clin North Am 8:155–166, 1995.
44. Shields JA, Parsons HM, Shields CL, Shah P: Lesions simulating retinoblastoma, J Pediatr Ophthalmol Strabismus 28:338–340, 1991.
45. Shields JA, Shields CL: Intraocular tumors: a text and atlas, Philadelphia, 1993, W.B. Saunders.
46. Shields JA, Shields CL: Atlas of intraocular tumors, Philadelphia, 1999, Lippincott. Williams & Wilkins.
47. Shields JA, Shields CL, Parsons HM: Differential diagnosis of retinoblastoma, Retina 11:232–243, 1991.
48. Shields JA, Shields CL, Honavar SG, Demirci H: Clinical variations and complications of Coats' disease in 150 cases: the 2000 Sanford Gifford Memorial Lecture, Am J Ophthalmol 131:561–571, 2001.
49. Shields JA, Shields CL, Honavar SG, et al.: Classification and management of Coats' disease: the 2000 Proctor Lecture, Am J Ophthalmol 131:572–583, 2001.
50. Goldberg MF: Persistent fetal vasculature (PFV): an integrated interpretation of signs and symptoms associated with persistent hyperplastic primary vitreous (PHPV). LIV Edward Jackson Memorial Lecture, Am J Ophthalmol 124:587–626, 1997.
51. Shields JA, Shields CL: Intraocular tumors: a text and atlas, Philadelphia, 1992, W.B. Saunders.
52. Broughton WL, Zimmerman LE: A clinicopathologic study of 56 cases of intraocular medulloepithelioma, Am J Ophthalmol 85: 407–418, 1978.
53. Shields JA, Eagle RC Jr, Shields CL, Potter PD: Congenital neoplasms of the nonpigmented ciliary epithelium (medulloepithelioma), Ophthalmology 103:1998–2006, 1996.
54. Kaliki S, Shields CL, Eagle RC Jr, et al.: Ciliary body medulloepithelioma: analysis of 41 cases, Ophthalmology 120(12):2552–2559, 2013.
55. Green WR, Iliff WJ, Trotter RR: Malignant teratoid medulloepithelioma of the optic nerve, Arch Ophthalmol 91:451–454, 1974.
56. O'Keefe M, Fulcher T, Kelly P, et al: Medulloepithelioma of the optic nerve head, Arch Ophthalmol 115:1325–1327, 1997.

ORBITAL TUMORS

Jurij R. Bilyk

CHAPTER 52

1. Should all orbital capillary hemangiomas be excised?

   No. Most capillary hemangioma (the preferred term is infantile hemangioma) will involute spontaneously over months and require no intervention. Periocular infantile hemangioma should be treated only if there is evidence of:
   - Amblyopia caused by refractive error (induced myopia or astigmatism) or
   - Ptosis causing visual obstruction or head tilt.

   Treatment options include:
   - Systemic or, in select superficial cases, topical β-blockers like propranolol. Note that use of systemic β-blockers requires close initial monitoring by a pediatric team for any cardiovascular side effects.
   - Corticosteroid injections or systemic therapy. The use of particulate suspension injection (e.g., triamcinolone) is often avoided because of the rare risk of vascular occlusion (ophthalmic artery, central retinal artery).
   - Excision, usually reserved for cases unresponsive to more conservative therapy or for isolated, well-circumscribed lesions of the anterior orbit.
   - Interferon α-2 therapy, especially in large localized or systemic cases. This therapy has largely been abandoned because of the risk of spastic diplegia and the success of β-blockers.[1–3]

2. What orbital tumors can mimic orbital cellulitis?

   In **both adults and children,** consider noninfectious inflammation (idiopathic orbital inflammation, thyroid eye disease, sarcoidosis, granulomatosis with polyangiitis).

   In **children,** consider:
   - Ruptured dermoid cyst, which causes a fulminant soft tissue inflammation
   - Rhabdomyosarcoma (RMS)
   - Lymphangioma, especially with rapid expansion from a blood-filled "chocolate cyst"
   - Neuroblastoma, which can present with a rapid onset of proptosis and ecchymosis

   In **adults,** consider:
   - Lymphoproliferative disease, including lymphoma. Although most lymphoma present in an indolent fashion, about 20% to 25% may present with inflammatory signs, especially if they are of an aggressive subtype.
   - Extrascleral spread and necrosis of an intraocular melanoma
   - Metastatic disease to the orbit

3. What are the most common causes of childhood proptosis?
   - Orbital cellulitis
   - Infantile hemangioma
   - Idiopathic orbital inflammation
   - Dermoid cyst
   - RMS
   - Lymphangioma

4. When and how does cavernous hemangioma usually present?
   - Cavernous hemangioma (CH) is the most common vascular orbital tumor in adults and the most common benign orbital tumor.
   - It is now characterized as a type of venous malformation of the orbit.
   - CH typically presents in the fourth and fifth decades of life.
   - It is well circumscribed on imaging (see question 16).
   - It is *not* the adult equivalent of infantile hemangioma. Not only are the lesions distinct histopathologically, but unlike infantile hemangioma, CH is a *slowly* proliferating entity.
   - Because of its slow growth, it is usually a well-tolerated lesion that causes few symptoms. Visual loss, if any, is slow and limited to lesions of the orbital apex.
   - Excision is curative.[4–6]

5. What are orbital fibrous histiocytoma and hemangiopericytoma?
   - Both lesions are so-called "spindle cell tumors" and should no longer be considered as distinct, separate entities. Advances in immunohistochemistry and molecular genetics have shown that both entities are now subsumed into the extrapleural solitary fibrous tumor (SFT) rubric.
   - SFTs are mesenchymal tumors with a spectrum of histopathologic findings and clinical behavior (as an example, hemangiopericytoma is now classified as "SFT with cellularity").

- Nuclear staining for Signal Transducer and Activator of Transcription 6 (STAT6) is helpful in making diagnosis of SFT.
- If surgery is indicated, complete excision is recommended to minimize the risk of recurrence, but this is often challenging because the tumors, albeit appearing well-circumscribed on imaging, often have infiltrating edges and can be adherent to normal orbital soft tissue anatomy.
- Even after presumed complete excision, patients need to be followed over the long term for recurrence and transformation into a more aggressive behavior, with possible regional or distant metastases. Fortunately, this occurs in only a minority of orbital SFTs.[7–9]

6. What about orbital schwannoma?
- Orbital schwannoma is a tumor of the Schwann cells that form the lining of peripheral nerves.
- Schwannomas do *not* arise from the optic nerve sheath.
- Within the orbit, most schwannomas arise from sensory nerve sheaths, which may explain their predilection for the superior orbit.
- Antoni A and B patterns are the classic histologic findings in schwannoma. The A pattern is characterized by abundant, tightly packed spindle cells, whereas the B pattern exhibits fewer cells within a myxoid matrix.[10–12]

7. How does one order orbital computed tomography?
- Newer multiscan computed tomography (CT) machines image patients in the axial plane but obtain three-dimensional data, allowing for coronal and parasagittal images with loss of resolution. Axial, coronal, and parasagittal images should be reviewed in all orbital studies (See IKey Points).
- Review both soft tissue and bone windows, as they provide complimentary information.
- Never order cuts greater than 3 mm. Emergency head CTs are often obtained with only axial planes and >3 mm width, with very limited views of the orbit.
- Intravenous contrast is helpful in cases of infection or inflammation. It is not necessary for trauma or in typical thyroid eye disease.
- Remember that CT requires the use of radiation, and multiple, serial CTs should be avoided in children to minimize the risk of secondary tumor formation in later years.[13–15]

8. How does one order orbital magnetic resonance imaging?
Very carefully, according to the following guidelines (See IKey Points):
- *Never* order magnetic resonance imaging (MRI) as the first imaging modality in trauma, unresponsive patients, or in poor historians. Occult metal within the magnetic field can move and cause severe soft tissue damage.
- Remember that brain MRI uses different imaging sequences compared with orbital MRI. If you want an orbital scan, *specifically order an orbital study*, and simply a brain MRI.
- Always review axial, coronal, and parasagittal views.
- Always include the cavernous sinus and paranasal sinuses.
- Always order gadolinium and fat suppression (Fig. 52.1).

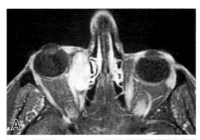
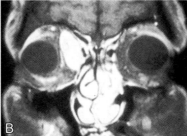

Fig. 52.1 A and **B,** T1-weighted magnetic resonance images of the orbit with fat suppression.

- In T1, orbital fat is bright and vitreous is dark.
- In T2, vitreous is brighter than fat.
- The majority of orbital masses are dark in T1 *before* gadolinium administration. Exceptions to this rule: lesions containing melanin (e.g., melanoma), lesions containing fat (e.g., lipoma, liposarcoma), lesions containing mucus (mucocele, dermoid cyst), and subacute blood (2–7 days old).[13,14]

KEY POINTS: IMAGING ORBITAL PROCESSES

1. Unilateral or bilateral proptosis usually requires imaging, especially if it is progressive.
2. Computed tomography (CT) of the orbit is generally easier to obtain and interpret than magnetic resonance imaging (MRI).
3. CT is the recommended imaging modality for trauma, infection, and thyroid eye disease.
4. MRI is recommended for soft tissue processes, for imaging of the orbital apex/cavernous sinus, skull base, and for suspected intracranial processes.
5. Well-tolerated, well-circumscribed lesions of the orbit can be followed conservatively with serial imaging alone in selected cases.

9. Discuss the histologic classification of orbital rhabdomyosarcoma.
Orbital RMS is histologically divided into the following four groups:
- Embryonal
- Alveolar
- Anaplastic (formerly pleomorphic)
- Spindle cell/sclerosing (which rarely affects the orbit)
    The average age of onset is 9 years, but the span is broad. RMS is thought to arise from pluripotential mesenchymal tissue within the orbit and *not* from extraocular muscle. There are many useful facts to remember about each group.
Embryonal
- This group is further subdivided into classic, botryoid, and not otherwise specified.
- This is the most common RMS subtype is found in children.
- The botryoid subtype is defined as an embryonal RMS abutting a mucosal surface (e.g., conjunctiva).
Alveolar
- Alveolar RMS appears to affect the inferior orbit most frequently and carries a worse prognosis than embryonal RMS.
- Fortunately, findings by the Intergroup Rhabdomyosarcoma Study (IRS) indicate that, with more aggressive therapy, the prognosis for alveolar RMS approaches the prognosis for the embryonal form.
Anaplastic
- This group of RMS occurs in older adults.[7,16,17]

10. How is orbital RMS best treated? What is the prognosis?
Much of what is known about the treatment of orbital RMS comes from the four IRSs.
- Treatment of orbital RMS consists of a combination of chemotherapy and radiation therapy.
- Radiation therapy in doses of 4000 to 6000 cGy definitely carries significant morbidity for the globe, but the third IRS concluded that it is still necessary for adequate treatment. Lower doses of radiation are currently under study.
- Orbital and genitourinary RMS carry the best prognosis for unclear reasons.
- Local spread from the orbit into the paranasal sinuses or cranial vault decreases survival rates.[7,16,17]

11. With regard to lacrimal gland lesions, what is "the rule of 50s"?
The "rule of 50s" summarizes the incidence of lacrimal gland tumors in an orbital referral practice.
- 50% of lacrimal gland lesions are nonepithelioid, consisting mostly of inflammatory and lymphoproliferative lesions, and 50% are of epithelial origin.
- 50% of the epithelial tumors are benign pleomorphic adenomas (benign mixed tumor), and 50% are various malignant types.
- 50% of the malignant tumors are adenoid cystic carcinomas.
- 50% of the adenoid cystic carcinomas are of the basaloid variant.
    The final rule is important clinically, because a basaloid histopathology for adenoid cystic carcinoma carries the worst prognosis.
    In a general ophthalmology practice, the rule of 50s does not apply. The incidence of infectious and noninfectious inflammatory dacryoadenitis is significantly higher than in an orbital referral practice.[18,19]

12. What factors help to distinguish benign and malignant epithelial lacrimal gland tumors?
See Table 52.1.

13. What is the most common metastatic tumor to the orbital soft tissue in men and women?
- **Men:** Lung.
- **Women:** Breast carcinoma (but the incidence of lung carcinoma is increasing).
  Note that the question asks specifically about orbital soft tissue. Otherwise, prostate carcinoma would be an acceptable alternative in men, depending on the clinical series. Metastatic prostate carcinoma has a propensity for orbital bone.
  Note: Metastatic lesions are approximately 10 times more common to the uvea than the orbit on autopsy studies. This may be caused by the high blood flow through the choroid, which may allow more facile metastatic seeding of uveal tissue.[20–22]

14. What is the appropriate workup for orbital lymphoma and lymphoid hyperplasia?
Regardless of the histopathology, any lymphoproliferative lesion of the orbit or ocular adnexa requires a systemic workup, as follows:
- Complete blood count.
- Serum protein electrophoresis and lactate dehydrogenase level.
- CT imaging of the neck, thorax, abdomen, and pelvis, which should be repeated every 6 months for at least 2 years, is performed. Alternatively, positron emission tomography (PET)/CT from the skull base to the midthighs may be performed.
- Bone marrow biopsy is now recommended on initial presentation in all cases of periocular lymphoma.[23–26]

15. What are the important facts about orbital lymphoproliferative lesions?
- Inflammatory orbital inflammation is *not* a lymphoproliferative disorder because, histopathologically, the reaction is not limited to lymphocytes. It is *not* a precursor for orbital lymphoma.
- Most orbital lymphomas are of non-Hodgkin, B-cell origin, usually of the so-called EMZL/MALT type (extranodal marginal zone lymphoma of mucosa-associated lymphoid tissue).
- The vast majority of lymphoid lesions, whether polyclonal (lymphoid hyperplasia) or monoclonal (lymphoma), are highly radiosensitive.
- The prognosis and treatment of orbital non-Hodgkin lymphoma (NHL) are highly dependent on the specific subtype—periocular NHL should never be approached as a generic, all-encompassing rubric of "lymphoma," but rather managed by the subtype and stage of disease (Tables 52.2 and 52.3).[23–26]

16. What are the differential diagnoses of a well-circumscribed orbital mass?
- CH (cavernous venous malformation)
- Schwannoma
- Neurofibroma
- SFT and its subtypes
- Dermoid cyst
- Lymphoma (about 50% are well circumscribed, especially when involving the lacrimal gland).

Table 52.1 Clinical Characteristics of Lacrimal Gland Lesions

	PLEOMORPHIC ADENOMA	ADENOID CYSTIC CARCINOMA
Duration	>1 year	<1 year
Pain	Rare	Common
Diplopia	Uncommon	Common
Computed tomographic findings	No bony destruction ± Fossa formation	Bony destruction common
Surgery	**Excisional biopsy**	**Incisional biopsy**
When in doubt, perform total excision of the mass.		
Postsurgical therapy	Clinical follow-up only	Controversial: Radiation, chemotherapy, radical excision

Data from Henderson JW: Adenoid cystic carcinoma of the lacrimal gland, is there a cure? *Trans Am Ophthal Soc* 85:312–319, 1987; Rose GE, Wright JE: Pleomorphic adenoma of the lacrimal gland. *Br J Ophthalmol* 76:395–400, 1992; and Wright JE: Factors affecting the survival of patients with lacrimal gland tumours. *Can J Ophthalmol* 17:3–9, 1982.

Table 52.2 Distribution of Most Common Systemic and Ocular Adnexal NHL Subtypes

SYSTEMIC LYMPHOMA (WHO DATA)	OCULAR ADNEXAL LYMPHOMA (N = 353 AND 797)
DLBCL (37%)	EMZL (52%–57%)
FL (29%)	FL (11%–23%)
EMZL (9%)	DLBCL (8%–15%)
CLL (12%)	MCL (5%–8%)
MCL (7%)	CLL/SCL (1%–4%)

CLL/SCL, Chronic lymphocytic leukemia/small cell lymphoma; *DLBCL*, diffuse large B cell lymphoma; *EMZL*, extranodal marginal zone lymphoma; *FL*, follicular lymphoma; *MCL*, mantle cell lymphoma; *NHL*, non-Hodgkin lymphoma; *WHO*, World Health Organization.
Data from Marey HM, Elmazar HF, Mandour SS, Khairy HA: Combined oral and topical beta blockers for the treatment of early proliferative superficial periocular infantile capillary hemangioma, *J Pediatr Ophthalmol Strabismus* 55:37–42, 2018; Al Dhaybi R, Superstein R, Milet A, et al.: Treatment of periocular infantile hemangiomas with propranolol: case series of 18 children, *Ophthalmology* 118:1184–1188; Harris GJ, Jakobiec FA: Cavernous hemangioma of the orbit: an analysis of 66 cases, *J Neurosurg* 51:219–228, 1979; and Schmitt E, Spoerri O: Schwannomas of the orbit, *Acta Neurochir* 53:79–85, 1980.

Table 52.3 Clinical Behavior and Management Strategies of the Most Common Ocular Adnexal NHL Subtypes

AGGRESSIVE LYMPHOMA	INDOLENT LYMPHOMA
DLBCL Mantle cell Burkitt	Follicular (Grades 1 and 2) EMZL/MALT CLL
Fatal if not cured	Incurable, indolent
Approach to cure	Chronic management

CLL, Chronic lymphocytic leukemia; *DLBCL*, diffuse large B cell lymphoma; *EMZL*, extranodal marginal zone lymphoma; *MCL*, mantle cell lymphoma.

REFERENCES

1. Marey HM, Elmazar HF, Mandour SS, Khairy HA: Combined oral and topical beta blockers for the treatment of early proliferative superficial periocular infantile capillary hemangioma, J Pediatr Ophthalmol Strabismus 55:37–42, 2018.
2. Al Dhaybi R, Superstein R, Milet A, et al.: Treatment of periocular infantile hemangiomas with propranolol: case series of 18 children, Ophthalmology 118:1184–1188.
3. Al-Haddad C, El Salloukh NA, El Moussawi Z: β-Blockers in the treatment of periocular infantile hemangioma, Curr Opin Ophthalmol 30:319–325, 2019.
4. Harris GJ, Jakobiec FA: Cavernous hemangioma of the orbit: an analysis of 66 cases, J Neurosurg 51:219–228, 1979.
5. McNab AA, Wright JE: Cavernous hemangioma of the orbit, Austr N Z J Ophthalmol 17:337–345, 1989.
6. Calandriello L, Grimaldi G, Petrone G, et al.: Cavernous venous malformation (cavernous hemangioma) of the orbit: current concepts and a review of the literature, Surv Ophthalmol 62:393–403, 2017.
7. Fletcher CDM, Bridge JA, Hogenddorn PCW, Mertens F: WHO classification of tumours of soft tissue and bone, ed 4, Lyon, 2013, IARC.
8. Ronchi A, Cozzolino I, Zito Marino F, et al.: Extrapleural solitary fibrous tumor: a distinct entity from pleural solitary fibrous tumor. An update on clinical, molecular and diagnostic features, Ann Diagn Pathol 34:142–150, 2018.
9. Smith SC, Gooding WE, Elkins M, et al.: Solitary fibrous tumors of the head and neck: a multi-institutional clinicopathologic study, Am J Surg Pathol 41(12):1642–1656, 2017.
10. Sweeney AR, Gupta D, Keene CD, et al.: Orbital peripheral nerve sheath tumors, Surv Ophthalmol 62:43–57, 2017.
11. Rootman J, Goldberg C, Robertson W: Primary orbital schwannomas, Br J Ophthalmol 66:194–204, 1982.
12. Schmitt E, Spoerri O: Schwannomas of the orbit, Acta Neurochir 53:79–85, 1980.
13. Dutton JJ: Radiology of the orbit and visual pathways, Philadelphia, 2010, Elsevier.
14. Bilaniuk L, Murchison MP, Bilyk JR: Imaging in pediatric orbital disease. In: Katowitz JA, Katowitz WR, editors: Pediatric oculoplastic surgery, ed 2, 2018, Springer, pp 551–622.
15. Pearce MS, Salotti JA, Little MP, et al.: Radiation exposure from CT scans in childhood and subsequent risk of leukaemia and brain tumours: a retrospective cohort study, Lancet 380(9840):499–505, 2012.
16. Malempati S, Hawkins DS: Rhabdomyosarcoma: review of the Children's Oncology Group (COG) Soft-Tissue Sarcoma Committee experience and rationale for current COG studies, Pediatr Blood Cancer 59(1):5–10, 2012.

17. Lane KA, Bilyk JR, Jakobiec FA: Mesenchymal, fibroosseous, and cartilagenous orbital tumors. In: Albert DM, Miller JW, editors: Principles and practice of ophthalmology, ed 4, Philadelphia, 2020, Saunders.
18. Font RL, Gamel JW: Epithelial tumors of the lacrimal gland: an analysis of 265 cases. In: Jakobiec FA, editor: Ocular and adnexal tumors, Birmingham, AL, 1978, Aesculapius Publishing, pp 787–805.
19. Font RL, Gamel JW: Adenoid cystic carcinoma of the lacrimal gland: a clinicopathologic study of 79 cases. In: Nicholson DH, editor: Ocular pathology update, New York, 1980, Masson Publishing, pp 277–283.
20. Font RL, Ferry AP: Carcinoma metastatic to the eye and orbit III. A clinicopathologic study of 28 cases metastatic to the orbit, Cancer 38:1326–1335, 1976.
21. Goldberg RA, Rootman J: Clinical characteristics of metastatic orbital tumors, Ophthalmology 97:620–624, 1990.
22. Shields CL, Shields JA, Peggs M: Tumors metastatic to the orbit, Ophthal Plast Reconstr Surg 4:73–80, 1988.
23. Swerdlow SH, Campo E, Harris NL, et al.: WHO classification of tumors of haematopoietic and lymphoid tissues, revised ed 4, Lyon, 2017, International Agency for Research on Cancer (IARC).
24. Olsen TG, Holm F, Mikkelsen LH, et al.: Orbital lymphoma—an international multicenter retrospective study, Am J Ophthalmol 199:44–57, 2019.
25. Olsen TG, Heegaard S: Orbital lymphoma, Surv Ophthalmol 64(1):45–66, 2019.
26. Murchison AP, Bilyk JR: Ocular adnexal lymphoproliferative disease. In: Black EV, Nesi FA, Calvano CJ, Gladstone GJ, Levine MR, editors: Smith and Nesi's ophthalmic plastic and reconstructive surgery, New York, 2020, C.V. Mosby.

INDEX

Note: Page numbers followed by "f" refer to illustrations; page numbers followed by "t" refer to tables; page numbers followed by "b" refer to boxes.

A

A wave, 29b
ABCDEF guide, 389
Abducens nerve palsy, 251
Abduction deficit, 223
Aberrant regeneration, 249, 252
Abetalipoproteinemia, 232
Abney effect, 25
Abscess
  orbital subperiosteal, 272
  subconjunctival, 237
Acanthamoeba, in corneal infections, 77, 82, 82f
Acanthamoeba keratitis, 87–88
AC:A ratio. *see* Accommodative convergence:accommodation
  (AC:A) ratio
Accommodation
  amplitude of, 11
    measurement of, 20
  range of, 11
Accommodative convergence, 241
Accommodative convergence:accommodation (AC:A) ratio, 225
Accommodative insufficiency, 229
Acetazolamide (Diamox), for cystoid macular edema, 215
Acetylcholine receptor antibody test, 287
Acetylcysteine, 110
Achromatopsia, 240
  electroretinographic evaluation of, 32
Acid burns, 71
Acne rosacea, 69
Acquired immunodeficiency syndrome (AIDS), ocular
  manifestations of, 305–309, 308b
Acquired periodic alternating nystagmus, 242
AcrySof IQ PanOptix IOL, 210
Acuity meters, false-positive readings with, 19
Acute acquired comitant esotropia, 226
Acute dacryocystitis, treatment for, 268
Acute primary angle closure (APAC), 155–156
Acute retinal necrosis (ARN) syndrome, 296t, 300
Acyclovir, 66–67, 93
  for herpes simplex keratitis, 85
Adaptometer, Goldmann-Weekers, 34
Adenoid cystic carcinomas, 399
Adenopathy, preauricular, 95
Adherence syndrome, 237
Adie's tonic pupil, test for, 246
Adolescents, myopia in, 130
Adrenergic agonist
  action of, 173
  for primary open-angle glaucoma, 173
  side effects of, 175, 175t
African Americans, glaucoma in, 143, 144–145

Afterimages, 25, 25f
Aggressive posterior ROP (AP-ROP), 343
Albinism, 240
Alcohol, anticoagulant effects of, 193
Alemtuzumab (Lemtrada), 257
Alexia, 263
Alkali burns, 71
Allergic reactions
  to ophthalmic medication, 65–66
  to penicillin, 97
  as ptosis cause, 288
  to topical medications, 179
Altitudinal defects, 53, 55f
Amaurosis
  fugax, 262, 354
  Leber's congenital
    electroretinographic evaluation of, 32
    keratoconus and, 122
Amblyopia, 218–1, 220b
  anatomic changes in, 218
  anisometropia and, 218
  anisometropic, 221
  classification of, 218
  in congenital esotropia, 224
  "critical" or "sensitive" period for, 218
  definition of, 218–222
  detecting, 219–220, 219f
  discontinuation of treatment for, 220
  orbital capillary hemangiomas and, 397
  photoscreening, 219–220
  prevalence of, 218
  treatment of, 221, 221b
    upper age limit for, 221
Aminocaproic acid
  adverse effects of, 194
  contraindications to, 194
  for hyphema, 194
Aminoglycosides, 96
Aminoguanidine, for glaucoma, 177
Amoxicillin, 97
Ampicillin, 97
Amplitude, in electroretinogram, 31
Amsler grids, 50, 335
Anesthesia
  for cataract surgery, 205–206
  retrobulbar injection of, 1
  for trabeculectomy, 182–183
Aneurysm
  Leber's miliary, 319
  telangiectatic-like, 319
  third-nerve palsy-associated, 248

Angiography
  computed tomography, 248
  fluorescein
    for age-related macular degeneration evaluation, 338
    for choroid visualization, 4
    for Coats disease diagnosis, 320
    for diabetic retinopathy evaluation, 348, 349f, 352
    for differentiation of choroidal melanoma from subretinal
      blood, 381
    findings in central serous chorioretinopathy, 44
    fovea on, 44
    neovascularization on, 44, 44f
    patterns of fluorescence on, 43, 43b, 43f
    phases of, 43
    of retinal vein occlusion, 362f
    technique of, 42
  indocyanine green, 45f
  magnetic resonance, 248
Angiomatosis retinae. *see* von Hippel-Lindau syndrome.
Angle recession, 191
  cyclodialysis and, 198
  gonioscopic appearance of, 198
  ocular trauma and, 198, 199f
Angular magnification, 16
Aniridia, 172
Aniseikonia, 248
Anisocoria, 245, 248
Anisometropia, 218
  as amblyopia cause, 220
  correction of, 221
  Prentice's rule of, 13
  symptomatic, alleviation of, 13b
Ankylosing spondylitis, 295, 295t
Annulus of Zinn, 1, 1f, 7
Anterior chamber
  after acute angle-closure attack, 162
  after trabeculectomy, 185, 186f
  angle of
    classification systems in, gonioscopic, 151
    gonioscopic appearance of, 3
    landmarks in, 151–156, 152f
    other methods of evaluating, 154
  blood in, 212
  cataract surgery-related, 211
  cell, in HSV infection, 66–67
  effect of pilocarpine on, 178
  flat
    differential diagnosis for, 189
    management of, 189–190
  lens of, 203
  reformation, for aqueous misdirection syndrome, 165
Anterior chamber tap, for endophthalmitis, 81
Anterior inferior cerebellar artery syndrome, 251t
Anterior membrane dystrophies, 112
Anterior segment
  blunt trauma to, 191
  ischemia of, 238
    surgery causing, 237
Antibiotics. *see also* names of specific antibiotics.
  as retinopathy cause, 315
  topical, 94–102, 99t
    and steroid combinations, 101t

Anticholinergic medications, contraindication in narrow-angle
  glaucoma, 163
Antifibrinolytic agents, for hyphema, 194
Antiglaucoma medications. *see* Glaucoma, medical treatment of;
  names of specific antiglaucoma medications
Antihistamines, for red eye treatment, 65
Antimetabolites
  indications for, in trabeculectomy, 186
  for orbital inflammation, 281
Anti–myelin oligodendrocyte glycoprotein (anti-MOG), 255
Antireflective coatings, on spectacle lens, 18
Anti-vascular endothelial growth factor, 338, 350
  for diabetic retinopathy, 352
Antiviral therapy
  for cytomegalovirus retinitis, 307
  resistance to, 306
Apert's syndrome, 228
Aphakia, 203, 208
Apoplexy, pituitary, 233
Apraclonidine, 175
  allergic reaction to, 179
  for glaucoma, 173
Apraxia, congenital ocular motor, 232
Aqueous layer, 5
Aqueous misdirection syndrome, 165
Aqueous tube shunts, for neovascular glaucoma, 166
Arden ratio, 33
Argon laser trabeculoplasty, 3
Arteritis, giant cell, 262, 356, 356b
Arthritis
  Lyme disease and, 299
  neonatal conjunctivitis and, 92b
  psoriatic, 295, 295t
A-scan ultrasonography, 35
Asian American, glaucoma in, 75–76
Aspergillus, as retinitis cause, 300
Aspiration, of subretinal exudates, 320
Aspirin, anticoagulant effects of, 193
Asthenopia, 20, 228
  convergence insufficiency-related, 252
Asthma, keratoconus and, 121–122
Astigmatism, 130, 216–217
  acquired, 19
  after corneal transplant, 140
  from contact lens, 121
  as diplopia cause, 248
  of oblique incidence, 15, 15f
  postkeratoplasty, 128
  treatment options for, 139–140, 140f
  with-the-rule or against-the-rule, 15
Astrocytoma, juvenile pilocytic, 272
Atopy, keratoconus and, 121–122
Atropine, 18, 184
Avellino dystrophy, 115
Axenfeld's anomaly, 172
Axial magnification, formula for, 16
Axial myopia, 11
Azithromycin, 99t

B
B wave, 29b
Bacillus cereus infections, 333

Bacitracin, 66, 92, 95, 99t
Bacterial resistance, 83
BAP1 gene, 389
BAP1 syndrome, 389
BAP-1 tumor predisposition syndrome, 384
Bartonella henselae, 300
Basal cell carcinoma, of eyelid, 289, 291f
  metastasis of, 290
  "rodent ulcer," 289
Basal cell nevus syndrome, 291
Bassen-Kornzweig syndrome, 232
Batten-Mayou (Vogt-Spielmeyer) disease, 355
Behçet's disease, 297t, 300
Bell's palsy, 103
Benedikt's syndrome, 251t
Benzalkonium chloride (BAK), 175
Bergmeister's papilla, 4
Besifloxacin, 99t
Best disease, 34
Betaxolol, 176
Bevacizumab, 364
Bezold-Brucke phenomenon, 24–25
Bietti's peripheral crystalline dystrophy, 114
Bifocals
  with low-vision aids, 17
  prismatic effect of, 14
Bimatoprost, 176–177
Binasal hemianopia, 55–56
Binocular diplopia
  causes of, 248
  nonsurgical approaches, 253
Biomicroscopy, ultrasound, 38, 38f
Biopsy
  conjunctival, 301
  corneal, 82
  fine-needle aspiration, of uveal melanoma, 382
  lacrimal, 301
  orbital, 280
  retinoblastoma and, 376
  of sebaceous gland carcinoma, 292
  of temporal artery, 8, 261
Birth control, as cause of dry eye, 104
Bitemporal field defect, simulation of, 259
Bleb needling, 189
Blebs, 182, 182f, 183f, 187f, 188–189
Blepharitis, 67–68, 68f, 104, 109, 110
  as cause of red eye, 65
  as cause of superficial punctate keratopathy, 67
  treatment of, 95
Blepharochalasis, as ptosis cause, 288
Blepharophimosis syndrome, 285, 285f
Blepharoplasty
  as cause of dry eye, 104
  in thyroid eye disease patients, 278
Blepharoptosis, topical steroids and, 98
Blepharotomy, transverse, 8
Blindness. *see also* Vision loss.
  cataract and, 201
  retinopathy of prematurity and, 343
Blind spot, physiologic, 50
Blink reflex, 103
Bloch-Sulzberger syndrome, 345t

β-blockers
  action of, 173
  for primary open-angle glaucoma, 173
  side effects of, 175–176, 175t
Blood-retinal barrier, 3
Blow-out fracture, orbital, 1–5
Blunt trauma, ocular, 191
Blurred vision
  chelating agents and, 316
  keratoconus and, 122
  near, convergence insufficiency-related, 228–229
  xanthopsia and, 314
Botulinum toxin (Botox), 110
  injections, as abducens nerve palsy treatment, 251
  as ptosis cause, 288
Bowman probe, 268
Bowman's layer, 3
  corneal dystrophies of, 113–114
"Boxcarring," 354
Branch retinal arterial obstructions (BRAOs), 354
Breast carcinoma, metastatic, 389, 400
Brightness, of colors, 24
Brimonidine, 175, 179
  contraindicated in children, 179
  for glaucoma, 173, 175
  during pregnancy, 179
Brimonidine tartrate, 74
Bromfenac (Prolensa), 65
Brow lift, 278
Brown, 24
Brown's syndrome, 229, 230b, 231f, 236
  differential diagnosis of, 230
  indications for surgery in, 236
  treatment of, 229–230
Bruch's membrane, 3, 3b
  tears of, 326–327
Bruckner test, 219, 219f
B-scan ultrasonography, 35
Burns
  phacoemulsification, 211
  ultraviolet, 67
Busacca nodules, 294, 295t

C

C wave, 29b
Calcification, on ultrasound, 37
Canaliculodacryocystorhinostomy (CDCR), 268
Canaliculus, obstructions, 267
Cancer therapy drugs, as toxic retinopathy cause, 316–317, 317f
Cannabinoids, for glaucoma, 178
Can-opener capsulotomy, 207–208, 208f
"Capsular bag," 203
Capsular rupture, vitreous loss after, 215
Capsular tension rings, 216
Capsulotomy, 207–208, 208f, 215
Carbonic anhydrase inhibitors, 215
  action of, 173
  for angle closure, 158
  side effects of, 175t, 176
Cataract(s), 201–204
  brunescent, 170
  Coats disease and, 319

Cataract(s) *(Continued)*
derivation of, 201–204
effect on electroretinographic findings, 32
extraction of
for acute primary angle closure, 161
with endocyclophotocoagulation, 162
in Fuchs' dystrophy patients, 117–119
with goniosynechialysis, 162
for pseudoexfoliation glaucoma, 168
Fuchs' heterochromic iridocyclitis and, 171
glassblowers', 202
morgagnian, 201
nonsurgical management of, 205
nuclear sclerotic, 201
"second sight" and, 201
symptoms of, 201
phacolytic, 201
phacomorphic, 202
posterior subcapsular, 201
radiation and, 291
removal of, basic steps of, 205
"ripe," 203
sympathetic ophthalmia and, 333
systemic findings in, 201
topical steroids and, 98–99
traumatic, 202
Cataract surgery
complications of, 211–217
intraoperative, 211b
postoperative, 212b
diabetes with, 215
extracapsular, 204, 206, 207f
future of, 209–210
indications for, 202, 205–210
intracapsular, 204, 206
patients with intraoperative floppy iris syndrome, 216
postoperative management of patients, 209
as retinal detachment risk factor, 367
significant trends in, 209
techniques of, 205–210
vision, restoration of, options for, 208
wound closure in, 209
Cat-scratch disease, as uveitis cause, 296t
Cavernous sinus syndrome, 251t
Cavernous sinus thrombosis, 233
Cecocentral lesion, 57
Cefazolin, 96
Ceftriaxone, 66, 92
Cellulitis
orbital, 272, 281, 397
in strabismus surgery, 237
Center-involving edema, 350
Central cloudy dystrophy of François, 115
Central nervous system, nystagmus and, 242
Central retinal arterial obstructions (CRAOs), 354
Central retinal artery, occlusion of, 4
electroretinographic evaluation of, 32
as giant cell arteritis cause, 262
Central retinal vein, occlusion of, electroretinographic evaluation
of, 32
Central vestibular instability nystagmus, 242
Cephalosporins, 96
Cephalosporium acremonium, 96

Cerebellopontine angle syndrome, 251t
Chalazion, 248, 292
Chalcosis, 332
as cause of open-angle glaucoma, 172
Chandler's syndrome, 172
Charcoal, color of, 26
Chelating agents, as maculopathy cause, 316
Chemical injuries, as cause of open-angle glaucoma, 172
Chemosis, 66, 95–96
Cherry-red spot, 355
Chest trauma, as fundus abnormalities cause, 333–334
Chiasm. *see* Optic chiasm
Chiasmal visual defects, differential diagnosis of, 259b
Child abuse, ocular manifestations in, 333–334
Children. *see also* Infants; Neonates.
amblyopia in, 218
amblyopia screening for, 219
astigmatism in, spectacle prescription for, 18
clinical techniques for checking in nonverbal children,
219, 219f
Coats disease in, 319
glaucoma medications for, 179–180
leukemia in, 305b
nonspecific orbital inflammation in, 279
open-angle glaucoma in, 172
optic nerve glioma, 272
orbital cellulitis in, 281
orbital tumors in, 397
retinoblastoma in, 303, 373
rhabdomyosarcoma in, 272
sarcoidosis in, 301
spontaneous hyphema in, 296
Chin-up position, 230
Chlamydia trachomatis, neonatal conjunctivitis from, 90
Chloramphenicol, 99t
Chlorolabe, 23
Chloroquine, 32, 259
in electroretinogram and electro-oculogram, 34
as retinopathy cause, 311
Chlorpromazine, as retinopathy cause, 313
Chorioretinitis, birdshot, 297t, 301
Choroid
detachment
drainage of, indication for, 190, 190f
detachment of, 37t
disciform lesion, 36t
fluorescein angiography visualization of, 4
hemangioma of, 36, 36t, 390, 390f
hemorrhage, 36t
leukemic infiltrate of, 304, 304f
melanoma of, 36, 36t, 383
acceptable method of treat, 383
melanosomes in, 3
neovascularization of, 337, 338
classic, 337, 337f
occult, 337, 337f
nevus of, 36t, 379, 379f
in optical coherence tomography, 42
rupture of, 326–327, 328f, 329, 329f, 330f
tumor of, 386
Choroidal effusions
filtering procedures-related, 3
trabeculectomy and, 190, 190f

Choroidal hemangiomas, 390
Choroiditis
    fungal, as uveitis cause, 296t
    multifocal, 301, 302
        as uveitis cause, 297t
    serpiginous, 297t, 302
    syphilis and, 300
    tuberculosis and, 300
Chromatic aberration, 15, 15f
Chronic progressive external ophthalmoplegia (CPEO), 232,
        233f, 285b
    diseases associated with, 232
Chronic relapsing inflammatory optic neuropathy (CRION), 258
Ciliary body
    gonioscopic appearance of, 3
    injury to, 199
    medulloepitheliomas of, 394
    melanoma of, 383, 383f
    swelling/anterior rotation of, angle closure glaucoma and,
        155
Ciliary body band, 151
Ciliary processes, blockage of trabeculectomy site by, 188
Ciliochoroidal effusions, 166–167
Cilioretinal arteries, 4
    in central retinal artery obstruction, 354
    occlusion of, oral contraceptives in, 316
Ciprofloxacin, 95, 96, 97, 98f, 99t
Circle of least confusion, 14, 14f
Clear corneal peripheral iridectomy, for acute primary angle clo-
        sure, 161
Clear lens extraction, 131, 141
Coats disease, 319–1, 320–322f, 323b, 394, 394f
    clinical characteristics of, 319
    common age at, 319
    differential diagnosis of, 39, 323t
    etiology of, 319
    exudate, 322
    eye with, 323
    fluorescein angiography, 320
    management, 320–322
    recurrence of, 323t
    retinal conditions, 323
    retinal vascular changes, 319
    subretinal exudates, 320
    treatment, 322
    unilateral *versus* bilateral, 319
Cocaine abuse, as retinopathy cause, 313
Cocaine test, for Horner's syndrome, 246
Cogan-Reese syndrome, 172
Cogan's eyelid twitch, 286
Collaborative Ocular Melanoma Study, 384, 385, 386
Collier's sign, 234
Coloboma, as bitemporal field defect, 259
Color
    attributes of, 24
    final determination of, 24
Color vision, 22–28, 28b
    amblyopia and, 221
    defects of, 27, 27t
Color wheel, 24
Coma, 15
Combigan, 177
Commotio retinae, 325

Complementary colors, 24
Computed tomography (CT)
    for calcification evaluation, 39
    for Coats disease diagnosis, 320
    for intraocular foreign body detection, 331–332, 332f
    of optic nerve lesions, 40
    of optic nerve sheath lesions, 40
    orbital, 39, 398
    of retinoblastoma, 376
    slices of, for foreign body or traumatic optic neuropathy
        evaluation, 39
Computed tomography (CT) angiography, 248
Computer vision syndrome, 266
Cone dystrophy, electroretinographic evaluation of, 32
    progressive, 32
Cones, 22, 30
    pigments of, 23
Confrontation fields, visual, 50
Congenital fibrosis syndrome, 231
Congenital hereditary endothelial dystrophy, 117
Congenital hypertrophy of the retinal pigment epithelium
        (CHRPE), 379, 384
Congenital obstructions, 268
Congenital ptosis, 283
Congenital rubella syndrome, 31
Congenital sixth nerve palsy, 223
Congenital stationary night blindness, electroretinographic
        evaluation of, 32
Conjunctiva
    follicular reaction in, in neonate, 90
    foreign body in, 70
    gonococcal, 66
    Kaposi's sarcoma of, 308f
    scarring of, as cause of dry eye, 103
    tarsal follicles of, 66
    traumatic hyphema and, 191
    viral, 66
Conjunctivitis
    bacterial, 71, 92, 95
    as cause of red eye, 65
    chlamydial inclusion, 72
    chronic, 72, 72f, 95, 289
    diffuse papillary, 95
    follicular, 289
    giant papillary, 69, 69f
    gonococcal, 83f, 92, 96
    herpes simplex, 93
    neonatal, 90, 91
    Parinaud's oculoglandular, 72
    toxic, 72
    vernal, keratoconus and, 122
    viral, 95
Connective tissue disorders, keratoconus and, 122
Contact lens, 208
    as cause of corneal ulcer, 69, 70b, 96
    as cause of dry eye, 104
    as cause of keratoconus, 121
    as cause of red eye, 69
    in corneal infection, 77
    corrective power of, 11
    deposits on, 69
    gas-permeable, 127
    for keratoconus treatment, 127

Contact lens *(Continued)*
nystagmus and, 241
as ptosis cause, 288
retinal detachment through, 326f
small peripheral infiltrates from, 80, 83f
steepening the fit of, 20, 20f
Contact lens warpage, 121
Continuous-curve capsulorrhexis, 207–208, 208f
Contrecoup mechanism, 325
Convergence insufficiency, 20, 228, 252
Copper foreign bodies, 332–333
Cornea
abrasion of
as cause of recurrent corneal erosions, 70
in neonates, 91
as red eye cause, 69
after acute angle-closure attack, 162
disease of, as cause of red eye, 65
dystrophies of, 70, 112–120
edema, after cataract surgery, 214, 214f
endothelial cells of, effects of refractive surgery on, 141
erosion of, 113
foreign bodies in, 70
in neonates, 91
infections of, 77–89
after LASIK, 86
after PRK, 85–86
gonococcal, 83, 83f
herpetic, 83–85, 83f
infiltrates of, 83
innervation of, 5
measured with keratometer, 17
opacity of
effect on electroretinographic findings, 32
as false-positive field defect cause, 51
in neonates, 5
perforation of, neonatal conjunctivitis and, 90
scarring of
from herpetic keratitis, 84
neonatal conjunctivitis and, 92b
scratches to, 69–70
thickness of, glaucoma and, 146
topography of, in refractive surgery patients, 130–131, 131f, 132f
traumatic hyphema and, 191
ulcers of. *see* corneal; Ulcers
Cornea guttata, 119
differentiated from Fuchs' dystrophy, 116
Corneal blood staining, 195
Corneal haze, after photorefractive keratectomy, 141
Corneal transplantation, 128
astigmatism after, 140, 140f
in Fuchs' dystrophy patients, 117–119
Corrected pattern standard deviation (CPSD), 51
Corticosteroids, 350
as glaucoma cause, 301
for orbital capillary hemangiomas, 397
for orbital inflammation, 281
topical
for corneal ulcers, 80–81
for herpes simplex keratitis, 85
for uveitis, 301
Cosopt, 177

Cotton-wool spots, 304, 305f, 333–334, 348, 359, 360f
Couching, 204, 206
Coumadin, anticoagulant effects of, 193
Covering test, 231
Cranial nerve palsies, as giant cell arteritis cause, 262
Cranial nerves
divisions of, 7
fifth, 233
fourth, 233
location within the superior orbital fissure, 1
third, 233
Crede prophylaxis, for neonatal conjunctivitis, 90
Critical angle, 11
Cross-fixation, 223
Crouzon syndrome, 228
Crowding phenomenon, 221
Cryotherapy
for basal cell carcinoma, 291
for blepharitis, 68
for retinopathy of prematurity, 343
Cryotherapy for Retinopathy of Prematurity (Cryo-ROP) study,
343, 343f
Cryptococcal meningitis, in AIDS patients, 308, 308f
Crystalens, 210
Cultures, for corneal infections, 78–79, 79t, 82
Cyanolabe, 23
Cyclodialysis, 191
angle recession and, 198
Cyclodialysis cleft, 198
Cyclogyl, 18
Cyclophotocoagulation
for acute primary angle closure, 161
laser, for neovascular glaucoma, 166
Cycloplegic agents
for aqueous misdirection syndrome, 165
for corneal ulcers, 80
length of effectiveness of, 18
as systemic intoxication cause, 18
Cyclosporine, for dry eyes, 110
Cyst
chocolate, 397
dermoid
ruptured, 397
Cystinosis, 114
Cystoid macular edema, treatment of, 215
Cytomegalovirus (CMV), AIDS and, 305

D

Dacryoadenitis, 280
Dacryocystitis, 72, 95
acute, 268
in neonates, 91
Dacryocystorhinostomy (DCR), 268
Dalen-Fuchs nodules, 301
Dark adaptation, 34, 34f
Decompression
optic nerve sheath, 261
orbital, 277
Decongestants, for red eye treatment, 65
Degenerations, differentiated from dystrophies, 112, 112b
Dehiscence, cataract surgery-related, 211
Dellen, 71

Dendrites
    corneal, herpes simplex in, 84, 84f
    of herpes simplex keratitis, 67f
    steroids and, 100
Dermatitis, radiation and, 291
Dermatochalasis, 283
    as false-positive field defect cause, 51
Descemet's membrane, 3
    corneal dystrophies of, 112
Descemet stripping only (DSO), 117, 118f
Deuteranopes, 27
Deuteranopia, 27
Dexamethasone phosphate, 99
Diabetes mellitus. *see also* Retinopathy; diabetic.
    as open-angle glaucoma risk factor, 143
    as retinal vein occlusion risk factor, 362
Diabetes, ophthalmologic examination for, 347
Diabetic retinopathy, 215
Diabetics, 215
Dialysis, retinal, 191
    inferotemporal, 368f
Dichromatism, congenital, 27
Diffuse unilateral subacute neuroretinitis, 32
Dilation, for anterior chamber angle visualization, 154
Diopters, 12
    relationship to meters, 11
Diplopia, 248–254
    binocular, 248
    definition of, 248
    intermittent, 252
    monocular, 18–19, 19b, 248
    myasthenia gravis and, 252
    proptosis-related, 270
Distortion, thick lens-related, 15
Divergence insufficiency, 229
Divergence paresis, 252
Dorsal midbrain syndrome. *see* Parinaud's syndrome
Dorzolamide, for glaucoma, 173
Double elevator palsy, 230, 232f
Double ring sign, 263f
Double vision. *see* Diplopia
Downbeat nystagmus, 4
Down syndrome, keratoconus and, 122
Doxycycline, 66, 92
Drusen, 335, 336f, 384
    optic nerve, 262
Dry eye questionnaire-5 (DEQ-5), 105, 105f
Dry eyes, 67f, 103–111, 110b
    as cause of red eye, 65
    definition of, 103–110
    signs of, 104
    symptoms of, 103–104
    treatments for, 108–109, 109b
    types of, 103
Duane's syndrome, 223, 229, 230f
    cause of, 229
    features associated with, 229
    strabismus surgery in, 236–237
Dye disappearance test, 267
Dyschromatopsia, 263
Dysphotopsia, positive and negative, 216
Dysproteinemias, 114

Dystrophy
    cone, 32
        progressive, 32
    corneal, 70, 112–120
    differentiated from degenerations, 112, 112b
    ocular pharyngeal, 232
    pattern, 34
    posterior polymorphous, 172

E

Ear, differentiated from eye, 24
Early receptor potentials (ERPs), 29b
Early Treatment Diabetic Retinopathy Study (ETDRS), 351, 351f
Early Treatment for Retinopathy of Prematurity (ETROP) study, 344
Ectasia, progressive corneal, 137
Ectropion, 267
    as cause of superficial punctate keratopathy, 67
    upper lid, 286–287
Eczema, keratoconus and, 121–122
Edema
    corneal, 85
        Fuchs' dystrophy and, 119
    of eyelid, 272
    macular
        acute, 19
        clinically significant, 350–351, 351f
        cystoid, 214f, 215, 314
        diabetic, 347, 352
        intravitreal injections, 350
        nicotinic acid and, 314
        refractory, 352
        retinal vein occlusion and, 360, 363
        treatment of, 364
        treatment options, 350
    of optic disc, 333–334, 361–362
    posterior polymorphous dystrophy-related, 172
Edinger-Westphal nucleus, 244
Edrophonium chloride, 252
Ehlers-Danlos syndrome, keratoconus and, 122
Elamipretide, 264
Electrolysis, for blepharitis, 68
Electromagnetic energy, 22, 22f
Electromagnetic spectrum, 22
Electro-oculogram (EOG), 33, 33f
    Arden ratio in, 33
    clinical uses for, 34
    electrical response in, generation of, 33
Electroretinogram (ERG), 30, 31, 32, 33, 34
    in age-related macular degeneration, 31
    clinical situations in, 31
    for congenitally decreased vision, 32
    extinguished, 32
    full-field, 29b, 30, 32
    parameters of, 31
    performing, 29
    in retinal ganglion cell disease, 31
    variations of, 33
    wave amplitude in, 31, 32–33
    in X-linked retinoschisis, 31
Elevated pigmented fundus lesion, differential diagnosis of, 380
Emboli, as retinal artery obstruction, 354
Embryonal medulloepithelioma, 394

Emmetropic eye
  far point for, 11
  secondary focal point for, 10
Endophthalmitis, 81
  after cataract surgery, 170
  after trabeculectomy, 181–182, 188f
  foreign bodies and, 332–333
  infectious, 213
  neonatal conjunctivitis and, 90
  postoperative, chronic, as uveitis cause, 296t
  posttraumatic, 333
    prophylactic antibiotics for, 333
  refractive surgery and, 141
  signs and symptoms of, 237
  vitreous of, 213
Endophthalmitis Vitrectomy Study, finding of, 213b
Enophthalmos, 271f, 284
Enterobacter, penicillin for, 97
Enterococcus faecalis, methicillin-resistant, 97
Entropion, 267
  as cause of superficial punctate keratopathy, 67
  involutional, 8–9
  radiation and, 291
Enucleation
  in Coats disease, 323
  for melanoma, 384
  as uveal melanoma treatment, 388
EOG. *see* Electro-oculogram (EOG)
Epicanthus inversus, 285f
Epikeratophakia, 128
Epi-LASIK, 137
Epiphora, congenital, treatment of, 268b
Episcleral venous pressure, elevated, 171
Episcleritis
  as cause of red eye, 65
  versus scleritis, 73, 73f
Epithelial basement membrane disease (EBMD), 112
Epithelial basement membrane dystrophy, 112
Epithelioid cells, 386
Epitheliopathy, acute posterior multifocal placoid pigment, 297t,
    300–301
ERG. *see* Electroretinogram (ERG).
Erythema migrans, 299
Erythema multiforme, 299
Erythema nodosum, 300
Erythema, orbital inflammation and, 280
Erythrolabe, 23
Erythromycin, 66, 91–92, 95, 99t
Esodeviations, 223
Esophoria, 223
Esotropia, 223, 226b
  accommodative, 224, 225f
    age of development, 224
    as amblyopia cause, 221
    age of development, 224
    early-onset, 224
    factors influence the development of, 225
    nonrefractive, 226
    partial or decompensated, 226
    relationship with congenital esotropia, 225–226
    treatment of partial or decompensated, 226
    types of, 225
  acute acquired comitant, 226

Esotropia *(Continued)*
  congenital, 221
    amblyopia before surgical correction of, 224
    binocular vision in children with, 224
    characteristics of, 223, 224f
    goals in treatment of, 224
    treatment of, 224
    vision evaluated in child with, 224
  cyclic, 226
  infantile, 223
  left, 223
  in the neurologically impaired, 224
  sensory, 224
Exenteration, of recurrent eyelid tumor, 291
Exercise, 178
Exfoliation syndrome, 202
Exodeviation, 229
Exophoria, 228
Exotropia
  constant, 221
  convergence insufficiency-related, 252
  differential diagnosis of, 228
  intermittent, 221, 228
  internuclear ophthalmoplegia and, 262
  sensory, 231
Expulsive choroidal hemorrhage, risk factors for, 212
External beam radiotherapy, for retinoblastoma, 378
Eye
  clinical anatomy of, 1–6
  differentiated from ear, 24
  schematic, 12, 13f
Eyedrops, 94–102. *see also* Topical medications.
  general rules for, 178
  for glaucoma, 148, 178
  improper administration of, 96
Eyelashes, misdirected, blepharitis and, 68
Eyelid crutches, 286
Eyelids
  anatomy of, 7–9
  crease of, 284, 284f
    height of, 286
  edema of, 272
  lag of, 271–272
  lesion of, benign and malignant, 289
  lower
    lacerations to, 8
    laxity of, 266
    retractors, 8
  malignancy
    patients with, 293
    prevention, 293
  muscle surgery affecting, 278
  proptosis and, 271f
  retraction of, 284
    thyroid eye disease, 275f
  rubbing of, as ptosis cause, 288
  schematic cross-section of, 2
  sensory nerve supply to, 8
  S-shaped deformity of, in orbital inflammation,
    280
  structures of, 8f
  surgery, for thyroid eye disease, 278
  swollen, 67–68

Eyelids *(Continued)*
  tear drainage path in, 265
  tears after leaving, 265
  tumors of, 289–293
  upper, fat pads of, 9
Eye rubbing, keratoconus and, 121

F

Facial trauma, orbital fractures, 253
Familial amyloid polyneuropathy type IV, 114
Far point, of eye, 11
Fat pads, of upper eyelid, 9
Femtosecond laser, 137
  in LASIK procedure, 134
Femtosecond laser-assisted cataract surgery, complications
    reported with, 216
Fetal alcohol syndrome, 314
Fetal hyaloid vasculature, 4
Fiber layer of Henle, 4
Fibrohistiocytoma, 273
Fibrosis syndrome, congenital, 231
Filters, neutral density, 221
Fingolimod (Gilenya), 257
Fistula
  arteriovenous, 233
  carotid, 171b
  dural, 171b
Fixation, eccentric, 221
Fixation errors, 51
Flat pigmented fundus lesion, 379–385
Fleischer ring, 124–126, 125f
Fleurettes, 392, 392f
Flexner-Wintersteiner rosettes, 376, 376f, 391–392,
    392f
Floaters, 306, 359
Flomax pupil, 203
Floppy eyelid syndrome, 288
  keratoconus and, 122
Floppy iris syndrome, intraoperative, 216
Fluorescein, 67
  in dry eye diagnosis, 104
  for retinal angiography, 44
  structures permeable to, 43
Fluorescein angiography, 4, 320
Fluorometholone, 100
Fluoroquinolones, 96, 98b
5-Fluorouracil, 186, 188, 188f
  mitomycin C and, 186
Follicular reaction, in neonate, 90
Forced ductions, 232, 235
Foreign bodies
  as cause of superficial punctate keratopathy, 67
  in conjunctiva, 70
  in cornea, 70
    in neonates, 91
  intraocular, 333b
    copper, 332–333
    detection of, 331–332
    iron, 316
    removal of, 332
    ultrasound findings with, 38
    as uveitis mimic, 303t, 305
  metallic, 70–71

Foreign-body sensation, 67, 69
  anterior membrane dystrophies and, 112–113
  corneal ulcer and, 96
Fovea
  anatomy of, 4
  in intraretinal hemorrhage, 359
Foville's syndrome, 251t
Fractures
  blow-out, 1–5
  medial wall, 228
Free radical scavengers, for glaucoma, 177
Frequency doubling technology (FDT), 51
Fuchs' endothelial dystrophy, 116, 117f
Fuchs' heterochromic iridocyclitis, 171, 294, 297t
Full-field light-evoked ERG, 30
Full-threshold testing, 50
Functio laesa, 279
Fundus
  pigmentation/pigmented lesions of, 3, 379–385
  trauma to, 325–334
Fundus autofluorescence (AF), 45–46, 45f
Fundus examination, in anterior uveitis patients, 294
Fungal infections, orbital, 281
Fungal keratitis, 78, 78f, 86–87
Fusion maldevelopment nystagmus, 242

G

β-galactosidase deficiency, 355
Ganciclovir, intraocular implant of, 306, 306f
Ganglion cell disease, retinal, 31
Gases, used inside eye, 371
Gass's theory, 5
Gatifloxacin, 99t
Gels, 94
Geneva lens clock, 17
Gentamicin, 99t
Germ-line mutation retinoblastoma, manifestation of, 373
Giant cell arteritis, 261, 262, 356, 356b
  biopsy in diagnosis of, 261
Ginkgo biloba, for glaucoma, 177
Girls, Coats disease in, 319
Glands of Krause, 4
Glands of Wolfring, 4
Glare/contrast sensitivity testing, 205
Glasses, thick aphakic, 208
Glaucoma, 143–150
  acute, as cause of red eye, 65
  alternative therapies or nontraditional medication for,
    177–178
  angle-closure, 151–167
    in Asian Americans, 75
    chronic, 156
    classification of, 155, 156t
    intermittent, 157
    primary, 155–156
    secondary to ocular inflammation, 166–167
    subacute, 157
    symptomatic acute, 156
    treatment of, 158–160, 159–160t
  angle-recession, 168, 198
    pathophysiology of, 199
    treatment for, 199
  as branch retinal vein occlusion risk factor, 359

Glaucoma *(Continued)*
  in cataract patient, 216
  central corneal thickness and, 146
  classification of, 143
  clinical presentation of primary open-angle, 143
  Coats disease and, 319
  common optic nerve findings in, 144b
  common visual-field defects in, 144b
  congenital, 91
  definition of, 143–149
  elevated episcleral venous pressure and, 171, 171b
  end-stage, 259
  filtering surgery for, failure of, 182, 182f
  genetics of primary open-angle, 143
  ghost-cell, 171
  hemolytic, 171
  high-tension, 149
  imaging in, 146
  initial treatment options for primary open-angle, 148
  low-tension, 148–149
  malignant, 171
    prevention of, 189b
  management of, commonly used agents for, 174t
  medical treatment of, 173–180
  melanomalytic, 304
  mesenchymal dysgenesis associated with, 172
  narrow-angle, medications contraindicated in, 163
  neovascular, 155, 166, 171, 357
    retinal vein occlusion and, 361
  normal-tension, 148–149
    treatment of, 149
  old records and, 145
  open-angle
    primary, 198–199
    secondary, 168–172
  optical coherence tomography for, 146–147, 147f
  pathogenesis of, 143
  phacoanaphylactic, 170
  postoperative, 171
  prevalence of, 143
  pseudoexfoliation, 168, 168b
  retinoblastoma with, 375
  risk factors for, 143
  surgery for, goal of, 181
  suspect of, 144
  sympathetic ophthalmia and, 333
  tests for, 149
  topical combination therapies for, 177, 177b
  topical steroids and, 98
  traumatic, 191–200
  treatment for
    algorithm, 197f
    factors affecting, 148
    primary goal of, 148
    treatment paradigm, 175
  true exfoliative, 168
  uveitis and, 301
  visual-field findings in, 57–59, 60f
Glaukomflecken, 162
Glioma, optic nerve, 272
Globe
  displacement of, 272
  loss of, Coats disease and, 323

Globe *(Continued)*
  perforation of, cataract surgery and, 211
  rupture of, 191, 330, 331b
    blunt trauma-related, 3
  scleral suture, 237
Glycerin, topical, for angle closure, 160
Goldenhar's syndrome, 263
Goldmann three-mirror lens, 151
Goldmann visual field, 50, 60, 62f
Goniolens, 151
Gonioscopy
  in acute primary angle closure, 157
  angle recession and, 198
  for anterior chamber angle visualization, 3
  determination of patients with narrow angles and,
    153–154
  for hyphema, 198
  kinds of, 151
  performance of, 152–153
Gonococcal conjunctivitis, 92, 96
Gonococcal infections, in cornea, 83, 83f
Gradenigo's syndrome, 251t
Graft rejection, in corneal transplantation, 128
Gram-negative organisms, in corneal infection, 78
Gram-positive organisms, in corneal infection, 77
Granular-lattice dystrophy, 115
Granulomatosis, Wegener's, 282, 302
Green light rays, refraction by plus lens, 16
Guarded filtering procedure, 166
Guillain-Barré syndrome, 233

H

HAART. *see* Highly active antiretroviral therapy (HAART)
Haemophilus influenza B (Hib), orbital cellulitis and, 281
Haemophilus influenzae
  as cause of conjunctivitis, 72
  as orbital cellulitis cause, 272
Hallervorden-Spatz disease, 355
Hallucinations, 263
Harada-Ito procedure, 250
Hay fever, keratoconus and, 121–122
Headaches, 259
  migraine, 285
Head injury, as fundus abnormalities cause, 333–334
Hemangioma
  capillary
    orbital, 397
  cavernous, 272f, 273, 397
  choroidal, 390f
    treatment of, 390
Hemangiopericytoma, 273, 397–398
Hemianopia, 264f
  binasal, 55–56
  bitemporal, 53, 54f, 57f
  definition of, 53
  double homonymous, 53, 55f
  types of, 53
Hemoglobin A_1C, 347
Hemorrhage
  of anterior segment, 191
  choroidal
    expulsive, 212
    ultrasound evaluation of, 36t

Hemorrhage *(Continued)*
   of optic disc, 148
   of optic nerve sheath, 211
   recurrent, 195
     increased risk of, factors associated with, 195
   retinal, 359
     artery obstruction and, 357
     vein occlusion and, 361–362
   retrobulbar, 211
   as risk for hemolytic glaucoma, 171
   significance of, 195
   subconjunctival, 70, 72–73, 191
     as cause of red eye, 65
   subretinal
     choroidal rupture and, 326–327
     differentiated from choroidal melanoma, 381
   suprachoroidal, after trabeculectomy, 186, 187f
   traumatic hyphema and, 195
   vitreous
     diabetic retinopathy and, 347, 352
     melanoma and, 304
     retinal vein occlusion and, 359
Hering's law, 286
Herpes simplex keratitis, 78, 83–84
Herpes simplex viral conjunctivitis, 93
Herpes simplex virus (HSV), 66–67
Herpesvirus infections
   as acute retinal necrosis syndrome cause, 300
   as uveitis cause, 296
Herpes zoster lesions, trigeminal nerve distribution of, 2
Herpes zoster ophthalmicus, 84, 84f
Herpes zoster virus, in corneal infections, 84–85
Heterochromia, 171
   of iris, 304
Highly active antiretroviral therapy (HAART), 306
High-risk characteristics (HRC), 351, 351b
Histamine₁ receptor antagonists, for red eye
     treatment, 65
Histiocytoma, fibrous, 397–398
Histoplasmosis, ocular, 296t, 299
Homatropine, 18
Homer Wright rosettes, 391–392, 391f
Homocystinuria, 202
Horner's syndrome, 246, 246f, 252, 287, 287b, 287f
   appropriate evaluation for patient with, 246–247
   causes of, 246
   pharmacologic testing in localization of lesion in, 246
   test for, 246
Horseshoe tears, retinal, 326, 367, 367f, 368f
Hruby lens, 18
Hue, 23
Human leukocyte antigen (HLA)-B27-associated conditions,
     295, 295t
Humphrey printout, 51
Humphrey visual field, 51, 311
Hutchinson's sign, 2
Hydrops, acute, 126, 126f
Hydroxychloroquine
   in electroretinogram and electro-oculogram, 34
   as retinopathy cause, 311
Hypercholesterolemia, 115, 289
Hyperemia, 95–96
Hyperlipidemias, 115

Hyperopia, 130
   absolute, 21
   accommodative requirements in, 16
   acquired, 19
   amplitude of accommodation, 11
   corrective lens for, 11
   cycloplegic refraction, 18
   direct ophthalmoscope image size in, 17
   facultative, 21
   far point in, 11
   latent, 21
   manifest, 20
   procedures for, 140–141
   round-top or flat-top reading lens for, 14
   secondary focal point for, 10, 10f
   total, 20
   undercorrection of, 20
Hyperopic person, with accommodative esotropia, 225
Hyperosmotic agents
   action of, 173
   for angle closure, 158
Hyperplasia, lymphoid, 400
Hypertension
   as branch retinal vein occlusion risk factor, 359
   as diabetic retinopathy risk factor, 347
   idiopathic intracranial. *see* Pseudotumor cerebri
   as open-angle glaucoma risk factor, 143
   as retinal vein occlusion risk factor, 362
Hyperthyroidism, 274
Hypertriglyceridemia, 115
Hypertropia
   differential diagnosis of, 229
   three-step test, 249
Hyphema, 191–1, 212
   after trabeculectomy, 185f
   causes of, 191
   classification of, 192t
   complications of, 195
   definition of, 191–199
   eight-ball, 195–196, 196f
     prognosis for, 196
     removal of, optimal time of, 196
   evacuation of, surgical techniques for, 196
   management of, 193, 193f
     medical, 193
   questions to ask patient with, 193
   secondary glaucoma and, 196, 198t
   spontaneous, in children, 296
   surgical intervention in, indications for, 195
   traumatic, 193b
     angle-recession glaucoma and, 198–199
     ocular injuries associated with, 191
     pathophysiology of, 191
   workup of patient with, approach to, 191–193
Hyphemectomy, for hyphema, 196
Hypopyon
   in infectious corneal ulcer, 81, 81f
   layered, 213f
Hyposecretive dry eye, 103
Hypothyroidism, 274
Hypotony, 186, 187f, 211
Hypotropia, 284, 285f
Hysteria, 260

I

Ice test, 252–253, 288
Idiopathic polypoidal choroidal vasculopathy, indocyanine green
and, 45
IgG4-related disease, 280
Image displacement, 14
Image jump, 14
Image point, 12
Imaging. *see also* Computed tomography (CT); Magnetic
resonance imaging (MRI); Ultrasonography.
orbital, for thyroid eye disease, 274
Immunohistochemistry (IHC), for uveal metastases, 389–390
Immunosuppressives, for uveitis, 302
Implicit time, in electroretinogram, 31
Incontinentia pigmenti, 345t
Indentation gonioscopy, 157
Indirect gonioscopy, 151, 152f
Indocyanine green (ICG), 45
Infantile nystagmus syndrome, 240
manifest latent nystagmus distinguished from, 242
sensory defects in, 241t
waveform of nystagmus in, 239
Infants. *see also* Neonates.
cataracts in, 201
Coats disease in, 319
myopia in, 130
nystagmus, 224
premature, retinopathy in, 341–1, 341b
strabismus in, 223
Infarction, vaso-occlusive, 248
Infection
after strabismus surgery, 237
of radial keratotomy incision, 133f
Infectious keratitis, 88
Infectious orbital cellulitis, 272
Inferior oblique overaction, 224, 225f
Inferior oblique palsy, 230
Inferior rectus, in thyroid eye disease, 281
Infiltrates, leukemic
choroidal, 304
of optic nerve, 304
Inflammation
definition of, 279
granulomatous, 333
of optic nerve. *see* Neuritis, optic
orbital, 279, 279b
nonspecific, 279, 281b
specific, 279
postoperative, 212–213
Inflammatory bowel disease, 295, 295t
Inflammatory signs, of melanoma, 304
Interferon, 315
Interferon-associated retinopathy, 315
Interferon α–2 therapy, 397
International Classification of Retinopathy of Prematurity
(ICROP), 341
International Committee for Classification of Corneal Dystrophies, 112
Internuclear ophthalmoplegia, 251–252, 262
causes of, 262
Intra-arterial chemotherapy, for retinoblastoma, 378, 378f
Intracameral administration, of anesthesia, 206
Intracorneal ring segments (Intacs), 131, 137
complications of, 138

Intracranial pressure, increased, 263
Intraocular implants, 213
Intraocular lens, 208
for aphakic patients, 208
calculation for, 16
common positions of, 209
complications related to, 215
composition of, 208
dislocation of, 202
multifocal, 203, 216
power of, determination of, 209
Intraocular lens implants
accommodative, 139
phakic, 131, 138f, 139
for hyperopia, 141
Verisyse, 139
Intraocular lens power, 203
Intraocular neoplasm, strategy for ordering imaging studies in, 39
Intraocular pressure
effect of corneal thickness on, 146
elevated
clogged trabecular meshwork and, 168
glaucoma and, 180
primary angle closure and, 157
steroids and, 168
in uveitis, 301
glaucoma and, 146
fluctuation in, 146
lowering of, nonmedical maneuver for, 157
measurement of, factors influencing, 146
normal, 144
optic nerves, 145f
resistant to damage, 148
persistent or recurrent, after peripheral iridotomy, 163
steroids and, 100
uncontrolled, 194
Intraocular retinoblastoma, management of, 376–377
Intraocular tumor, as cause of open-angle glaucoma, 171
Intraoperative floppy iris syndrome, 203, 216
Intraretinal and subretinal exudation, 319
Intravenous chemotherapy (chemoreduction), for retinoblastoma,
377, 377f
Intravitreal chemotherapy, for retinoblastoma, 378
Iodine, radioactive, 274
Iridectomy, during trabeculectomy, 184
Iridocorneal endothelial syndrome, 117, 155, 172
Iridocyclectomy, as ciliary body melanoma treatment, 384
Iridocyclitis, Fuchs' heterochromic, 171, 294, 297t
Iridodialysis, 191
Iridozonulohyalovitrectomy, for aqueous misdirection syndrome, 165
Iris
in acute primary angle closure, 157
after acute angle-closure attack, 162
atrophy of
as diplopia cause, 248
essential, 172
melanomas of, 389
neovascularization of, 357
in diabetes, 352
retinal vein occlusion and, 363
prolapse, cataract surgery-related, 211–212
sphincter tears of, 191
trabeculectomy site blockage by, 188

Iritis, 294
    bilateral chronic granulomatous, 301
Iron, as siderosis cause, 332
Iron intraocular foreign body, 316
Irrigation, eye, 66
    for lye burns, 71
Ischemia
    anterior segment, 238
    in retinal artery obstruction, 354
    retinal vein occlusion and, 359, 363
Ischemic optic neuropathy, nonarteritic and arteritic, 261t
Isolated cranial neuropathies, 249, 249t

J

Jackson cross, 20
Jones dye test, primary or secondary, 267
Jones, Lester, 9
Juvenile idiopathic arthritis (JIA), 296, 297t

K

Kaiser Fleischer ring, 332–333
Kamra corneal inlay, 139, 139f
Kawasaki syndrome, 297t
Kearns-Sayre syndrome, 232, 233f
Kellman, Charles, 206
Keratectomy
    photorefractive, 131, 134f
        drugs in, 141
        hyperopic excimer laser, 141
        versus LASIK, 135
    phototherapeutic, 113
Keratic precipitates, 77, 294, 295f, 295t
Keratitis
    Acanthamoeba, 78
    bacterial, 83
    from contact lens, 78
    diffuse lamellar, 86, 86f, 137
    fungal, 78, 78f, 86–87
    gonococcal, 83
    herpes simplex, 78, 83–84, 85b
    herpetic, steroids for, 100
    infectious, 88
    sicca, radiation and, 291
Keratoacanthoma, 289, 290f
Keratoconjunctivitis
    atopic, keratoconus and, 121–122
    sicca. *see* Dry eyes
    superior limbic, 73, 73f
Keratoconus, 119, 121–129
    atrophy, as diplopia cause, 248
    as contraindication to refractive surgery, 130
    diagnosis of, 122, 122b
    forme fruste, 137
    heredity in, 121
    histopathology of, 126
    prevention of, 127
    surgical options for, 127–128
    symptoms of, 122
    topographic signs of, 122–123, 123f
    treatment of, 127–128
Keratometer, 17
Keratometry, 16

Keratomileusis, laser in situ (LASIK)
    as cause of dry eye, 104
    complications of, 135, 136f
    contraindications to, 135b
    corneal infections after, 86, 86f
    definition of, 134
    Epi-LASIK, 137
    hyperopic, 141
    wavefront ablations and, 135
Keratopathy
    exposure, proptosis-related, 270
    infectious crystalline, 78
    neurotrophic, 77
    superficial punctate, 67
        Thygeson's, 67
Keratoplasty
    conductive, 140
    deep anterior lamellar, 115, 116f
    Descemet stripping endothelial, 117, 118f, 119
    lamellar (partial thickness), 127–128
    penetrating, 116f, 127
Keratosis
    actinic, 289, 290f
    seborrheic, 289, 289f
Keratotomy
    astigmatic, 139–140
    radial, 131, 133f
        complications of, 133, 133f
        versus LASIK, 135
Keratouveitis
    chronic, 85
    herpetic, 100, 101
Knapp's rules, 249
Koeppe gonioscope, 151
Koeppe nodules, 294, 295t
Kollner's rule, 27–28
Krukenberg spindle, 169–170, 169f

L

Lacrimal bone, 265
Lacrimal gland
    accessory, 4
    lesions of, 399
        benign and malignant, 400, 400t
        "rule of 50s" for, 399
Lacrimal pump mechanism, 9
Lacrimal sac, obstructions, 267
    evaluation of, 267
Lacrimal stenosis, radiation and, 291
Lacrimal system
    obstructions of, 267
        eyelid portion, 268
    tearing and, 265–269
Lacrisert, 109
Lagophthalmos, 4
    red eye and, 67
Laser (light amplification by stimulated emission of radiation), 204
    for angle closure, 160–161, 161f
    for aqueous misdirection syndrome, 165
    in corneal dystrophy treatment, 113
    definition of, 20
    femtosecond, 137, 208
    for macular degeneration, 338

Laser (light amplification by stimulated emission of radiation) *(Continued)*
  as macular edema treatment, 360
  in photocoagulation
    as age-related macular degeneration treatment, 338
    differentiated from photodynamic therapy, 339
  in photorefractive keratectomy, 133
  as retinal vein occlusion treatment, 360
  as retinopathy of prematurity treatment, 344, 344f, 345b
  use in capsulotomy, 215
  use in cataract surgery, 208
Laser in situ keratomileusis (LASIK). *see* Keratomileusis, laser in situ (LASIK)
Laser iridoplasty, for acute primary angle closure, 161
Laser peripheral iridectomy, for pigmentary dispersion, 170
Laser peripheral iridoplasty, for plateau iris syndrome, 164
Laser peripheral iridotomy
  complications of, 161
  open angles after, 165
  for plateau iris syndrome, 164
Latanoprost, 176–177
Latanoprostene bunod (Vyzultza), 175
Latent nystagmus, 242
Lateral canthal tendon, 266
  insertion of, 9
Lateral inhibition, 25
Lattice corneal dystrophy, 114
Lattice degeneration, 367, 367f
"Leash effect", 229
Leber's congenital amaurosis
  electroretinographic evaluation of, 32
  keratoconus and, 122
Leber's hereditary optic neuropathy, 264, 264f
Leber's miliary aneurysm, 319
Leber's neuroretinitis, 300
Lens. *see also* Spectacles, lens of.
  after acute angle-closure attack, 162
  angle closure glaucoma and, 155
  binocular high-power single-vision, adjustment of, 17
  corrective, power of, 11
  dislocated, 202, 202b
  extraction of, for aqueous misdirection syndrome, 165
  Hruby, 18
  innervation of, 5
  opacity of, as false-positive field defect cause, 51
  refractive function of, 11
  retained material, 212
  subluxation of, 155, 191, 202b
  Volk 90 D, 18
Lesion
  causative of internuclear ophthalmoplegia, 234
  causing afferent pupillary defect, 244–245
Leukemia, 303t, 304
Leukemic infiltrates
  of choroid, 304
  of optic nerve, 304, 304f
Leukocoria
  imaging studies of, 39
  retinoblastoma with, 374, 374f
Levator muscle
  aponeurosis dehiscence of, 288
  maldevelopment of, 283
  in ptosis, 283
    function measurement of, 286

Levofloxacin, 99t
Lifitegrast (Xiidra), 110
Light
  fluorescent, 26
  incandescent, 26
  spectrum of, 22
  transmission to the brain, 23, 23f
  wavelengths of, 18
Light/near dissociation, 247
Light rays
  refraction by plus lens, 16
  refractive index-related bending of, 11, 12f
  vergence of, 12
Light reflex test, 231
Limbus
  rectus-muscle insertions from, 1–2
  surgical, 3
Lipid layer, 5
Lissamine green stains, 67
  in dry eye diagnosis, 104
Liver, as uveal melanoma metastasis site, 388
Loratadine (Claritin), 65
Loteprednol, 65, 100
Loupes, as low-vision aids, 17
Lower lid retractors, 8
Low penetrant retinoblastoma, 373
Low-tension glaucoma, 148–149
Low-vision aids, 17, 339
Lubricating ointments, 109
Lung carcinoma, metastatic, 389, 400
Lye burns, 71
Lyme disease, 255, 296t, 299
Lymphadenopathy, 300
Lymphangioma, 397
Lymphatics, absence of, from the orbit, 2
Lymphocyte function-associated antigen (LFA-1), 110
Lymphoma
  orbital, 273, 400
  as papilledema cause, 308
  primary intraocular, 304, 304f
  as retinitis cause, 300
  as uveitis mimic, 303t
Lymphoproliferative lesions, orbital, 400, 401t
Lysergic acid diethylamide (LSD), 263

M
Macropsia, 335
Macula
  anatomy of, 4
  cherry-red spot of, 355
  edema of, effect on potential acuity readings, 19
  optical coherence tomography of, 350
  scar, as amblyopia cause, 218
  vertically displaced, 231
  in visual cortex, 5
Macular degeneration
  age-related, 335–1, 336f
    clinical findings in, 336b
    dry, 335, 337f
    electroretinographic evaluation of, 31
    exudative (wet), 335, 336f
    nonexudative (dry), 335, 337f
    wet, 335, 336f
    indocyanine green and, 45

Macular hole formation, stages of, 5
Macular sparing, 53, 263
Macular splitting, 53
Maculopathy
　bull's eye, 311, 312f
　ischemic, 359, 363
　pentosan polysulfate, 317, 317f
　poppers, 316
Magnetic resonance imaging (MRI)
　indications for, 39
　of intraocular foreign bodies, 331–332
　metallic foreign body as contraindication to, 332
　multiple sclerosis development in, 256, 256f
　of normal ocular and orbital tissues, 40, 41t
　in nystagmus, 240–241
　ocular, 39
　ocular lesions, 39
　of optic nerve lesions, 40
　of optic nerve sheath lesions, 40
　orbital, 38, 39, 398–399, 398f
　orbital lesions, 39
　postcontrast, 38–39
　of retinoblastoma, 376
　for third-nerve palsy, 248
Magnifiers, handheld, 17
Malingering, 260
Manifest latent nystagmus (MLN), 242
Marcus Gunn's jaw-winking syndrome, 287
Mare's tail sign, 113f
Marfan's syndrome, 202
Marginal reflex distance, 286
Masquerade syndromes, 302–305
Mast cell inhibitors, 65
Maxillary bonc, 265
Maxillary nerve, 8
McLean, Ian, 386
Mean deviation (MD), 51
Medial wall fracture, 228
Medulloepitheliomas, 394
Meesmann's dystrophy, 112
Meibomian gland disease, 109
Meibomian gland dysfunction (MGD), 68
Meibomian glands, 103
Meibomianitis, 69
Melanocytoma, 383, 384f
Melanocytosis
　congenital ocular, 383
　oculodermal, 383
Melanoma, 386, 387f
　cell types in, 386, 387f
　choroidal, 383, 388–389
　　acceptable method of treat, 383
　　characteristic features of, on ultrasound, 36, 36f
　　clinical and imaging signs, 382, 382t
　　diagnosis of, 381
　　differentiated from subretinal hemorrhage, 381
　　metastasis, 388–389
　　"To Find Small Ocular Melanoma Using Helpful Hints Daily"
　　　mnemonic for, 388
　　ultrasound evaluation of, 36, 36t
　of ciliary body, 383, 383f
　common treatment for, 384
　of eyelid, 292
　inflammatory signs of, 304

Melanoma (Continued)
　of iris, 389
　malignant, 386
　prognosis of, 384
　retinoblastoma with, 374–375
　shape of, 386
　uveal, 382, 383, 384, 386, 388b
　　BAP-1 tumor predisposition syndrome, 384
　　Callender classification of, 386
　　enucleation of, 388
　　genes in, 389
　　malignant, 386
　　metastatic, 388
　　posterior, 388
　　predilection for age, race, or sex, 383
　　prognostic factors in, 388b
　　route of distant spread, 383
　　special tests for, 387–388
　　staging of, American Joint Commission on Cancer (AJCC)
　　　Cancer Staging Manual in, 386
　　treatment of, 388
　　versus uveal metastasis, 384
　as uveitis mimic, 303t
Memantine, for glaucoma, 178
Meningioma, 233
　of olfactory groove, 53
Meningitis
　cryptococcal, 308, 308f
　neonatal conjunctivitis and, 92b
Meniscus
　low tear, 67, 73
　normal, 67
Meretoja's syndrome, 114
Metallosis, 32
Metals, ocular toxicity of, 332
Metamorphopsia, 248, 335
Metastasis
　uveal, 386, 389
　　common site of, 389
　　immunohistochemistry, 389–390
　　primary tumors, 389
Methylphenidate hydrochloride, as retinopathy cause, 314
Meyer's loop, 263
Microaneurysm, diabetic retinopathy and, 348
Micropsia, 335
Migraine, 143, 149
　ophthalmoplegic, 245, 285
Mild steroids, 109
Millard-Gubler syndrome, 251t
Minus cylinder form, 14
Miotics
　action of, 173
　for angle closure, 158–160
　as contraindication in clogged trabecular meshwork, 168
　for narrow-angle glaucoma, 163
　for pigmentary dispersion, 170
　for primary open-angle glaucoma, 173
Mitomycin C, 186, 187f
　5-fluorouracil and, 186
　in photorefractive keratectomy, 141
Mittendorf's dot, 4
Möbius syndrome, 224, 231
MOG-IgG syndrome, 257
Mohs' lamellar resection, 291

Molluscum contagiosum, 72, 289
Motility disorders, associated with congenital esotropia, 224
Moxifloxacin, 99t
Mucin, as tear composition, 266
Mucocele, 233
Mucoid layer, 5
Mucormycosis, 233
Müller's muscle contraction, in ptosis, 286
Multiple evanescent white dot syndrome, 297t
Multiple sclerosis (MS)
    developing after optic neuritis, 256
    development of, 256
    neuromyelitis optica and, 257
    ocular adverse effects, 257
    optic neuritis as risk factor for, 255, 256
    as uveitis cause, 300–301
Muscle surgery, for thyroid eye disease, 277
Mushroom-shaped fundus lesion, 381, 381f
MuSK antibodies, 287
Myasthenia gravis, 228, 253b
    as abduction deficit cause, 251
    diagnosis of, 287
    hypertropia and, 229
    ptosis and, 284
    signs and symptoms of, 285–286, 286b
    weakness of orbicularis muscle in, 286
    workup for, 252
Mycobacterium avium, AIDS and, 305
Mycotic Ulcer Treatment Trial 1 (MUTT), 87
Mydriasis, 191
Myeloma, 114
Myopia, 3
    acquired, 19
    age and, 130
    amplitude of accommodation, 11
    axial, 11
    corrective lens for, 11
        power of, 11
    definition of, 130
    direct ophthalmoscope image size in, 17
    far point in, 11
    LASIK for, 135
    as open-angle glaucoma risk factor, 143
    photorefractive keratectomy for, 133, 134f
    radial keratotomy for, 133, 133f
    refractive, 11
    residual, after refractive surgery, 140
    as retinal detachment risk factor, 367
    round-top or flat-top reading lens for, 14
    secondary focal point for, 10, 10f
    surgical treatment of, 131, 139
Myositis
    as diplopia cause, 248
    orbital, 280
Myotonic dystrophy, 32

N

Nanophthalmos, 166, 188
Nasolacrimal duct, 267
    blockage of, 268
    obstruction of, 268
        in neonates, 91
        signs of, 268

Nasopharyngeal carcinoma, 233
Near point, 11
Near reflex, spasm of, 248
Nearsightedness. *see* Myopia
Necrosis
    progressive outer retinal, 307, 307f
    retinal, 296t, 300
Neisseria gonorrhoeae, 66
    neonatal conjunctivitis from, 90
Neisseria species, in corneal ulcers, 81
Neomycin, 99t
    toxicity of, 97
Neonates
    conjunctivitis in, 90, 91
    corneal opacification in, 5
    retinopathy of prematurity in, 341–346
Neo-Synephrine test, 287
Neovascular glaucoma, 166
Neovascularization
    anterior-segment, 363
    of choroid, 337, 338
        classic, 337, 337f
        occult, 337, 337f
        on fluorescein angiography, 44, 44f
    of iris
        in diabetes, 352
        retinal vein occlusion and, 363
    retinal, 359, 360
        diabetic retinopathy and, 347
        retinal arterial obstruction and, 357
        retinal vein occlusion and, 359, 360
        talc and, 314
Nepafenac (Nevanac, Ilevro), 65
Nerve palsy
    localizing symptom, 251t
    third, 245, 247b
Netarsudil/latanoprost (Rockalatan), 175
Neuritis, optic, 255–258
    clinical findings in, 255
    clinical test for patients with, 255
    definition of, 255
    field defects found in patients with, 255
    natural history of, 255
    ONTT conclusions regarding treatment of, 256
    recurrence of, 257
    retrobulbar, in AIDS patients, 308
    visual outcome for, 255
    workup and treatment for patients with, 257
Neurofibroma, 273
Neurofibromatosis, 172, 272
Neuroimaging test, 271
Neurologic disturbances, 259–264
Neuromuscular junction disorders, as diplopia cause, 248
Neuromyelitis optica, 257
Neuromyelitis optica spectrum disorders (NMOSDs), 255
Neuropathy, optic
    ischemic, 260
    Malingering, 260f
    metabolic, 259
    miscellaneous, 259–264
    radiation and, 291
    syphilis and, 300
Neuroretinitis, diffuse unilateral subacute, 296t

Nevus
  choroidal, 36t, 379, 379f
    rate of transformation, 382t
    risk factors for, 382t
  of Ota, 383
Nicotinic acid, as cystoid macular edema cause, 314
Night blindness, stationary, congenital, 32
  electro-oculographic evaluation of, 34
  electroretinographic evaluation of, 32
Night vision, 23
Nodal point (np), of schematic eye, 13f
Noncompliance, 179
Nonhealing corneal epithelial defects, 352
Nonsteroidal anti-inflammatory drugs (NSAIDs), 65
  anticoagulant effects of, 193
  in photorefractive keratectomy, 141
  for scleritis, 75
Norfloxacin, 99t
Normal-tension glaucoma, 148–149
Nucleus, phacoemulsified, 208
Null point, in nystagmus, 240
Nystagmus, 239–243
  associated with specific ocular pathology, 242
  blockage syndrome, 240
  classifications of, 239, 239t
  congenital esotropia-related, 224
  congenital periodic alternating, 242
  contact lenses and, 241
  definition of, 239
  downbeat, 4
  evolution of different movements, 240, 240t
  latent, 242
  mirror, 240
  nonsurgical treatment of, 241
  null point in, 240
  patients, 239–240
    oscillopsia and, 240
  patients without pathologic disease, 239
  periodic alternating, 242
  photophobia and, 240
  refraction with, 242b
  surgical treatment options for, 241–242
  syndrome, 240
  time cycle of periodic, 242
  upbeat, 262
  vertical, 242
  vision, 241
  well-adapted, 240
Nystagmus blockage syndrome, 224

O

Obesity, as pseudotumor cerebri cause, 263b
Oblique muscles, in strabismus surgery, 235
Occipital lobe lesions, 263
Ocular deviations, miscellaneous, 228–234
Ocular fundus, pigmented lesions of, 379–385
Ocular ischemic syndrome, as uveitis mimic, 303t
Ocular surface disease index (OSDI), 105, 107f
Oculocerebrorenal syndrome, 172
Oculomotor synkinesis, 249
Ofloxacin, 96, 99t
Oguchi's disease, 33
Oil paints, 26

Ointments, 94
Older patients, steroid-resistant panuveitis in, 304
Olfactory groove, meningioma of, 53
Onchocerciasis, 296t
Opacities, media, false-positive field defect cause, 51, 53b
Ophthalmia neonatorum, 90
  causes of, 90b, 91t
    Gram and Giemsa stain findings with, 91t
  reduction of incidence of, 93
  sequelae of, 92t
Ophthalmia, sympathetic, 297t, 301
Ophthalmic artery, occlusion of, 32
Ophthalmic medication, allergic reaction to, 65–66
Ophthalmic nerve, 8
Ophthalmicus, herpes zoster, 84, 84f
Ophthalmoplegia
  chronic progressive external (CPEO), 232, 233f
  internuclear, 234
Ophthalmoscope/ophthalmoscopy
  direct, 17
  indirect, 18, 331–332, 331f, 370
Opsin, 23
Optical coherence tomography (OCT), 5, 40, 146–147, 215, 337f, 338, 350, 350f
  for anterior chamber angle evaluation, 154
  basic principles of, 40
  for glaucoma, 146–147, 147f
  indications for, 41, 42f
  retinal layers on, 40, 41f
  time-domain and spectral (or Fourier)-domain, 40
Optical coherence tomography angiography (OCTA), 46, 46f
  clinical disorders imaged with, 47
  disadvantages of, 46
  in high-risk diabetic retinopathy, 47
  potential advantages of, 46
  principles of, 46
Optic atrophy
  homonymous hemianopia without, 53
  sympathetic ophthalmia and, 333
Optic canal, structures pass through, 7
Optic chiasm, crossed and uncrossed fibers in, 4
Optic disc
  edema of, 333–334, 361–362
  glaucoma-like, differential diagnosis of, 149t
  hemorrhages in, 148
  pallor, 260f
  tilted, as false-positive field defect cause, 51, 53b
Optic nerve
  after acute angle-closure attack, 162
  avulsion of, 325, 325f
  compression of, 270, 277
  cup of, elongation of, 148, 148f
  decompression of
    complications of, 277
    patients requiring, 277
  drusen, 262
  examination of, glaucoma and, 144
  glioma, 272
  hypoplasia, 263
  injury to, glaucoma-related, 144–145, 145f
  intraocular pressure damage resistant, 148
  irradiation of, 276–277
    candidates for, 276–277

Optic nerve *(Continued)*
  lesions of, differentiated from optic nerve sheath
      lesions, 40
  leukemic infiltrates of, 304, 304f
  melanocytoma of, 384f
  papillitis of, 308, 308f
  retinoblastoma invasion of, 375
Optic nerve sheath
  hemorrhage from, 211
  lesions of, differentiated from optic nerve sheath lesions, 40
Optic Neuritis Treatment Trial (ONTT), 255
Optics, 10–21
Optic-tract syndrome, 57, 59f
Optociliary shunt vessels, 262b
Oral contraceptives, as retinal arterial occlusion cause, 316
Oral medications, for basal cell carcinoma, 291
Orbicularis oculi muscle
  in involutional entropion, 8–9
  in lacrimal pump mechanism, 9
  three portions of, 9
Orbit
  adnexal trauma to, 329
  anatomy of, 7–9, 7f
  anterior, schematic cross-section of, 2f
  bones of, 1
  cellulitis of, 281
  fat/fat pads of, 2
  infections of, 281b
  inflammatory conditions of, 279, 279b
      nonspecific, 279, 281b
      specific, 279
  lymphoma of, 273, 400, 401t
  lymphoproliferative lesions of, 400
  thyroid eye disease, 274
  trauma to, 229
  tumors of, 273, 397–402
  vasculitis of, 282
  weakest bone within, 7
Orbital apex syndrome, 280
Orbital granulomatosis, with polyangiitis, 282
Orbital imaging, findings, thyroid eye disease, 274
Orbital inflammatory diseases, 279–282
Orbital inflammatory pseudotumor, 228, 272
Orbital mass, 400
Orbital processes, imaging, 399b
Orbital rim, weak spots of, 7
Orbital schwannoma, 398
Orthophoria, 231
Oscillatory potentials, 29b, 29f
Oscillopsia, 240
Osteosarcoma, 374–375
Otitis, neonatal conjunctivitis and, 92b
Oxalosis, secondary, drugs that cause, 314

P

Pachymeters, 18
Pain
  with optic neuritis, 255
  orbital, 280
Paints, unpredictable results of mixing, 26
Palpebral fissure width, in ptosis, 286
PanOptix, 139
Panuveitis, 294
  steroid-resistant, 304

Papilledema, 262f, 308, 308f
  differentiated from pseudopapilledema, 262
Papillitis, 308, 308f
Paracentesis, 184, 356
  during trabeculectomy, 184
Paramagnetic agents, 38
Parasitic infections, orbital, 281
Parinaud's oculoglandular conjunctivitis, 72
Parinaud's syndrome, 234, 247, 300
  cause of, 234
Pars plana, vitrectomy of, 370
Pars planitis
  treatment of, 298
  as uveitis cause, 297t
  vision loss and, 298
Partial homonymous hemianopia, 53
Patching
  part-time compared with full-time, 220
  for recurrent corneal erosions associated with anterior
      membrane dystrophies, 113
  steps in, 220
Pattern deviation, 51
Pattern standard deviation (PSD), 51
Penalization, steps in, 220
"Pencil push-ups," 229
Penicillin, allergy to, 97
Pentosan polysulfate maculopathy, 317, 317f
Perfect Lens, 210
Peribulbar injection, of anesthesia, 206
Perimetry
  kinetic, 50
      using of, 50
  short wavelength automated, 51
  static, 50
Periorbitopathy, prostaglandin-associated, eyelid position and, 288
Peripheral iridectomy, for hyphema, 196
Peripheral vision, loss of, 144
Phacodonesis, 202
Phacoemulsification, 206, 207f
Phenothiazines, 32
  as retinopathy cause, 313
Phimosis, of eyelid, 285f
Photocoagulation
  in darkly pigmented fundi, 3
  laser in
      as age-related macular degeneration treatment, 338
      differentiated from photodynamic therapy, 339
      as macular edema treatment, 360
      as retinal vein occlusion treatment, 360
      as retinopathy of prematurity treatment, 344f
  panretinal, 351f, 352
      as constricted visual field cause, 259
      side effects of, 352
  as retinopathy of prematurity treatment, 344
Photodynamic therapy, for macular degeneration, 339
Photons, 22–28
  physical properties of, 22
Photophobia
  anterior membrane dystrophies and, 112–113
  in anterior uveitis, 75
  corneal ulcer and, 96
  in HSV infection, 66–67
  nystagmus and, 240
  in superior limbic keratoconjunctivitis, 73

Photoreceptor response, associated with stimulus conditions, 30, 30f, 30t
Photoreceptors, 22, 26, 367
  fragmentation of, 325
Photorefractive keratectomy (PRK), corneal infections after, 85–86
Phthisis bulbi, 284, 319
Physiologic blind spot, 50
Physostigmine, 18
"Pie-in-the-sky" lesion, 57, 58f
"Pie-on-the-floor" lesion, 57, 58f
Pigmentary dispersion, treatment of, 170
Pigments, 26
Pilocarpine
  for angle-closure glaucoma, 179
  symblepharon and, 179
Pinealoblastoma, 374
Pinguecula, 71
Pinhole diameter, most effective, 18
"Pink eye," 95
Pituitary tumors, 259
Plateau iris, 155, 163–165, 164f
Plateau iris syndrome, 164
Plus cylinder form, 14
Plus disease, 342–343, 343f
Pneumonitis, neonatal conjunctivitis and, 92b
Polycoria, as diplopia cause, 248
Polyhexamethylene biguanide, 87
Polymyxin B, 95, 99t
Polymyxin, toxicity of, 97
Polyneuropathy, familial amyloid type IV, 114
Polypoidal choroidal maculopathy, 339
Polysporin, 95
Poor visual outcome, in optic neuritis, 255
Posner lenses, 151
Posner-Schlossman syndrome, 170
Posterior capsule
  cataract surgery-related rupture, 212, 213f
  incidence of, 212
  opacification of, 204
Posterior chamber, lens of, 203
Posterior crocodile shagreen, 115
Posterior membrane corneal dystrophies, 112, 116t
Posterior polymorphous dystrophy, 117
  as cause of open-angle glaucoma, 172
Posterior vitrectomy, for aqueous misdirection syndrome, 165
Postkeratoplasty astigmatism, 128
Postoperative iris prolapse, 212
Power, of schematic eye, 13f
Preauricular node, 65
Prednisolone acetate, 100
Prednisone, 256
Pregnancy
  as aminocaproic acid contraindication, 194
  diabetic retinopathy during, 347
  glaucoma medications in, 179
  tetracycline on, 92
Prematurity, retinopathy of, 231, 341–346
  complications of, 345, 345f
  differential diagnosis of, 319, 345, 345t
  posterior, 344
  stages of, 342, 342f
  zones of, 341, 342f
Prentice's rule, 13, 13f

Presbyopia, 130
  surgical treatment of, 139
Pressure patch, for corneal abrasion, 69–70
Primary angle closure (PAC), 155–156
  acute
    other laser treatments for, 161
    signs or exam findings seen in, 157, 157b
    symptoms of, 156
    treatment of, 160b
  anatomic characteristics of, 157
  attack
    broken, 162
    short- and long-term sequelae to structures of the eye after, 162, 163b
  epidemiology of, 156–163
Primary angle closure glaucoma (PACG), 155–156
Primary angle closure suspect (PACS), 155–156
Primary colors, 24
Primary focal point (f), 10–21, 10f, 13f
Prince rule, 20
Principal plane, of schematic eye, 13f
Prismatic effect, alleviation of, 13
Prisms
  base-in, 229
  break of, 23
  calculation of power of, 12
  for thyroid eye disease, 277
Progression of cataract, 352
Progressive outer retinal necrosis, 307, 307f
Progressive supranuclear palsy, 233, 252
Prolactinoma, 259
Prophylactic laser PI, 162
Propionibacterium acnes, 296
Proptosis, 270–273
  bilateral, 2, 270
  causes of, 270
  childhood, 397
  computed tomographic scan of, 270f
  definition of, 270
  diagnosis of, 270
  etiology of, 271
  and eyelid retraction, 271f
  magnetic resonance imaging evaluation of, 40
  thyroid eye disease with, 274, 275f
  unilateral, 2, 270
Prosopagnosia, 263
Prostaglandin analogs, 168
  action of, 173
  for primary open-angle glaucoma, 173
  side effects of, 173, 175t, 176–177
Prostaglandin-associated periorbitopathy (PAP), 177
Prostaglandins, in photorefractive keratectomy, 141
Proteinuria, as diabetic retinopathy risk factor, 347
Proteus spp., penicillin for, 97
Pseudoabduction deficit, distinguished from true abduction deficit, 223
Pseudoesotropia, 223
Pseudoexfoliation, 202
Pseudoexfoliation syndrome, 168
Pseudo-Foster Kennedy syndrome, 264
Pseudohypertropia, 231
Pseudohypopyon, 304, 304f
Pseudomembranes, 66
Pseudomonas infections, in cornea, 78

Pseudomonas sp.
  as cause of red eye, 69–70
  penicillin for, 97
  treatment for, 96
Pseudopapilledema, papilledema differentiated from, 262
Pseudophakia, 203
Pseudoproptosis, causes of, 271
Pseudoptosis, 284
Pseudostrabismus, 228
Pseudotumor
  as diplopia cause, 248
  orbital, 279
Pseudotumor cerebri, 263b
Pseudoxanthoma elasticum, 3
Pterygium, 71, 71f
Ptosis, 283–288
  acquired, 283, 283f, 288
  after intraocular surgery, 284
  aponeurotic, 283–284, 284b
  bilateral, 231, 285f
  classification of, 283
  congenital, 283, 284f
  as false-positive field defect cause, 51, 53b
  in Horner's syndrome, 246, 246f
  myogenic causes of, 285
  neurologic conditions associated with, 285
  nonsurgical correction of, 286
  orbital capillary hemangiomas and, 397
  preoperative examination of, 286
  surgical correction of, 286
    complications of, 286–287
    types of, 288
  unilateral, producing amblyopia, 220
Punctal obstructions, 267
Punctal occlusion
  for dry eyes, 110
  in topical antibiotics and steroids delivery, 94
  topical medication administration and, 178
Pupil, 244–247
  Adie's tonic, 228, 246
  afferent defect of, 221, 244, 245f
  Argyll Robertson, 299
  Flomax, 203
  innervation of, 244
  nonreactive, 248
  in oculomotor nerve palsies, 248–249
  small, as false-positive field defect cause, 51,
    52f, 53b
  sparing, in third-nerve palsy, 245
  sympathetic innervation of, 244
  unilateral dilated, poorly reactive, 245
Pupillary block
  angle closure glaucoma and, 155
  relative, pathophysiologic mechanism of, 157, 158f
Pupillary dilation, for cataract, 205
Pupillary light reflex, 244
Pupillary parasympathetic fibers, 248

Q

Quadrantanopia
  crossed, 53
  homonymous, 53

Quinine intoxication, 33
Quinine sulfate, as retinopathy cause, 313, 314f

R

Radiation
  for basal cell carcinoma, 291
  complications of, 291–292, 292b
  treatments, as cause of dry eye, 104
Ranibizumab (Lucentis), for diabetic macular edema, 352
Rapid immunoassay test strips, 66
Raynaud's phenomenon, 143
Recess-resect procedure, 235
Rectus muscles
  inferior, entrapment of, 230
  medial, restricted, 251
  recession of, 1–2, 231
  slipped or lost, 231
  in strabismus surgery, 235
  in thyroid eye disease, 276f
Red eye, 65–76, 68b
  retinal vein occlusion and, 361
  treatment of, 95
Red light rays, refraction by plus lens, 16
Reflection
  critical angle of, 11, 12f
  total internal, 11
Refraction, 10–21
  in against-the-rule astigmatism, 15
  for cataract, 205
  cycloplegic, 18
  plus cylinder conversion to minus cylinder form, 14
Refractive components, of eye, 130–141
Refractive errors, types of, 130
Refractive indices, 13f
Refractive surgery, 130–142
  for anisometropic amblyopia in children, 221
  contraindications to, 130
  drugs in, 141
  goals of, 130
Refsum's disease, 232
Reis-Bücklers corneal dystrophy, 113
Reiter's disease, 295, 295t
Relative luminosity curves, 25
Retina
  after acute angle-closure attack, 162
  anatomic layers of, 3
  attachment of, 367
  breaks/tears of, 325, 367–368, 369b. *see also* Retinal
    detachment.
    atrophic hole, 368
    blunt trauma and, 326, 329b
    dialysis and, 325, 326f, 368, 368f
    horseshoe, 326, 367, 367f, 368f
    operculated, 368
  cells of, 3
  degenerative diseases of, 31
  imaging of, key modalities for, 46b
  infiltrates of, 304
  microvasculopathy of, AIDS and, 305
  necrosis of, 300, 307, 307f
  neovascularization of
    diabetic retinopathy and, 347, 352

Retina *(Continued)*
  retinal arterial obstruction and, 357
  retinal vein occlusion and, 359, 360
  talc and, 314
  pigmentation of, 23
    in Kearns-Sayre syndrome, 232
  separation from ora serrata, 191
Retinal arterial obstruction, 354–1, 357b
  as altitudinal defect cause, 60–63
  branch, 354
    symptoms of, 354, 355f
  causes of, 354, 355f
  central, 354, 357
    emergency treatment of, 357
    symptoms of, 354
  differentiated from retinal venous obstruction, 357
  prevention of, 356–357
  systemic diseases associated with, 355–356
  treatment of, 356–357
Retinal arterial occlusion, oral contraceptives and, 313
Retinal arteries, central, structure of, 5
Retinal arterioles, structure of, 5
Retinal detachment, 366–372
  acute retinal necrosis syndrome and, 300
  after cataract surgery, 215
  AIDS-related, 307
  in children, imaging studies of, 39
  chronic, *versus* retinoschisis, 369b
  Coats disease and, 319, 323
  definition of, 366
  extinguished electroretinogram in, 32
  exudative, 300, 366
  infectious retinitis and, 307
  peripheral, as uveitis mimic, 303t
  repair of, 369, 371, 371f
  retinal dialysis and, 325
  retinopathy of prematurity and, 342
  rhegmatogenous, 366, 366f, 368b, 369, 370
    diabetes and, 352
    uveitis and, 304
  scleral buckle for, 370f
  sympathetic ophthalmia and, 333
  tractional, 366, 371, 371f, 372f
    diabetes and, 352
  traumatic hyphema and, 191
  ultrasound features of, 37t
  visual-field defects associated with, 60–63
Retinal ganglion cells (RGCs), 244
Retinal pigment epithelial cells, in retinal attachment, 367
Retinal pigment epithelium
  congenital hypertrophy of, 379, 379f
  thioridazine and, 312–313
Retinal veins
  occlusions, branch-type, 4
  tortuous, 361f
Retinal venous occlusive disease, 359–365
  branch, 359–361, 359b, 360f, 361b, 364f
    ischemic, treatment of, 361
  central, 361–365, 361f, 362b, 362f, 363f, 364b, 364f
    ischemic, treatment of, 365

Retinitis
  cytomegalovirus, in AIDS patient, 305, 305f
  necrotizing, 305
  syphilitic, 300
Retinitis pigmentosa, 32
  as bitemporal field defect, 259
  Coats disease and, 323
  as constricted visual field cause, 259
  electroretinographic evaluation of, 31, 32f
  keratoconus and, 122
  as uveitis mimic, 303t, 305
  X-linked, electroretinographic evaluation of, 31
Retinoblastoma, 373–379, 375b, 386, 390, 393b
  age in, 374
  bilateral, 374, 393
  causes of, 373
  on chromosome, 393
  classification of, 376, 376t
  clinical features of, 303
  clinical growth patterns of, 375
  Coats disease and, 319
  definition of, 373
  diagnosis of, 390
  diseases confused with, 393
  endophytic, 375
  exophytic, 375, 390, 391f
  familial, 393
  fatal, 392
  fleurettes in, 392, 392f
  genetic mutation associated with, 373
  genetic testing in, 375
  germ-line mutation, 373
  gross appearance of, 390
  high-risk, 375
  histopathologic risk factors of, 392
  laterality of, 373
  lesions simulating, 374
  low-magnification light microscopy of, 390–391
  low penetrant, 373
  magnetic resonance imaging of, 39
  management of, 377b
  occurrence of, 373
  prognostic features of, 392
  rosettes in, 391
  second cancers associated with, 374–375
  small, management of
    anterior to equator of eye, 377
    posterior to equator of eye, 377
  somatic mutation, 374
  spontaneous regression of, 375
  sporadic, 393
  survival rate with, 375
  syndrome associated with, 373
  trilateral, 374, 393
  on ultrasound, 376
  unifocal, 393
  unilateral, 373, 393
  as uveitis mimic, 303t
Retinoblastoma gene, 393
Retinochoroiditis, necrotizing, 298–299
Retinocytoma, 375
Retinoma, 375

Retinopathy
  cancer-associated, 32
  crystalline, 314
  decompression, 162
  diabetic, 347–353
    after cataract surgery, 215
    differential diagnosis of, 352
    proliferative, 352, 371, 371f
  interferon, 315
  nonproliferative, 347, 348f
  of prematurity, 231, 341–353
    Coats disease and, 319
    complications of, 345, 345f
    differential diagnosis of, 345, 345t
    posterior, 344
    stages of, 342, 342f
    zones of, 341, 342f
  proliferative, 347, 348f
  radiation, 291
  tacrolimus-associated, 316, 316f
  toxic, 311–346
Retinopexy, pneumatic, 369, 371
Retinoschisis
  degenerative, 369
  X-linked, 345t
    juvenile, electroretinographic evaluation of, 32
Retinoscopy, "with" movement during, 18
Retrobulbar hemorrhage, treatment of, 211
Retrobulbar injection, of anesthesia, 205, 206f
Retrobulbar tumors, 171b
Rhabdomyosarcoma, 272, 397
  histologic classification of, 399
  treatment for, 399
Rhinophyma, 69
Rhodopsin, 23
Rho kinase inhibitors, 173
Ridley, Sir Harold, 208
Rieger's anomaly, 172
Rifabutin, ocular toxicity of, 309
Rim defects, as false-positive field defect cause, 51, 52f, 53b
Ritalin, as retinopathy cause, 314
"Rodent ulcer," 289
Rods, 22, 30
Rose bengal stain, 67f
  in dry eye diagnosis, 104
Rosettes, in retinoblastoma, 391
Rubella, congenital, 172
"Rule of 50s," 399

S

Sampaolesi's line, 168, 169f
"Sand in eyes," 67–68
"Sands of the Sahara syndrome," 86
Sarcoidosis, 168
  associated with optic neuritis, 255
  diagnosis of, 301
  features of, 301
  as uveitis cause, 296, 301
Sarcoma, retinoblastoma with, 374–375
Saturation, of colors, 24
Schaffer system, of anterior chamber angle classification, 154, 154t
Scheie system, of anterior chamber angle classification, 154, 154t

Schirmer's test, 67, 104, 266
Schlemm's canal, 151
  blood in, 171
Schnyder's crystalline dystrophy, 114–115, 115f
Schwalbe's line, 3, 151, 168, 169f
Schwannoma, 273, 398
Sclera
  blunt trauma to, 325
  rupture of, 330
  thinnest area of, 3
Scleral buckling, 369, 370, 370f
Scleral flap, 183
Scleral spur, 151
Scleritis
  as cause of red eye, 65–76
  versus episcleritis, 73, 73f
  necrotizing anterior, 74
  nodular, 74, 74f
  posterior, 75
  systemic disease and, 75
Scleromalacia perforans, 74f, 75
Scopolamine, 18
Scotoma
  bilateral arcuate, 55–56
  cecocentral, 58f
  central, 60–63, 63f
    bilateral, 259
    centrocecal, 259
  definition of, 51
  junctional, 57, 59f, 259
    anatomic explanation for, 57
  macular, 19
  paracentral, 314
  parafoveal, 311
  ring, 60, 62f
Sebaceous cell carcinoma, 68
Sebaceous gland carcinoma, 292
Secondary focal point (f'), 10, 10f, 13f
Secondary membrane, 215
"Second sight," 201
Sepsis, neonatal conjunctivitis and, 92b
Septum, of orbit, 2, 2f
Severe conjunctival chemosis, 271f
Short-term fluctuation (SF), 51
Short-wavelength automated perimetry (SWAP), 51
Sickle cell disease, hyphema and, 194, 194b
Siderosis, as cause of open-angle glaucoma, 172
Siderosis bulbi, 332
Sildenafil (Viagra), as retinopathy cause, 313
Silent sinus syndrome, 253
Silver nitrate drops, for neonatal conjunctivitis, 90
Simbrinza, 177
Sjögren syndrome, 104
Skew deviation, 229, 252
Sky, color of, 26–27
Slab-off, 13
Slipped muscle, 237
Slit lamp
  dilation with, 154
  findings, on keratoconus, 123–124, 124f, 125f
Small incision lenticule extraction (SMILE), 131, 136
  advantages and disadvantages of, 136
  versus LASIK, 136

Small incision lenticule extraction *(Continued)*
  myopia for correction of, 136
  potential complications of, 136–137
  potential contraindications to, 137b
Smears, for corneal infections, 78–79, 79t
Smoking, as environmental factor affecting thyroid eye
    disease, 274
Snellen eye chart, for visual acuity, 17, 20
Snell's law, 12f
Solutions, 94
Somatic mutation retinoblastoma, manifestation of, 374
Sonidegib (Odomzo), 291
Spaeth system, of anterior chamber angle classification, 154
Spasmus nutans, 242
Spectacles
  aphakic, 203
  bifocal, with low-vision aids, 17
  for children with astigmatism, 18
  corrective power of, 11
  lens of
    antireflective coatings on, 18
    bifocal, 17
    high-power single-vision, 17
    as low-vision aids, 17
    minus, 11
    plus, 14
    for ptosis correction, 286
    strabismic deviation measurement of, 14
    thick, aberrations of, 15
  new, patients complain with, 19
  options for astigmatism, 20
  power of
    comparison with contact lens, 11
    lensmeter measurement of, 18
  refractive accommodative esotropia treatment, 225
  vertex distance and, 18
Spectral-domain optical coherence tomography (SD-OCT),
    311
Spherical aberration, of thick lens, 15
Spherical equivalent, 14
Sphingolipidosis, 355
Spindle cells, 386
Spiral of Tillaux, 2
Squamous cell carcinoma, 292, 292f
SRK formula, for intraocular lens implant calculation, 209
Standard automated perimetry (SAP), 51
Standard patient evaluation of eye dryness (SPEED),
    105, 106f
Staphylococcal hypersensitivity infiltrates, 83, 83f
Staphylococcus aureus
  as cause of blepharitis, 68
  as cause of conjunctivitis, 72
  as cause of orbital cellulitis, 281
  endophthalmitis and, 333
  methicillin-resistant, 97
  penicillin-resistant, 97
  in vitreous of endophthalmitis patients, 213
Staphylococcus aureus, methicillin-resistant, 97
Staphylococcus epidermidis, penicillin-resistant, 97
Steroids. *see also* Corticosteroids.
  after trabeculectomy, use of, 184–185
  as giant cell arteritis treatment, 261
  for glaucoma, 171

Steroids *(Continued)*
  low-dose, as red eye treatment, 65
  subconjunctival injection of, 75
  systemic, 276
  as thyroid eye disease treatment, 275
  topical, 94–102, 101t
    for angle closure, 158
    and antibiotic combinations, 101t
    in photorefractive keratectomy, 141
    side effects of, 98–99
Stevens-Johnson's reaction, 299
Strabismus
  alternating, 223
  as amblyopia cause, 218
  cycloplegic refraction in, 18
  horizontal or vertical, 235
  in infants, 223
  measurement of, Prentice's rule of, 14
  retinoblastoma with, 374
  surgery, 235–238
    in amblyopia patients, 222
    complications of, 237b
  A and V patterns of, 236, 236f
Streptococci, as cause of orbital cellulitis, 281
Strokes, occipital, 259
Stromal corneal dystrophies, 112, 114, 114f, 114t
STUMPED mnemonic, of neonatal cloudy corneas, 5
Sturge-Weber syndrome, 171b, 172
Subretinal exudates, 320
Sulfacetamide, 95, 99t
Sulfur hexafluoride, 371
Sunset, color of, 27
Superior oblique palsy, 249
Superior orbital fissure, 1, 7
Superior orbital fissure syndrome, 251t
Superior vena cava syndrome, 171b
Superotemporal quadrant, of retina, 4
Suprathreshold testing, 50
Surgical limbus, 3
Suspensions, 94
Sussman four- or six-mirror lenses, 151
Sutures
  adjustable, 235
  releasable, 184
  scleral, 235
  spatulated needle, 235
  type of needle in, 235
Swedish interactive threshold algorithm (SITA), 51
Swinging flashlight test, 244
Sympathetic ophthalmia, 297t, 301, 333
Synechiae
  peripheral anterior, 294
  posterior, 168, 294
Syphilis
  associated with optic neuritis, 255
  ocular, 299
    in AIDS patient, 307–308
    retinitis and, 300
    uveitis and, 296t, 300
  tertiary, Argyll-Robertson pupil and, 247
Syphilitic uveitis, diagnostic tests for, 299
Systemic lupus erythematosus, 255
Systemic thyroid imbalance, 274

T

Talc, as retinopathy cause, 314, 315f
Tamoxifen, as retinopathy cause, 315
Tamsulosin (Flomax), 203, 216
Tarsal conjunctival follicles, 66
Tay-Sachs disease, 355
Tear breakup time, measurement of, 104
Tear film
  components of, 103
  layers of, 5, 103
  normal, 103
Tear Film and Ocular Surface Society (TFOS), 108–109
Tearing, causes of, 265
Tear pump, 265
Tear replacement therapy, 108–109
Tears
  artificial, 95
  chronic
    causes of, 265b
    testing patients with, 267b
  composition of, 266
    inadequate, 266
  dry eyes and, 266
  preservative-free, 109
  probing, 268–269
Tecnis Z9000, 210
Telangiectasia, 69
  retinal, Coats disease and, 319
Telecanthus, 285
Telescope, 16–17
Temporal artery
  biopsy of, 8, 261
  superficial, surgical landmarks of, 8
Temporal lobe, "pie-in-the-sky" defect of, 263
Tenon's capsule, in strabismus surgery, 235
Tensilon test, 252
Teprotumumab, 278
Teratoid medulloepithelioma, 394, 394f
Testing, ophthalmic and orbital, 29–49, 40b
Tetracycline, 69, 92, 99t
Thermokeratoplasty, 128
  holmium laser, 140
Thiel-Behnke corneal dystrophy, 113
Thioridazine (Mellaril), as retinopathy cause, 312–313, 313f
Third-nerve palsy, 248, 248b, 285b
  isolated
    pupillary involvement, 245–246
    pupil-sparing, 245, 248–249
  workup of pupil-involving, 248
13q deletion syndrome, 373
Three-step test, 249, 250f
Thromboembolic events, drugs causing, 316
Thrombophlebitis, Behçet's disease and, 300
Thrombus, as retinal artery obstruction cause, 354
Thyroid disease, 230
Thyroid eye disease, 274–1, 277b
  causes of, 274
  definition of, 274
  development of, 275
  environmental factors affecting, 274
  hyperthyroidism and, 274
  irradiation as treatment for, 276
  kinds of surgery in patients with, 277

Thyroid eye disease (Continued)
  orbital irradiation affecting, 276
  orbit change in, 275
  risk for, 274
  signs of, 274
  surgery in, 277
  teprotumumab for, 278
  treatment of, 275
  workup for, 274
Thyroid ophthalmopathy
  as cause of elevated episcleral venous pressure, 171b
  in proptosis, 271
Thyroid orbitopathy, 2
Thyroid-stimulating hormone receptors, 2, 274
Tight lens syndrome, 69
Timolol, 100–101
  for glaucoma, 173
TINU syndrome, 297t
Tobramycin, 97, 99t
Tolosa-Hunt syndrome, 233
Topical anesthesia, for cataract surgery, 206
Topical medications
  allergic reactions to, 179
  antibiotics. see Antibiotics; topical
  penetration of, 95b
  for red eye treatment, 65
  steroids. see Steroids; topical
Topiramate, for angle closure, 166–167
Topographic mapping, for keratoconus diagnosis, 122b
Torticollis, 242
Total deviation, 51
Total homonymous hemianopia, 53
Toxic anterior segment syndrome (TASS), 214
  causes of, 214
Toxocariasis, ocular, 231
  as uveitis cause, 296t
Toxoplasmosis, ocular
  AIDS and, 305
  management of, 298–299
  as papilledema cause, 308
  as retinitis cause, 299
  as uveitis cause, 296t
Trabecular meshwork
  anterior, nonpigmented, 151
  inflammatory cell blockage of, 168
  obstruction of, 196
  posterior, pigmented, 151, 152f
  tear in, 191
Trabeculectomy, 181–190
  for acute primary angle closure, 162
  anesthesia for, 182–183
  antimetabolites in, indications for, 186
  complications of, how to avoid, 186b
  failure of, 182, 182f
  flaps in, 183
  fornix *versus* limbal-conjunctival approach to, 182, 182f, 183f
  indications for, 181–190
  for neovascular glaucoma, 166
  risks of, 181–182
  size of internal blocks and, 184
  success rate in, improving, 189b
  wound leak after, 185–186
Trabeculectomy site, blocked, 188

Trabeculoplasty, argon laser, 3
Trachoma, 72
Tranexamic acid, 194
Transillumination, of uveal melanoma, 382
Transposition procedure, 236
Transsynaptic degeneration, 33
Transverse magnification, formula for, 16
Trapdoor orbital fracture, 253
Trauma
    angle-recession glaucoma and, 168
    ocular
        angle recession and, 198, 199f
        blunt, 191
        to fundus, 325–334
        initial examination of, 330
        treatment algorithm for, 197f
        ultrasound evaluation of, 38
    operative, 212
Traumatic macular holes, 326, 327f
Travoprost, 176–177
Triamcinolone, 360, 364
Trichiasis, blepharitis and, 68
Trichromatism, anomalous, 27
Trichromats, 27
Trigeminal nerve, herpes zoster lesions of, 2
Trimethoprim, 95
Trochlear nerve, 7
Trochlear nerve palsy, 249, 251
Trophozoites, 82
Tropicamide (Mydriacyl), 18
Tuberculosis, ocular
    features of, 300
    as uveitis cause, 296t
Tumors
    ocular, 386–396
    of eyelid, 289–293
    orbital, 397–402
        soft tissue, 400

U
Ulcers
    Behçet's disease and, 300
    corneal, 77–82, 82b
        antibiotics for, 80
        biopsy of, 82
        from contact lens, 69
        infectious, 77
        perforated, 82, 82f
        ptosis surgery and, 286–287
        sequelae of, 82
        smears and cultures of, 78–79, 79t
        sterile, 77, 78f
        topical antibiotics and steroids for, 98b
        topical corticosteroids for, 80–81
    dendritic, 66–67, 67f
    genital, 300
    oral, 300
Ultrasonography, ophthalmic
    biomicroscopy method in, 38, 38f
    of calcification, 37
    of choroidal hemangioma, 36, 36t
    of choroidal melanoma, 36, 36t
    for Coats disease diagnosis, 320
    color-Doppler, 38

Ultrasonography, ophthalmic (Continued)
    display of, 35, 35f
    of foreign bodies, 332
    frequency used for, 34
    indications for, 34
    of intraocular foreign bodies, 38
    of intraocular tumors, 36
    lesion features evaluated in, 35, 35f
    of ocular trauma, 38
    of orbital lesions, 40
    for preoperative cataract evaluation, 36
    principles of, 34
    of retinal detachment, 37, 37f
    of uveal melanoma, 382
Ultrasound biomicroscopy (UBM), 171
    for anterior chamber angle evaluation, 154
Urochrome pigment, 201
Uveal melanoma, 382, 383, 384, 386
    BAP-1 tumor predisposition syndrome, 384
    predilection for age, race, or sex, 383
    route of distant spread, 383
    versus uveal metastasis, 384
Uveitis, 294–310
    anterior, 75, 76b, 294
        granulomatous, 294, 295t, 296
        nongranulomatous, 294, 295t
    as cause of red eye, 65–76
    definition of, 294
    glaucoma and, 301
    granulomatous, 294
    in immunocompetent patient, 294
    infectious causes of, 296t
    intermediate, 294, 298
    masquerade syndromes and, 302–305, 303t, 305b
    most common forms of, 302b
    nongranulomatous, 294
    noninfectious causes of, 297t
    orbital inflammation and, 280
    phacoanaphylactic, 297t
    posterior, 294, 300–302
        Behçet's disease and, 300–302
    postoperative, 212
    syphilitic, 299
    treatment of, 301–302
Uveitis-glaucoma-hyphema syndrome, 171
Uveoscleral outflow enhancers, for angle closure, 158

V
Valsalva maneuver, 73
Valve of Rosenmüller, 265
Vancomycin, 97
van Herick technique, 153–154
Varicella zoster virus infection, 84
Vascular endothelial growth factor, 338
Vasculitis
    orbital, 282
    rheumatoid arthritis-associated, 302
Vasoconstrictor, as red eye cause, 74
Vaso-occlusive nerve palsies, with aberrant regeneration, 252
Vergence
    of convex mirrors, 17
    formula for, 12
    of parallel light rays, 12
Vertex distance, 18

Vertical deviation, dissociated, 224
Vertical rectus transposition, 236
Vidarabine, 66–67, 93
Video-angiography, indocyanine, 338
Vigabatrin retinotoxicity, 313–314
Viscoelastic, retained, 171
Vision
  compromised, papillitis and, 308
  normal field of, 50
  sympathetic ophthalmia and, 333
Vision loss
  in diabetic retinopathy, 347, 347b
  glaucoma-related, 144
  macular degeneration and, 338
  pars planitis and, 298
  retinal vein occlusion and, 360
Vismodegib (Erivedge), 291
Visual acuity
  in amblyopia, 220
  in infants, 4–5
  in nystagmus, 241
  20/20, 4
Visual cortex, location of, 4
Visual fields, 50–64
  constricted, 259–260
  defects of
    congruous, 53
    description of, 53
    false, 51
    general depression of, 60
    glaucoma and, 59–60, 61f, 144b
    homonymous, 53
    neuro-ophthalmologic disorders-related, 55, 56f, 56t
    visual acuity and, 56
  right eye *versus* left eye in, 50
  10-2 tests, 64
Visual field testing
  false-negative errors in, 51
  false-positive errors in, 51
  future for, 64
  monocular, 53
  types of, 50
Visual impairment, preoperative tests for, 205, 205b
Visual pathway, 54
Visual pigments, 23
Vitamin A aldehyde, 23
Vitamin A deficiency, 259
Vitamin B$_{12}$ deficiency, 259
Vitamin E, for glaucoma, 177
Vitamins, for macular degeneration, 339
Vitelliform dystrophy, 34
Vitrectomy
  as diabetic retinopathy treatment, 352
    complications of, 352
  "dry," 186
  for endophthalmitis, 81

Vitrectomy (*Continued*)
  for foreign body removal, 332
  pars plana, 370
    retinoblastoma and, 376
Vitreoretinal surgery, 323
Vitreoretinopathy
  familial exudative, 345t
    Coats disease and, 319
  proliferative, 371
Vitreous
  loss of
    cataract surgery-related, 215
    posterior capsule rupture-related, 212
    during trabeculectomy, 186
  opacity of, as false-positive field defect cause, 51
  persistent hyperplastic primary, 394
  posterior, detachment of, ultrasound features of, 37t
Vitreous tap, for endophthalmitis, 81
Vitritis
  steroid-resistant panuveitis and, 304
  syphilis and, 300
Vogt-Koyanagi-Harada syndrome, 297t, 300
Volk 90 D lens, 18
von Hippel-Lindau syndrome, 319

W

Waldenstrom's macroglobulinemia, 114
"Wall-eyed," 228
Warfarin, anticoagulant effects of, 193
Wavefront ablations, 135
Weber's syndrome, 252
Wegener's granulomatosis, 282, 302
White-dot syndrome, retinal, 300
Whitnall's ligament
  in ptosis, 287
  superior suspensory, bony attachments, 9
Willebrand's knee, 4, 57
Women, optic neuritis in, 255
Wound burn, cataract surgery-related, 211
Wound leak, cataract surgery-related, 211

X

Xanthelasma, 289, 290f
Xanthogranuloma, juvenile, 296, 297f, 297t
Xanthopsia, 314

Y

YAG capsulotomy, 204
Yellow vision, 314

Z

Zeiss goniolens, 151, 152f
Zonules
  after acute angle-closure attack, 162
  tears in, 191